SMITH'S RECOGNIZABLE PATTERNS OF HUMAN DEFORMATION

EDITION 5

JOHN M. GRAHAM, JR., MD, SCD

Consulting Medical Geneticist
Harbor-UCLA Medical Center
Torrance, California

Professor Emeritus
Departments of Pediatrics and Biomedical Sciences
Guerin Children's at Cedars-Sinai Medical Center
Los Angeles, California

Professor Emeritus
Department of Pediatrics
David Geffen School of Medicine at UCLA
Los Angeles, California

PEDRO A. SANCHEZ-LARA, MD, MSCE, FAAP, FACMG

Director, Pediatric Medical Genetics
Associate Clinical Professor
Department of Pediatrics
Guerin Children's at Cedars-Sinai Medical Center
Los Angeles, California

Associate Clinical Professor
Department of Pediatrics
David Geffen School of Medicine at UCLA
Los Angeles, California

Adjunct Professor
Center for Craniofacial Molecular Biology
Ostrow School of Dentistry
University of Southern California
Los Angeles, California

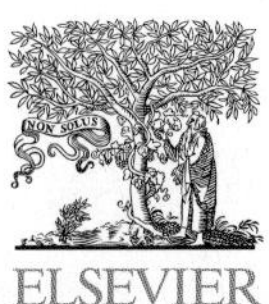

ELSEVIER

Elsevier
1600 John F. Kennedy Blvd.
Ste 1800
Philadelphia, PA 19103-2899

SMITH'S RECOGNIZABLE PATTERNS OF HUMAN DEFORMATION, FIFTH EDITION ISBN: 978-0-443-11414-4

Content Strategist: Sarah E. Barth
Content Development Specialist: Angie Breckon
Publishing Services Manager: Shereen Jameel
Project Manager: Maria Shalini
Design Direction: Bridget Hoette

Printed in India

Last digit is the print number: 9 8 7 6 5 4 3 2 1

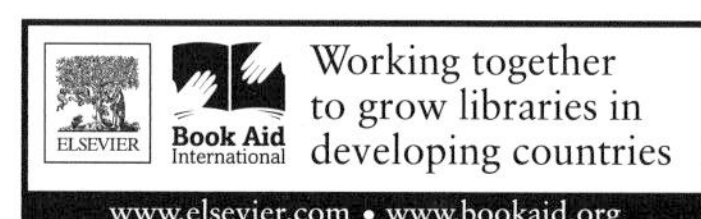

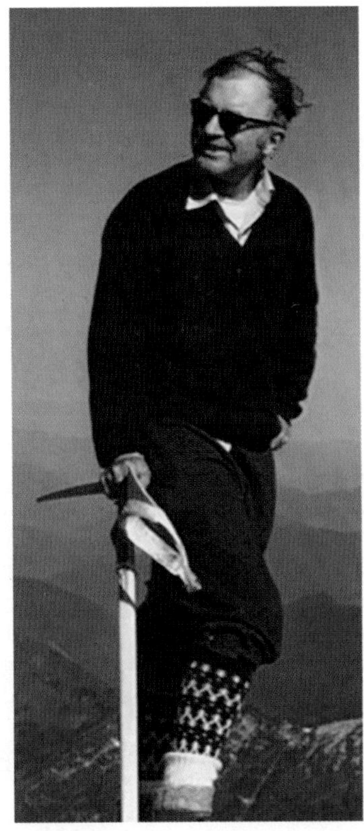

I was inspired and trusted by David W. Smith, MD (1926-1981) to continue this work.

His favorite saying was: "Far better it is to dare mighty things, to win glorious triumphs, even though checkered by failure...than to rank with those poor spirits who neither enjoy nor suffer much, because they live in a gray twilight that knows not victory nor defeat." By Teddy Roosevelt. I simply say, God loves runners who don't quit on hills.

I still remember when Dave Smith packed a trunk of resources and notes and headed off to Whidbey Island in the Puget Sound, north of Seattle, Washington. The island's rugged terrain spans beaches, hills, and farmlands. This is where he wrote the first edition of *Recognizable Patterns of Human Deformation* in 1980, and I promised to continue his work and advance knowledge concerning human deformations.

I would like to dedicate this book to my family, most especially my wife Elizabeth, and my three sons and their wives: George and Mary, Zack and Nicole, and John and Amanda. I am especially proud of my six grandchildren: Oliver and Amelia, Viola and Sebastian, and Alyssa and Evan. They are our future, and they will all accomplish great things.

I am passing this work along to my fellow, friend, and colleague, Pedro A. Sanchez-Lara, MD, who will continue on in the tradition of Teddy Roosevelt and Dave Smith.

John M. Graham

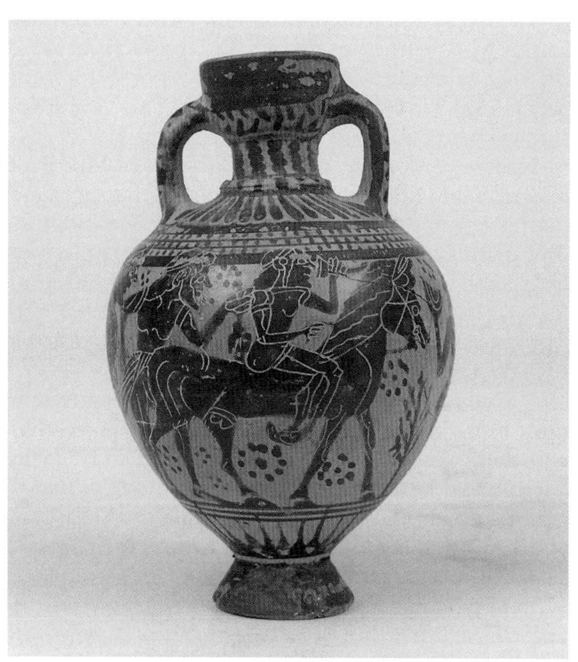

To all the students, residents, and future pediatric and genetic colleagues, I hope this book reminds you to think outside the box and remember that not all congenital anomalies have a genetic origin.

To my patients, their parents, and all those who care for people that are differently abled, This picture is of the Greek god Hephaestus; born different from all other gods and with a congenital foot deformation.

He is best known as the god of fire, metalworking, invention, and creativity. When learning about Hephaestus, some may think that his story is of hardship, struggle, and tragedy, but every story has two sides: it also includes a story of kindness, forgiveness, and the incredible benefits of raising all children in a supportive and nurturing environment. Being differently abled didn't stop Hephaestus from finding his strengths and becoming the greatest blacksmith, inventor, and craftsman of all Olympian gods. He forged Zeus' thunderbolts, Helios' chariot, Poseidon's trident, the armor for the heroes such as Achilles and Hercules, and many other essential items such as the knife of Perseus that beheaded Medusa. He even crafted his own wheelchair and invented automatons (the first robots!).

Find the good, change the narrative, and change the world.

Pedro A. Sanchez-Lara

PREFACE

Since Peter Dunn and David Smith presented the basic concepts of deformation in 1975–1976, it has become accepted that unusual mechanical forces are responsible for a wide variety of structural birth defects. The impact of mechanical forces on form not only has provided an understanding of extrinsic constraint deformations, but it has also led to the appreciation that many malformation sequences can be interpreted as arising from an initiating malformation that results in altered mechanical forces and a cascade of intrinsic deformations. This biomechanical perspective provides a better understanding of the importance of mechanical forces in normal morphogenesis.

The major emphasis of *Smith's Recognizable Patterns of Human Deformation* is on extrinsic constraint deformations that are secondary to crowding in utero. These should, to the extent possible, be distinguished from malformations with or without secondary intrinsic deformations. Not only are there major differences in the etiology, prognosis, management, and recurrence risk for extrinsic deformations, but also there are profound differences in the prognosis that can be conveyed to the child's parents. The child with extrinsic deformation can usually be interpreted as normal, and the parents can look forward to the restoration of normal form. This attitude toward considering extrinsic deformations as a separable category of birth defects is also critical in providing better answers relative to etiology and prevention. The etiologic factors that cause extrinsic deformation are obviously very different from those that cause malformation problems, which is a critical distinction that has not always been appreciated in epidemiologic studies. The preventive measures for extrinsic deformations are also different and entail such considerations as external cephalic version for fetal malpresentation and/or possible surgical reconstruction of a malformed uterus. Furthermore, because extrinsic deformations are more common in infants of primigravida mothers and in larger fetuses, it is quite reasonable to anticipate that the incidence of extrinsic deformations might increase because of smaller families and/or larger babies.

The basic principles of extrinsic deformation are simple. The magnitude and direction of force have a direct impact on form. These same simple precepts are relevant to the management of deformations. With rare exceptions, correction can be accomplished by the rational application of subtle forces. Over the course of the last 43 years, since collecting the data for the first edition of this book (1981), this knowledge has become an integral part of medicine because extrinsic deformations are common, and these basic concepts have become well established. The overall concepts that relate to the developmental pathology, diagnosis, and management of extrinsic deformations are simple and easily understood by primary care providers and subspecialists, as well as by parents. In recent times there has been a tendency to look for more complex answers of a biochemical, molecular, or physiologic nature, and to bypass the simple mechanistic approaches. Hence this book is dedicated to bringing the mechanical aspects of morphogenesis and deformation into the mainstream of medicine, where they belong.

Very few studies of extrinsic deformation in experimental animals have been done. One reason is that few creatures other than humans tend to outgrow the uterus before birth and to have constraint deformations at birth. Most other animals are born at a much more mature state of development, ready to stand and run away from predators; however, humans are unable to stand and run for almost a year after birth. Humans spend much of their infancy in a recumbent position, which may lead to deformation if the infant's resting position is not purposefully varied. This is one price the slowly aging, rapidly growing, large-brained human must pay for his or her present level of evolvement. One major aspect of human evolution is the prolonged period necessary to complete human brain development, such that the human brain continues to grow slowly over a much longer time than that necessary for other primates. It takes 6 months of postnatal growth for the human brain to reach the proportions found in a chimpanzee at birth. Thus, human gestation would take an additional 7 to 8 months if human neonates were to be born at the same stage of maturity as other primate infants. This continued growth of the human brain appears to leave the human cranium much more vulnerable to mechanical forces than that of other species. To accommodate this continued growth of the brain, the cranial sutures remain open for decades, while the plates of cranial bone continue to afford protection to the developing brain.

Congenital deformations are common, with most resolving spontaneously within the first few days of postnatal life. When such prompt resolution does not take place, further evaluation may be necessary to plan therapeutic interventions and prevent long-term negative consequences. This book provides a rational approach for the diagnosis and management of such deformations. Information concerning unusual intrauterine positions should be transmitted to physicians caring for such newborns in the nursery. When such data are properly interpreted, it can guide further evaluation and therapy and be vastly reassuring to the parents. Prompt treatment of deformations leads to prompt resolution of such problems, whereas delays in treatment sometimes lead to permanent alterations and residual deformations, which can have long-term implications.

ACKNOWLEDGMENTS

In the acknowledgment section of the first edition of this book (1981), Dr. David W. Smith indicated that he was strongly influenced by neonatologist Dr. Peter Dunn of Bristol, England, who recommended a clear distinction between defects caused by mechanical constraint forces (deformation) and those caused by poor formation (malformation). After Dunn first published his observations on fetal deformation, Dr. David Smith and his colleagues expanded many of these concepts, and this book would not be possible without those contributions. After completing the first edition of this book, Dr. Smith died on February 21, 1981, and he requested that I continue his work and revise this book.

Bill Pollard from Medical Illustrations at Cedars-Sinai Medical Center prepared many of the figures for the third edition of the book, and Tim Littlefield of Cranial Technology provided updated figures for the plagiocephaly and brachycephaly chapters. I've also appreciated the assistance of my own students, nurses, colleagues, and fellows at Cedars-Sinai Medical Center, as well as an expert review by pediatric orthopedist Dr. Robert Matthew Bernstein at Cedars-Sinai Medical Center in Los Angeles. Many of the radiologic images came from the International Skeletal Dysplasia Registry at Cedars-Sinai Medical Center, which was established by Drs. David L. Rimoin and Ralph Lachman, who both provided support and guidance.

I express my deepest personal gratitude to my loving wife, Elizabeth, and my two sons, Zachary and George Graham, without whom none of this work would have been possible. They have endured the spread of research files, figures, and partially written texts to virtually every flat surface in our home, where the past 40 years have tested many of the concepts advanced by David W. Smith in the first edition of this book, and these concepts have clearly stood the test of time.

John M. Graham

I am immensely grateful to my teacher, friend, and lifelong mentor, Dr. John M. Graham, Jr., for extending his invitation to contribute to the 5th edition of *Smith's Recognizable Patterns of Human Deformation*. It has always been an honor and privilege to have him impart the art and science of dysmorphology.

I extend my heartfelt appreciation to my clinical, laboratory, and research colleagues, as well as the patients who have entrusted me with their care, for their invaluable contributions to my knowledge and understanding of pediatric developmental disorders. In particular, I would like to thank Karla Haynes, RN, MPH, CPNP, Yvonne Gutierrez, MD, Eugene S. Kim, MD. David L. Skaggs, MD, MMM, Robert Kay, MD, Kenneth Illingworth, MD, Nina Lightdale-Miric, MD, Sheryl Lewin, MD, Victor Chien, MD, Jeffrey A. Hammoudeh, MD, DDS and Mark M. Urata, MD, DDS, for their diligent review and constructive feedback on our chapters, and for their assistance in updating the figures. I owe special thanks to Drs. Yang Chai, DDS, PhD, Tim R. Rebbeck, PhD, Harold C. Slavkin, DDS, PhD, Nancy B. Spinner, PhD, and Elaine H. Zackai, MD for their mentorship, guidance and enduring inspiration to advance science, education and patient care.

I would like to express my gratitude to Angie Breckon at Elsevier, who dedicated her time and expertise to edit and format the content of this 5th edition. Her dedication and professionalism have greatly enhanced the quality of this work.

Most importantly, I wish to extend my deepest thanks to my loving wife Esther, and our children, Zen, Karina, and Joaquin: please know that your unwavering love and support provides me with limitless inspiration and motivation to transcend beyond any perceived boundaries. Thank you for sacrificing all those evenings and weekends and making sure I never ran out of snacks (and coffee) while I edited this book. You are the pillars that sustain me and bring immeasurable joy to my life.

Pedro A. Sanchez-Lara

CONTENTS

VIDEO CONTENTS

Section I
Introduction

CHAPTER 1

Clinical Approach to Deformation Problems

Malformations, Deformations, Disruptions, and Dysplasias

KEY POINTS

- This text is primarily concerned with extrinsic deformations produced by unusual or excessive constraint of an otherwise normal fetus.
- Individual deformations in this book are presented in an atlas format along with deformation sequences.
- *Deformations* are structural defects that represent a normal response of a tissue to an external mechanical force.
- Deformations are usually attributed to intrauterine molding and termed *positional defects*.
- The mechanical pressure causing the molding can either be intrinsic (e.g., neuromuscular imbalance) or extrinsic (e.g., fetal crowding).
- A *deformation sequence* refers to the manifold molding effects of a given deforming situation, such as the oligohydramnios sequence.
- A clear distinction between deformation and malformation is critical for prognosis, management, and recurrence risk counseling.

Mechanical forces play an important role in both normal and abnormal morphogenesis. Anomalies that represent the normal response of a tissue to unusual mechanical forces are termed *deformations*, in contrast to *malformations*, which denote a primary problem in the morphogenesis of a tissue, and *disruptions*, which represent the breakdown of previously normal tissues. A fourth category of problems, termed *dysplasias*, results in abnormal structure because the tissues from which individual structures are formed are abnormal (Fig. 1.1). An isolated structural defect can arise through any of these four basic categories of morphogenesis, and clarifying the nature of the underlying defect is necessary to provide proper counseling. An isolated malformation, such as an idiopathic talipes equinovarus (rigid clubfoot), can arise as a localized error in morphogenesis with a multifactorial recurrence risk and differences in birth prevalence among various racial groups and between genders. Prevalence ranges from a high of 6.8 per 1000 live births in Hawaiian and Maori people, to 1.2 per l000 in White people, to 0.74 per 1000 in US Black and Hispanic people, to 0.39 per 1000 in Chinese populations.[1] Bilateral cases occur slightly more frequently than unilateral cases, and males are affected twice as frequently as females. Such variations in race and sex predilection occur for many different multifactorial defects, emphasizing the importance of differences in genetic background. If a clubfoot arises as part of a broader pattern of defects, it can do so through any one of these underlying categories of abnormal morphogenesis, and the recurrence risk is based on the cause of the overall pattern of abnormal morphogenesis.

A multiple *malformation syndrome* results in a primary developmental anomaly of two or more systems in which all of the structural defects are caused by a single underlying etiology, which can be genetic, chromosomal, or environmental (teratogenic). In some cases the cause may be unknown, but as mechanisms of abnormal morphogenesis become better understood, the number of syndromes in this category has been diminishing. Multiple structural defects can also result from a *sequence* in which a single primary defect in morphogenesis produces multiple abnormalities through a cascading process of secondary and tertiary problems in morphogenesis. During the evaluation of a child with multiple anomalies, it is extremely important from the standpoint of recurrence risk counseling

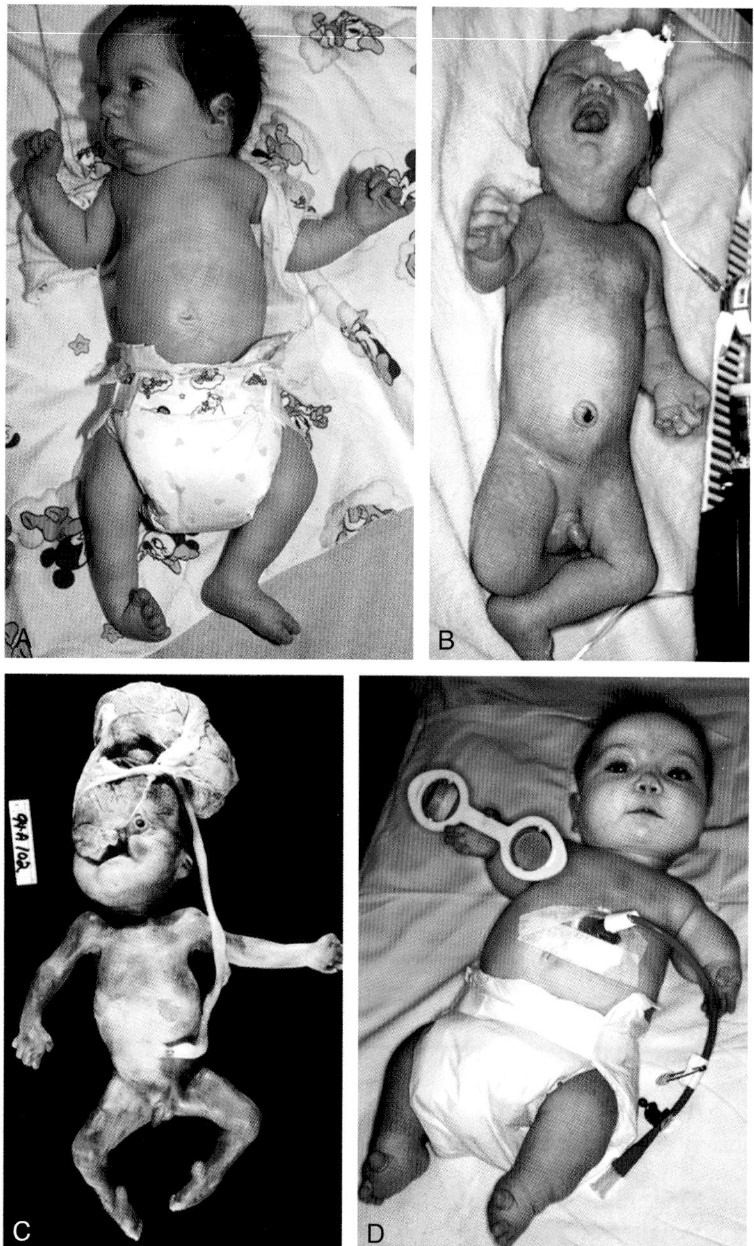

FIGURE 1.1 The four major types of problems in morphogenesis: malformation, deformation, disruption, and dysplasia. **A,** An infant with camptomelic dysplasia syndrome, which results in a multiple malformation syndrome caused by a mutation in *SOX9*. **B,** An infant with oligohydramnios deformation sequence caused by premature rupture of membranes from 17 weeks of gestation until birth at 36 weeks; the infant was delivered from a persistent transverse lie. **C,** A fetus with early amnion rupture sequence with attachment of the placenta to the head and resultant disruption of craniofacial structures with distal limb contractures. **D,** An infant with diastrophic dysplasia caused by inherited autosomal recessive mutations in a sulfate transporter protein.

to distinguish a malformation syndrome from multiple defects that arose from a single localized error in morphogenesis, such as spina bifida malformation sequence (when a failure in neural tube closure results in neurogenic clubfeet and bladder/bowel problems). Examples of different types of structural defects are discussed in the next paragraph.

In Fig. 1.1A, an infant with campomelic syndrome has a cleft palate, hypospadias, abnormal skeletal development, and talipes equinovarus because of a mutation in *SOX9*, which resulted in a malformation syndrome. In Fig. 1.1B, an infant was born at 36 weeks after amniotic membranes ruptured prematurely at 26 weeks, resulting in oligohydramnios deformation sequence. This may have occurred spontaneously or it could have been caused by an underlying genetic connective tissue disorder such as Ehlers-Danlos syndrome, which predisposes the fetus toward early amnion rupture, ligamentous laxity, and hernias. The fetus in Fig. 1.1C has been affected by the disruption of previously normal structures because of early amnion rupture during the first trimester, resulting in strands of amnion damaging facial structures. The infant in Fig. 1.1D has an autosomal recessive skeletal dysplasia (diastrophic dysplasia) that resulted in cleft palate, malformed pinna with calcification of ear cartilage, hitchhiker thumbs, symphalangism, and talipes equinovarus with progressive scoliosis, which is particularly refractory to treatment. This condition results from a mutant sulfate transporter protein gene, which is inherited from each parent, with no signs evident in the carrier parents. To offer appropriate genetic counseling, it is important to distinguish such underlying malformation syndromes, skeletal dysplasias, and genetic connective tissue disorders from isolated defects that resulted solely from fetal disruption or late gestational constraint. Syndromes and dysplasias often have a genetic basis.

Deformations often involve either the craniofacial region or the limbs, and they are usually attributed to intrauterine molding and termed *positional defects*. The mechanical pressure causing the molding can either be intrinsic (e.g., neuromuscular imbalance) or extrinsic (e.g., fetal crowding). When a prolonged decrease in fetal movement occurs resulting from either type of problem, joints may develop contractures because joints require movement to form in a normal way. Thus there are predominantly two types of deformational problems: those in which the causative forces are caused by an intrinsic problem within the developing fetus (e.g., a neuromuscular insufficiency or a central nervous system developmental defect) and those in which the deformation was produced by mechanical forces that were extrinsic to an otherwise normal fetus.

The two predominant types of deformations are depicted in Fig. 1.2, and the distinctions between these two types are based on historical and physical findings. In Fig. 1.3, the overall pattern of intrinsic deformation due to neuromuscular insufficiency is quite similar for both congenital myotonic dystrophy (Fig. 1.3A), an autosomal dominant disorder with a 50% recurrence risk, and Pena-Shokeir syndrome (Fig. 1.3B), an autosomal recessive disorder with a 25% recurrence risk. Myotonic dystrophy results from amplification of a trinucleotide repeat in the 3′ untranslated region of a protein kinase gene on chromosome 19. Normally, there are 5–30 copies of this repeat. When there are 50–80 repeats, the result is mild disease; when there are more than 2000 repeats, infants are severely affected with congenital myotonic dystrophy, as depicted in Fig. 1.3A. This severe pattern is seen in the offspring of affected women only and becomes more likely as the mutant allele is transmitted through successive generations, a phenomenon termed *anticipation*.

The pattern of intrinsic neuromuscular deformation is recognizably different from the pattern seen with extrinsic deformation resulting from oligohydramnios deformation sequence, as demonstrated in Fig. 1.1B. In Fig. 1.3C, the facial effects of intrinsic deformation caused by Möbius sequence (deficient cranial nerve VI and VII function) also differ from the extrinsic facial deformations seen in Fig. 1.3D, in which prolonged oligohydramnios and a persistent transverse lie resulted in marked facial compression. Disruptive defects occur when a previously normally formed structure is partly or completely destroyed. This can result from either amniotic bands (see Fig. 1.1C) or an interruption of blood supply (Fig. 1.4A–B); in some cases of early amnion rupture, both mechanisms may occur (Fig. 1.4C). When one monozygotic, monochorionic twin dies in utero, interruption of blood supply to fetal structures can lead to infarction, necrosis, hypoplasia, and/or resorption of tissues distal to a point at which thromboembolic debris lodge in the circulation of the surviving twin (see Fig. 1.4A).

Extrinsic forces may result in a single localized deformation, such as a positional foot deformation, or they may cause a deformation sequence. A *deformation sequence* refers to the manifold molding effects of a given deforming situation. A good example of one such deformation sequence is the oligohydramnios sequence, in which oligohydramnios is responsible

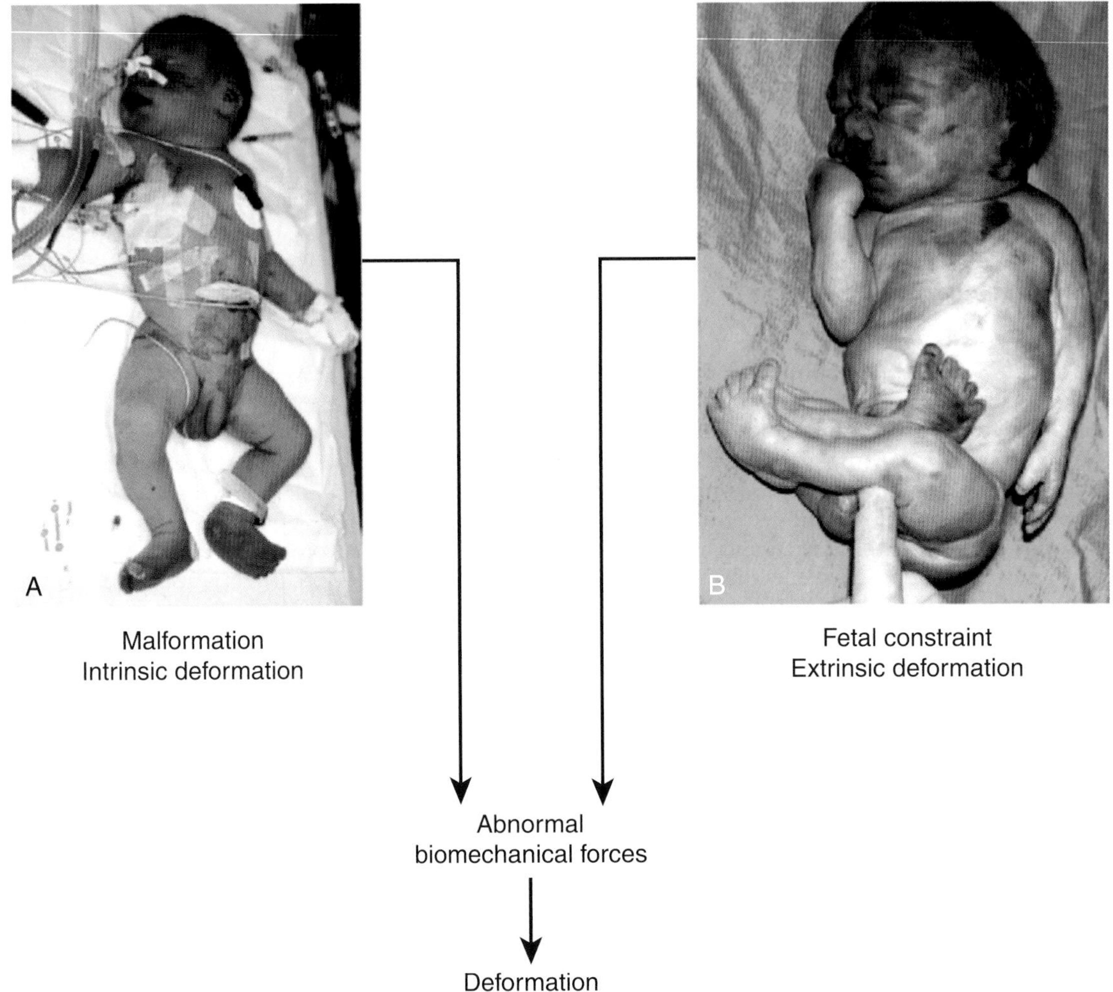

FIGURE 1.2 Unusual mechanical forces resulting in deformation may be the consequence of extrinsic constraint of a normal fetus, or they may be the result of an intrinsic malformation of the fetus. **A,** An infant with oligohydramnios deformation sequence caused by bilateral renal agenesis. **B,** An infant with oligohydramnios deformation sequence caused by prolonged leakage of amniotic fluid. Both infants died shortly after birth from associated pulmonary hypoplasia.

for a number of associated deformations (see Figs. 1.1B, 1.2B, and 1.3D). The major cause of such deformations is uterine constraint of the rapidly growing, malleable fetus in late gestation. Most of these molded deformations have an excellent prognosis once the fetus is released from the constraining environment. However, they usually merit prompt treatment at the appropriate time to achieve the best result (usually the earlier, the better). Such treatment often involves the use of gentle mechanical forces to attempt to reshape the deformed structure into a more normal form.

A clear distinction between deformation and malformation is critical to providing parents with a clear understanding of their infant's problem and its prognosis, management, and recurrence risk. Such a clear distinction may not always be possible, and the study of structural defects in twins demonstrates the complexity of making such distinctions. Twin studies represent a unique approach to understanding both genetic and environmental etiologic contributions to the development of congenital anomalies.[2,3] Twins share identical intrauterine environments, but their genetic constitutions are either homogeneous, as in

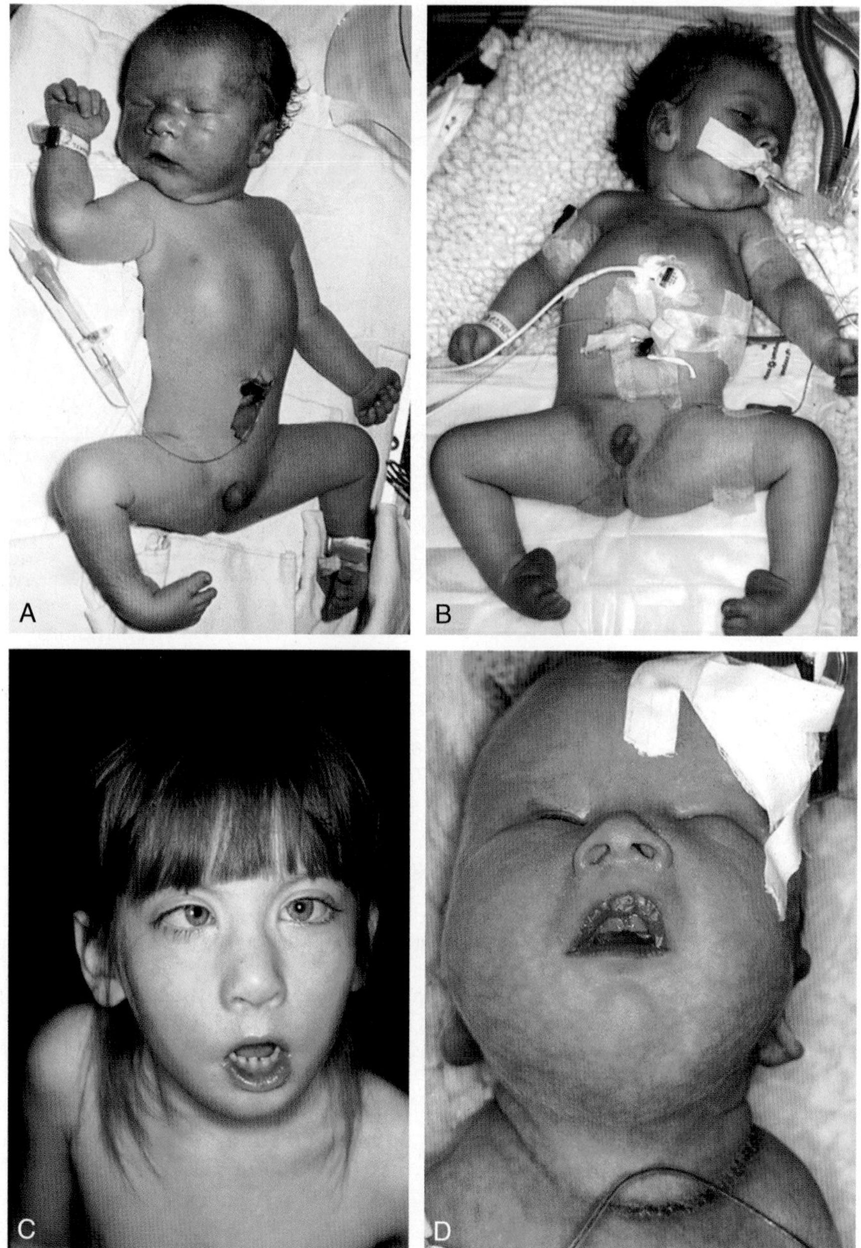

FIGURE 1.3 The overall pattern of intrinsic deformation caused by neuromuscular insufficiency is quite similar for both congenital myotonic dystrophy (**A**), an autosomal dominant disorder with a 50% recurrence risk, and Pena-Shokeir syndrome (**B**), an autosomal recessive disorder with a 25% recurrence risk. In **C**, note the facial effects of intrinsic deformation caused by Möbius sequence (deficient cranial nerve VI and VII function), which differ from the extrinsic facial deformations seen in **D**, in which prolonged oligohydramnios and a persistent transverse lie resulted in marked facial compression.

monozygotic twins, or heterogeneous, as in dizygotic twins. Monozygotic twins often share the same placenta and placental vasculature, which makes them more vulnerable to vascular disruption. Late fetal crowding makes deformations much more common in twins, and deformations are equally likely in both types of twinning. Because the fetal head accounts for much of the volume in late gestation, it is particularly

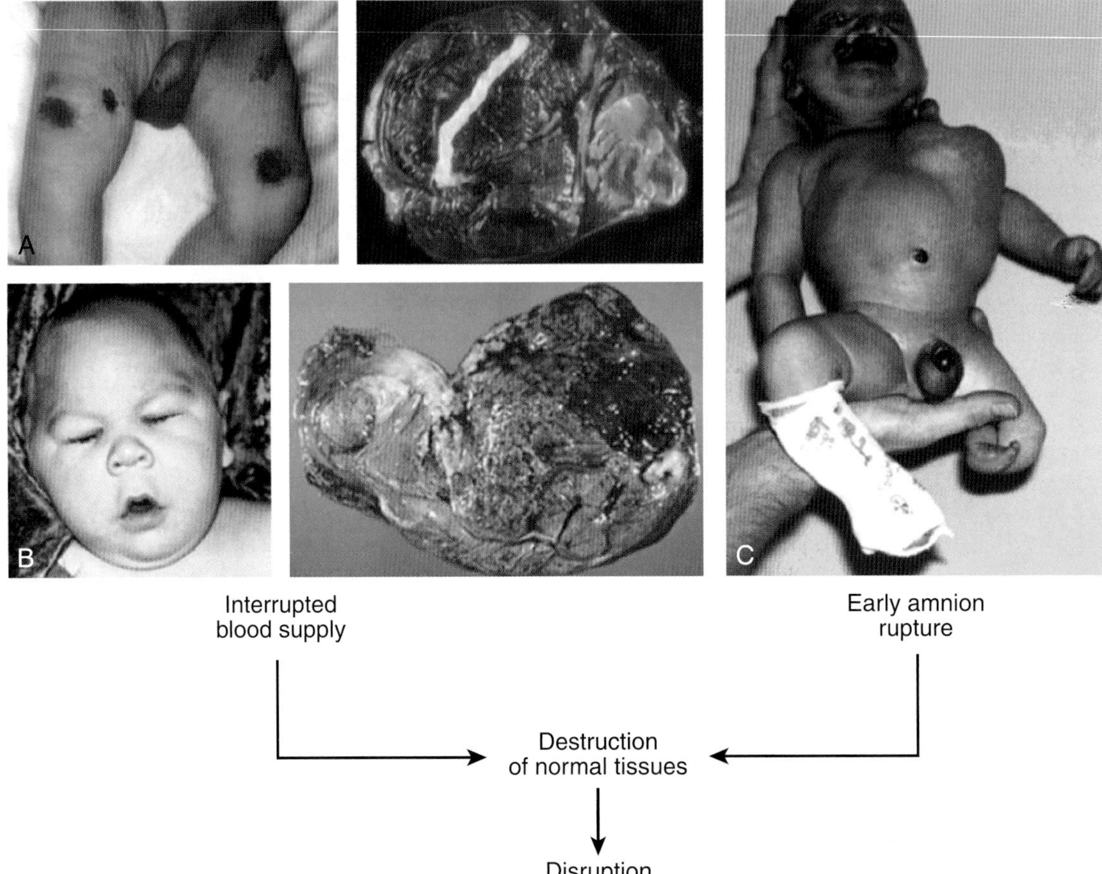

FIGURE 1.4 The two predominant types of fetal disruptions are demonstrated. Disruptive defects occur when there is destruction of a previously normally formed part. This can result from interruption of blood supply (**A** and **B**) or from amniotic bands. In some cases of early amnion rupture, both mechanisms may occur (**C**). When one monozygotic, monochorionic twin dies in utero, interruption of blood supply to fetal structures can lead to infarction, necrosis, hypoplasia, and/or resorption of tissues distal to where thromboembolic debris lodges in the circulation of the surviving co-twin (**A** and **B**). A deceased co-twin is evident on examination of the placentas for an infant born with cutis aplasia over the knees (**A**) and an infant with hydranencephaly (**B**).

susceptible to extrinsic, constraint-related deformations. Among 801 infants with deformational plagiocephaly who were treated with an external orthotic device, 69 (8.6%) were of multiple-birth origin.[4] Because there is less space within the lower portion of the uterus, the bottom twin in vertex presentation is most likely to develop torticollis-plagiocephaly deformation sequence (Fig. 1.5).

Monozygotic twinning results when a fertilized zygote splits into two embryos during the first 14 days after fertilization; this splitting process is associated with an increased likelihood of early malformations, many of which lead to the threefold higher mortality rate seen in monozygotic twins compared with dizygotic twins or singletons.[2] Among craniofacial anomalies, structural defects of the malformative or disruptive type occur more frequently in monozygotic twins compared with dizygotic twins. Malformations are often concordant, whereas disruptions and deformations are not. Among 35 twin pairs in which one or both twins exhibited craniofacial anomalies, 21 pairs were monozygotic and 14 pairs were dizygotic.[3] Malformations were more common among monozygotic twins compared with dizygotic twins, and concordance occurred predominantly in the monozygotic group, with seven of eight pairs being concordant. Among 20 twin pairs with discordant anomalies for whom there was information

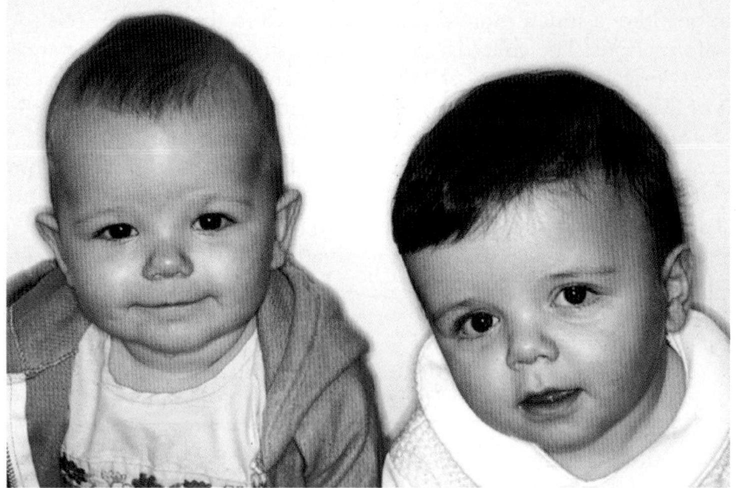

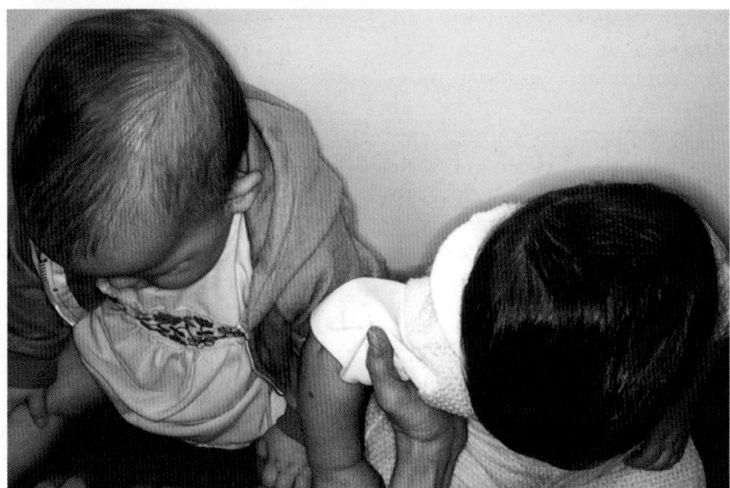

FIGURE 1.5 Torticollis-plagiocephaly deformation sequence is more frequent in twins, and it is usually the bottom-most twin who is most likely to develop torticollis and secondary craniofacial deformation. The twin on the right was on the bottom and has residual plagiocephaly at age 10 months because of untreated torticollis and an asymmetric postnatal resting position.

regarding fetal position, the affected infant was usually vertex and inferior in the pelvis, and deformational craniofacial anomalies were often associated with early fetal head descent during the third trimester.[3]

Monozygotic twins with placental vascular interconnections may be predisposed toward vasculodisruptive defects in the surviving twin when one twin dies in utero (termed *twin disruption sequence*). Among monochorionic twin pregnancies with one dead twin (see Fig. 1.4A–B), only 57% of the co-twin survivors were unaffected, with 19% of the co-twins dying in utero or during the neonatal period and 24% surviving with serious sequelae (e.g., cerebellar infarcts, porencephaly, hydranencephaly, microcephaly, spinal cord infarcts, hemifacial microsomia, gastroschisis, limb-reduction defects, renal cortical necrosis, atresia of the small bowel, and cutis aplasia).[5] Among 18 twins with twin disruption sequence, most deaths occurred in the second or third trimester, and intrauterine death in the first trimester rarely caused damage to the surviving co-twin. Survivors had a poor prognosis resulting from microcephaly, spastic tetraplegia, severe intellectual disability, and therapy-resistant epilepsy.[6]

In general, deformations have a much more favorable prognosis than malformations. The collective frequency of all types of extrinsic deformations of late fetal origin is about 2% of live births.[7–9] This frequency is based on the work of neonatologist Dr. Peter Dunn, who correlated clinical records of 4754 infants born in the Birmingham Maternity Hospital (United Kingdom) with maternal medical history and infant follow-up. This population study documented a 3.6% incidence of malformation, with or without deformation, and among the malformed infants in Dunn's sample, 7.6% were also deformed.[7–9] The deformation rate was 26.7% for infants with urinary tract malformations and 100% for those with bilateral renal agenesis. Of 11 infants born to mothers with premature rupture of membranes, none were malformed but 10 were deformed. Among the group of infants with postural deformations, Dunn noted that 33% had two or more deformations and that there were significant associations between facial deformity, plagiocephaly, mandibular asymmetry, muscular torticollis, scoliosis, developmental dysplasia of the hip (DDH), and talipes equinovarus.[9] About one-third (32%) of the deformed infants had been in breech presentation. First-born infants were significantly more likely to be deformed than subsequently born infants (54% vs. 35%). Thus it is particularly important to look for deformations in the infants of primigravida mothers and in infants with malpresentation.

In a study of 1,455,405 Spanish infants born alive between 1976 and 1997, 26,290 (1.8%) had major or minor anomalies detected at birth; of this group, 3.67% also had deformations. Deformations were found four times more frequently (14.62%) among stillborn infants with anomalies.[10] These authors distinguished three distinct patterns of deformations. One pattern featured polyhydramnios, thin skin without dermal ridges, and multiple deformations resulting from fetal akinesia-hypokinesia sequence caused by various intrinsic neuromuscular defects. A second pattern resulted in oligohydramnios with redundant thick skin and multiple deformations caused by intrinsic renal or urinary tract defects, or due to extrinsic loss of amniotic fluid. A third pattern of deformation was associated with normal amounts of amniotic fluid and was caused by various types of extrinsic fetal compression.[10] Differences between the 0.07% frequency of extrinsic deformations in this latter study and the 2% frequency noted by Dunn reflect major differences in the classification of minor postural deformations. In Dunn's earlier studies, 90% of the postural deformations he observed resolved spontaneously, and such transient defects were probably not counted in the Spanish study. Alternatively, with more accurate gestational dating and size determination, the incidence of large-for-gestational-age and postmature infants has been decreasing, thereby lowering the risk for late gestational constraint.

This text is primarily concerned with extrinsic deformations produced by unusual or excessive constraint of an otherwise normal fetus. Individual deformations in this book are presented in an atlas format along with deformation sequences. Because it may sometimes be difficult to exclude an underlying connective tissue dysplasia, examples of such problems are also discussed as part of the differential diagnosis. Because the major emphasis of this text is extrinsic deformations caused by uterine constraint, this category will be considered first. Next, consideration will be given to the interaction between extrinsic and intrinsic factors in the genesis of some deformations. Finally, intrinsic deformations caused by a fetal neuromuscular insufficiency are discussed.

EXTRINSIC DEFORMATIONS CAUSED BY UTERINE CONSTRAINT

The presumption in this category is that there is no primary problem within the fetus and that the deformations are secondary to extrinsic forces that have deformed an otherwise normal fetus. The most common cause of extrinsic deformation is uterine constraint. About 2% of babies are born with an extrinsic deformation, 90% of which resolve spontaneously; hence, these are relatively common problems.[7–10] Usually the amount of amniotic fluid is adequate to cushion the fetus, allowing for normal growth and mobility before 36–37 weeks of gestation. Thus one of the major functions of the amniotic fluid is to distend the uterus and enable the fetus to move freely and to grow with equal pressure in all regions with no excessive or localized constraint.[11] As the fetus becomes more crowded within the uterus during late gestation, it will usually settle into a position in which the largest moving fetal parts, the relatively bulky legs, have more room in the upper portion of the uterus. Thus the fetus tends to assume a vertex presentation. The implication that most extrinsic deformations are produced during late fetal life is supported by the observations of Nishimura, who found that both hip dislocation and clubfoot are rare findings in aborted fetuses before 20 weeks of gestation.[12]

After about 35–38 weeks of gestation, the human fetus tends to grow out of proportion to the size of

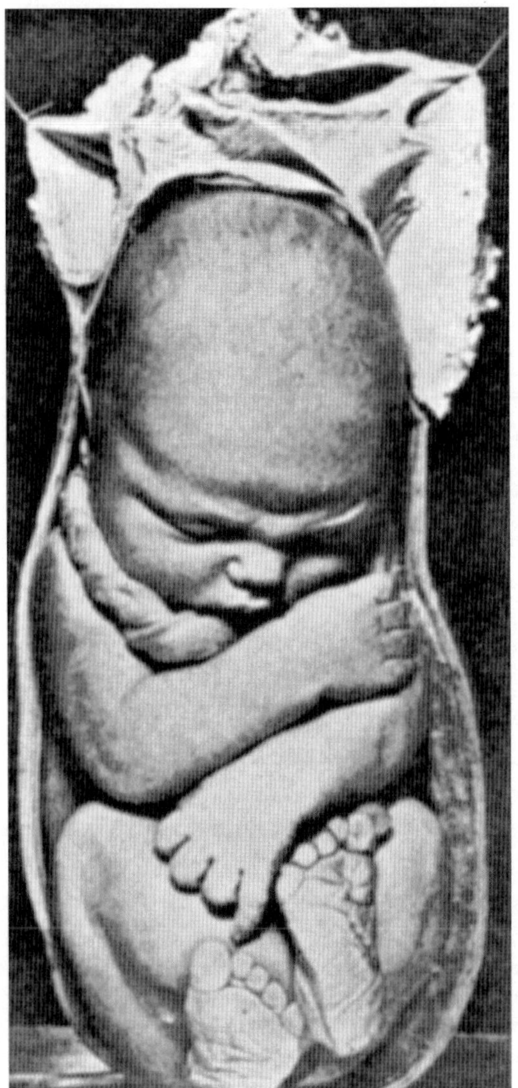

FIGURE 1.6 A primigravida's term fetus in breech position illustrates the uterine constraint that is a feature of late fetal life and this mode of presentation. The mother was killed in a motor vehicle accident, and the fetus was dead on arrival at the hospital. (Courtesy of Peter Dunn, Southmead Hospital, Bristol, United Kingdom.)

the uterine cavity (Fig. 1.6). During this period of rapid late fetal growth, the relative proportion of amniotic fluid decreases, causing the fetus to become increasingly constrained. Uterine constraint of rapidly growing, malleable fetal structures may result in mechanically induced deformations. Because the cause of one deformation may often have led to other constraint-related problems in the pliable fetus, there may be a nonrandom occurrence of more than one deformation in the same child. Dunn[8] found that 33% of newborn infants with one deformation problem had additional deformations (Fig. 1.7). In this text, the combination of multiple deformations resulting from the same extrinsic cause is termed a *deformation sequence*.

Uterine constraint tends also to reduce the rate of late fetal growth and is one cause of prenatal growth deficiency.[13,14] Such newborn babies frequently show deformational evidence of uterine constraint other than growth deficiency alone. Any situation that tends to overly distend the uterus may be associated with early onset of labor and premature birth. This is a major concern for multiple-gestation infants, who simply distend the uterus prematurely, and also for the woman with uterine structural malformations or extensive uterine myomas. When fetal growth has been constrained during late gestation, catch-up growth is usually initiated promptly after delivery so that most term fetuses reach their genetically determined growth percentiles by 6–8 months of age.[15]

If the basic type of deformation is not clearly determined at the time of birth, then the early postnatal course usually provides valuable clues as to whether the deformations noted at birth are extrinsic or intrinsic in causation. The otherwise normal infant who has been constrained in late fetal life tends to show progressive improvement in growth and form after being released from the deforming situation upon delivery. If growth has been slowed by constraint in late fetal life, the infant tends to show catch-up growth toward their genetic potential in early infancy, beginning within the first 2 months. If the growth of particular structures has been restrained, they tend to show catch-up growth toward normal form, such as with the nasal and mandibular growth restriction seen following prolonged face presentation. Joints that have been externally constrained prenatally tend to show progressive increases in their range of motion after birth, often showing more dramatic resolution with neonatal physical therapy. This is clearly evident with positional torticollis or positional foot deformations but not with structural neck malformations (e.g., Klippel-Feil malformation) or rigid clubfoot. If there is a lack of catch-up growth and/or little or no return toward normal form after birth, then further evaluation is indicated to search for a more intrinsic problem that might be responsible for the deformation(s).

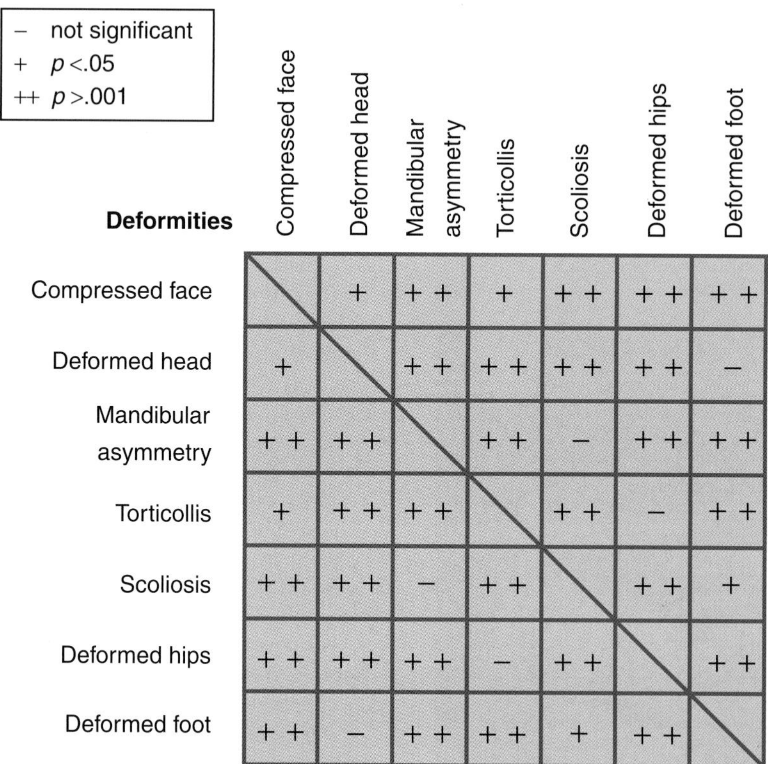

–	not significant
+	p<.05
++	p>.001

Deformities	Compressed face	Deformed head	Mandibular asymmetry	Torticollis	Scoliosis	Deformed hips	Deformed foot
Compressed face		+	+ +	+	+ +	+ +	+ +
Deformed head	+		+ +	+ +	+ +	+ +	–
Mandibular asymmetry	+ +	+ +		+ +	–	+ +	+ +
Torticollis	+	+ +	+ +		+ +	–	+ +
Scoliosis	+ +	+ +	–	+ +		+ +	+
Deformed hips	+ +	+ +	+ +	–	+ +		+ +
Deformed foot	+ +	–	+ +	+ +	+	+ +	

FIGURE 1.7 The nonrandom clinical association among deformations. (Adapted from Dunn PM. Congenital postural deformities: further perinatal associations. *Proc R Soc Med*. 1972;65:735.)

Historical Perspective

As long ago as Hippocrates, it was known that uterine constraint could cause fetal deformation. Aristotle carried out experiments demonstrating that crowding of development caused limb deformations in chicks; however, little was written about constraint deformations until the Renaissance era. In 1573 Ambroise Paré[16] of France wrote:

> *Narrowness of the uterus produces monsters by the same manner that the Dame of Paris carried the little dog in a small basket to the end that it didn't grow.*

In 1921, von Reuss's text *Diseases of the Newborn* contained an entire chapter on postural deformations,[17] but modern texts about the newborn have more limited coverage of this subject. Full understanding of the mechanisms and types of fetal deformations is vitally important for clinicians who deal with problems of aberrant morphogenesis. A number of investigators have made major contributions to the knowledge and understanding of extrinsic deformations during the past century. A few brief summations and quotations from representative investigators will serve to emphasize some of their important observations and interpretations.

Thompson[18]: This Scottish naturalist and mathematician held the Chair of Natural History in St. Andrews for 64 years. He wrote:

> *We are ruled by gravity. ... There is freedom of movement in the plane perpendicular to gravitational force. ... Gravity affects stature and leads to sagging of tissues and drooping of the mouth.*

von Reuss[17]: This early Viennese neonatologist made the following statement about contractural deformities:

> *...the deformities occur probably most frequently from pressure on the part of the uterine wall; sometimes marks of pressure may be observed on the skin.*

Chapple and Davidson[19]: These pediatricians noted that the "position of comfort" of the deformed infant soon after birth tends to be that which had existed in utero, and repositioning the baby into the "position of comfort" might allow the clinician to more readily deduce the causative compressive factors that resulted in the deformation.

Browne[20,21]: Denis Browne, an orthopedist at Great Ormond Street Children's Hospital in London, recognized that deformed infants were often the product of an "uncomfortable" pregnancy, implying uterine constraint. He emphasized the need for controlled forces, using functional growth, in the correction of such deformations.

Dunn[7–9]: This English neonatologist was responsible for resurrecting and extending knowledge regarding the importance of extrinsic deformation. He stated that:

> *Intrauterine forces capable of moulding the fetus increase throughout pregnancy as the infant grows, the mother's uterus and abdominal wall are stretched, and the volume of amniotic fluid diminishes. At the same time the ability of the infant to resist deformation increases as the rate of fetal growth slows, the skeleton ossifies, and leg movements become more powerful. All these factors are, of course, themselves directly or indirectly under the influence of heredity and are involved in a dynamic interplay throughout fetal life. Nature plays her hand to the limit. The price paid for a larger and more mature infant at birth, better able to withstand the stresses of extra uterine life, is a 2% incidence of deformities.*

Factors That Enhance Fetal Constraint in Utero

Box 1.1 summarizes some of the factors that increase the likelihood of fetal constraint in utero; these factors are presented in more detail in this section.

BOX 1.1 RISK FACTORS FOR FETAL CONSTRAINT

Maternal Risk Factors
Primigravida
Small maternal size
Small uterus
Uterine malformation
Uterine fibromata
Small maternal pelvis

Fetal Risk Factors
Oligohydramnios
Large fetus
Multiple fetuses
Malpresentation (e.g., breech or transverse lie)

Primigravida

The first fetus usually experiences more constraint than later offspring because it is the first to distend the mother's muscular uterus and abdominal wall. As a consequence, constraint-related deformations are more common in infants born to primigravida mothers than to multigravidas. Fig. 1.8 shows the form of the uterus in a primigravida compared with a multigravida, emphasizing the difference in shape and size of the structures surrounding the fetus. The greater magnitude of late fetal constraint in the primigravida is one major reason why the first-born infant is normally smaller at birth than later-born offspring. Even though the first-born infant tends to be 200–300 g smaller than later offspring at birth, they are of comparable size by 1 year of age. Thus the mild late fetal growth deficiency in the offspring of a primigravida is transient, and such infants tend to catch up to their genetically determined rate of growth within the first few months after birth.[13–15] The first-born infant is also more likely to become constrained in an unusual position, such as a breech presentation, and to have consequent deformations relating to malpresentation.

Small Maternal Size

The smaller the mother in relation to fetal size, the greater the likelihood will be of deforming uterine constraint in late fetal life. Deformations are more common in offspring born to small women than in those born to larger women. This impact is readily evident in terms of birth size. Maternal size has a much greater impact on birth size than does paternal size; however, by 1 year of age, the length of the infant relates equally to maternal and paternal stature. Much of this maternal impact on birth size appears to relate to the transient effect of small maternal size in restraining late fetal growth. After birth, the infant moves into their own genetic pace of growth, which is usually evident by 6–8 months of age.[15] The effect of maternal size on prenatal growth is illustrated in Figs. 1.9 and 1.10. Many infants born with torticollis-plagiocephaly deformation sequence are born to parents with obvious size discrepancies (i.e., small mothers and large fathers).

Uterine Malformation

Limitation in the capacity of the uterus to accommodate a term-size fetus may result in early miscarriage, stillbirth, prematurity, and/or offspring who survive

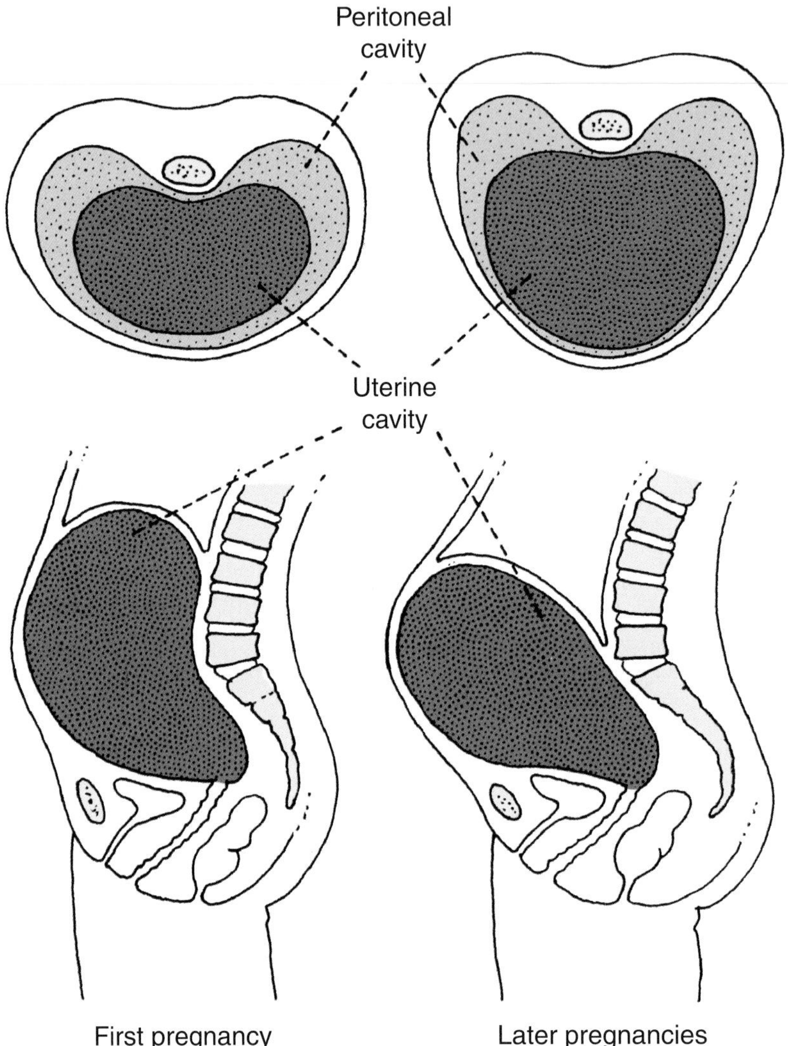

FIGURE 1.8 Transverse and sagittal section diagrams of the abdomens of primigravida and multigravida women illustrate the impact of unstretched abdominal muscles on the shape of the uterine cavity during the later weeks of pregnancy. (Adapted from Dunn PM. Perinatal observations on the etiology of congenital dislocation of the hip. *Clin Orthop*. 1976;119:11.)

to be born with sufficient constraint to give rise to deformation(s). Such reproductive problems are particularly likely to occur with uterine malformations such as a bicornuate or unicornuate uterus. About 1%–2% of women have a uterine malformation, and the likelihood of a deformation problem in a fetus reared in a bicornuate uterus has been crudely estimated to be about 30%.[22] Many of the genetic factors that result in a bicornuate uterus also affect renal morphogenesis, which leads to renal dysplasia and resultant oligohydramnios, further increasing the likelihood of fetal deformation. The recognition that a malformation of the mother's uterus has caused a fetal problem may lead to corrective surgery on that uterus, thus

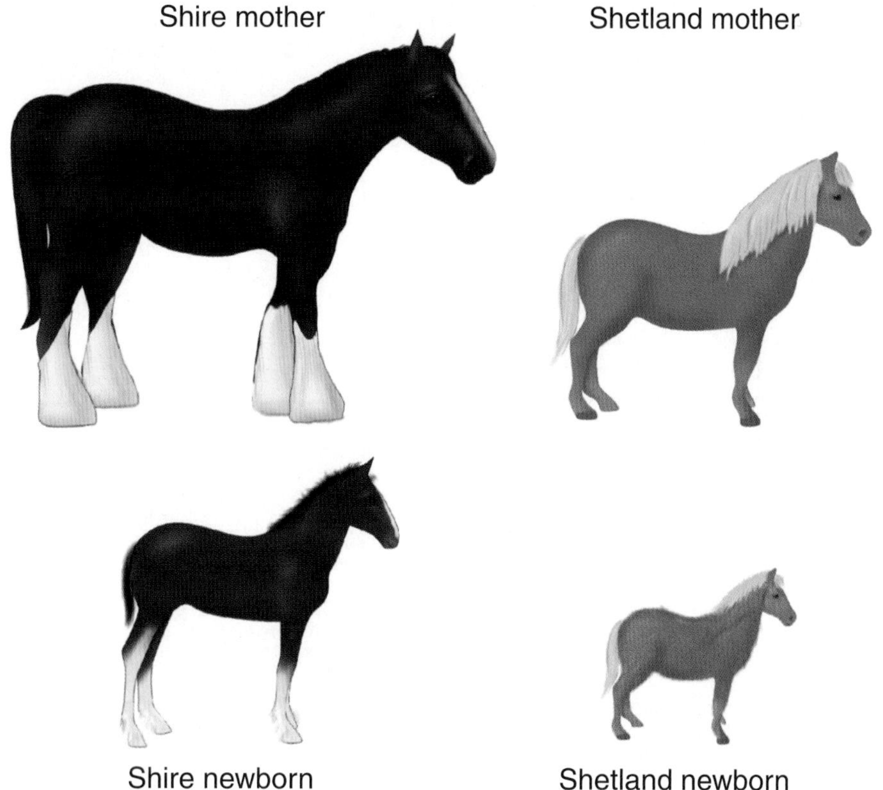

FIGURE 1.9 The cross between a shire horse and a Shetland pony dramatically illustrates the influence of maternal size on the size of the offspring at birth. Although the genetic situation is the same, the foal of the small mother is much smaller at birth than that of the large mother, presumably because of the smaller space within which to rear this fetus. (From Walton A, Hammond J. The maternal effects on growth and conformation in shire horse-Shetland pony crosses. *Proc R Coc Lond.* 1938;B125:311-335. http://doi.org/10.1098/rspb.1938.0029.)

providing a better opportunity for the next fetus to grow without as much constraint.

Uterine Fibromata

A large fibroid of the uterus may limit intrauterine space and therefore have a gestational impact similar to that of a bicornuate uterus. Surgical removal of the fibroid may allow for better fetal space, and this merits consideration if it will not weaken the structure of the uterus. Fortunately, most uterine fibromata develop relatively late in reproductive life and are an infrequent cause of fetal deformation; however, a small fibroma may grow rapidly during gestation under the influence of increased levels of maternal estrogen.

Small Maternal Pelvis

Vaginal delivery through a pelvic outlet that is small in relation to the size of the fetus may result in appreciable molding of the craniofacial region. This molding is usually transient; however, if there has been prolonged engagement of the fetal head the degree of molding can be severe, and there may be a slower resolution toward normal form after birth. Early treatment via appropriate positioning can facilitate a more complete return to normal form.

Early Pelvic Engagement of the Fetal Head

During labor, the fetal head usually engages in an occiput transverse position as the head enters and passes through the pelvic inlet. In the typical female

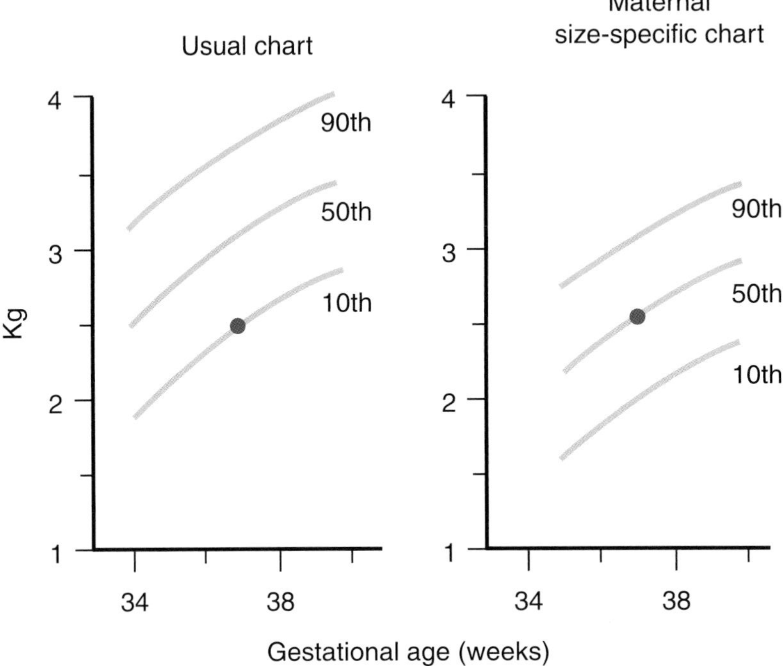

FIGURE 1.10 The weight of a 2.3-kg newborn baby born to a small mother with a weight of 40 kg and height of 150 cm, plotted on the usual growth chart *(left)* and on one that is specific for maternal size *(right)*. (Adapted from Winick M. Biologic correlations. *Am J Dis Child.* 1970;120:416. Standards for the chart on the right are from Thomson AM, Billewicz WZ, Hytten FE, et al. The assessment of fetal growth. *J Obstet Gynecol Br Comm.* 1968;75:903.)

pelvis (gynecoid), this results more commonly in a left-oriented occiput position than in a right-oriented position (58.5% vs. 40.5%).[23-25] Progressive descent of the fetal head occurs as it traverses the pelvic inlet with the sagittal suture in the transverse diameter of the pelvic inlet and the biparietal diameter parallel to the anteroposterior diameter of the pelvic inlet. With progressing descent of the fetal head, internal rotation occurs, and the fetal head usually passes the ischial spines in an occiput anterior or posterior position. As the head descends, it encounters resistance from the cervix, the walls of the pelvis, and/or the pelvic floor, resulting in further flexion of the fetal head. Engagement of the fetal head is considered to have occurred when the biparietal diameter, the largest transverse diameter of the fetal head, has traversed the pelvic inlet. In nulliparous patients, engagement may occur by 36 weeks, but most nulliparous women present in labor without the fetal head engaged; in multiparous patients, engagement occurs significantly later and often only intrapartum.[26]

Early descent of the fetal head into the maternal pelvis is an unusual event often accompanied by maternal symptoms of marked pelvic pressure and pubic discomfort that sometimes include pain radiating down the back of the legs. It is very unusual for the fetal head to descend more than 6 weeks before term, and it rarely does so more than 1 month before delivery. Early fetal head descent is more common in the primigravida. When the symptoms are severe, pain may make it difficult for the mother to walk during late gestation. Fetal head descent usually takes place shortly before birth, and the head in vertex presentation rotates into the left occiput transverse position in 58.5% of cases so as to pass through the mother's pelvis (Fig. 1.11). Consequences of early fetal head descent can include congenital muscular torticollis, craniotabes, craniosynostosis, and persistent vertex molding.[27] The fetal head is particularly susceptible to deforming forces because it is a relatively large and rapidly growing structure. One manifestation is vertex craniotabes secondary to prolonged compression of the top of the calvarium, resulting in poorly mineralized, malleable bone in the region of compression.[28] Another potential consequence is lateral constraint of the fetal head, resulting in a lack of growth stretch

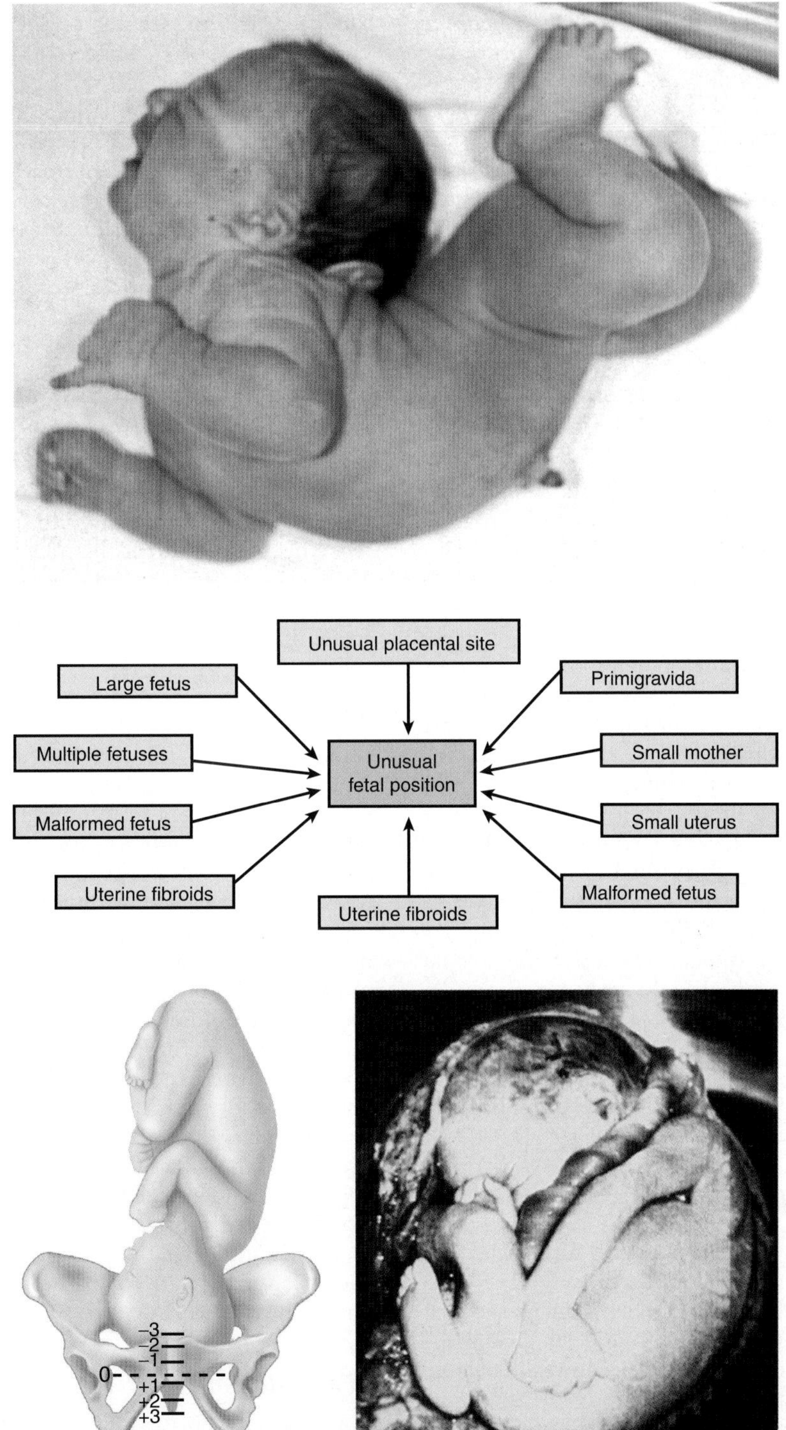

FIGURE 1.11 This drawing shows the left occiput transverse position, which occurs most commonly in vertex presentations. The top figure and the bottom right figure show aberrant fetal positions that can result from any of the factors shown in this diagram. *(Courtesy Jan Norbisrath, Medical Illustrator, Dept. of Obstetrics and Gynecology, University of Washington School of Medicine, Seattle.)*

across the sagittal suture. If there is a lack of growth stretch across a given suture then that suture can become ossified, resulting in craniosynostosis.[27,29] The most common problem after early fetal head descent is congenital muscular torticollis, which can lead to deformational plagiocephaly without appropriate therapy. Some degree of transient vertex head molding occurs in most infants in cephalic presentation, but this usually resolves within a few days. It is rare, even with prolonged engagement of the fetal head, for such molding to persist, and corrective postnatal positioning can facilitate a return to normal head shape.

Fetal Position

Before 36–37 weeks, when the fetus usually has adequate room for movement in its aquatic environment, it is not unusual for the fetus to be in varying positions, most commonly breech presentation. As the fetus becomes more crowded, they tend to shift into the vertex presentation position, there being more room in the fundal portion of the uterus for the bulkier legs. Unusual late fetal position in utero may result from all the factors that increase the risk for fetal constraint (see Fig. 11.1), as well as from a primary fetal neuromuscular problem or malformation, which limits the ability of the fetus to move (Fig. 1.12). The most common reason for an aberrant position is fetal constraint that has limited the capacity of the fetus to move into a vertex presentation. Abnormal fetal position during late fetal life may result in unusual constraint forces that significantly affect craniofacial structures. Examples include breech presentation, face presentation, brow presentation, and transverse lie. Breech presentation, although occurring in only 4% of pregnancies, was associated with 32% of all extrinsic deformations in Dunn's early studies.[7–9]

Large Fetus With Rapid Growth

The fetus normally manifests a rapid rate of growth. For example, it normally doubles in weight between 28 and 34 weeks of gestation. The faster the growth rate, the larger the fetus becomes, and the greater the likelihood of all types of external constraint-related deformations. In a prospective study of 801 pregnancies that resulted in the birth of an infant weighing 4100 g or more, shoulder dystocia and perinatal lacerations were related to increasing birth weight. Difficult deliveries leading to clavicular fractures, brachial plexus injuries, or facial trauma resulted in an 11.4% perinatal morbidity rate. Asphyxia was observed in 7.7% and hypoglycemia in 5.2%, suggesting a need for close surveillance of infants of obese or diabetic mothers.[30] The male is normally larger and grows more rapidly in late fetal life than does the female.[15] Many extrinsic deformations are more common in the male than in the female, with the exceptions of DDH and other similar joint-dislocation deformations that appear to be related to greater connective tissue laxity in females. Although torticollis-plagiocephaly deformation sequence is more common in males, this does not appear to result from size differences at birth.[31] The effects of relaxing hormones and hormone receptors in the female fetus may affect their connective tissues to allow for cervical dilatation, increase their susceptibility to congenital hip dislocation, and protect them from torticollis. Testosterone may also accentuate muscular development in males, increasing susceptibility to torticollis and protecting them from hip dislocation.

Multiple Fetuses

Multiple fetuses fill out the uterine cavity more quickly than a singleton fetus would, and the average uterus can handle a maximum of 4 kg of fetal mass. For twins, this combined size is usually achieved by approximately 34 weeks of gestation, after which there tends to be a slowing in growth as the uterine cavity becomes filled,[32] as shown in Fig. 1.13. Postural deformations and transient growth deficiency are more common in twins, especially malpositioning of the feet and molding of the cranium.[4,21,31,32] Torticollis-plagiocephaly deformation sequence occurs particularly frequently in multiple births, and usually the bottom-most twin is more likely to develop torticollis and secondary craniofacial deformation (see Fig. 1.5). Because of these factors, monozygotic twins may not appear to be identical at the time of birth. One twin may have been constrained in a different manner and to a different degree than the other twin. Some differences also may relate to aberrant fetal positioning in one of the twins.

Oligohydramnios

A deficit of amniotic fluid in late fetal life may result from a variety of causes such as early rupture of the amnion with chronic leakage of amniotic fluid, lack

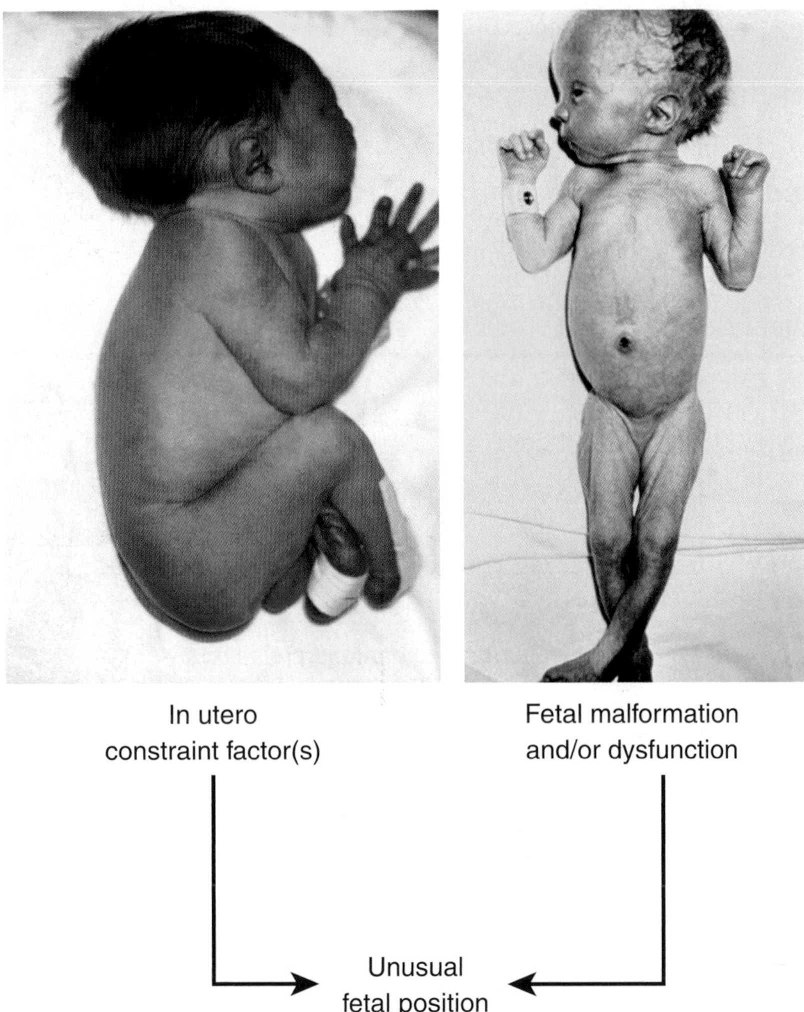

FIGURE 1.12 An unusual fetal position in utero may be the result of constraint factors to a normal fetus (prolonged breech presentation, left fetus), or it may be the consequence of a primary fetal malformation and/or neuromuscular dysfunction, such as the right fetus with Trisomy 18.

of urine flow into the amniotic space, or maternal hypertension. Regardless of the cause, a lack of amniotic fluid tends to give rise to an unusual degree of uterine constraint, which adversely affects fetal growth and pulmonary maturation and results in craniofacial and limb deformations.[33] The consequences of a prolonged deficit of amniotic fluid are referred to as the *oligohydramnios deformation sequence*. The impact of oligohydramnios versus polyhydramnios on birth size is shown in Fig. 1.14.

Management, Prognosis, and Counsel

When a deformation is caused by external constraint in late fetal life in an otherwise normal infant, the prognosis for a return to normal form is usually excellent, but this does not imply that the clinician caring for such infants should do nothing. The management of extrinsic deformations varies with the cause and type of deformation, and early treatment is the key to a successful outcome. Sometimes it is worthwhile to observe the neonate

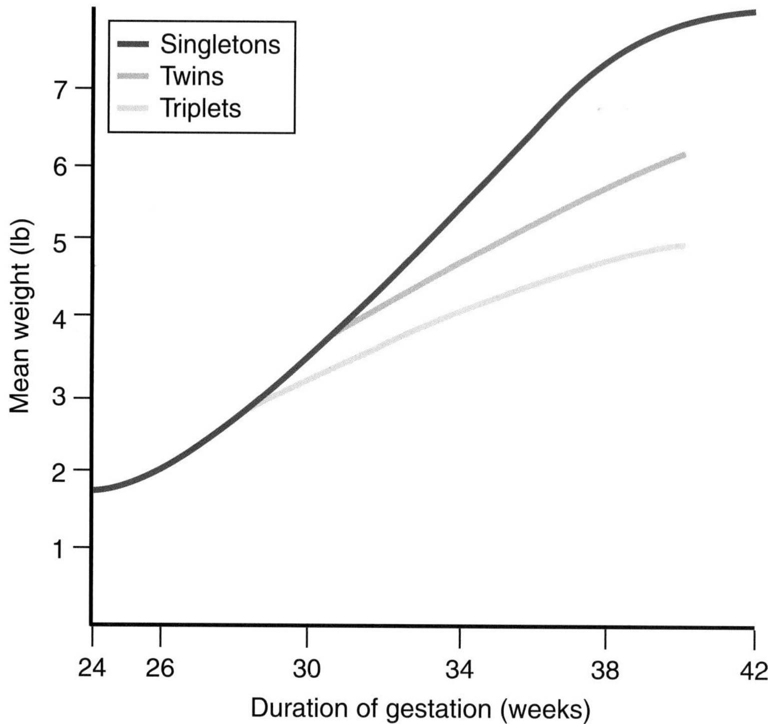

FIGURE 1.13 The mean fetal weights of singletons compared with twins and triplets. Although the initial growth rate is the same, the combined size of twins or triplets leads to earlier uterine constraint and late fetal slowing of growth. (Adapted from Bulmer MG. *The Biology of Twinning in Man.* Oxford, UK: Clarendon Press; 1970.)

for spontaneous changes for several days after birth before deciding whether any further therapy is indicated. Treatment often uses corrective mechanical forces like those that gave rise to the deformation, in an effort to reshape the deformed structures into a more normal form. When possible, this mechanical therapy should take advantage of the normal rapid rate of postnatal growth. This is particularly true for torticollis-plagiocephaly deformation sequence. When deformational plagiocephaly cannot be corrected with repositioning, use of orthotic management while the head is still growing rapidly has repeatedly been documented to correct deformational cranial asymmetry in otherwise normal infants.[31,33–36]

The precise modes of management for constraint-related deformations may vary appreciably and yet accomplish the same purpose. Simple manual manipulation with molding and stretching toward a normal form may be all that is needed. This is a common practice in India, where "massage women" are employed to mold and shape the neonate's head and extremities. These women come to the infant's home daily for the first few months or as long as indicated. By massage with oil and stretching, they form the baby into a normal shape and remove any extrinsic deformations that may have been present at birth. In a similar fashion, parents can be instructed to accomplish such molding or stretching at home. Reshaping forces can be applied to foot deformations by frequent adhesive taping, resulting in gradual improvement in form. When such benign measures do not adequately correct the deformation, more rigorous means of molding and stretching, such as casting of the limbs or orthotic molding of the head, may be used. The current epidemic of torticollis-plagiocephaly deformation sequence is caused by failure to recognize signs of positional torticollis at birth and institute corrective measures of physical therapy of the neck and repositioning of the infant's head in a timely manner.[31] When a joint is seriously dislocated or malpositioned and conservative measures have not been successful in correcting the joint into normal alignment, surgical intervention may

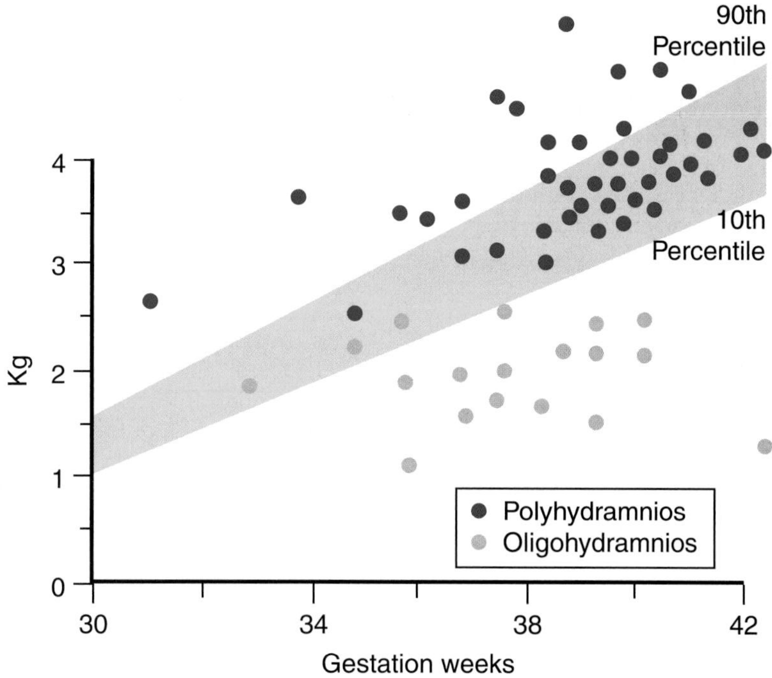

FIGURE 1.14 Impact on birth weight in kilograms of oligohydramnios caused by renal insufficiency versus polyhydramnios. (Adapted from Dunn PM. Growth retardation of infants with congenital postural deformities. *Acta Med Auxol.* 1975;7:63.)

be indicated. Ideally this should be done as soon as it is established that conservative measures are not working. The tendency toward earlier surgery for such defects is especially important for DDH and for severe equinovarus deformity in which the calcaneus and talus are at least partially dislocated. Proper bony alignment is necessary to foster normal subsequent joint development.

The counseling given to parents of a baby with an extrinsic deformation problem can usually be quite optimistic. With rare exceptions, the parents may be counseled in the following manner:

> *I believe your baby is normally formed. He/she became crowded in the uterus before birth, and this resulted in some unusual features at birth. Having been released from this constraint, the baby's features should return toward normal with proper neonatal management. It is for this reason that I say your baby is normal but requires some consistent management.*

Any treatment that is merited should be explained to the parents, and appropriate demonstrations of how to manage the infant should be provided. This is particularly important when it comes to infant sleeping positions and the early, frequent establishment of "tummy time" while the infant is awake and under observation. The switch from a prone to supine infant sleep position has decreased the frequencies of sudden infant death syndrome (SIDS), tibial torsion, and in-toeing while increasing the frequency of deformational plagiocephaly and brachycephaly, which is usually preventable.[31] The recurrence risk depends on the cause of the extrinsic deformation. For most deformations, the recurrence risk is low. However, it may be quite high if the cause is a persisting one, such as a uterine malformation. Obviously, it is important to distinguish extrinsic deformation from intrinsic deformation, which may be secondary to a genetic neuromuscular problem, because this distinction has a major impact on the prognosis and management of the child and on the recurrence risk for the parents.

Prevention

The prevention of extrinsic deformation seems an unlikely possibility because of the immaturity, pliability, and size of the human fetus. However, several examples of preventive measures already exist, and more may be developed in the future. Surgical repair of a malformed uterus that has previously resulted in serious deformation problems and decreased fetal survival may result in a greatly improved prognosis for normal offspring. The prevention of pulmonary hypoplasia by instilling replacement fluid for leaking amniotic fluid or by fetal surgery for diaphragmatic hernia or urethral obstruction malformation sequence may lead to improved fetal viability.

External cephalic version (ECV) of a fetus in an abnormal presentation is now an accepted mode of therapy in maternal-fetal medicine. This is usually accomplished between 35 and 37 weeks from conception. After 37 weeks, it is more difficult to accomplish ECV of the fetus into the vertex presentation, and before 35 weeks, the fetus may revert to a breech presentation. The most common indication for ECV is breech presentation, and use of ECV for term fetal malpresentation reduces the rate of noncephalic births and cesarean sections. Overall, pooled data from included studies showed a statistically significant and clinically meaningful reduction in noncephalic birth (seven trials, 1245 women; risk ratio [RR] 0.46; 95% confidence interval [CI] 0.31–0.66) and cesarean section (seven trials, 1245 women; RR 0.63; 95% CI 0.44–0.90) when ECV was attempted.[37] Because breech presentation was responsible for about one-third of the extrinsic deformations and one-half of the cases of dislocation of the hip in Dunn's series, any reduction in the frequency of breech presentation at term would have a significant impact on the frequency of deformations. Contraindications to ECV include multiple pregnancy, placenta previa, malformation of the uterus, and gross obesity. ECV is accomplished by gently manipulating the fetus through the abdominal wall and uterus while monitoring the fetal heart.

Prevention of more serious problems secondary to constraint deformation merits additional commentary. One example is the dolichocephalic head with prominent occiput that may develop following prolonged breech presentation in late fetal life.[38] Breech head deformation sequence is itself usually a benign deformation that tends to resolve after birth. However, the contour of this head can pose serious problems during vaginal delivery because it tends to become arrested during the second stage of labor. This complication increases the likelihood of damage to the brachial plexus and cervical spinal cord during vaginal delivery. Detection of the breech head by ultrasonography is now an indication for cesarean section delivery of a fetus in breech presentation. Thus prenatal detection of such a deformation may influence management toward the prevention of serious birth trauma.

INTERACTIONS BETWEEN EXTRINSIC AND INTRINSIC FACTORS

A given deformation might relate to both extrinsic and intrinsic factors, representing an interaction between the two categories. One example is congenital hip dislocation (Fig. 1.15). Most instances of DDH are secondary to external constraint, which forces the head of the femur out of its socket and stretches the joint capsule and ligamentum teres. DDH is more common in females because of increased connective tissue laxity in females resulting from the impact of relaxing hormones and the relative deficiency of testosterone during the perinatal period.[39] DDH also may result from an intrinsic abnormality in the fetus with unusually lax connective tissues caused by a genetic connective tissue dysplasia, such as Ehlers-Danlos syndrome or a malformation syndrome such as Larsen syndrome. Ehlers-Danlos syndrome can be suspected clinically by noting laxity in multiple joints and/or detecting joint laxity in a parent.

Another example of the interaction between intrinsic and extrinsic factors in creating a deformation is the fetus that has an intrinsic neuromuscular abnormality that limits the ability of the fetus to turn into the vertex position before birth. Such a fetus is more likely to be caught in the breech position and to be born with such problems as breech head, DDH, and other deformations that occur more frequently in the fetus presenting in breech position.

INTRINSIC CAUSATION OF DEFORMATION

Intramembranous bones are usually flat, and they primarily comprise the bones in the cranial vault and facial region. They arise directly from mesenchyme and differ from endochondral bones, which are formed initially from cartilage models.[40] The axial and appendicular skeletal bones form primarily through endochondral ossification and are of mesodermal origin, whereas some membranous bones originate from the neural crest and others originate from the mesoderm.[40] The clavicle is formed through a combination of both endochondral and intramembranous ossification. Type I and XI collagens are involved in bone formation, and type II, IX, X, and XI collagens are involved in cartilage

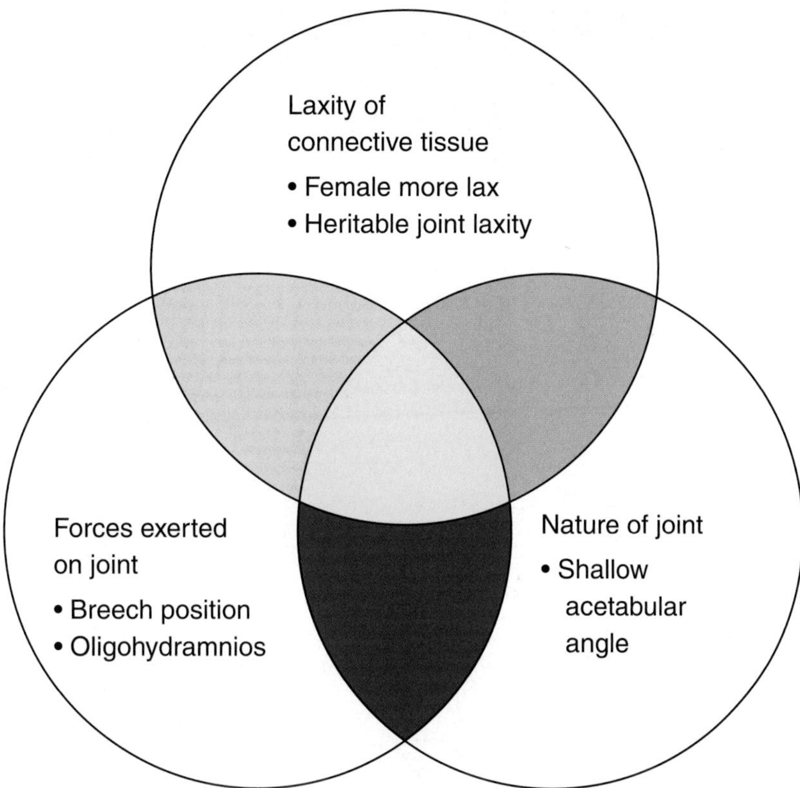

FIGURE 1.15 Interacting factors may relate to the likelihood of developing a deformation such as developmental dysplasia of the hip.

formation.[41] In addition to these structural proteins, other genes play critical roles in osteogenesis, such as transcription factors and various growth factors and their receptors. Mutations in these genes account for a wide variety of genetic connective tissue disorders, many of which are associated with an increased risk of deformation.[41] The cause of a given deformation may result from altered mechanical forces that are the consequence of a more primary problem within the fetus, such as a malformation. Although these intrinsic deformations are not the main subject of this text, it is important to consider them in the differential diagnosis of extrinsic deformations. Some deformations may be caused by either extrinsic or intrinsic factors. For example, the same type of malposition of the foot may result from external constraint, a neurologic deficit, or a muscle disorder. The judgment of the clinician is required to determine the primary causation of such deformations. The overall diagnosis, prognosis, and recurrence risk for a child with a malpositioned foot may differ widely if the deformation is secondary to uterine constraint rather than the result of a primary neuromuscular problem. Several types of intrinsic fetal problems may result in altered mechanics and thereby give rise to deformation of otherwise normal tissues. Examples include neuromuscular disorders, aberrant growth of a tissue, and obstruction of a hollow organ. Examples of each are described in this section.

Neuromuscular Problems

Any deficit of neuromuscular function may result in multiple deformations. When the primary problem is neural, a secondary loss of muscle mass may occur (Fig. 1.16). As a consequence of diminished movement, there may be joint fixations, and with a lack of stress, the bone grows more slowly in breadth, tending to become slenderer and more fragile. This phenotype has been termed *fetal akinesia deformation sequence*.[42,43] Sites of muscle attachment to bone, which are normally prominent, may be less prominent or even lacking because of such neuromuscular

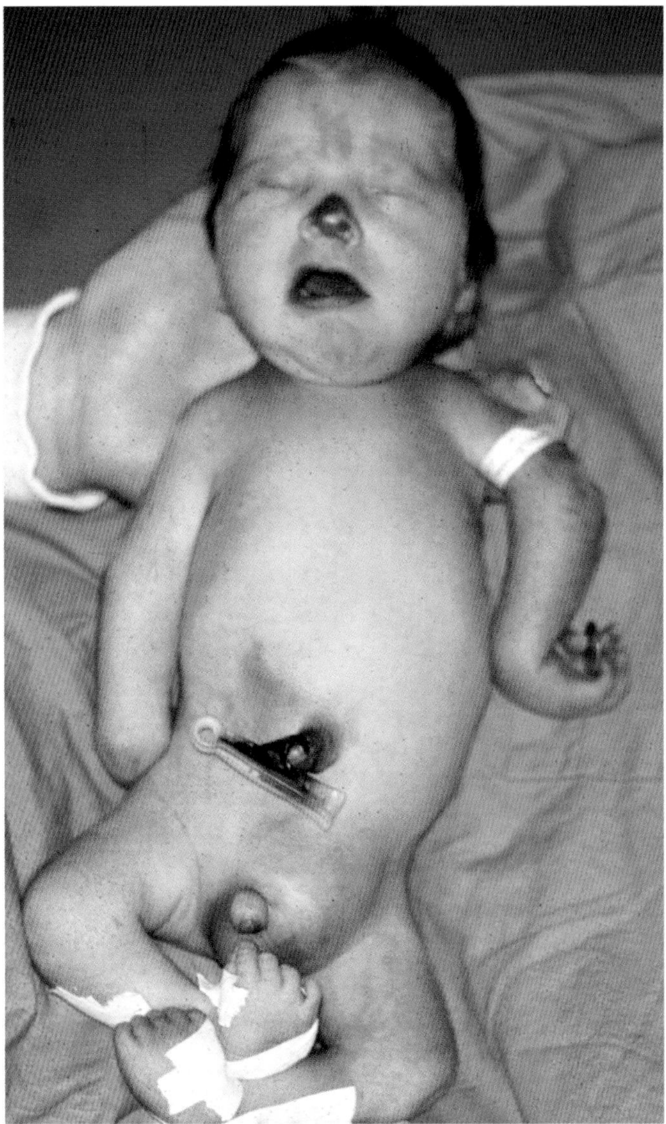

FIGURE 1.16 This infant with the amyoplasia form of arthrogryposis experienced early loss of motor nerve function to the limbs (possibly because of disruption of blood supply to the spinal cord), resulting in replacement of muscle with fibrous tissue and fat, and causing joints to become fixed in an early fetal position.

deficiency. Excessive neuromuscular function, such as that seen with spasticity, may give rise to an unusual magnitude and direction of muscle forces with consequent mechanical effects on the spine, hips, and feet. These unusual neuromuscular forces may require repeated injections of neuromuscular toxins such as botulinum toxin or orthopedic surgical management to reduce the magnitude of the excessive neuromuscular forces.

Localized Growth Deficiency

Localized growth deficiency within one tissue may give rise to subsequent deformational problems in adjacent tissues, as can be seen with localized growth deficiency of the mandible. If this occurs during early morphogenesis, it tends to place the tongue in a posterior location in the oropharynx (termed *glossoptosis*). If this happens before 9–10 weeks of gestation, before closure of the posterior palate, the tongue may obstruct posterior palatal closure, yielding a U-shaped palatal defect. Once the baby is born, there may be upper airway obstruction secondary to the retroplaced tongue. These combined findings are referred to as the *Pierre Robin malformation sequence*.[44] Deficient mandibular growth may result from any of the types of abnormal morphogeneses described in Fig. 1.1. Beyond the initiating malformation of a small mandible, the remaining features are the consequences of altered biomechanics engendered by the small mandible. When the mandibular growth deficiency occurs as part of a malformation syndrome or connective tissue dysplasia, it carries a much worse prognosis than does isolated Pierre Robin sequence (PRS). Isolated PRS is associated with twinning in 9% of cases and is usually discordant.[45] PRS affects approximately up to 1 in 14,000 newborns a year. PRS can occur in isolation but is more often associated with other syndromes. In roughly 70% of cases of PRS, placing the neonate in a prone or side position relieves airway obstruction, but if the neonate desaturates then a nasopharyngeal tube can be placed to bypass upper airway obstruction. Patients with mild airway obstruction managed conservatively are at risk for failure to thrive due to feeding difficulties, gastroesophageal reflux, and aspiration. In such cases placing a gastrostomy tube until they achieve catch-up growth may help prevent the above complications. In acute severe airway obstruction, the patient must undergo an emergent tracheostomy to bypass the compromised airway. After initial stabilization of the patient, procedures such as tongue lip adhesion and mandibular distraction osteogenesis can correct glossoptosis, lengthen the mandible, and relieve glossoptosis.[46]

Localized Overgrowth

Localized overgrowth may cause mechanical problems in the adjacent region. This is apparent with many tumors. One example is a cervical teratoma, which can obstruct palatal closure and partially occlude the upper airway, yielding deformational features like those noted for PRS.[47]

Obstruction of a Hollow Viscus

Obstruction of a hollow organ will result in altered mechanical forces, with increased pressures causing deformations or disruptions of the expanded tissue, as well as distortion of tissues that surround the enlarging hollow structure. Examples include obstructive hydrocephalus, intestinal obstruction, and obstruction in the urogenital system. One dramatic illustration is the urethral obstruction sequence shown in Fig. 1.17, which has been more commonly termed *prune belly syndrome*.[48,49] Usually the primary malformation is an obstruction in the development of the penile urethra. This results in massive enlargement of the bladder and the ureters, and the backpressure adversely affects renal morphogenesis. The enlarging bladder distends the abdomen, causing diminished abdominal musculature. It also prevents full rotation of the gut resulting in malrotation; obstructs the descent of the testes; and may compress vessels to the legs resulting in hypoplastic legs.[49] The horrendous compressive effects of the distended bladder are usually lethal in early fetal life unless the bladder is decompressed, either by rupturing an obstructing urethral valve or by draining through a patent urachus (which tends to remain patent as a consequence of the pressure). Once the bladder is decompressed, the fetus is left with a lax abdomen and redundant folds of excess skin, the so-called prune belly. Thus all these deformations are secondary to one primary intrinsic malformation, early urethral obstruction. There were 31 cases of prune belly syndrome in Finland between 1993 and 2015, 15 of which were live born and 16 were elective terminations. The total prevalence was 1 in 44,000 births. Three patients (20%) died during infancy.[50] Perinatal mortality is related to the severity of pulmonary hypoplasia as a result of oligohydramnios from reduced fetal urine production from renal dysplasia and urinary tract abnormalities. There may also be a high prevalence of prostate and seminal vesicle abnormalities, which can affect fertility.[51] Similar distension and muscular thinning of the abdomen can be seen with congenital ascites, which may result from a variety of causes.

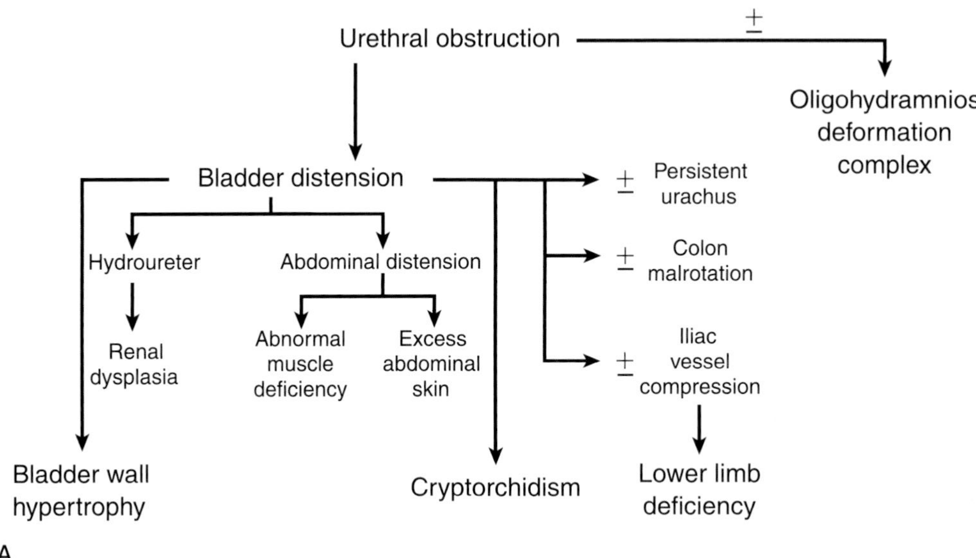

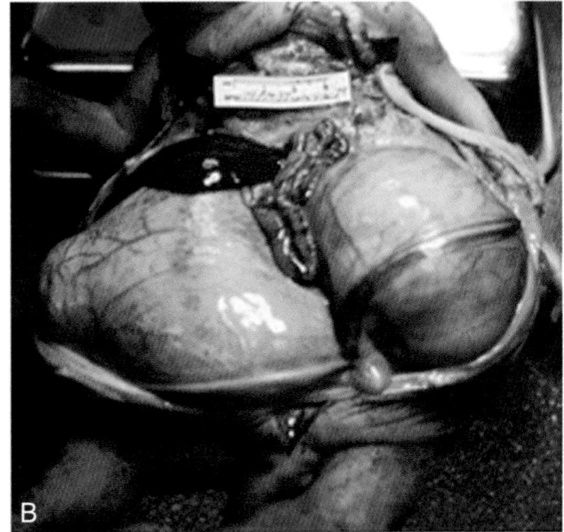

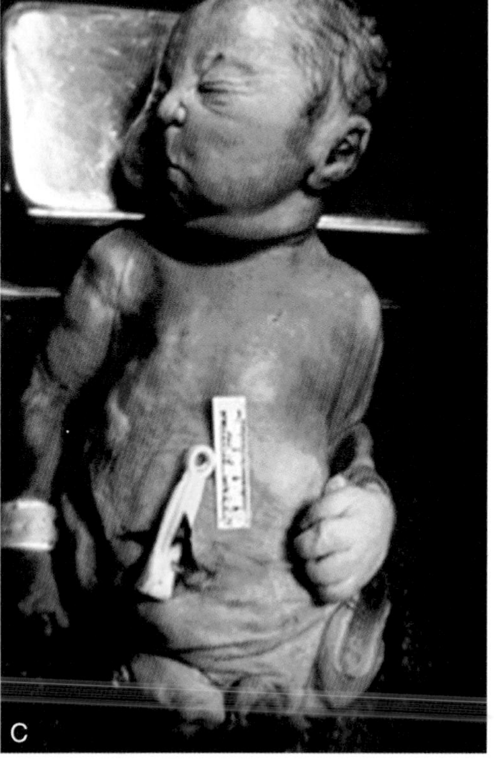

FIGURE 1.17 **A,** Urethral obstruction malformation sequence stems from the initiating malformation of urethral obstruction, which usually occurs at the level of the prostatic urethra (hence, it is nine times more frequent in males than females). Most of the other features are deformations caused by the back pressure in the urinary system. Sometimes the distended bladder (**B**) disrupts iliac vessel blood flow to the legs. To survive to a term birth, the distended bladder must decompress, thus yielding the "prune belly" abdomen (**C**). (**A** from Pagon RA, Smith DW, Shepard TH. Urethral obstruction malformation complex: a cause of abdominal muscle deficiency and the "prune belly." *J Pediatr*. 1979;96:900-906.)

References

1. Moorthi RN, Hashmi SS, Langois P, et al. Idiopathic talipes equinovarus (ITEV) (clubfeet) in Texas. *Am J Med Genet.* 2005;132A:376–380.
2. Schinzel AA, Smith DW, Miller JR. Monozygotic twinning and structural defects. *J Pediatr.* 1979;95:921–930.
3. Keusch CF, Mulliken JB, Kaplan LC. Craniofacial anomalies in twins. *Plast Reconstr Surg.* 1991;87:16–23.
4. Littlefield TR, Kelly KM, Pomatto JK, et al. Multiple-birth infants at higher risk for development of deformational plagiocephaly. *Pediatrics.* 1999;103:565–569.
5. Nicolini U, Poblete A. Single intrauterine death in monochorionic twin pregnancies. *Ultrasound Obstet Gynecol.* 1999;14:297–301.
6. Zankl A, Brooks D, Boltshauser E, et al. Natural history of twin disruption sequence. *Amer J Med Genet.* 2004;127A:133–138.
7. Dunn P. Congenital postural deformities: perinatal associations. *Proc R Soc Med.* 1974;67:1174–1178.
8. Dunn P. Congenital postural deformities: further perinatal associations. *Proc R Soc Med.* 1972;65:735–738.
9. Dunn PM. Congenital postural deformities. *Br Med Bull.* 1976;32:71–76.
10. Martinez-Frias ML, Bermejo E, Frias JL. Analysis of deformations in 26,810 consecutive infants with congenital defects. *Am J Med Genet.* 1999;84:365–368.
11. Harrison RG, Malpas P. The volume of human amniotic fluid. *J Obstet Gynaec Br Emp.* 1953;60:632–639.
12. Nishimura H. Etiological mechanism of congenital abnormalities. In: Fraser FC, McKusick VA, eds. *Congenital Malformations (International Congress Series.* no. 204. Amsterdam: Excerpta Medica; 1970:275.
13. Alkalay AL, Graham Jr JM, Pomerance JJ. Evaluation of neonates born with intrauterine growth retardation: review and practice guidelines. *J Perinatol.* 1998;18:142–151.
14. Moh W, Graham Jr JM, Wadhawan I, et al. Extrinsic factors influencing fetal deformations and intrauterine growth restriction. *J Pregnancy.* 2012:750485.
15. Harvey MA, Smith DW, Skinner AL. Infant growth standards in relation to parental stature. *Clin Pediatr.* 1979;18(602-603):611–613.
16. Tarruffi C. *Storia della Teratologia [History of Teratology].* Bologna: Regia Tipografia; 1881.
17. von Reuss AR. *The Diseases of the Newborn.* New York: William Wood; 1921.
18. Thompson DW. *On Growth and Form. A New Edition.* Cambridge, UK: Cambridge University Press; 1942.
19. Chapple CC, Davidson DT. A study of the relationship between fetal position and certain congenital deformities. *J Pediatr.* 1941;18:483–493.
20. Browne D. Talipes equinovarus. *Lancet.* 1934;224: 969–974.
21. Browne D. Congenital deformities of mechanical origin. *Arch Dis Child.* 1955;30:37–41.
22. Miller ME, Dunn PM, Smith DW. Uterine malformation and fetal deformation. *J Pediatr.* 1979;94:387–390.
23. Caldwell WE, Moloy HC, D'Esopo DA. A roentgenologic study of the mechanism of engagement of the fetal head. *Am J Obstet Gynecol.* 1974;28:824–841.
24. Sherer DM, Miodovnik M, Bradley KS, et al. Intrapartum fetal head position I: comparison between transvaginal digital examination and transabdominal ultrasound assessment during the active stage of labor. *Ultrasound Obstet Gynecol.* 2002;19:258–263.
25. Sherer DM, Miodovnik M, Bradley KS, et al. Intrapartum fetal head position II: comparison between transvaginal digital examination and transabdominal ultrasound assessment during second stage of labor. *Ultrasound Obstet Gynecol.* 2002;19:264–268.
26. Sherer DM, Abulafia O. Intrapartum assessment of fetal head engagement: comparison between transvaginal digital and transabdominal ultrasound determinations. *Ultrasound Obstet Gynecol.* 2003;21:430–436.
27. Graham Jr. JM. Craniofacial deformation. *Balliere's Clinical Paediatrics.* 1998;6:293–315.
28. Graham JM, Smith DW. Parietal craniotabes in the neonate: its origin and relevance. *J Pediatr.* 1979;95:114–116.
29. Graham JM, deSaxe M, Smith DW. Sagittal craniostenosis: fetal head constraint as one possible cause. *J Pediatr.* 1979;95:747–750.
30. Golditch IM, Kirkman K. The large fetus: management and outcome. *Obstet Gynecol.* 1978;52:26–30.
31. Graham Jr JM, Gomez M, Halberg A, et al. Management of deformational plagiocephaly: repositioning versus orthotic therapy. *J Pediatr.* 2005;146:258–262.
32. Graham Jr JM, Kneutzman J, Earl D, et al. Deformational brachycephaly in supine-sleeping infants. *J Pediatr.* 2005;146:258–262.
33. Thomas IT, Smith DW. Oligohydramnios, cause of the nonrenal features of Potter's syndrome, including pulmonary hypoplasia. *J Pediatr.* 1974;84:811–814.
34. Littlefield TR, Beals SP, Manwarring KH, et al. Treatment of craniofacial asymmetry with dynamic orthotic cranioplasty. *J Craniofacial Surg.* 1998;9:11–17.
35. Kelly KM, Littlefield TR, Pomatto JK, et al. Importance of early recognition and treatment of deformational plagiocephaly with orthotic cranioplasty. *Cleft Palate Craniofac J.* 1999;36:127–130.
36. Mulliken JB, Vander Woude DL, Hansen M, et al. Analysis of posterior plagiocephaly: deformational versus synostotic. *Plast Reconstr Surg.* 1999;103:371–380.
37. Hofmeyr GJ, Kuller R. External cephalic version for breech presentation at term. *Cochrane Database Syst Rev.* 2012;10:CD000083.
38. Haberkern CM, Smith DW, Jones KL. The "breech head" and its relevance. *Am J Dis Child.* 1979;133:154–156.
39. Fernando J, Arena P, Smith DW. Sex liability to single structural defects. *Am J Dis Child.* 1987;132:970–972.
40. Cohen MM. Merging the old skeletal biology with the new. I. Intramembranous ossification, endochondral ossification, ectopic bone, secondary cartilage, and pathologic considerations. *J Craniofac Genet Dev Biol.* 2000;20:84–93.

41. Cohen MM. Merging the old skeletal biology with the new. II. Molecular aspects of bone formation and bone growth. *J Craniofac Genet Dev Biol*. 2000;20:94–106.
42. Moessinger AC. Fetal akinesia deformation sequence: an animal model. *Pediatrics*. 1983;72:857–863.
43. Hall JG. Analysis of the Pena-Shokeir phenotype. *Am J Med Genet*. 1986;25:99–117.
44. Hanson JW, Smith DW. U-shaped palatal defect in the Robin anomalad: developmental and clinical relevance. *J Pediatr*. 1975;87:30–33.
45. Holder-Espinasse M, Abadie V, Cormier-Daire V, et al. Pierre Robin sequence: analysis of 117 consecutive cases. *J Pediatr*. 2001;139:588–590.
46. Hegde N, Singh A. *Anesthetic consideration. Pierre-Robin Sequence*. Treasure Island (FL): StatPearls Publishing; 2022.
47. Kerner B, Flaum E, Mathews H, et al. Cervical teratoma: prenatal diagnosis and long-term follow-up. *Prenatal Diagnosis*. 1998;18:51–59.
48. Pagon RA, Smith DW, Shepard TH. Urethral obstruction malformation complex: a cause of abdominal muscle deficiency and the "prune belly. *J Pediatr*. 1979;94:900–906.
49. Perez-Aytes A, Graham Jr JM, Hersh JH, et al. The urethral obstruction sequence and lower limb deficiency: evidence for the vascular disruption hypothesis. *J Pediatr*. 1993;123:398–405.
50. Pakkasjärvi N, Syvänen J, Tauriainen A, et al. Prune belly syndrome in Finland - a population-based study on current epidemiology and hospital admissions. *J Pediatr Urol*. 2021;17(5):702.e1–702.e6.
51. Lopes RI, Tavares A, Dénes FT, Cocuzza M. Gonadal function and reproductive system anatomy in post-pubertal prune-belly syndrome patients. *Urology*. 2020;145:292–296.

Section II
Patterns of Deformation

CHAPTER 2

Foot Deformations

Foot Contractures and Positional Foot Abnormalities

KEY POINTS BOX

- Prolonged immobilization of a joint tends to give rise to joint fixation with contracture.
- When fixations of multiple joints are present at birth, the term *arthrogryposis* is used.
- Amyoplasia is a clinically recognizable form of arthrogryposis, representing about one-third of individuals with arthrogryposis surviving the newborn period.
- Postural foot deformations are common and are often considered physiologic variations in foot shape; these include metatarsus adductus, calcaneovalgus, and flexible flatfeet.
- Congenital club foot and vertical talus require early and aggressive treatment.
- Several modes of management to restore the foot to a normal position are summarized.

Prolonged immobilization of a joint tends to give rise to joint fixation with contracture. This can arise from immobilization due to external constraint, intrinsic neuromuscular problems, defects in the formation of the joint, or joints formed from abnormal connective tissue (Figs. 2.1 and 2.2). When the problem is the result of external constraint, the position of a given joint reflects the nature of the forces that resulted in the deformation. The most common region affected is the foot, although fixations of other joints may also occur. The differential diagnosis of foot anomalies includes the following: metatarsus adductus (deformation or malformation), talipes equinovarus (deformation or malformation), talipes calcaneovalgus (deformation), pes planus (often associated with connective tissue dysplasia), and vertical talus (malformation).[1–3] Hall has reviewed the deformations associated with arthrogryposis.[4]

Foot deformation usually originates during fetal life, but in China the practice of foot binding in young girls became widespread during the 12th century (Fig. 2.3). This practice was initiated around age 3 years, when all toes but the first toes were broken and bound with tight cloth over the next 2 years so as to keep the feet less than 10 cm in length with a marked concavity of the sole.[5] After contact with Western cultures, this practice ceased at the beginning of the 20th century, but even as late as 1997 in the Chinese population, 38% of women older than 80 years and 18% of women between ages 70 and 79 years had their feet bound. An additional 17% of women older than 70 years had their feet bound, but the binding was released early. Women with deformed feet resulting from such foot binding are more prone to falling, are less able to rise from a chair, are unable to squat, and suffer severe, lifelong disability.[5]

When fixations of multiple joints are present at birth, the term *arthrogryposis* is used (Fig. 2.4). This term designates a descriptive category and should not be considered a diagnosis. Arthrogryposis is a sign that can be associated with many specific conditions or syndromes.[6] Decreased fetal movement results in arthrogryposis, although the cause of such *fetal akinesia* may not always be known with certainty. Multiple congenital contractures (arthrogryposis) occur in 1 in 3000 live births, and in 1 in 200 newborns there is some form of joint contracture, with clubfeet (1 in 500) and dislocated or subluxing hips (1 in 200 to 1 in 500) being most frequent.[7] The decreased fetal movements that result in arthrogryposis can be caused by either fetal abnormalities or maternal abnormalities, and the earlier the onset of decreased fetal movement, the more severe the resultant contractures. Hall has delineated six major causes of decreased fetal movements[6]:

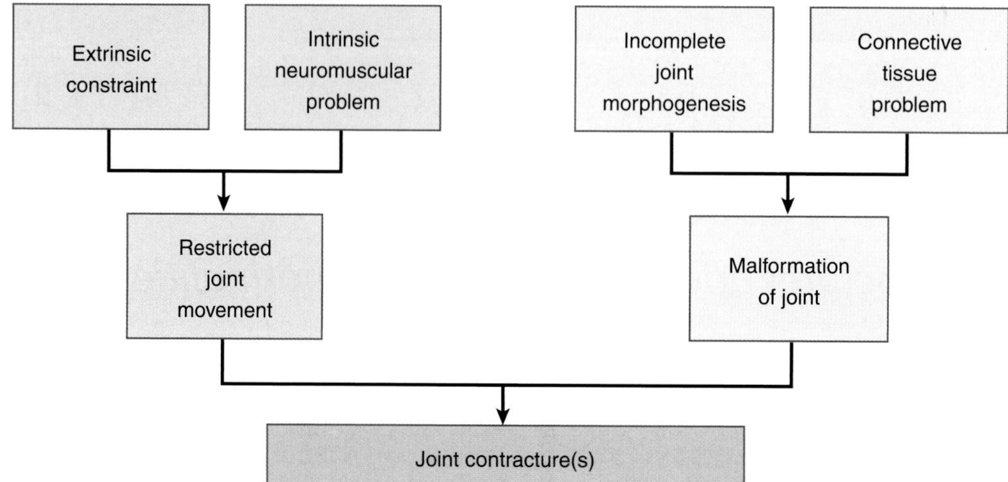

FIGURE 2.1 Joint contracture at birth may be the consequence of a number of modes of developmental pathology, of which in utero constraint is the most common.

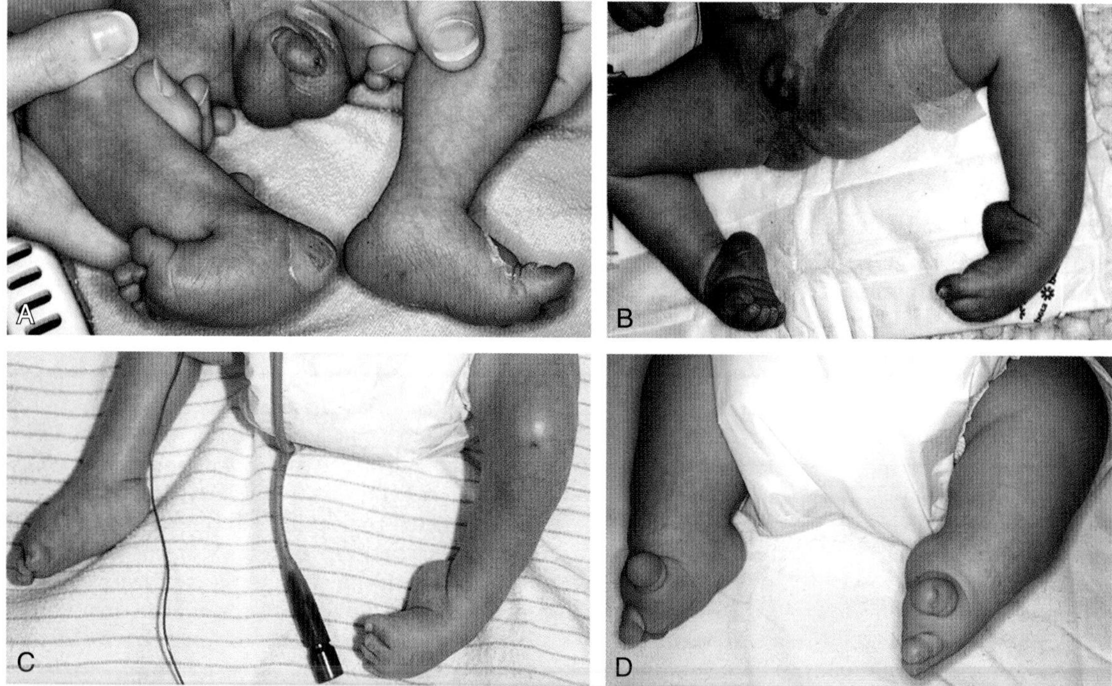

FIGURE 2.2 A, This infant has bilateral equinovarus foot deformations caused by prolonged oligohydramnios resulting from leaking amniotic fluid from 17 weeks of gestation until birth. This is an example of extrinsic deformation. B, This infant with type I Pena-Shokeir syndrome demonstrates bilateral equinovarus foot deformities caused by fetal akinesia deformation sequence (intrinsic deformation). C, Neurogenic clubfeet caused by an unknown neuromuscular disorder. D, These equinovarus feet resulted from a connective tissue abnormality in an infant with diastrophic dysplasia. This is an example of a connective tissue dysplasia that has given rise to malformation of a joint.

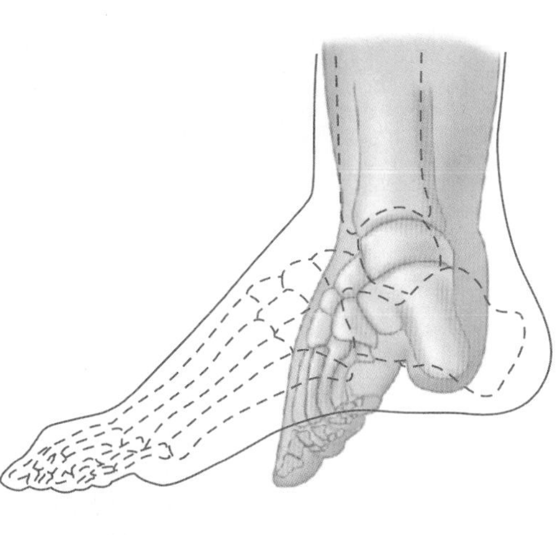

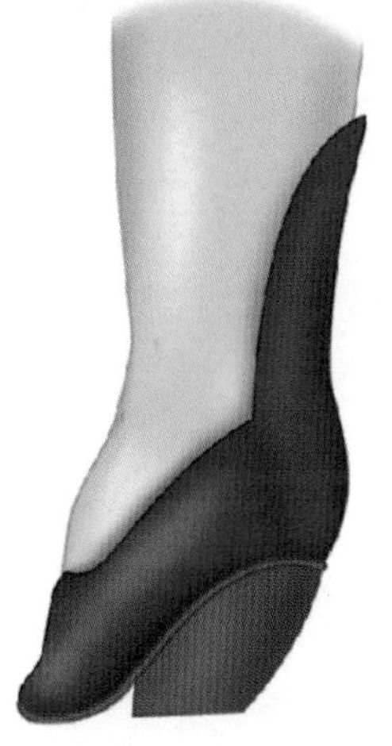

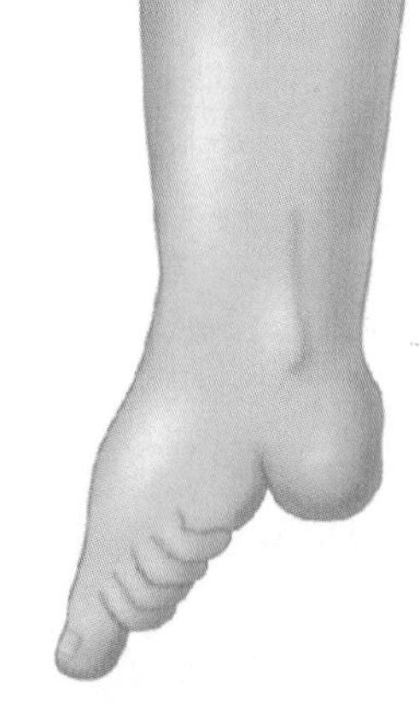

FIGURE 2.3 For almost 1500 years, certain young Chinese girls were subjected to the harrowing experience of foot binding for several years so as to produce the desired small feet, which were considered physically attractive. The form into which the deformed feet were molded is shown, along with the special shoes and resultant foot position. (From Levy HS. *Chinese Footbinding*. New York: Walton Rawls; 1966.)

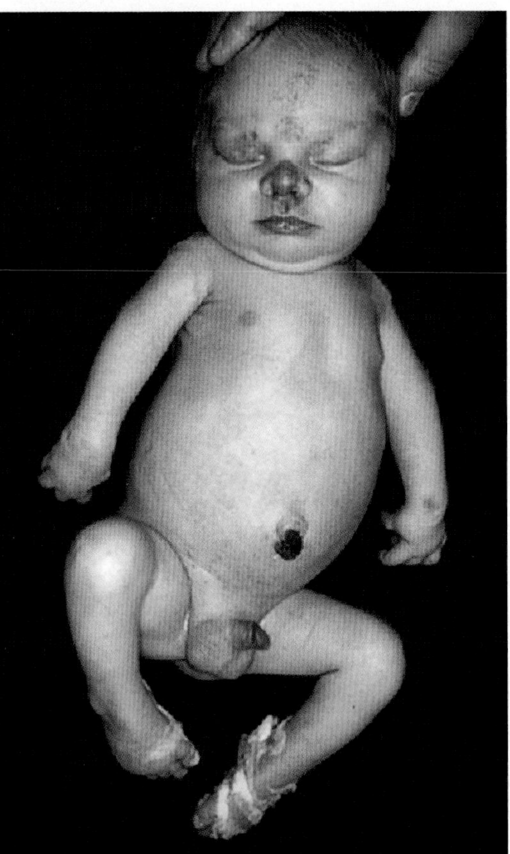

FIGURE 2.4 This infant has the amyoplasia form of arthrogryposis, a sporadic condition attributed to spinal cord damage (possibly with a vascular basis) in early gestation. Fetal movement is limited, with joint ankylosis and absent flexion creases. The posture of this condition is quite characteristic, with the hands fixed in external rotation and extension of the elbows (the "policeman's tip" position). This is an example of intrinsic deformation caused by vascular disruption.

1. Neuropathic abnormalities (e.g., spina bifida)
2. Muscular abnormalities (see Fig. 2.5, Marden-Walker syndrome)
3. Abnormalities of connective tissue (e.g., diastrophic dysplasia [see Fig. 1.1D])
4. Space limitations (e.g., multiple gestation, uterine structural abnormalities)
5. Vascular disruption (e.g., amyoplasia [see Figs. 1.16 or 2.4])
6. Maternal diseases (e.g., multiple sclerosis or myasthenia gravis)

Sorting of presentations into three major categories can be helpful in identifying underlying conditions or syndromes: (1) disorders with mainly limb involvement (e.g., amyoplasia or distal arthrogryposis); (2) limbs plus other body areas (e.g., multiple pterygium syndrome or diastrophic dysplasia); and (3) limbs plus central nervous system dysfunction (e.g., trisomy 18 [see Fig. 1.12, right image]) or Pena-Shokeir syndrome (see Fig. 1.3B).[6]

There are over 400 discrete diagnoses that can lead to a child being born with arthrogryposis multiplex

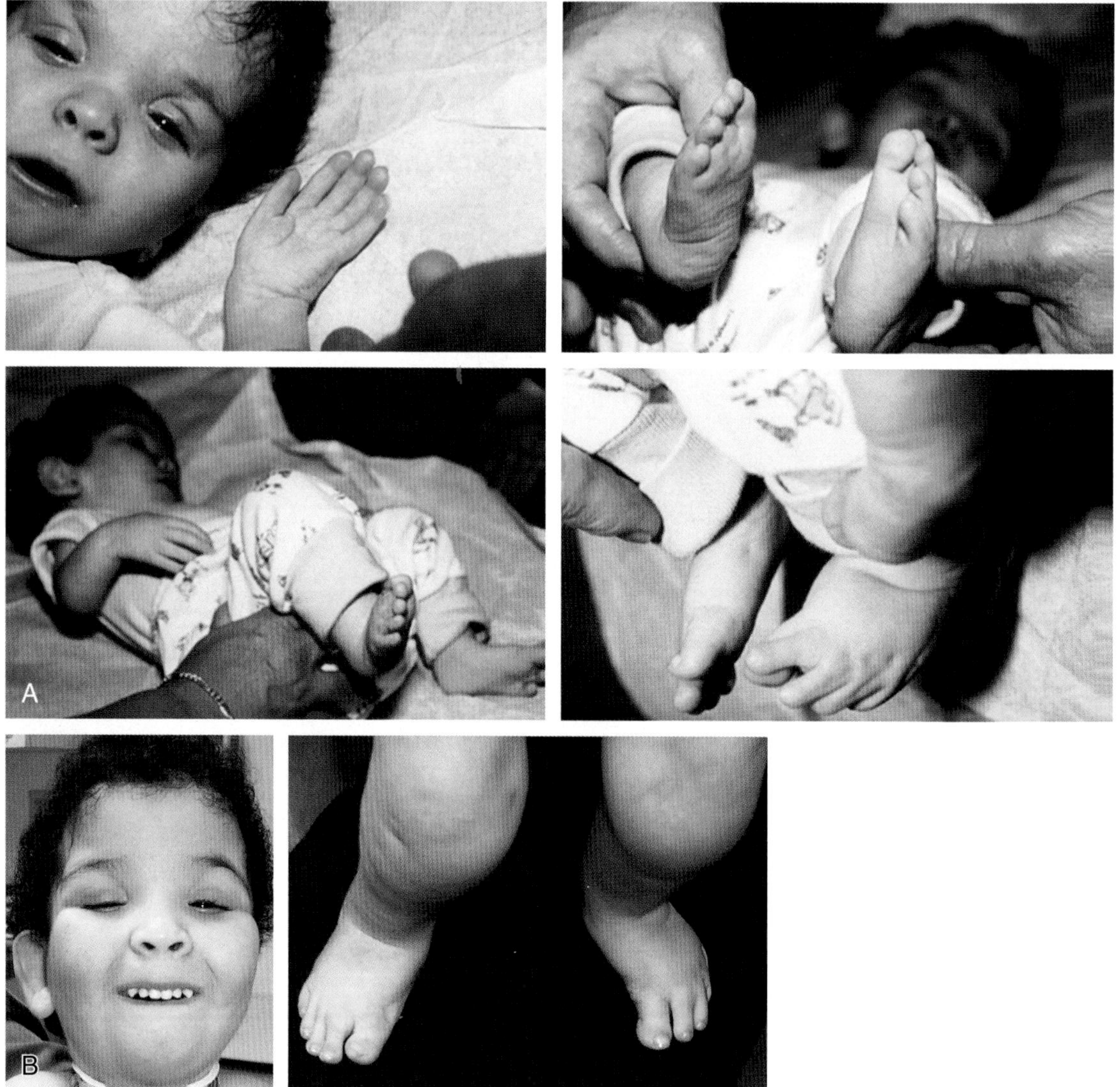

FIGURE 2.5 This infant has Marden-Walker syndrome caused by a de novo heterozygous mutation in *PIEZO2*, which encodes a transmembrane protein responsible for mechanically or stretch-activated ion channels found in many tissues. This gene is also mutated in the allelic disorders Gordon syndrome and distal arthrogryposis type 5. **A,** He was born with severe congenital contractures, Dandy-Walker malformation, cleft palate, blepharophimosis, tethered spinal cord, and severe growth and developmental delay. Note diminished finger creases from lack of movement in utero. **B,** By age 6 years, the child's contractures had responded well to early intermittent splinting to reduce contractures and physical therapy, followed by surgical correction.

congenita (AMC).[8] The two biggest categories of conditions are amyoplasia and distal arthrogryposis, which combined make up approximately 50–65% of all diagnoses within the AMC subset. Amyoplasia, the most common AMC condition, seems to be a nongenetic syndrome, leading to very characteristic upper and lower limb contractures. The distal arthrogryposes, in contrast, have an underlying genetic abnormality that in many cases seems to target the fast twitch muscles of the developing fetus.[8] Among 2500 cases of arthrogryposis, 30 cases (1.2%) were associated with longstanding oligohydramnios, Potter syndrome facial features, and compressive skin changes. No case had renal agenesis or renal disease, and 22 cases (73%) had a history of known rupture of membranes.[9]

AMC is defined as congenital contractures of at least two joint levels, and such joint contractures are always secondary to diminished fetal movement, which can have numerous causes that affect joint function at multiple levels such as the central nervous system, the anterior horn cell, the nerve, the neuromuscular junction, the muscle, or the joint itself. Genetic sequencing studies and chromosomal microarray analysis in patients with intellectual disability and AMC should be utilized as first-tier investigations over electromyography and muscle biopsy.[10]

Amyoplasia is a nongenetic, specific, clinically recognizable form of arthrogryposis, representing about one-third of individuals with arthrogryposis surviving the newborn period. There is an increased number of individuals with amyoplasia who are one of spontaneous monozygotic (MZ) twins, with the other twin being normal. Thus amyoplasia is associated with and may be caused by MZ twinning, and the twin–twin transfusion that is found in MZ twins may play an etiologic role in producing amyoplasia.[11]

According to Ruth Wynne-Davies, congenital malposition of the foot occurs with a frequency of about 4.0–5.6 per 1000 live births.[7,12] The most serious subtype is talipes equinovarus (clubfoot), which is difficult to treat, manifests a tendency to recur within families, and occurs with a frequency of 1.2–1.3 per 1000 live births (males, 1.6 per 1000; females, 0.8 per 1000).[8,12] Postural talipes equinovarus occurs in 0.5 per 1000 live births (males, 1.6 per 1000; females, 0.8 per 1000); talipes calcaneovalgus occurs in 1.1 per 1000 live births (males, 0.1 per 1000; females, 0.3 per 1000); and metatarsus varus occurs in 1.2 per 1000 live births (males, 1.0 per 1000; females, 0.2 per 1000).[5] Many congenital malpositions of the foot represent deformations resulting from external constraint in utero, and the treatment prognosis is much better for postural deformations than for other types of congenital joint contractures.

Evaluation of the foot includes determination of the full range of its mobility, inspection of its usual position or posture with notation of unusual skin creases, and palpation of the dorsalis pedis pulse because the anterior tibial vascular tree is often poorly developed in children with neuromuscular clubfoot.[13] Radiographs are of little value in early infancy because feet are best evaluated radiographically when bearing weight and the bones are not sufficiently ossified to allow for the relevant assessment; however, magnetic resonance imaging has been used in congenital talipes equinovarus.[14,15] In a prospective study of 2401 newborns, 4% were found to have foot contractures, of which three-fourths were various forms of adductus anomalies. These children were followed through age 16 years, when they were examined by dynamic foot pressure and gait analysis. Only those children with clubfeet showed persistent abnormalities. By age 6 years, 87% of adductus anomalies had resolved, and by age 16 years, 95% had resolved.[16] Congenital clubfoot and congenital vertical talus tend to persist and cause disability unless treated aggressively; thus early referral and treatment are extremely important. Such joint contractures may be released operatively in the first year of life. Among the associated anomalies that tend to occur with postural equinovarus or calcaneovalgus types of foot deformities are joint laxity (10%) and inguinal hernia (7%). These findings suggest that minor connective tissue problems may enhance the tendency toward positional deformation of the foot. Postural deformations that began in utero may be perpetuated by prone sleeping postures in early infancy. Consequently, the incidence of these postural deformations has decreased in cultures using supine sleeping positions. Hence, consideration of sleeping posture and whether it is augmenting or ameliorating the deformation may be an important part of the infant's initial evaluation.

Postural foot deformations are common and are often considered physiologic variations in foot shape; these include metatarsus adductus, calcaneovalgus, and flexible flatfeet. Similar physiologic variations affecting the shape of the legs include genu varum, genu valgum, femoral anteversion, and tibial torsion. On the other hand, cavus feet are usually a manifestation of muscle imbalance from an underlying neuromuscular disorder, which might be static (cerebral palsy), recurrent after initial stabilization (spina bifida), or progressive (Charcot-Marie-Tooth disease). Several modes of management have been used in the attempt to restore the foot to its usual position, which are summarized in Table 2.1. In infants who are born prematurely, contractures can be splinted using silicone rubber dental-impression material, which is held in place with Velcro strips (Fig. 2.6).[17] Such splints can easily be removed for passive stretching exercises or intravenous access and then replaced just as easily. Each type of foot contracture should be considered individually regarding both prognosis and management. For example, the prognosis for calcaneovalgus with manipulative stretching alone is usually excellent, whereas at least half the cases of equinovarus contracture resist correction by conservative measures. In general, initial corrective surgery is accomplished through soft tissue releases to align the joints

Table 2.1 MANAGEMENT STRATEGIES FOR FOOT CONTRACTURES

Method	Comment
Manual stretching	Performed at each feeding and diaper change
Adhesive taping	Sometimes alternated with physical therapy to increase joint range of motion
Splinting	Devices such as the Denis-Browne splint and reversed-last shoes may be used, particularly at night, to maintain desired position. Newer, lightweight fiberglass splints may be used with physical therapy
Plaster cast	Used initially with stretching and taping to correct position and facilitate surgery. Also used after surgery to maintain position
Surgery	Merits consideration if more conservative measures have not resulted in improvement of foot position during early infancy

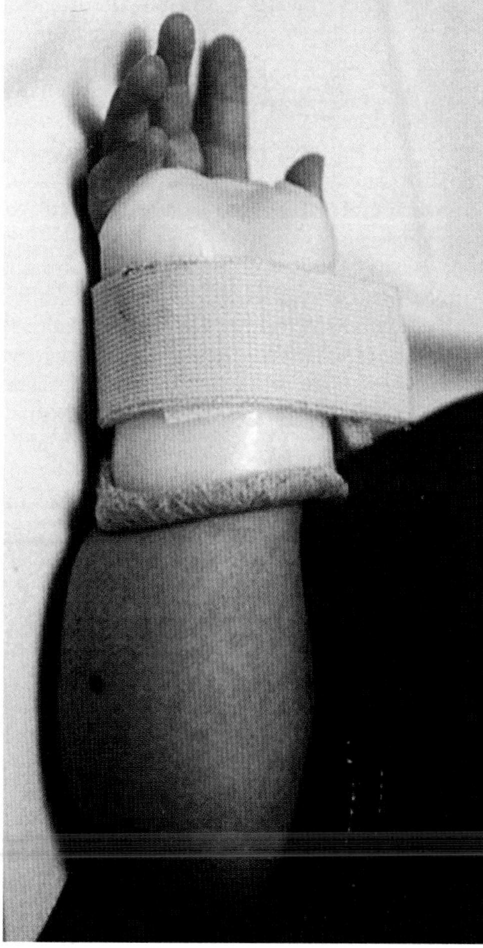

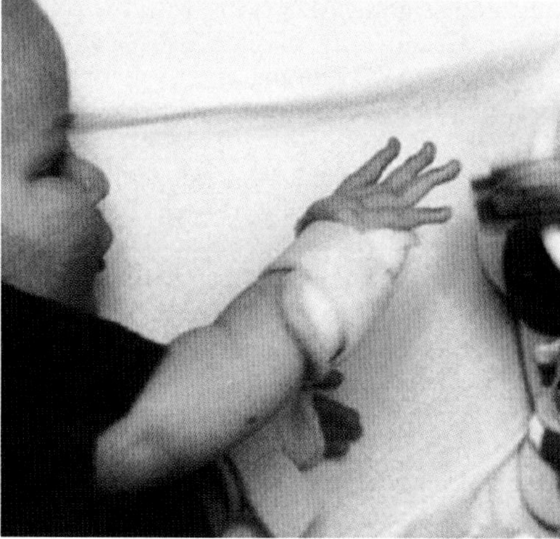

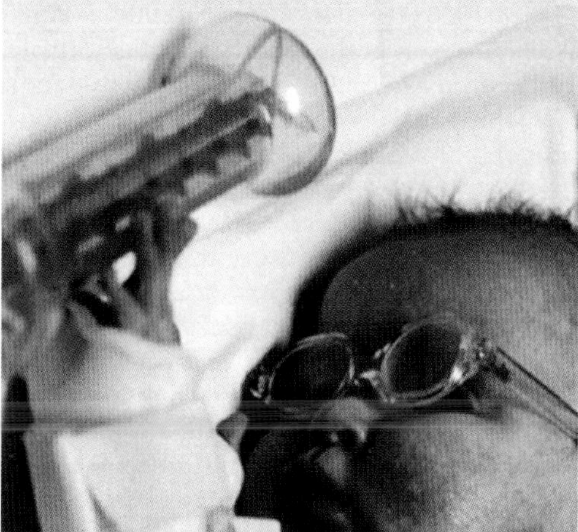

FIGURE 2.6 Use of custom hand splints held in place with Velcro fasteners in a child with congenital contractural arachnodactyly caused by Beals syndrome. Fingers are left free to encourage their use in grasping and reaching, and the splints can be removed for physical therapy.

and osteotomies to correct residual deformities, with arthrodesis reserved for the older child or adult with established degenerative arthrosis of a joint, or with severe problems that cannot be corrected with releases and osteotomies. For the child with arthrogryposis, additional management strategies are overviewed and comprehensively illustrated in a patient-oriented text by Staheli et al.[18]

References

1. Furdon SA, Donlon CR. Examination of the newborn foot: positional and structural abnormalities. *Adv Neonatal Care*. 2002;2:248–258.
2. Gore AI, Spencer JP. The newborn foot. *Am Fam Physician*. 2004;69:865–872.
3. Sass P, Hassan G. Lower extremity abnormalities in children. *Am Fam Physician*. 2003;68:461–468.
4. Hall JG. Deformations associated with arthrogryposis. *Am J Med Genet A*. 2021;185(9):2676–2682.
5. Cummings SR, Ling X, Stone K. Consequences of foot binding among older women in Beijing, China. *Am J Pub Health*. 1997;87:1677–1679.
6. Hall JG. Arthrogryposis multiplex congenita: etiology, genetics, classification, diagnostic approach, and general aspects. *Part B, J Pediatr Orthop*. 1997;6:159–166.
7. Wynne-Davies R. Family studies and aetiology of clubfoot. *J Med Genet*. 1965;2:227–232.
8. Hall JG, Kimber E, van Bosse HJP. Arthrogryposis 2017 Supplement: Genetics and Classifications. *J Pediatr Orthop*. 2017;37(Suppl 1):S4–S8.
9. Hall JG. Oligohydramnios sequence revisited in relationship to arthrogryposis, with distinctive skin changes. *Am J Med Genet A*. 2014;164A(11):2775–2792.
10. Dieterich K, Le Tanno P, Kimber E, Jouk PS, Hall J, Giampietro P. The diagnostic workup in a patient with AMC: overview of the clinical evaluation and paraclinical analyses with review of the literature. *Am J Med Genet C Semin Med Genet*. 2019;181(3):337–344.
11. Hall JG. The mystery of monozygotic twinning I: what can Amyoplasia tell us about monozygotic twinning and the possible role of twin-twin transfusion? *Am J Med Genet A*. 2021;185(6):1816–1821.
12. Boo NY, Ong LC. Congenital talipes in Malaysian neonates: incidence, pattern and associated factors. *Sing Med J*. 1990;31:539–542.
13. Muir L, Laliotis N, Kutty S, et al. Absence of the dorsalis pedis pulse in the parents of children with clubfoot. *J Bone Joint Surg Br*. 1995;77:114–116.
14. Downey DJ, Drennan JC, Garcia JF. Magnetic resonance image findings in congenital talipes equinovarus. *J Pediatr Orthop*. 1992;12:224–228.
15. Grayhack JJ, Zawin JK, Shore RM, et al. Assessment of calcaneocuboid joint deformity by magnetic resonance imaging in talipes equinovarus. *Part B, J Pediatr Orthop*. 1995;4:36–38.
16. Widhe T. Foot deformities at birth: a longitudinal prospective study over a 16-year period. *J Pediatr Orthop*. 1997;17:20–24.
17. Bell E, Graham EK. A new material for splinting neonatal limb deformities. *J Pediatr Orthop*. 1995;15:613–616.
18. Staheli LT, Hall JG, Jaffe KM, et al. *Arthrogryposis: a text atlas*. Cambridge: Cambridge University Press; 1998.

CHAPTER 3

Calcaneovalgus Feet

> **KEY POINTS**
> - Calcaneovalgus deformation is usually the result of extrinsic deformation.
> - The foot is usually quite flexible and should return to normal without intervention.
> - If not resolved after several months, consider the use of external splints.

GENESIS

Calcaneovalgus deformation has a reported frequency of 1.1 per 1000 live births,[1] although some authors indicate that more than 30% of newborns have calcaneovalgus deformity of both feet.[2] It is usually the result of uterine constraint having forced the foot into a dorsiflexed position against the lower leg and is especially common after prolonged breech position with extended legs. Associated congenital hip dislocation occurs in 5–6% of patients with calcaneovalgus[1,3] and should be searched for in any newborn with this foot deformity. Congenital hip dislocation is more frequent among infants in breech presentation (0.9%), and minor anomalies comprising the breech head deformation complex are also much more frequent with breech presentation, regardless of the mode of delivery.[4,5] Among infants with frank breech presentation, the extended leg is particularly susceptible to calcaneovalgus foot deformation and genu recurvatum of the knee. Calcaneovalgus is more common in first born infants, with 75% of affected infants being primiparous,[6] and it is much more common in females than in males (4:1).[1] More joint laxity occurs in females, which may explain this finding. There is also a 2.6% frequency of this deformity in parents and siblings by history.[1]

FEATURES

Calcaneovalgus is usually the result of extrinsic deformation where the foot is dorsiflexed toward the fibular side of the lower leg (Figs. 3.1 and 3.2). This often results in posterior displacement of the lateral malleolus in association with pressure-induced deficiency of subcutaneous adipose tissue at the presumed site of folding compression. In unusual cases the heel may be in valgus position relative to the ankle, but the bones of the foot itself are usually in normal alignment. Posteromedial bowing of the tibia is sometimes associated with calcaneovalgus foot deformity (Fig. 3.3). It is important to rule out congenital vertical talus (Fig. 3.4), which is a malformation resulting in a rigid congenital flatfoot.

MANAGEMENT, PROGNOSIS, AND COUNSEL

The foot is usually flexible, and, with no therapy or with passive stretching toward a normal position, there should be a rapid return toward normal form. If the improvement is not rapid, then taping may be used. If the situation has not resolved within the first few postnatal months, then the use of splinting, night braces, and/or casting merits consideration. Therefore, serial examinations are useful to confirm the progress of resolution. When casted, the foot is positioned in an equinovarus position with a mold placed under the arch to relax the plantar ligaments and posterior tibialis muscle, which repositions the foot in normal alignment and allows the stretched ligaments to tighten.[7] Calcaneovalgus was diagnosed in 13 (0.5%) of 2401 examined newborns, and all 13 had normal feet at age 16 years. Dynamic foot pressure showed no tendency to planus or increased outward rotation of the feet.[8] When associated posterior medial bowing occurs, it usually resolves during postnatal life, suggesting intrauterine fracture or fetal deformation as the cause; thus

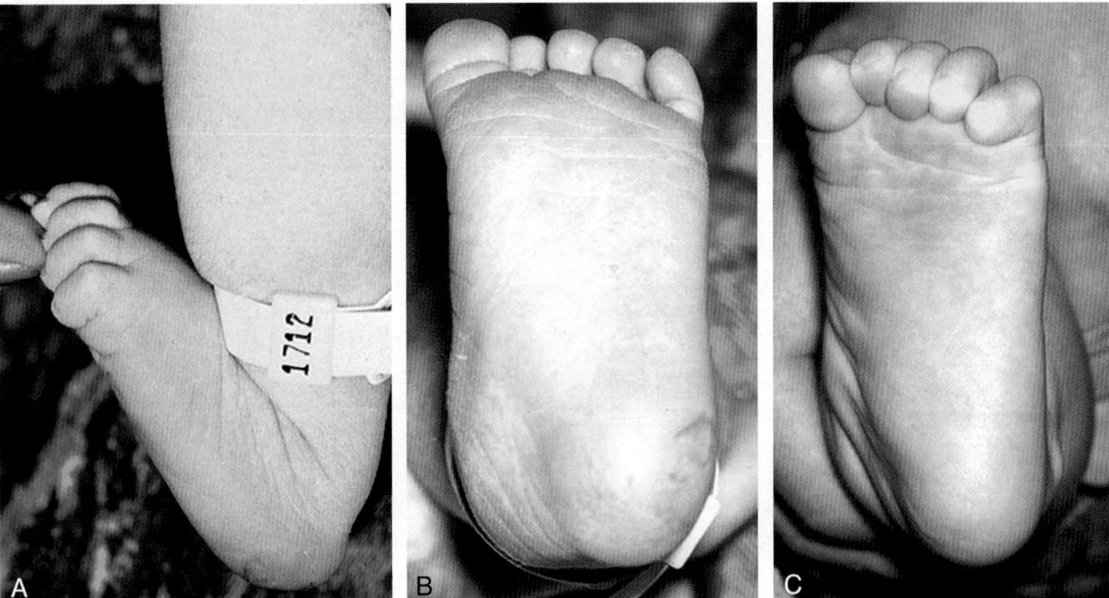

FIGURE 3.1 A, Gentle pressure recreates the presumed in utero position of this foot, which engendered the calcaneovalgus positioning. The foot dorsiflexes quite easily at birth because of a stretched elongated heel cord. B, The valgus deviation of the heel is evident in this view, and the heel deviates laterally. C, The same foot, treated with simple manipulation, at age 12 weeks.

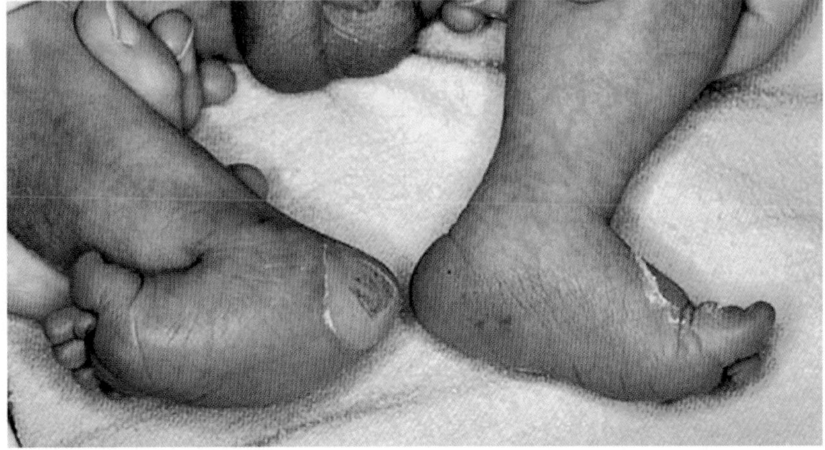

FIGURE 3.2 Bilateral calcaneovalgus feet (more significant in the right foot than the left) after prolonged oligohydramnios because of prolonged leakage of amniotic fluid.

corrective osteotomy should be delayed to allow for spontaneous correction. The prevalence of pes planus was 10.3% in Iranian children aged 7–14 years, but this prevalence decreased with age.[9] In a cross-sectional study of pes planus in Chinese children, prevalence decreased from 39.5% at 6 years to 11.8% at 12 years and reached a plateau at 12–13 years.[10] Children with a high BMI were more likely to have pes planus.[9-11] A Cochrane systematic review of the effect of custom foot orthotics (high cost) or prefabricated foot orthotics (low cost) on pain and function suggested the use of high-cost custom foot orthotics for healthy children with flexible flat feet had no supporting evidence.[12] Although the posteromedial bowing usually corrects, there may be a 2–5-cm leg length discrepancy at maturation (with the degree of shortening proportional

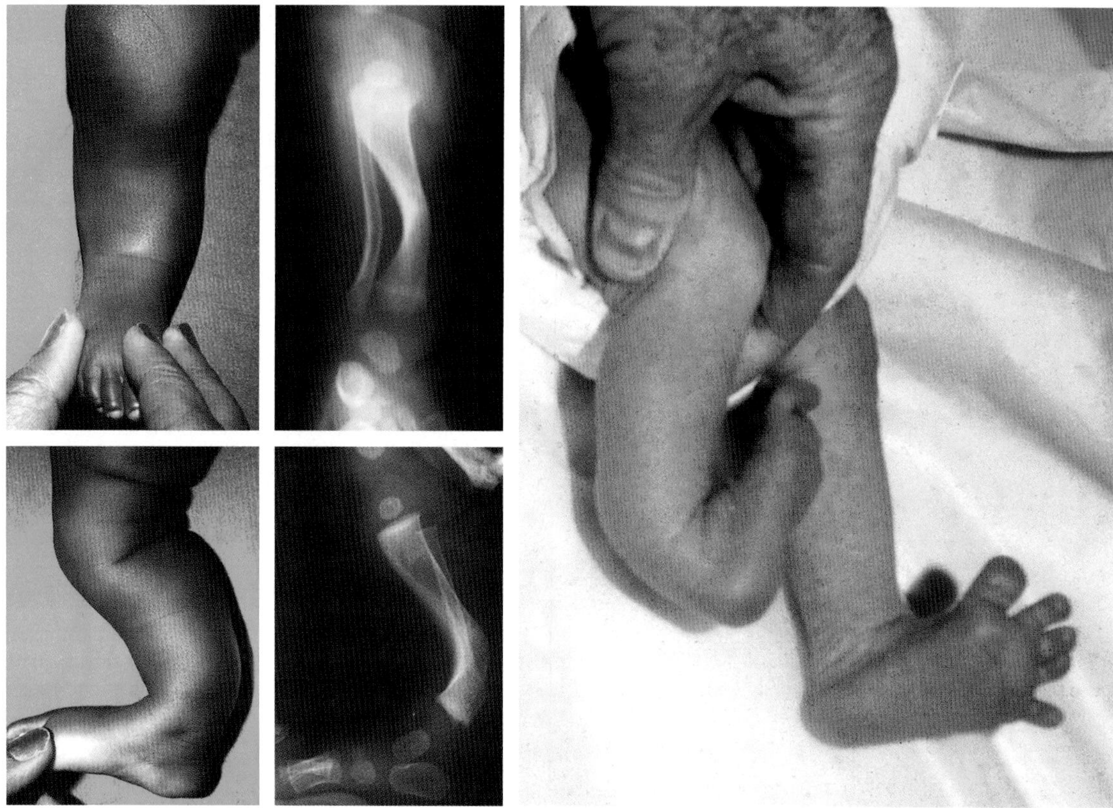

FIGURE 3.3 Posteromedial bowing of the tibia can be associated with calcaneovalgus foot deformation and usually corrects spontaneously, although it may lead to a clinically significant leg length discrepancy requiring epiphysiodesis of the opposite proximal tibia prior to maturation. (Courtesy Saul Bernstein and Robert M. Bernstein, Cedar Sinai Medical Center, Los Angeles.)

to the initial deformity). Hence this deformity may require epiphysiodesis of the opposite proximal tibia before full-growth attainment to result in equalization of leg length by adulthood.

DIFFERENTIAL DIAGNOSIS

Pes planus is common in infants and children, and often resolves by adolescence. Thus flatfoot is described as physiologic because it is usually flexible, painless, and of no functional consequence. In rare instances, flatfoot can become painful or rigid, which may be a sign of underlying foot pathology, including arthritis or tarsal coalition. Surgery is only indicated when nonoperative interventions have failed to resolve symptoms. In symptomatic pes planus patients, surgery is associated with a manageable complication profile and results in a satisfactory long-term clinical as well as radiological outcome.[13]

Congenital vertical talus is a rare malformation, occurring 1 in 150,000 births, that may yield a foot in similar position to calcaneovalgus at birth, but this defect is associated with muscle atrophy and the foot is stiff with a concave outer border, compared with the flexible flatfeet of calcaneovalgus foot deformity (see Fig. 3.4), with at least 50% of cases associated with genetic neuromuscular disorders.[14] With congenital vertical talus, the calcaneus is in equinus and the forefoot is in dorsiflexion, resulting in a midfoot break. The definitive abnormality is fixed dorsal dislocation of the navicular on the neck of the talus. The term *vertical talus* refers to the classic radiographic appearance of the affected foot in lateral view, which results in a rocker-bottom foot when viewed from the side. Congenital vertical talus can be inherited as a variable autosomal

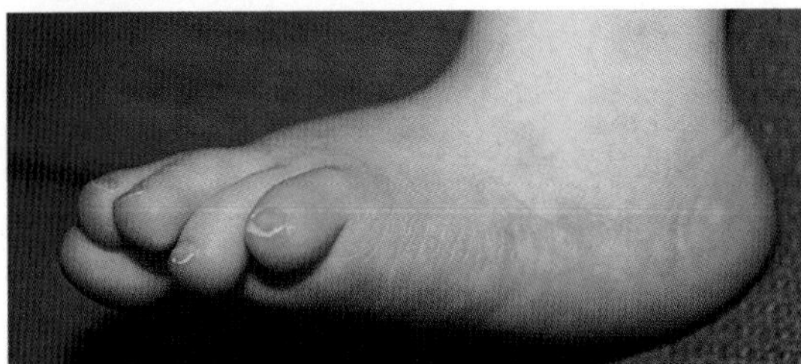

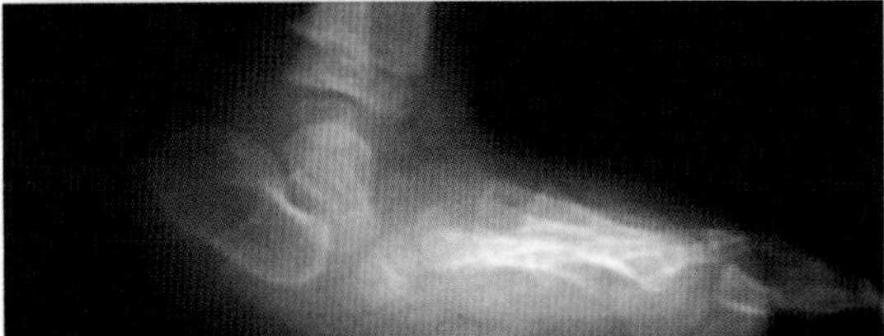

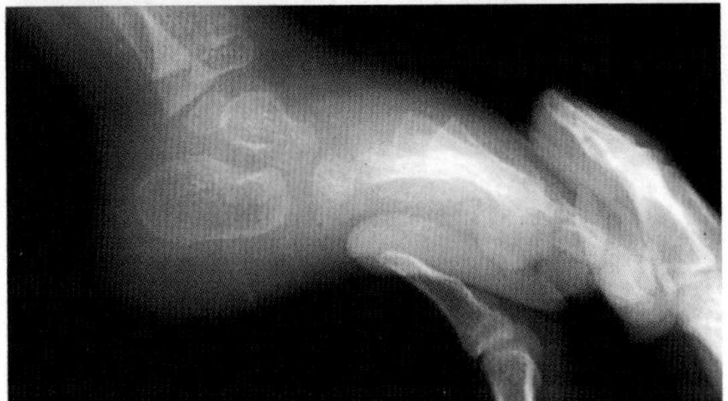

FIGURE 3.4 Congenital vertical talus results in a rigid flatfoot with a rocker-bottom appearance, and the head of the talus is palpable medially in the foot. In the calcaneovalgus foot, plantar flexion reduces the navicular on the talus, but in these radiographs of congenital vertical talus, the relationship of the dorsally displaced talus is not changed and the navicular remains in its dislocated position on the dorsum of the talus. (Courtesy Robert M. Bernstein, Cedar Sinai Medical Center, Los Angeles.)

dominant trait with no evidence of associated malformations or neuromuscular disease. One family spanning four generations included 11 individuals with isolated congenital vertical talus evident at infancy; during their teenage years, a few of these individuals developed cavo-varus foot deformities that resembled Charcot-Marie-Tooth disease.[15] This family was found to have a *HOXD10* mutation segregating with this foot malformation,[16] but this appears to be a rare cause of idiopathic clubfeet or vertical talus.[17] Other associated congenital anomalies often occur, such as arthrogryposis, myelodysplasia, sacral agenesis, trisomy 18, or 18q22q23 deletion syndrome (Fig. 3.5).[18] Congenital vertical talus is particularly common in patients with distal arthrogryposis, and a novel mutation in *TNNT3* was found to segregate with vertical talus in a Chinese family with Sheldon-Hall syndrome (Fig. 3.6).[19] Although mutations in *MYH3*, *TNNT3*, and *TPM2* are frequently associated with distal arthrogryposis syndromes, they were not present in patients with familial vertical talus or clubfoot.[20] Different types of distal arthrogryposis (nonprogressive congenital contractures of two or more body areas) are caused by mutations in different genes that encode proteins of the contractile machinery of fast-twitch myofibers. These neuromuscular problems are extremely difficult to treat, and recent studies of congenital vertical talus suggest correction can be obtained by serial casting followed by a minimally invasive reduction of the talonavicular joint.[21,22]

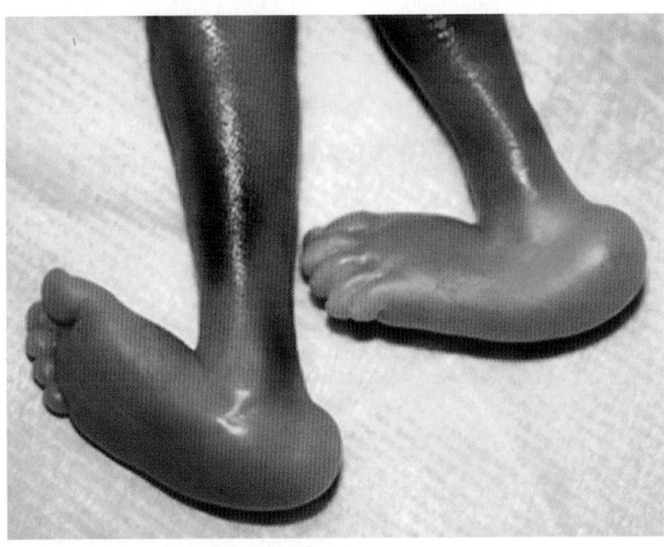

FIGURE 3.5 Bilateral congenital vertical talus in a fetus with trisomy 18.

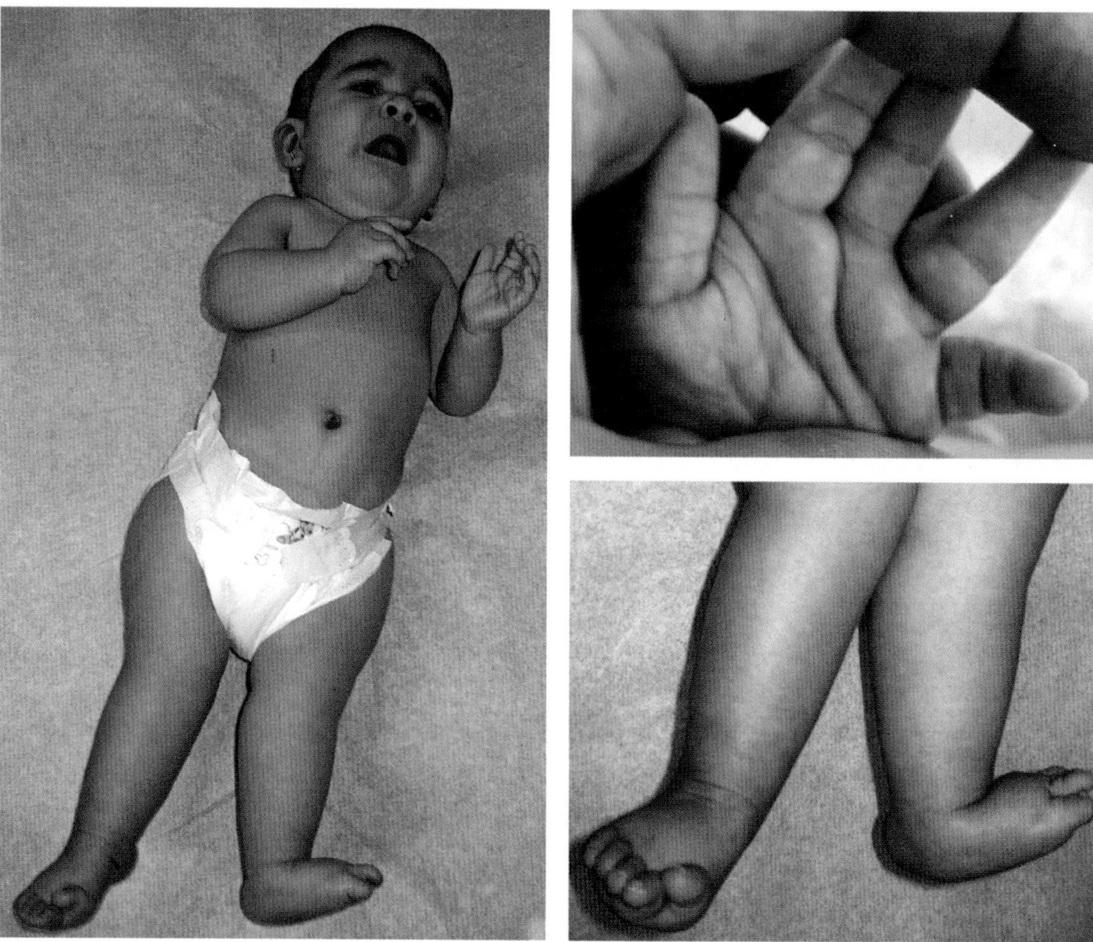

FIGURE 3.6 This child has congenital vertical talus rather than talipes equinovarus, and she demonstrates classic features of distal arthrogryposis. Note the rocker-bottom feet with hand contractures and absent distal finger flexion creases; these features underline the fact that congenital vertical talus can be part of a broader pattern of defects caused by an underlying neuromuscular disorder, such as distal arthrogryposis.

References

1. Wynne-Davies R. Family studies and aetiology of clubfoot. *J Med Genet.* 1965;2:227–232.
2. Sullivan JA. Pediatric flatfoot: evaluation and management. *J Am Acad Orthop Surg.* 1999;7:44–53.
3. Håberg Ø, Foss OA, Lian ØB, Holen KJ. Is foot deformity associated with developmental dysplasia of the hip? *Bone Joint J.* 2020;102-B(11):1582–1586.
4. Gunther A, Smith SJ, Maynard PV, et al. A case-control study of congenital hip dislocation. *Public Health.* 1993;107:9–18.
5. Hsieh Y-Y, Tsai F-J, Lin C-C, et al. Breech deformation complex in neonates. *J Reprod Med.* 2000;45:933–935.
6. Aberman E. The causes of congenital clubfoot. *Arch Dis Child.* 1965;40:548–554.
7. Furdon SA, Donlon CR. Examination of the newborn foot: positional and structural abnormalities. *Adv Neonatal Care.* 2002;2:248–258.
8. Widhe T. Foot deformities at birth: a longitudinal prospective study over a 16-year period. *J Pediatr Orthop.* 1997;17:20–24.
9. Sadeghi-Demneh E, Melvin JMA, Mickle K. Prevalence of pathological flatfoot in school-age children. *Foot (Edinb).* 2018;37:38–44.
10. Molina-Garcia P, Miranda-Aparicio D, Ubago-Guisado E, et al. The impact of childhood obesity on joint

alignment: a systematic review and meta-analysis. *Phys Ther*. 2021;101(7):pzab066.
11. Yin J, Zhao H, Zhuang G, et al. Flexible flatfoot of 6-13-year-old children: a cross-sectional study. *J Orthop Sci*. 2018;23(3):552–556.
12. Evans AM, Rome K, Carroll M, Hawke F. Foot orthoses for treating paediatric flat feet. *Cochrane Database Syst Rev*. 2022;1(1):CD006311.
13. Smolle MA, Svehlik M, Regvar K, Leithner A, Kraus T. Long-term clinical and radiological outcomes following surgical treatment for symptomatic pediatric flexible flat feet: a systematic review. *Acta Orthop*. 2022;93:367–374.
14. Tileston K, Baskar D, Frick SL. What is new in pediatric orthopaedic foot and ankle. *J Pediatr Orthop*. 2022;42(5):e448–e452.
15. Levinsohn EM, Shrimpton AE, Cady RB, et al. Congenital vertical talus and its familial occurrence: an analysis of 36 patients. *Skeletal Radiol*. 2004;33:649–654.
16. Shrimpton AE, Levinsohn EM, Yozawitz JM, et al. A *HOX* gene mutation in a family with isolated congenital vertical talus and Charcot-Marie-Tooth disease. *Am J Hum Genet*. 2004;75:92–96.
17. Gurnett CA, Keppel C, Bick J, et al. Absence of *HOXD10* mutations in idiopathic clubfeet and sporadic vertical talus. *Clin Orthop Rel Res*. 2007;462:27–31.
18. Mark PR, Radlinski BC, Core N, et al. Narrowing the critical region for congenital vertical talus in patients with interstitial 18q deletions. *Am J Med Genet Part A*. 2013;161A:1117–1121.
19. Zhao N, Jing M, Han W, et al. A novel mutation in *TNNT3* associated with Sheldon-Hall syndrome in a Chinese family with vertical talus. *Eur J Med Genet*. 2011;54:351–353.
20. Gurnett CA, Alaee F, Desruisseau D, et al. Skeletal muscle contractile gene (*TNNT3, MYH3, TPM2*) mutations not found in vertical talus or clubfoot. *Clin Orthop Rel Res*. 2009;467:1195–2000.
21. Hafez M, Davis N. Outcomes of a minimally invasive approach for congenital vertical talus with a comparison between idiopathic and syndromic feet. *J Pediatr Orthop*. 2021;41:249–254.
22. Tan JHI, Tan SHS, Lim AKS, Hui JH. The outcomes of subtalar arthroereisis in pes planus: a systemic review and meta-analysis. *Arch Orthop Trauma Surg*. 2021;141(5):761–773.

CHAPTER 4

Metatarsus Adductus (Metatarsus Varus)

KEY POINTS

- Metatarsus adductus is the most common pediatric foot deformation related to intrauterine constraint.
- The feet turn inward, but the ankle and heel are generally in normal position with a flexible heel cord.
- In mild and flexible cases, manipulative stretching of the tight medial soft tissues and avoidance of sleeping postures that tend to augment the deformity may be all that are required.
- When metatarsus adductus is accompanied by heel cord rigidity and varus positioning of the heel, the most likely diagnosis is talipes equinovarus (clubfoot), which requires prompt referral to a pediatric orthopedist.

GENESIS

Compression of the forefoot with the legs flexed across the lower body in late gestation is a frequent cause of metatarsus adductus (also known as *metatarsus varus*), which occurs in about 1.2 per 1000 live births and has an 80% predilection for males.[1,2] Metatarsus adductus is associated with congenital hip dislocation in 5–10% of infants, further implicating fetal constraint as an important etiologic factor.[3,4] In a large group of children treated for idiopathic early-onset scoliosis, there was a high prevalence of commonly associated deformational conditions such as hip dysplasia, torticollis, plagiocephaly, metatarsus adductus, and clubfoot.[5] Such fetal constraint takes place late in gestation, and metatarsus adductus is rarely found in premature infants delivered before 30 weeks of gestation.[6] Metatarsus adductus is the most common pediatric foot deformation related to intrauterine constraint. Although most cases may resolve spontaneously, moderate and severe cases may cause future discomfort and are therefore often treated. Common treatment alternatives include stretching, serial casting, and orthoses. Surgery is reserved for severe cases that are unresponsive to conservative management.[7]

FEATURES

Metatarsus adductus may be caused by either deformation or malformation. The predominant feature is adduction of the forefoot, often with some supination and inability to abduct the forefoot past neutral. The feet turn inward, but the ankle and heel are generally in normal position with a flexible heel cord (Fig. 4.1). Metatarsus adductus with significant hindfoot valgus is termed *skew foot* or *serpentine foot*; however, this is a rare condition. Normally the lateral border of the foot is straight, but in metatarsus adductus the lateral border of the foot is convex, with a concave inner border (i.e., kidney bean–shaped) when viewed from the sole with the infant lying prone with the knees flexed. The adduction occurs at the tarsal-metatarsal joint, leaving a wider space between the first and second toes, and often resulting in a deep crease on the medial midfoot (see Fig. 4.1). The shape and direction of the sole of the foot can be detected by projecting a line along the longitudinal axis of the foot. Normally a line bisecting the heel should traverse the space between the first and second toes. In patients with metatarsus adductus, this line is directed toward the lateral toes. The line passes through the third toe with mild deformity and between the fourth and fifth toes with severe deformity. This deformation can be aggravated by the infant sleeping on his or her abdomen with the knees tucked up and the lower legs and feet rolled inward (Fig. 4.2); hence, its frequency is reduced in supine sleeping infants. To discriminate between positional metatarsus adductus and structural metatarsus adductus, try to abduct the forefoot past midline without using excessive pressure or causing pain. Structural metatarsus adductus is fixed and does not abduct beyond neutral, making it difficult to distinguish from talipes equinovarus.[8]

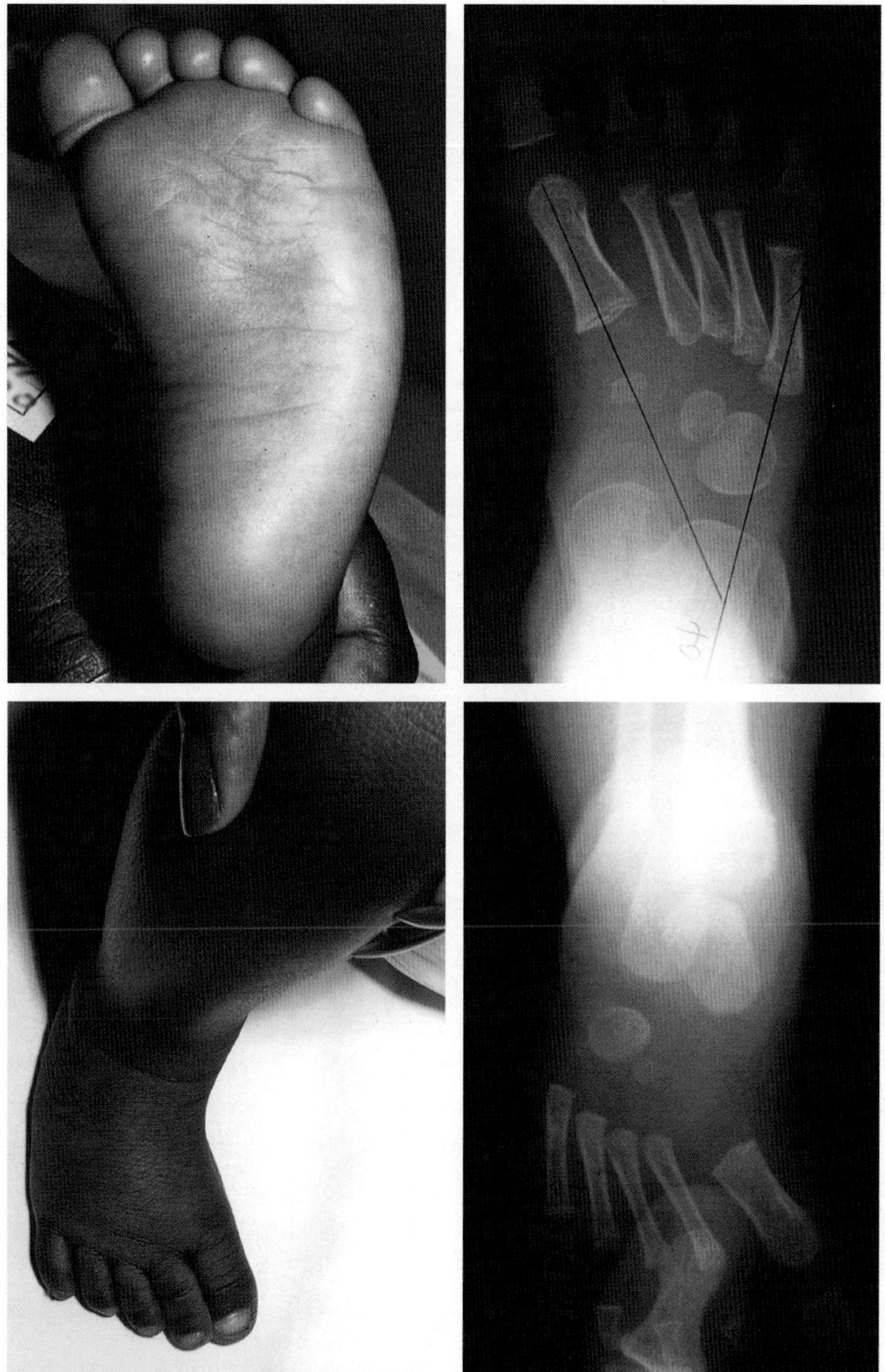

FIGURE 4.1 The normal lateral border of the foot is straight, but in metatarsus adductus the lateral border of the foot is convex, with a concave inner border, when viewed from the sole with the infant lying prone with the knees flexed. This results in a kidney bean–shaped sole. Forefoot adduction occurs at the tarsal-metatarsal joint, leaving a wider space between the first and second toes and often resulting in a deep crease on the medial midfoot. When a line is projected along the longitudinal axis of the foot from the heel, it should traverse the space between the first and second toes, but in metatarsus adductus this line is directed toward the lateral toes. (Courtesy Saul Bernstein and Robert M. Bernstein, Cedar Sinai Medical Center, Los Angeles.)

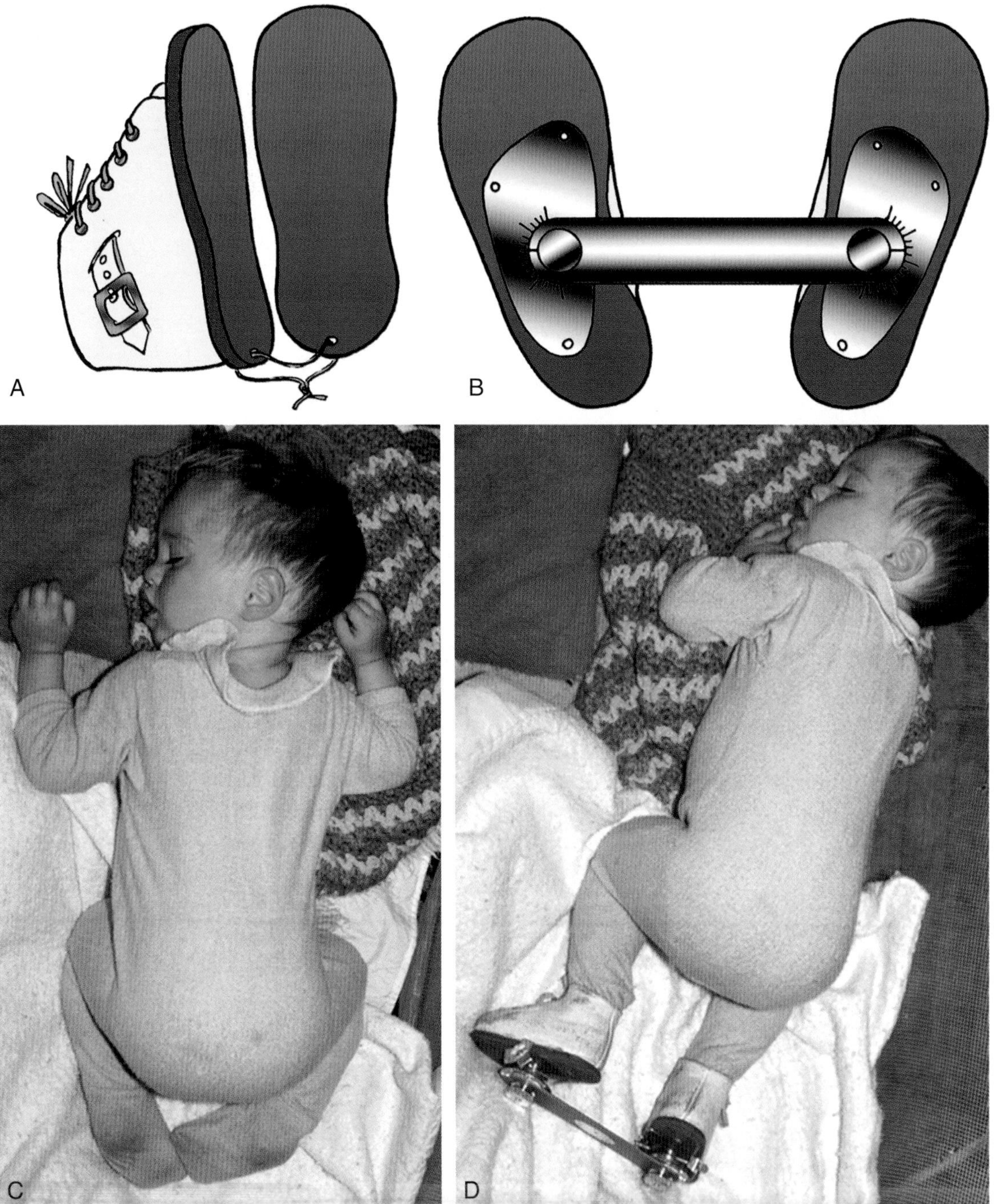

FIGURE 4.2 Simple methods for controlling sleeping posture by using open-toed, straight-last shoes and tying the heels together with a shoelace through holes punched in the heels (A) and a Denis-Browne splint (B) placed on sleeping shoes to prevent the deforming sleeping posture. C, This infant characteristically slept on their stomach with their knees flexed and toes turned inward, accentuating metatarsus adductus. D, Management was directed toward trying to correct the sleeping posture by turning the feet out with a Fillauer bar.

MANAGEMENT, PROGNOSIS, AND COUNSEL

Approximately 85–90% of cases resolve without treatment, and treatment is based on the severity of the condition (Fig. 4.3).[8,9] In mild and flexible cases, manipulative stretching of the tight medial soft tissues and avoidance of sleeping postures that tend to augment the deformity may be all that are required. If the sleeping posture is perpetuating the deformation, then attempts to change this posture may be of value. Several practical suggestions may be useful. One is putting the child in a heavy sleeper garment, which keeps the child warm and causes him or her to sprawl rather than tuck in the legs. The leggings of the sleeper may be pinned or sewn together at the knees, making it difficult to achieve the deforming posture. If this garment is not helpful, a pair of open-toed, straight-last shoes with the heels tied together may be placed on the child. If simpler measures fail, then reversed-last, open-toed shoes tied at the heels may be tried for nighttime wear, or the shoes may be connected by a short Denis-Browne or Fillauer splint to provide mild outward rotation (see Fig. 4.2). It may be necessary to augment this by early reversed-last shoes to maintain the corrected form.

If the foot cannot be passively placed in the neutral position, it is advisable to achieve initial correction by very careful casting. If there is associated internal tibial torsion, as frequently happens, a long leg cast may be used; however, if there is no internal tibial torsion, a short leg cast is usually adequate. The hindfoot and midfoot should be carefully maintained in their neutral positions during the casting. Early management may be critical because the metatarsus adductus tends to become less flexible with time, and excessive compensation at the level of the mediotarsal joint can lead to the development of bunions, hammer toes, and other conditions.[9] In severe, rigid cases, surgical treatment such as anteromedial soft tissue release may be needed. The presence of hallux valgus complicates surgical treatment, and identification and careful analysis

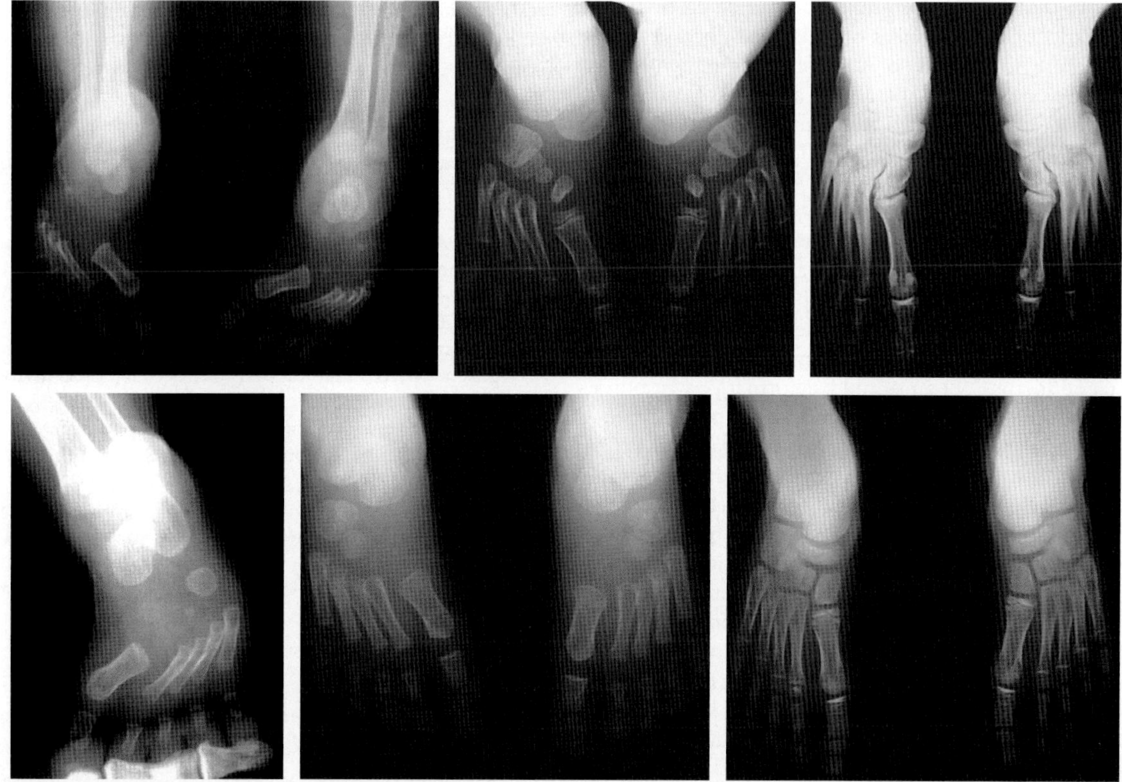

FIGURE 4.3 Serial radiographs from two individuals with spontaneous correction of metatarsus adductus without casting or bracing. (Courtesy Saul Bernstein and Robert M. Bernstein, Cedar Sinai Medical Center, Los Angeles.)

of these combined deformities are very important. The inability to completely correct hallux valgus and an increased incidence of recurrence have been established when metatarsus adductus deformity is present.[10,11]

One study evaluated treatment of metatarsus adductovarus with a hinged, adjustable shoe orthotic during infancy and reported that 96% of the 120 cases resolved with use of the orthotic alone, 3% required additional casting, and 1% required both a bar and shoes for complete correction.[12] Another study of 795 patients used a straight metal bar and attached reversed-last shoe protocol and reported that 99% achieved full correction, with surgery necessary in less than 1% of cases.[13] A long-term study of patients who received either no treatment or serial manipulation and application of plaster holding casts during infancy showed uniformly good results in adulthood, with no need for surgery.[14] In another long-term study of 2401 infants, 3.1% were found to have adductus deformities. By 6 years of age, 87% of adductus anomalies had resolved, and by 16 years of age, 95% had resolved.[15] Dynamic foot pressure and gait analyses at 16 years of age showed no differences between the group with adductus deformities and the group with normal feet at birth. Radiologic examination can be particularly important for the diagnosis of mild cases, because various radiologic methods of angular measurement have been developed for the diagnosis and classification of metatarsus adductus.[16] Thirteen articles were reviewed using the National Health and Medical Research Council levels of evidence and guidelines for clinical practice. Conservative treatment options reported on included the following: no treatment, stretching, splinting, serial casting, sitting and sleeping positions, and footwear/orthotics. There was strong evidence supporting no treatment in the case of flexible metatarsus adductus. Some limited evidence was found for the treatment of semirigid metatarsus adductus.[17] Because mild deformations respond well to simple observation or minimal treatment with a home program of stretching, it is important to make this diagnosis early. Resistant cases may need a more aggressive approach such as serial casting or special bracing, and when clinical outcomes were compared prospectively for serial casting versus orthoses for resistant metatarsus adductus, there was no statistical difference between casting and orthotics. Both groups showed improvement in footprint and radiographic measurements after treatment, without worsening of heel valgus, but cost analysis revealed that orthotic treatment was about half the cost of casting.[18] Metatarsus adductus is considered to be a multifactorial defect and the recurrence risk in first-degree relatives is 1.8%.[1]

DIFFERENTIAL DIAGNOSIS

When metatarsus adductus is accompanied by heel cord rigidity and varus positioning of the heel, the most likely diagnosis is talipes equinovarus (clubfoot), which requires prompt referral to a pediatric orthopedist if early treatment is to be maximally effective before soft tissue contractures become fixed and more resistant to treatment. Another common cause of in-toeing is internal tibial torsion, which occurs when the tibia is medially rotated on its long axis at birth; however, this may not be noticed until the child begins to walk. This condition tends to spontaneously resolve by 2–3 years of age unless accentuated by sleeping in the prone, in-toed position or sitting in the "reverse tailor" position. Neither special shoes nor shoe modifications alter the course of internal tibial torsion resolution. Another common cause of in-toeing is femoral anteversion, which results from medial rotation of the femur at birth. This condition is at its peak in children aged 1–3 years, and it resolves spontaneously by late adolescence. Use of special shoes or bracing does not hasten this process, but continuation of adverse sleeping or sitting positions will slow or prevent resolution. Surgery is usually only contemplated in skeletally mature individuals with insufficient spontaneous correction.

References

1. Wynne-Davies R. Family studies and aetiology of clubfoot. *J Med Genet.* 1965;2:221–232.
2. Rocca G, De Venuto A, Colasanto G, Zielli SO, Mazzotti A, Faldini C. Congenital metatarsus varus: early diagnosis and conservative treatment in 112 patients. *Musculoskelet Surg.* 2022. https://doi.org/10.1007/s12306-022-00751-0.
3. Kumar SJ, MacEwen GD. The incidence of hip dysplasia with metatarsus adductus. *Clin Orthop.* 1982;164:234–235.
4. Håberg Ø, Foss OA, Lian ØB, Holen KJ. Is foot deformity associated with developmental dysplasia of the hip? *Bone Joint J.* 2022;102-B(11):1582–1586.
5. Talmage MS, Nielson AN, Heflin JA, D'Astous JL, Fedorak GT. Prevalence of hip dysplasia and associated conditions in children treated for idiopathic early-onset scoliosis-don't just look at the spine. *J Pediatr Orthop.* 2020;40(1):e49–e52.
6. Katz K, Naor N, Merlob P, et al. Rotational deformities of the tibia and foot in preterm infants. *J Pediatr Orthop.* 1990;10:483–485.
7. Panski A, Goldman V, Simanovsky N, Lamdan M, Lamdan R. Universal neonatal foot orthotics: a novel treatment of infantile metatarsus adductus. *Eur J Pediatr.* 2021;180(9):2943–2949.

8. Furdon SA, Donlon CR. Examination of the newborn foot: positional and structural abnormalities. *Adv Neonatal Care*. 2002;2:248–258.
9. Gore AI, Spencer JP. The newborn foot. *Am Family Physician*. 2004;69:865–872.
10. McAleer JP, Dayton P, DeCarbo WT, et al. A systematic approach to the surgical correction of combined hallux valgus and metatarsus adductus deformities. *J Foot Ankle Surg*. 2021;60(5):1048–1053.
11. Conti MS, Caolo KC, Ellis SJ, Cody EA. Radiographic and clinical outcomes of hallux valgus and metatarsus adductus treated with a modified lapidus procedure. *Foot Ankle Int*. 2021;42(1):38–45.
12. Allen WD, Weiner DS, Riley PM. The treatment of rigid metatarsus adductovarus with the use of a new hinged adjustable shoe orthosis. *Foot Ankle*. 1993;14:450–454.
13. Pentz AS, Weiner DS. Management of metatarsus adductovarus. *Foot Ankle*. 1993;14:241–246.
14. Farsetti P, Weinstein SL, Ponseti IV. The long-term functional and radiographic outcomes of untreated and non-operatively treated metatarsus adductus. *J Bone Joint Surg Am*. 1994;76:257–265.
15. Widhe T. Foot deformities at birth: a longitudinal prospective study over a 16-year period. *J Pediatr Orthop*. 1997;17:20–24.
16. Dawoodi AI, Perera A. Radiological assessment of metatarsus adductus. *Foot Ankle Surg*. 2012;18:1–8.
17. Williams CM, James AM, Tran T. Metatarsus adductus: development of a non-surgical treatment pathway. *J Paediatr Child Health*. 2013;49:E428–433.
18. Herzenberg JE, Burghardt RD. Resistant metatarsus adductus: prospective randomized trial of casting versus orthosis. *J Orthop Sci*. 2014;19:250–256.

CHAPTER 5

Talipes Equinovarus (Clubfoot)

KEY POINTS

- Over the past 25 years there has been a dramatic shift away from extensive surgical releases to manipulative methods with serial casting.
- The term *idiopathic talipes equinovarus* is used to describe the most common type of isolated clubfoot that is not part of a syndrome.
- Structural talipes equinovarus can be either isolated or syndromic (termed *complex* when there are associated malformations).
- The forefoot is inverted, as are the heel and the whole foot, which is in plantar flexion, with a characteristic single posterior skin crease and a medial midfoot crease.
- Congenital vertical talus, or rocker-bottom foot, is a severe malformation that results in a rigid foot with a convex plantar surface rather than a cavus arch and with a deep crease on the lateral dorsal side of the foot.
- Neonates with talipes equinovarus should be referred immediately to an experienced pediatric orthopedist for corrective serial casting during the first week to take advantage of residual neonatal ligamentous laxity.

GENESIS

Talipes equinovarus (TEV; clubfoot) is often a serious foot defect, but predicting severity and response to treatment in the newborn has been notoriously difficult. Over the past 25 years there has been a dramatic shift away from extensive surgical releases to manipulative methods with serial casting (primarily the Ponseti method), in which a series of manipulations and weekly casts are used to bring the foot into a corrected position, followed by the use of splinting and orthotics to maintain the corrected position. In general, the stiffer the foot, the more difficult it will be to correct by manipulation, but early treatment shortly after birth with manipulations and serial casting is extremely important, and relapse is strongly correlated with noncompliance with orthotic bracing. The term *idiopathic talipes equinovarus* is used to describe the most common type of isolated clubfoot that is not part of a syndrome. The birth prevalence varies among racial groups, averaging 1.12 per 1000 live births among Caucasians; it is lowest among Chinese (0.39 per 1000) and highest among Hawaiian and Maori people (6.8 per 1000).[1-4] In a study of the birth prevalence of clubfoot in low- and middle-income countries, the birth prevalence ranged from 0.51 per 1000 in China, to 1.11 per 1000 in the Africa region, to 1.74 per 1000 in the Americas, to 1.21 per 1000 in Southeast Asia, to 1.21 per 1000 in India, to 1.19 per 1000 in the Eastern Mediterranean region, to 2.03 per 1000 in Turkey.[5] Males are affected twice as often as females among all ethnic groups, and bilateral involvement occurs slightly more often than unilateral involvement, with the right side more frequently involved than the left side.[2-4] Postural equinovarus occurs in 0.5 per 1000 live births and is two to three times more common among females than males.[1-4] TEV can be either a positional deformation or a structural malformation resulting from a wide variety of causes (intrauterine compression, abnormal myogenesis, neurologic abnormalities, vascular insufficiency, and/or genetic factors).[2]

Structural TEV can be either isolated or syndromic (termed *complex TEV* when there are associated malformations), and such syndromes can result from genetic, chromosomal, or teratogenic causes. Whenever TEV occurs as part of a broader pattern of altered morphogenesis, strong consideration should be given to various genetic connective tissue disorders and skeletal dysplasias that affect the tissues forming the foot (e.g., Larsen syndrome, diastrophic dysplasia, camptomelic dysplasia), neuromuscular disorders that result in diminished foot movement (e.g., spina bifida or distal arthrogryposis), and various types of vascular disruptions as possible causes. Isolated TEV is seen more frequently in large-for-gestational-age infants, as is congenital hip subluxation.[6] TEV also occurs 3.1 times more frequently in infants born to obese diabetic women than in those born to nonobese, nondiabetic women.[7] A population-based study of 6139 cases of clubfoot born in 10 US states from 2001 through 2005 reported strong associations between male sex, preterm birth, low birth weight, primiparity, and breech presentation, as well as dose-related associations with maternal smoking and both pregestational and gestational diabetes.[8] A three-state case-control study of 677 cases of clubfoot revealed cases were more likely to be male and born to primiparous mothers and obese mothers. These associations were greatest in isolated and bilateral cases. Positive associations with high body mass index were confined to cases with a marker of fetal constraint (oligohydramnios, breech delivery, bicornuate uterus, plural birth), inheritance (family history in a first-degree relative), or vascular disruption (early amniocentesis, chorion villus sampling, plural gestation with fetal loss).[9] It is not always possible to determine whether idiopathic TEV is caused by constraint-related foot deformations, and a multifactorial cause encompassing both environmental and genetic factors seems most likely. Positional TEV can result from uterine constraint owing to factors such as oligohydramnios, multiple gestation, or breech presentation (Figs. 5.1 and 5.2).

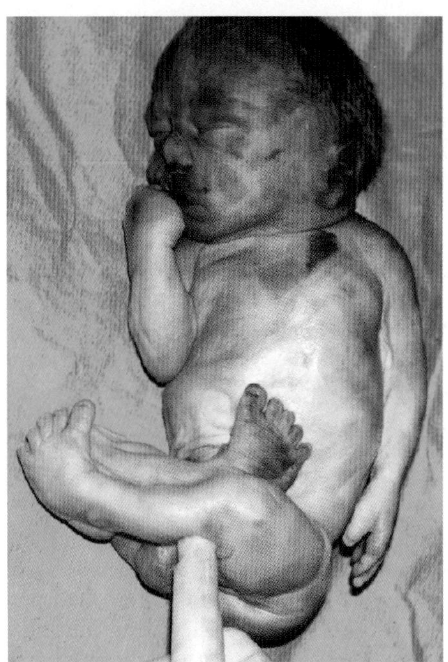

FIGURE 5.1 This term newborn died from pulmonary hypoplasia following 6 weeks of oligohydramnios caused by premature rupture of membranes. He was in complete breech presentation with breech head deformation sequence and oligohydramnios deformation sequence. When folded into his in utero position of comfort, his feet demonstrate bilateral positional equinovarus foot deformations.

TEV should be regarded as a multifactorial disorder resulting from a combination of genetic and environmental factors. TEV is positively associated with Hox family genes, collagen family genes, GLI3, N-acetylation genes, T-box family genes, apoptotic pathway genes, and muscle contractile family genes, as well as with maternal smoking.[10,11] Among 785 individuals with TEV from the United Kingdom and The Netherlands, the male:female ratio was 2.3:1, 58% were affected bilaterally, and 11% had a first- to second-degree family history.[12] One study of Pacific Island people noted a positive family history for idiopathic TEV in 24.4% of all patients studied, and in 20.8% pedigrees studied, parent-to-child transmission occurred.[13] There is also evidence that the anterior tibial vascular tree is poorly developed in children with clubfoot, with a significantly greater prevalence of absence of the dorsalis pedis pulse in the parents of such children.[14] Among 192 patients with 279 clubfeet, using vascular imaging the dorsalis pedis was most frequently reported as absent (21.5%) and the anterior tibial artery was most frequently reported as hypoplastic (18.3%), with 61% of patients noted to have a dominant supply from the posterior tibial artery. Therefore routine Doppler ultrasound (US) imaging is recommended prior to operative

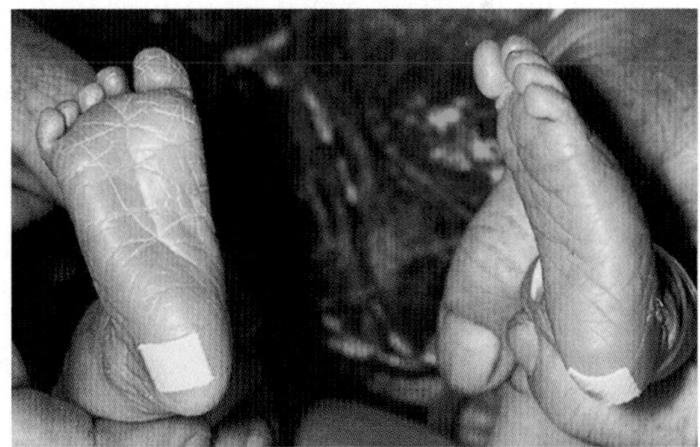

FIGURE 5.2 This flexible equinovarus left foot was associated with a maternal bicornuate uterus.

intervention.[15] Parental smoking is a known risk factor for this multifactorial defect,[16,17] and a family history of a first-degree relative with TEV, combined with maternal smoking, increases the risk for isolated TEV, thereby suggesting a gene/environment interaction.[17] Oligohydramnios and early amnion rupture are associated with TEV, and there is a higher incidence of TEV with early amniocentesis at 11–12 weeks of gestation (1.3%) compared with second-trimester amniocentesis at 15–17 weeks (0.1%).[18,19] This may relate to the relatively larger proportion of total amniotic fluid volume withdrawn for early amniocentesis (15.7% vs. 7.3% at mid-trimester) at a time when the fetal foot is assuming its normal position from a previous physiologic equinus position. This period may be unusually sensitive to constraint and/or vascular disruption. Amniotic fluid leakage before 22 weeks was the only significant factor associated with clubfoot, there being a 15% risk with leakage but only a 1.1% risk without leakage (Fig. 5.3). No case of clubfoot had persistent leakage at 18–20 weeks. Such a transient fluid leak suggests that a disruptive process might have resulted in a developmental arrest of the foot as it moved from the normal equinus position at 9 weeks to the neutral position at 12 weeks. Vascular disruption may be a final common pathway for environmentally induced TEV, which has also been caused by maternal hyperthermia.[20] The use of misoprostol, as well as other unsuccessful early pregnancy termination attempts that result in vascular disruption and hypoxic-ischemic insults to the spinal cord and brainstem, can result in structural TEV, arthrogryposis, Möbius sequence, and cranial nerve damage.[21] Neuromuscular toxins administered during gestation or neuromuscular defects such as arthrogryposis, spinal muscular atrophy, meningomyelocele, and sacral dysgenesis are all associated with structural TEV.

FEATURES

Idiopathic TEV, or true clubfoot, is an isolated congenital deformity of the foot and lower leg resulting in fixation of the foot into four positional components: cavus and adduction of the forefoot, along with varus and equinus positioning of the hindfoot, which are associated with concomitant soft tissue abnormalities. The forefoot is inverted, as are the heel and the whole foot, which is in plantar flexion, with a characteristic single posterior skin crease and a medial midfoot crease (Figs. 5.4–5.8). Clubfoot is characterized by the inability to dorsiflex, medial deviation of the heel, and a sole that is kidney shaped when viewed from the bottom. There is often a varus deformation of the neck of the talus and a medial shift of the navicular on the head of the talus. The calf muscles may be deficient with shortening and tapering. The fibrous capsule of the joint may be thickened on the lateral aspect of the foot. If there has been a long-term compression over the lateral margin of the foot, that site may have thin skin with deficient subcutaneous tissue. The depth of skin creases on the medial side of the foot is indicative of the severity of the deformity, and the more rigid the foot, the poorer the prognosis. TEV is unilateral in 45% of cases and more commonly affects the right foot.

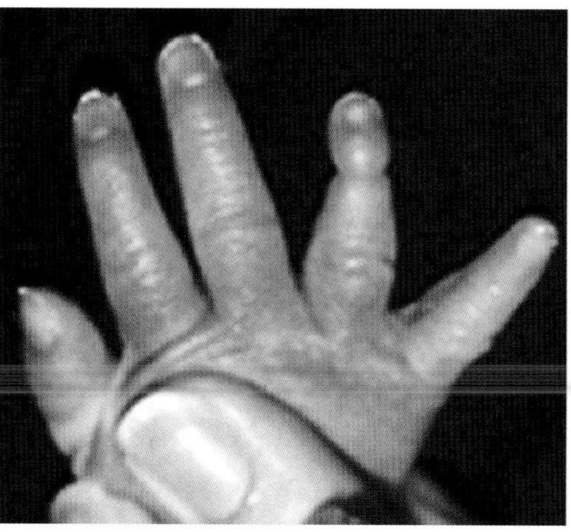

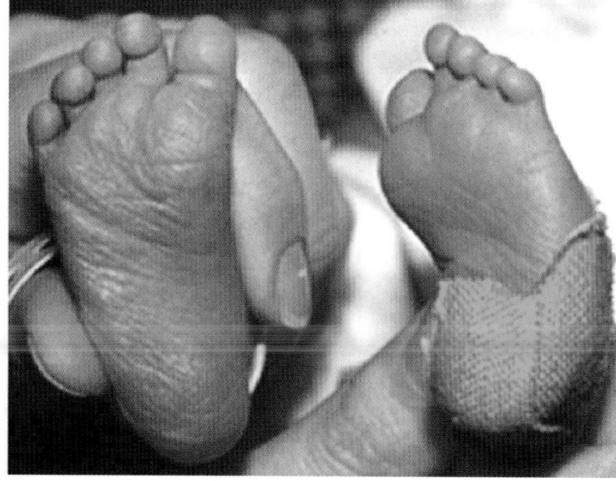

FIGURE 5.3 This rigid equinovarus left foot deformity was associated with an amniotic band around the fourth finger and a history of amniotic fluid leakage at 11–12 weeks.

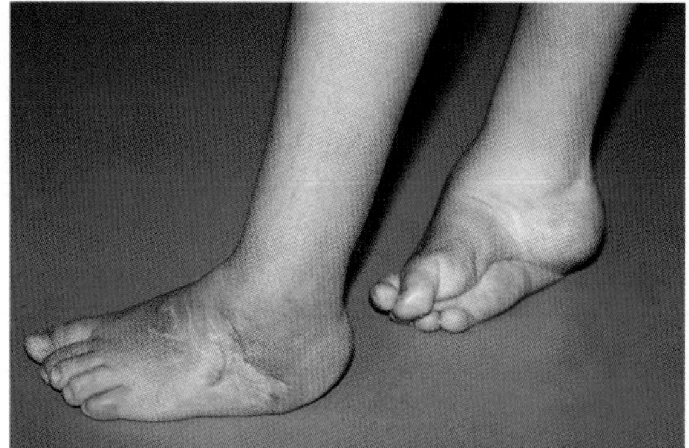

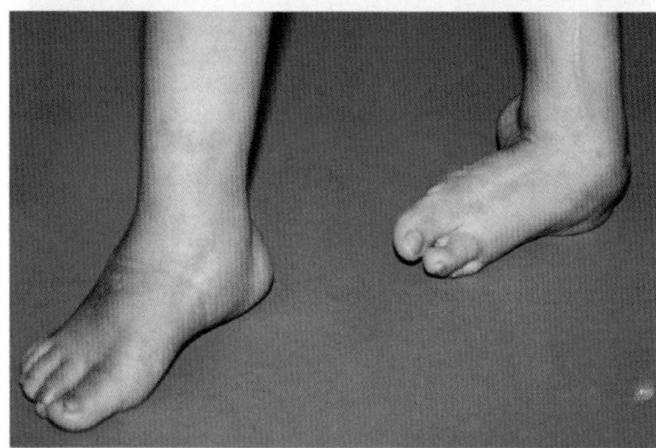

FIGURE 5.4 This rigid left equinovarus foot in an 18-year-old individual was untreated, resulting in the individual walking on the outside edge of this foot. (Courtesy Robert M. Bernstein, Cedar Sinai Medical Center, Los Angeles.)

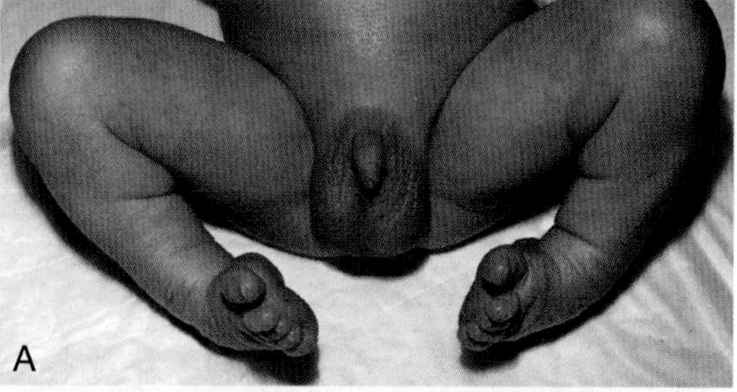

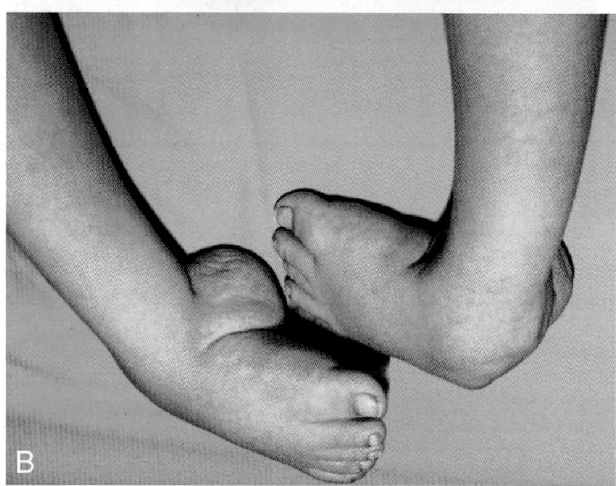

FIGURE 5.5 Bilateral talipes equinovarus feet at birth (A) and later in childhood (without treatment) (B). Note the heel varus (medial deviation) and rigid foot posture with inability to dorsiflex. (Courtesy Robert M. Bernstein, Cedar Sinai Medical Center, Los Angeles.)

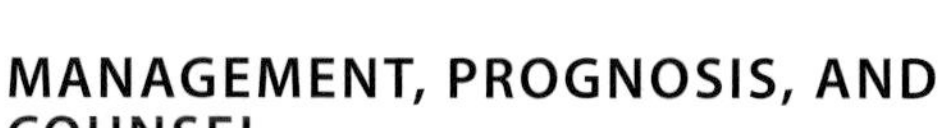

MANAGEMENT, PROGNOSIS, AND COUNSEL

Neonates with TEV should be referred immediately to an experienced pediatric orthopedist for corrective serial casting during the first week to take advantage of residual neonatal ligamentous laxity. If there is flexibility to the foot, initial manipulation and stretch taping toward dorsiflexion of the foot with eversion of the heel should be attempted (Fig. 5.9). Maintenance of the corrected position may sometimes need to be fostered by casting and/or Denis-Browne splints in order to prevent a lapse toward the deformed position. The Ponseti method is now considered the gold standard of treatment for primary clubfoot. Long-term results of manipulation and serial casting using the Ponseti method suggest that when properly performed, surgical release is indicated in less than 1% of cases, primarily those with a short, rigid forefoot or with severe deformity that does not respond to proper manipulation.[22] Reviews have shown that the Ponseti method provides excellent results, with an initial correction rate of around 90%. Noncompliance with bracing is the most common cause of relapse. This suggests that the best practice for treatment of TEV is the original Ponseti method, with hyperabduction of the foot in the final cast and the need for longer term bracing for up to 4 years.[23-25] Clinically important variations in results are due to deviations from the classic Ponseti approach to clubfoot management regarding manipulation, casting, percutaneous Achilles tenotomy, use of the bar-connected brace, and indications for relapse recognition. It is strongly recommended that clinicians follow the Ponseti method as initially described without deviation to optimize treatment outcomes.[25]

Prognostic classification in older studies was usually based on the reducibility of the equinovarus deformity by manipulation. Mild TEV that can be manipulated to or beyond neutral had an 89% success rate with serial casting compared with 46% for

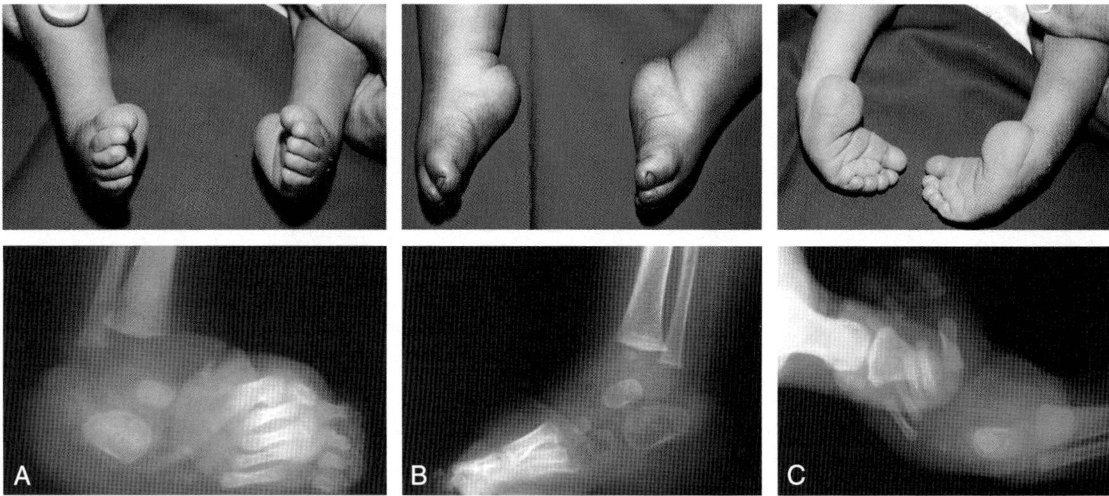

FIGURE 5.6 These neurogenic equinovarus feet resulted from a lumbosacral meningomyelocele. Note varus deformation (A), equinus position (B), and adductus deformation (C). (Courtesy Robert M. Bernstein, Cedar Sinai Medical Center, Los Angeles.)

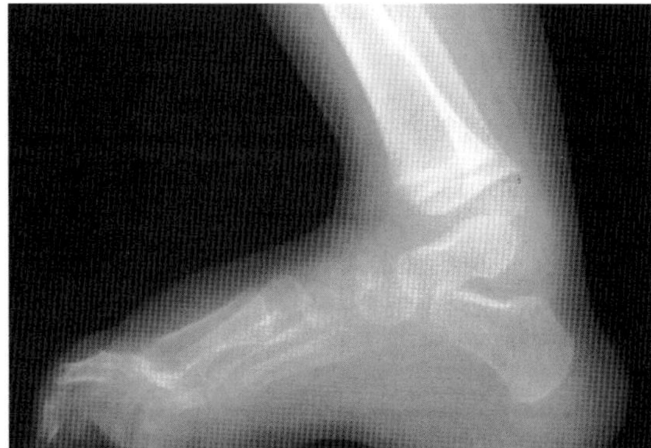

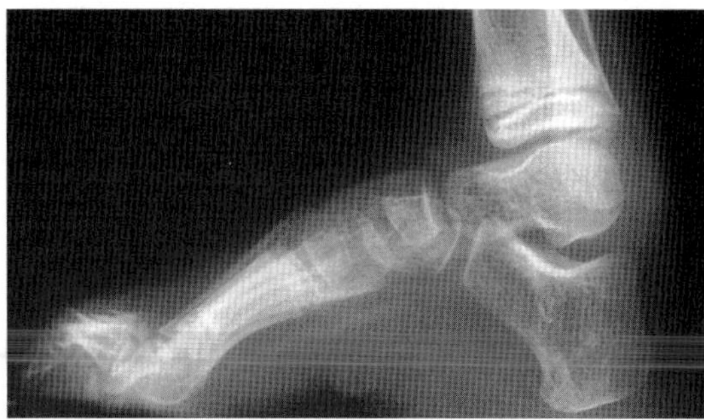

FIGURE 5.7 Cavus foot deformity can result from muscular imbalance due to deficient gastrocnemius function in spina bifida. (Courtesy Saul Bernstein and Robert M. Bernstein, Cedar Sinai Medical Center, Los Angeles.)

moderate deformity that could only be manipulated to within 20 degrees of neutral and 10% for more severe deformity.[25] The initial treatment is usually nonsurgical regardless of severity, with serial casting favored in North America and vigorous physical therapy with splinting favored in Europe. This latter approach has reported good results in as many as 77% of cases.[26] Early correction usually begins distally and is accomplished in the following order: adduction, varus, and then equinus. Good results were also reported in most cases in a prospective study of congenital equinovarus foot among 20,000 neonates.[27] A case-control study of individuals treated for clubfoot at two separate institutions with different methods of treatment between 1983 and 1987 compared the results of 18 adults treated with the Ponseti method with 24 adults treated via comprehensive clubfoot release. The Ponseti group fared better than the surgically treated group owing to increased range of motion observed upon physical examination and greater strength during gait evaluations, and less arthritis.[28]

Because of the previous association between TEV and developmental dysplasia of the hip (DDH), there has been a recent debate as to whether to routinely screen patients with TEV for DDH. Among 614 infants screened between 1996 and 2006, there were 436 cases of postural TEV, 60 of congenital fixed TEV, 93 of congenital talipes calcaneovalgus (CTCV), and 25 of metatarsus adductus. The overall risk of ultrasonographic dysplasia or instability was 1:27 in postural TEV, 1:8.6 in congenital talipes equinovarus (CTEV),

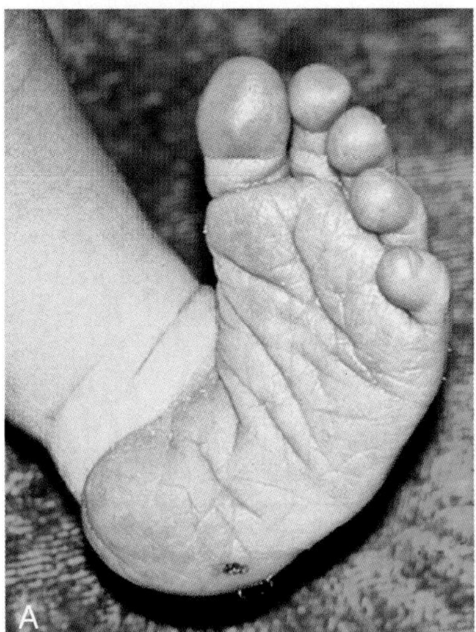

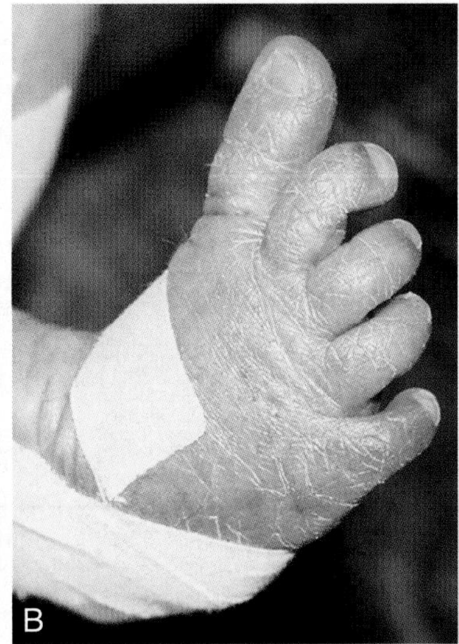

FIGURE 5.8 A, Plantar view of an equinovarus foot. Note the inward rotation of the heel and forefoot with the whole foot deviated inward at the ankle. B, At the site of in utero compression over the left lateral ankle, the skin was very thin, erythematous, and stretched as a result of prolonged pressure. Outward pressure on the heel and forefoot via taping resulted in partial correction toward a neutral foot position. Taping and manipulation alone corrected this foot.

1:5.2 in CTCV, and 1:25 in metatarsus adductus. The risk of type IV instability of the hip or irreducible dislocation was 1:436 (0.2%) in postural TEV, 1:15.4 (6.5%) in CTCV, and 1:25 (4%) in metatarsus adductus. There were no cases of hip instability (type IV) or irreducible dislocation in the fixed TEV group. Therefore routine screening for DDH in cases of postural TEV and CTEV was discouraged, whereas ultrasonographic imaging and surveillance of hips in infants with CTCV and possibly those with metatarsus adductus seemed warranted,[29] and a second study of 119 infants with TEV noted DDH in 1 in 17 infants and also supported selected screening.[30] An epidemiologic study of 677 TEV patients and 2037 normal controls noted 5/677 (0.74%) patients with clubfoot and 5/2037 (0.25%) controls being treated with a brace or harness for hip problems ($P = .134$). Of the patients with clubfoot, two of them did not need treatment for their DDH and two would have been discovered by standard hip screening. A follow-up study at 3.3 years of age found no serious late hip dysplasia. The authors concluded that routine hip US or radiographic screening of idiopathic clubfoot patients is not necessary unless indicated by standard infant hip screening,[31] and this view was supported in another recent study of 101 patients with TEV in which only one child required treatment for DDH.[32]

In a 2008 retrospective study of 20,663 pregnant women who underwent routine US scanning at 18–22 weeks of gestation, 42 cases of congenital clubfoot were diagnosed (incidence: 0.2%); 28 of them (66.6%) were isolated and 14 (33.3%) were complex (other structural or chromosomal abnormalities present), of which 3 (7.1%) had an abnormal karyotype and 11 (26.2%) had an associated structural anomaly. The false-positive rate was 2.3% (1 out of 32 liveborns).[33] When counseling women regarding prenatally diagnosed isolated clubfoot, it is important to tell them that approximately 10% of individuals will have a normal foot or positional foot deformity requiring minimal treatment. Conversely, 10–13% of prenatally diagnosed cases of isolated clubfoot will have complex clubfoot postnatally, based on findings of additional structural or neurodevelopmental abnormalities. A review of the literature indicated a risk for associated chromosomal abnormalities of 1.7–3.6%, with a predominance of sex chromosome aneuploidy.[34] Among 174 prenatally identified TEV cases in 2011, outcome data were available for 88.5% (154/174), 83 cases (47.7%) were isolated, and 91 cases (52.3%) were associated with additional abnormalities. Bilateral abnormality tended to be more severe, a high caesarean section rate was noted overall, and a high preterm delivery rate was seen in the isolated group. In this study, the aneuploidy rate was 30% in the nonisolated cohort compared with 1.2% in the isolated group. The three most associated structural abnormalities were brain (35/91, 19.5%), skeletal (22/91, 24.2%), and

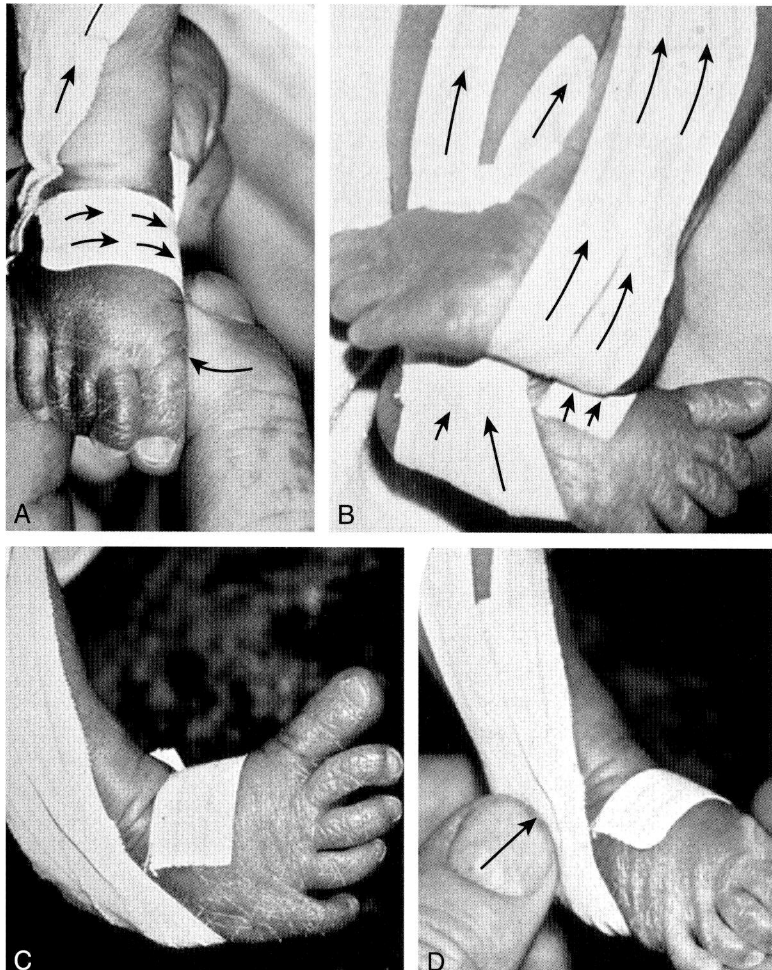

FIGURE 5.9 A, After manipulating the foot of this patient into a more normal position, several layers of adhesive tape are applied (tincture of benzoin on the skin), starting over the dorsum of the foot and bringing the tape medially under the sole and up the lateral aspect of the leg. B, After taping, the feet tend to return partially to their pretaped position. When the foot is taped and partially corrected, it is possible for the parents to manipulate the foot repeatedly toward the ideal position (C and D), a mode of management that is not possible when the foot is in a cast.

heart (21/91, 23.1%), with spina bifida evident in 13 cases (14.3%).[35] Among 44 fetuses for which prenatal imaging included both US and magnetic resonance imaging (MRI), isolated TEV was found in 19/44 (43.2%) fetuses and complex TEV in 25/44 (56.8%). The two most associated abnormalities were central nervous system/spinal abnormalities in 13/25 (52.0%) fetuses and musculoskeletal abnormalities in 7/25 (28.0%). Isolated TEV on US may not be an MRI indication, whereas MRI may be useful in cases of complex TEV.[36]

Among 83 fetuses with a prenatal diagnosis of at least one clubfoot, 67 had a clubfoot documented at birth (false-positive rate 19%) in a 2010 study.[37] A foot classified as "mild" on prenatal US was significantly less likely to be a true clubfoot at birth than when a "moderate" or "severe" diagnosis was given. If "mild" clubfoot patients were removed from the analysis, the false-positive rate was 7%; thus an isolated "mild" clubfoot diagnosed on a prenatal sonogram is less likely to be a clubfoot at birth.[37] In a 2021 metaanalysis of studies reporting prenatal diagnoses of clubfoot made through US and MRI from January 2010 to June 2021, US was the primary diagnostic instrument. Thirteen of the studies used

US exclusively, while three used MRI in addition to US, and seven performed karyotyping after US diagnosis. Thus US is the instrument of choice for the prenatal diagnosis of clubfoot.[38] A 2021 retrospective observational cohort study of fetuses with a prenatal diagnosis of isolated TEV between 2004 and 2018 was treated by the Ponseti method and children were followed-up postnatally for at least 2 years, with a specific focus on neurodevelopmental outcome.[39] This cohort included 81 fetuses with a prenatal diagnosis of TEV confirmed postnatally in 86.4% of cases. Concordance between prenatal and postnatal assessment was good for both laterality and degree of severity. Within the most severe group, although there had not been a clear separation of postural TEV from other types of TEV, the rate of relapse was 11% and the rate of major surgery was 6%. The postnatal outcome was normal in 68.6% of newborns, while 14% of cases had a diagnosis of minor additional findings and 17% had an impairment of neurological development. The accuracy of prenatal US for isolated TEV was 86% with a false-positive diagnosis of 14%. The grade of TEV assigned prenatally correlated to postnatal severity and longer orthopedic rehabilitation in terms of number of casts and need for surgery.[39] The prognosis for restoration toward normal form is much better when the cause is uterine constraint in an otherwise normal child. The general recurrence risk for an equinovarus defect is 2%, and when only postural equinovarus cases are considered, the recurrence risk is 3%.[1] If the propositus is male, the recurrence risk for siblings is 6.3%; if the proposita is female, the recurrence risk for siblings is 1.9%, with 4.2% of patients having an affected first-degree relative.[2]

DIFFERENTIAL DIAGNOSIS

Congenital vertical talus, or rocker-bottom foot, is a severe malformation that results in a rigid foot with a convex plantar surface rather than a cavus arch and with a deep crease on the lateral dorsal side of the foot (see Fig. 5.4). The forefoot is abducted (turned outward) and dorsiflexed, while the heel is also turned outward with the toes pointing down, resulting in the "rocker-bottom foot" configuration. With congenital vertical talus, the talus is rigidly fixed in a vertical position in plantar flexion, and the forefoot cannot be plantar flexed. There is dorsal dislocation of the navicular on the talus, and the calcaneocuboid joint is irreducible. The Achilles tendon is contracted, and hypoplasia of the talar head can be palpated on the medial sole. Early casting to stretch soft tissues and tendons starts at birth and continues until surgical reconstruction, but the foot usually remains abnormal. Congenital vertical talus can be isolated or part of a broader pattern of malformation due to chromosomal or neuromuscular disorders (see Figs. 3.5 and 3.6).

Pronounced tightness of the Achilles tendon, with very little dorsiflexion, differentiates TEV from metatarsus adductus. The etiology for idiopathic TEV, which has a predilection for males and varies in racial incidence, is unknown, but it tends to be more rigid than constraint-induced deformation, with more associated atrophy of calf muscles. The talus tends to be hypoplastic and altered in form, and there is some question as to whether the primary defect is in talonavicular development, possibly on a vascular basis. When TEV is a feature of intrinsic deformation, the prognosis for achieving a normal foot form is usually poor. TEV may accompany certain neurologic deficiencies, especially those affecting the spinal cord, and as such occurs frequently with meningomyelocele. An infant with TEV should be checked for spinal defects, and the lower spine should be closely inspected for hemangiomata, hairy nevus, or other subtle clues that might suggest occult spinal dysraphism. A neurologic evaluation is also indicated, because partial degrees of equinovarus position occur in many neuromuscular and cerebral palsy disorders. Deficiency of the tibia (tibial hemimelia) often results in an equinovarus foot defect, and amniotic bands around the leg, proximal to the foot, may also result in TEV. This defect may also be part of an arthrogrypotic disorder such as amyoplasia, in which the inward rotation of the hands and shoulders may allow an overall diagnosis (see Fig. 2.4) or indicate distal arthrogryposis syndrome (see Fig. 2.5). Talectomy is an effective procedure for salvaging arthrogrypotic TEV. Supplementation of the procedure by a simplified Ilizarof fixator was associated with more satisfactory morphological and functional results, particularly in older children.[40] TEV may also be one feature of a skeletal dysplasia such as diastrophic dysplasia, an autosomal recessive genetic connective tissue dysplasia (see Figs. 1.1D, and 2.2D). This represents an example of an underlying connective tissue dysplasia leading to malformation of a joint.

References

1. Wynn-Davies R. Family studies and aetiology of clubfoot. *J Med Genet.* 1965;2:227–232.
2. Moorthi RN, Hashmi SS, Langois P, et al. Idiopathic talipes equinovarus (ITEV) (clubfeet) in Texas. *Amer J Med Genet.* 2005;132A:376–380.
3. Chung CS, Nemechek RW, Larson IJ, et al. Genetic and epidemiological studies of clubfoot in Hawaii. *Hum Hered.* 1969;19:321–342.
4. Lochmiller CL, Johnston D, Scott A, et al. Genetic epidemiology study of idiopathic talipes equinovarus. *Amer J Med Genet.* 1998;79:90–96.
5. Smythe T, Kuper H, Macleod D, Foster A, Lavy C. Birth prevalence of congenital talipes equinovarus in low- and middle-income countries: a systematic review and meta-analysis. *Trop Med Int Health.* 2017;22(3):269–285.
6. Lapunzina P, Camelo JS, Rittler M, et al. Risks of congenital anomalies in large for gestational age infants. *J Pediatr.* 2002;140:200–204.
7. Moore LL, Singer MR, Bradlee ML, et al. A prospective study of risk of congenital defects associated with maternal obesity and diabetes mellitus. *Epidemiology.* 2000;11:689–694.
8. Parker SE, Mai CT, Strickland MJ, et al. Multistate study of the epidemiology of clubfoot. *Birth Defects Research (Part A).* 2009;85A:897–904.
9. Werler MM, Yazdy MM, Mitchell AA, et al. Descriptive epidemiology of idiopathic clubfoot. *Am J Med Genet A.* 2013;161A:1569–1578.
10. Yong BC, Xun FX, Zhao LJ, Deng HW, Xu HW. A systematic review of association studies of common variants associated with idiopathic congenital talipes equinovarus (ICTEV) in humans in the past 30 years. *Springerplus.* 2016;27(5(1)):896.
11. Pavone V, Chisari E, Vescio A, Lucenti L, Sessa G, Testa G. The etiology of idiopathic congenital talipes equinovarus: a systematic review. *J Orthop Surg Res.* 2018;22(13(1)):206.
12. Cardy AH, Sharp L, Torrance N, et al. Is there evidence for aetiologically distinct subgroups of idiopathic congenital talipes equinovarus? A case-only study and pedigree analysis. *PLoS One.* 2011;6:e17895. https://doi.org/10.1371/journal.pone.0017895.
13. Chapman C, Stott NS, Port RV, et al. Genetics of clubfoot in Maori and Pacific people. *J Med Genet.* 2000;37:680–683.
14. Muir L, Laliotis N, Kutty S, et al. Absence of the dorsalis pedis pulse in the parents of children with clubfoot. *J Bone Joint Surg.* 1995;B77:114–116.
15. Puri AMC, Hughes KP, Stenson KM, Gelfer Y, Holt PJE, Patterson BO. Variations in arterial pedal circulation in idiopathic congenital talipes equinovarus: a systematic review. *J Pediatr Orthop B.* 2021;30(1):59–65.
16. Hackshaw A, Rodeck C, Boniface S. Maternal smoking in pregnancy and birth defects: a systematic review based on 173,687 malformed cases and 11.7 million controls. *Human Reproduction Update.* 2011;17:589–604.
17. Honein MA, Paulozzi LJ, Moore CA. Family history, maternal smoking, and clubfoot: an indication of a gene-environment interaction. *Am J Epidemiol.* 2000;152:658–665.
18. Farrell SA, Summers AM, Dallaire L, et al. Clubfoot, an adverse outcome of early amniocentesis: disruption or amniocentesis? *J Med Genet.* 1999;36:843–846.
19. Tredwell SJ, Wilson D, Wilmink MA. Review of the effect of early amniocentesis on foot deformity in the neonate. *J Pediatr Orthop.* 2001;21:636–641.
20. Graham JM Jr, Edwards MJ, Edwards MJ. Teratogen update: gestational effects of maternal hyperthermia due to febrile illnesses and resultant patterns of defects in humans. *Teratology.* 1998;58:209–221.
21. Gonzales CH, Marques-Dias MJ, Kim CA, et al. Congenital abnormalities in Brazilian children associated with misoprostol misuse in first trimester of pregnancy. *Lancet.* 1998;351:1624–1627.
22. Ganesan B, Luximon A, Al-Jumaily A, Balasankar SK, Naik GR. Ponseti method in the management of clubfoot under 2 years of age: a systematic review. *PLoS One.* 2017;20(12(6)):e0178299.
23. Jowett CR, Morcuende JA, Ramachandran M. Management of congenital talipes equinovarus using the Ponseti method: a systematic review. *J Bone Joint Surg Br.* 2011;93:1160–1164.
24. Zhao D, Li H, Zhao L, et al. Results of clubfoot management using the Ponseti method: do the details matter? A systematic review. *Clin Orthop Relat Res.* 2014;472:1329–1336.
25. Harold AJ, Walker CJ. Treatment and prognosis in congenital clubfoot. *J Bone Joint Surg Br.* 1983;65:8–11.
26. Souchet P, Bensahel H, Themar-Noel C, et al. Functional treatment of clubfoot: a new series of 350 idiopathic clubfeet with long-term follow-up. *J Pediatr Orthop B.* 2004;13:189–196.
27. Vadivieso-Garcia JL, Escassi-Gil A, Zapatero-Martinez M, et al. Prospective study of equinovarus foot in 20,000 live newborn infants. *An Esp Pediatr.* 1988;28:325–326.
28. Smith PA, Kuo KN, Graf AN, et al. Long-term results of comprehensive clubfoot release versus the Ponseti method: which is better? *Clin Orthop Relat Res.* 2014;472:1281–1290.
29. Paton RW, Choudry Q. Neonatal foot deformities and their relationship to developmental dysplasia of the hip: an 11-year prospective, longitudinal observational study. *J Bone Joint Surg Br.* 2009;91:655–658.
30. Perry DC, Tawfiq SM, Roche AJ, et al. The association between clubfoot and developmental dysplasia of the hip. *Bone Joint Surg Br.* 2010;92:1586–1588.
31. Mahan ST, Yazdy MM, Kasser JR, et al. Is it worthwhile to routinely ultrasound screen children with idiopathic clubfoot for hip dysplasia? *J Pediatr Orthop.* 2013;33:847–851.
32. Chou DT, Ramachandran M. Prevalence of developmental dysplasia of the hip in children with clubfoot. *J Child Orthop.* 2013;7:263–267.

33. Canto MJ, Cano S, Palau J, et al. Prenatal diagnosis of clubfoot in low-risk population: associated anomalies and long-term outcome. *Prenat Diagn*. 2008;28:343–346.
34. Lauson S, Alvarez C, Patel MS, et al. Outcome of prenatally diagnosed isolated clubfoot. *Ultrasound Obstet Gynecol*. 2010;35:708–714.
35. Sharma R, Stone S, Alzouebi A, et al. Perinatal outcome of prenatally diagnosed congenital talipes equinovarus. *Prenat Diagn*. 2011;31:142–145.
36. Nemec U, Nemec SF, Kasprian G, et al. Clubfeet and associated abnormalities on fetal magnetic resonance imaging. *Prenat Diagn*. 2012;32:822–828.
37. Glotzbecker MP, Estroff JA, Spencer SA, et al. Prenatally diagnosed clubfeet: comparing ultrasonographic severity with objective clinical outcomes. *J Pediatr Orthop*. 2010;30:606–611.
38. Ruzzini L, De Salvatore S, Longo UG, et al. Prenatal diagnosis of clubfoot: where are we now? Systematic review and meta-analysis. *Diagnostics (Basel)*. 2021;11(12):2235.
39. Fantasia I, Dibello D, Di Carlo V, et al. Prenatal diagnosis of isolated clubfoot: diagnostic accuracy and long-term postnatal outcomes. *Eur J Obstet Gynecol Reprod Biol*. 2021;264:60–64.
40. Atef A, El-Rosasy M, El-Tantawy A. Talectomy for the management of resistant talipes equinovarus deformity; does adding Ilizarov external fixator provide extra advantages? *J Foot Ankle Surg*. 2021;60(2):307–311.

CHAPTER 6

Deformed Toes

KEY POINTS

- Constraint of the feet while the legs are in a flexed and folded position can result in medial overlapping of the toes, especially the fifth, fourth, and third toes.
- Congenital curly toes are relatively common, asymptomatic soft tissue abnormalities of the lateral toes.

GENESIS

Constraint of the feet while the legs are in a flexed and folded position can result in medial overlapping of the toes, especially the fifth, fourth, and third toes.

FEATURES

The fifth, fourth, and third toes tend to overlap medially with mild to moderate incurvature (Fig. 6.1). There may be accentuated longitudinal creasing in the sole of the foot, where the sole has been "folded" by external compression. Congenital curly toes are relatively common, affecting 2.8–3.26% of the population.[1,2] They are generally asymptomatic soft tissue abnormalities of the lateral toes, of which the third and fourth toes are most often affected.

MANAGEMENT AND PROGNOSIS

Most cases of curly toes resolve spontaneously in early childhood with normal ambulation, and manipulative lateral stretching and/or taping may not be particularly effective.[3,4] Rarely is surgery necessary, except in the most severe cases, where tenotomy may be performed on the affected toes (Figs. 6.2 and 6.3).[5,6]

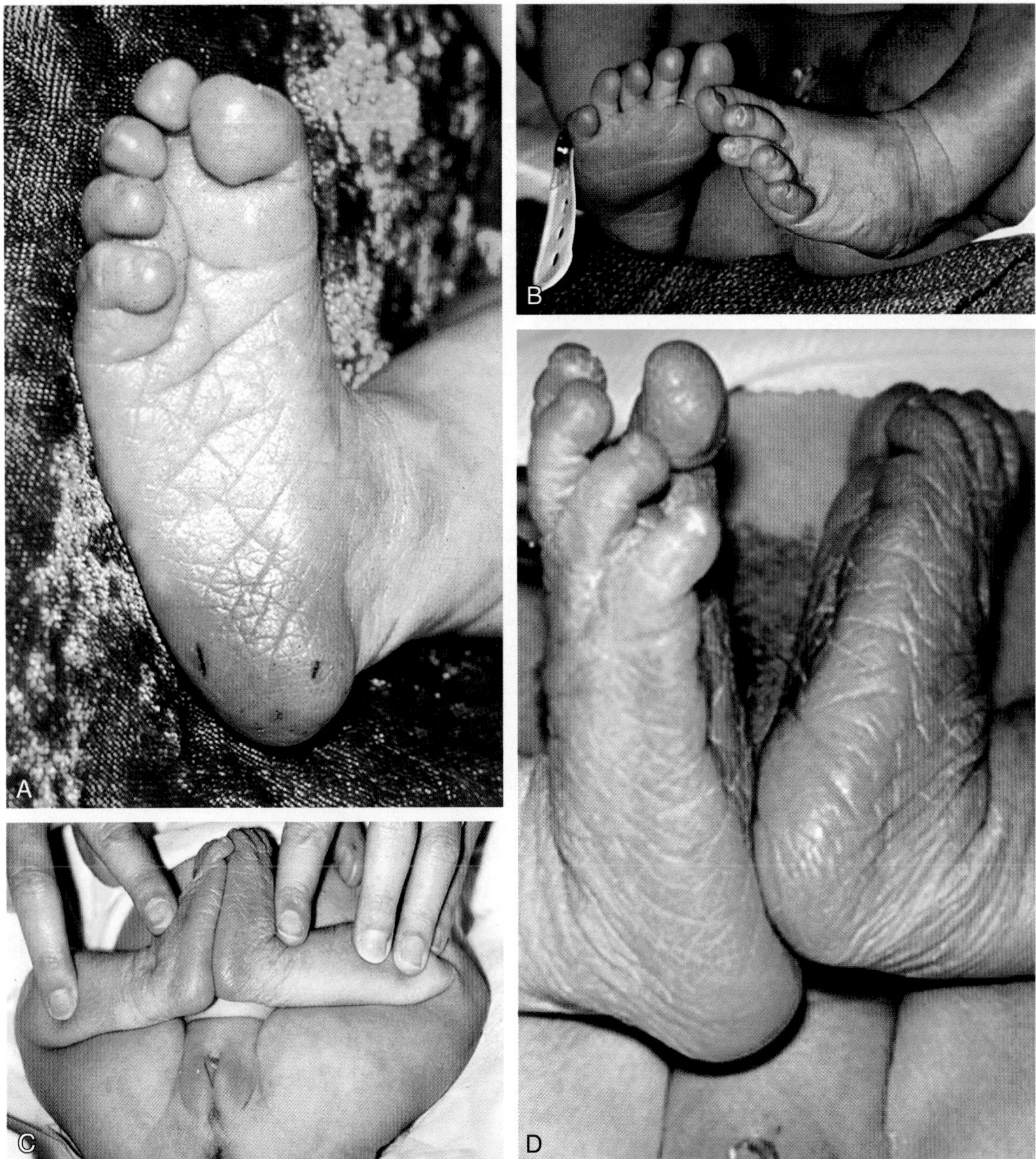

FIGURE 6.1 A, Deformed toes. B, Presumed position in utero, in which uterine constraint from oligohydramnios compressed the forefoot, resulting in overlapping of the toes. C, Presumed positioning in utero, in which uterine constraint compressed the feet, yielding unilateral, partially folded forefoot and deformation of toes. D, Note the thin, wrinkled skin over the lateral malleolus *(left)*, which is a strong clue that constraint induction of the deformation occurred.

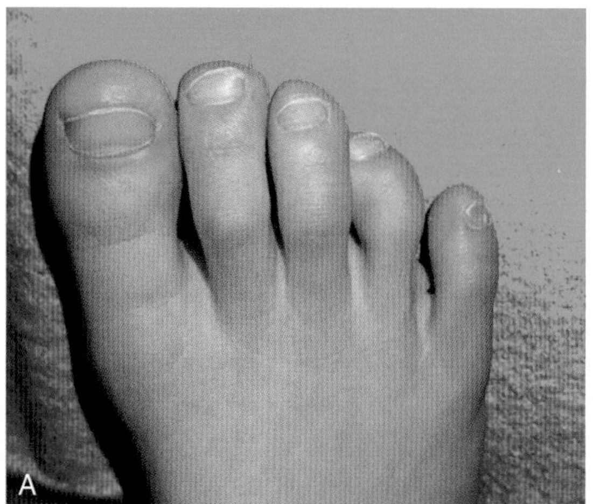

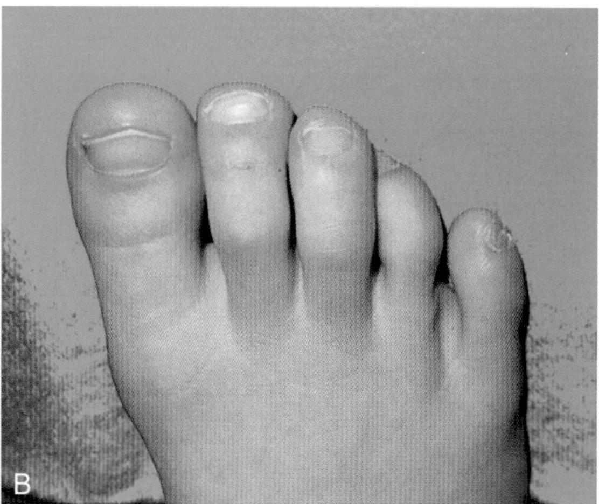

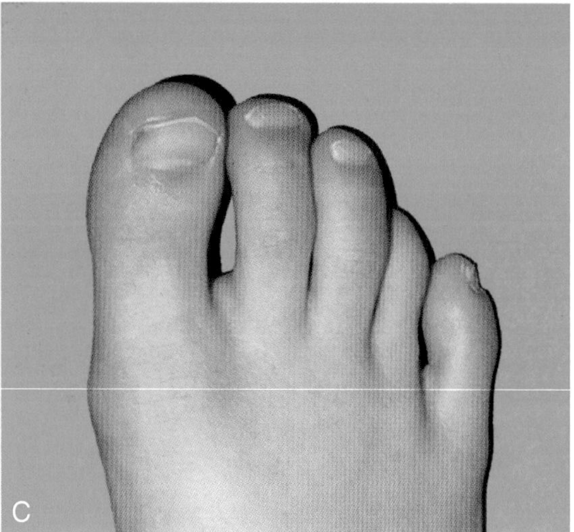

FIGURE 6.2 Curly toe deformations of the right fourth toe by appearance. A, Grade 1, mild curl with the whole nail visible. B, Grade 2, moderate curl with part of the nail underlapping the third toe. C, Grade 3, severe curl with the nail not visible. (Satake H, Kura H, Naganuma Y, et al. Assessment of the severity of curly toe. *J Orthop Sci.* 2022;27(6):1278-1282.)

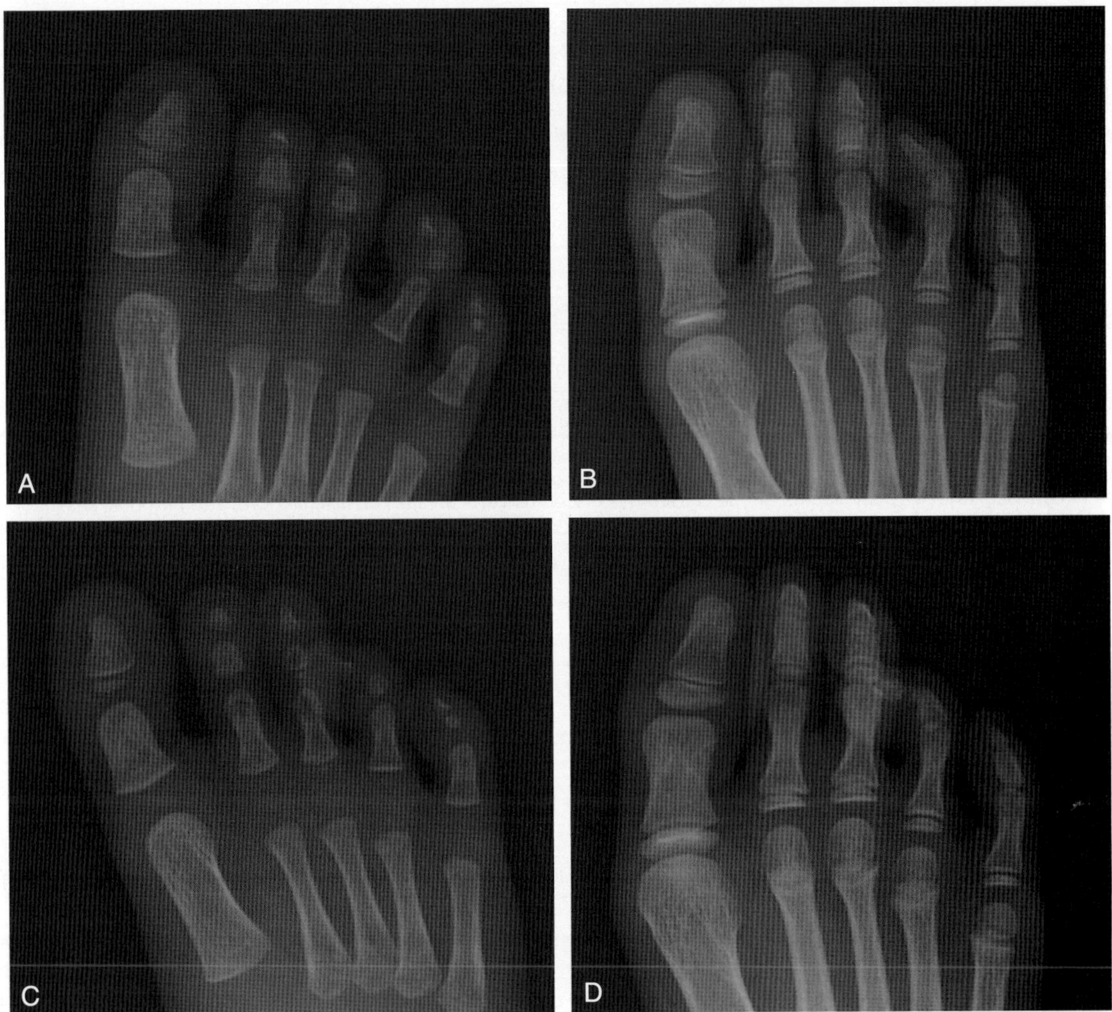

FIGURE 6.3 Curly deformations of the right fourth toe by X-ray. A, Type 0, no overlapping. B, Type 1, soft tissue of the fourth toe overlapping the third toe. C, Type 2, soft tissue of the fourth toe overlapping the phalanx of the third toe. D, Type 3, distal phalanx of the fourth toe overlapping the phalanx of the third toe. (Satake H, Kura H, Naganuma Y, et al. Assessment of the severity of curly toe. *J Orthop Sci.* 2022;27(6):1278-1282.)

References

1. Smith WG, Seki JT, Smith RW. Prospective study of noninvasive treatment for two common congenital toe abnormalities. *Paediatr Child Health.* 2007;12(9):755–759.
2. Cho JY, Park JH, Kim JH, Lee YH. Congenital curly toe of the fetus. *Ultrasound Obstet Gynecol.* 2004;24(4):417–420.
3. Turner PL. Strapping of curly toes in children. *Aust N Z J Surg.* 1987;57(7):467–470.
4. Brucato MP, Lin DY. Pediatric forefoot deformities. *Clin Podiatr Med Surg.* 2022;39(1):73–87.
5. Satake H, Kura H, Naganuma Y, et al. Assessment of the severity of curly toe. *J Orthop Sci.* 2022;27(6):1278–1282.
6. Tokiko K, Nakatsuka T, Tsuji S, Ishida K, Obana K, Osawa K. Surgical correction for curly toe using open tenotomy of flexor digitorum brevis tendon. *J Plast Reconstr Aesthet Surg.* 2007;60(12):1317–1322.

CHAPTER 7

Flexible Flatfoot

KEY POINTS

- Flexible flatfoot is common in children and influenced by age, weight, and gender.
- This deformity usually becomes evident with weight bearing and is often caused by ligamentous laxity and strongly associated with genetic connective tissue disorders.
- Treatment of flexible flatfeet is controversial as to whether corrective shoes or orthotics provide demonstrable benefit.
- Rigid pediatric pes planovalgus can be caused by congenital vertical talus, tarsal coalitions, and peroneal spastic flatfoot without coalition.

GENESIS

Flexible flatfoot is common in children and influenced by age, weight, and gender.[1] This deformity usually becomes evident with weight bearing and is often caused by ligamentous laxity; hence it is strongly associated with genetic connective tissue disorders such as Marfan syndrome and Ehlers-Danlos syndrome. When flexible flatfeet are part of such a broader pattern of connective tissue dysplasia, there is usually hyperextension of fingers, elbows, and knees with a positive family history because such disorders are often genetic. The prevalence of flexible flatfeet in 3-year-old children is 54%, whereas in 6-year-old children it is 24%[1] and 15% in 10-year-olds.[2] Overall in the 3–6-year age group, the prevalence is 44% (52% in boys and 36% in girls), with pathologic flatfoot present in less than 1%. Overweight boys have a 55.6% prevalence of flatfeet.[1] Children with flexible flatfeet are generally asymptomatic as adults, and the development of the arch occurs with growth and is not related to the use of external supports or shoes.[2,3] There is a higher prevalence of flatfeet in children who wear shoes versus those who wear no shoes at all, and closed-toe shoes inhibit development of the arch more than do slippers and sandals.[4] The support of the longitudinal arch is primarily ligamentous, with muscle supporting and stabilizing the arch during heavy loading.[3]

FEATURES

All children have a minimal arch filled with fatty tissue at birth, but more than 30% of neonates have a calcaneovalgus deformity of both feet that is not painful and usually resolves without treatment.[3] The arch develops slowly by about age 4–5 years, and most children presenting to an orthopedist for evaluation of flatfeet have flexible flatfeet that only became apparent after the child began to walk.[3,4] Ligamentous laxity allows the foot to collapse medially with weight bearing, and the heel rolls into a medially deviated valgus position. The ankle and foot are sufficiently strong, and the child with flexible flatfeet can form a good arch when asked to stand on tiptoe and when the heel goes into mild varus (Fig. 7.1). The ability to stand on the heel implies that the heel cord is not excessively tight. The ability to stand first on the outer border of the foot and then on the inner border of the foot implies normal function of the posterior tibialis, anterior tibialis, and peroneal musculature, with normal subtalar function. Foot muscle strength and passive range of motion of the ankle and subtalar joint are examined in the seated position.[3] Examination of shoe wear can yield important clues. Normally there is heel wear on the lateral aspect, with no heel wear implying tight heel cords. Wear on the medial portion of the heel may be associated with a pronated flexible flatfoot. An abnormal gait may suggest a skeletal dysplasia or neuromuscular disorder. Radiographs

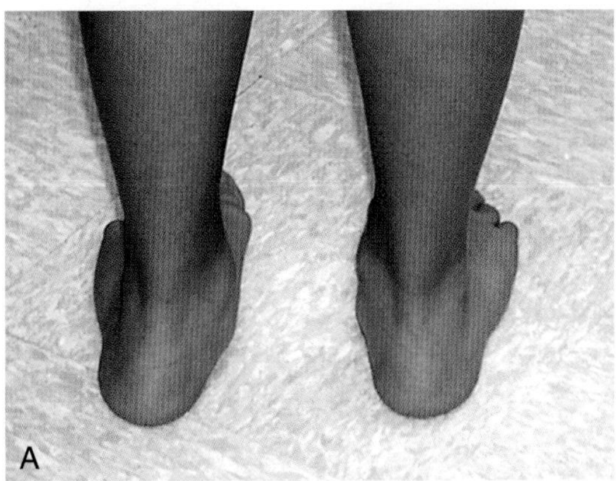

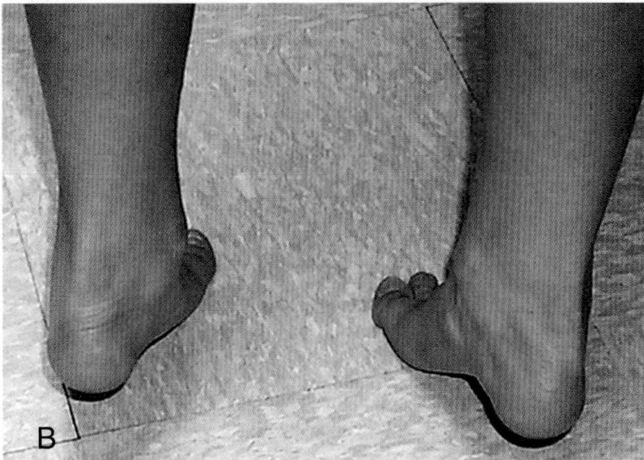

FIGURE 7.1 A, Ligamentous laxity allows the foot to collapse medially with weight bearing; the heel rolls into a medially deviated valgus position and the arch disappears. B, The ankle and foot are sufficiently strong and the child with flexible flatfeet can form a good arch when asked to stand on tiptoe, when the heel goes into mild varus. (Courtesy Robert M. Bernstein, Cedar Sinai Medical Center, Los Angeles.)

are indicated when the flatfoot is symptomatic and painful, particularly if a skeletal dysplasia is suspected. Up until 10 years of age the medial column of the foot is developing, and only 4% of 10-year-old children have a persistent or progressive deformity. Beyond the age of 10 years there is a danger of deformity decompensation as well as an increased rigidity. Only a minority of children develop some pain (<2%). A clear risk factor for persistent pediatric flat foot is obesity (62% of 6-year-old children with flat foot are obese).[5]

MANAGEMENT, PROGNOSIS, AND COUNSEL

Treatment of flexible flatfeet is controversial as to whether corrective shoes or orthotics provide demonstrable benefit. Recent systematic reviews concur that the evidence supporting the use of orthotics in pediatric flexible flatfeet lacks clarity and uniformity in terms of outcomes for pediatric flexible flat feet.[2,5–10] Some physicians recommend the use of running or basketball shoes with good arch support and a shoe design that is straight with adequate room for the toes; special shoes are used only for cases with severe deformity or persistent pain.

It is critical to differentiate flexible from rigid flatfeet and to assess for associated Achilles contracture with a careful history, physical examination, and initial radiographs. Rigid pediatric pes planovalgus refers to a condition of the foot in which the medial longitudinal arch height is abnormally decreased along with a significant loss of midfoot and hindfoot motion. Known causes for this condition are well documented and consist of congenital vertical talus, tarsal coalitions, and peroneal spastic flatfoot without coalition. Rigid flatfeet in infants may be attributable to a congenital vertical talus, whereas in older children and adolescents they may be due to an underlying tarsal coalition. Children with asymptomatic rigid flatfeet may not require treatment, whereas those with pain or functional deficits may benefit from orthotics, osteotomies, or fusions. Initial treatment options include activity modification, proper shoes and orthotics, exercises, and medication. Although there are limited data, nonsurgical management of symptomatic flatfeet, both flexible and rigid, should be exhausted before considering surgical intervention. If patients fail conservative treatment, surgical management with joint-preserving, deformity-corrective techniques can be used for pediatric flexible flatfeet in conjunction with deformity-specific soft tissue procedures.

Arthroereisis is a technique for treating flexible flatfoot by means of inserting a prosthesis into the sinus tarsi. Comorbidities such as obesity and ligamentous laxity should be identified and managed, if applicable. When all nonsurgical treatment options fail, surgery can be considered. Multiple studies have recently reported on the results of surgical procedures for symptomatic flat feet. A systematic review of 10 studies of surgical outcomes in 846 pediatric patients aged 6–14 years with 1536 symptomatic flexible flatfeet revealed a manageable complication profile with satisfactory long-term clinical and radiological

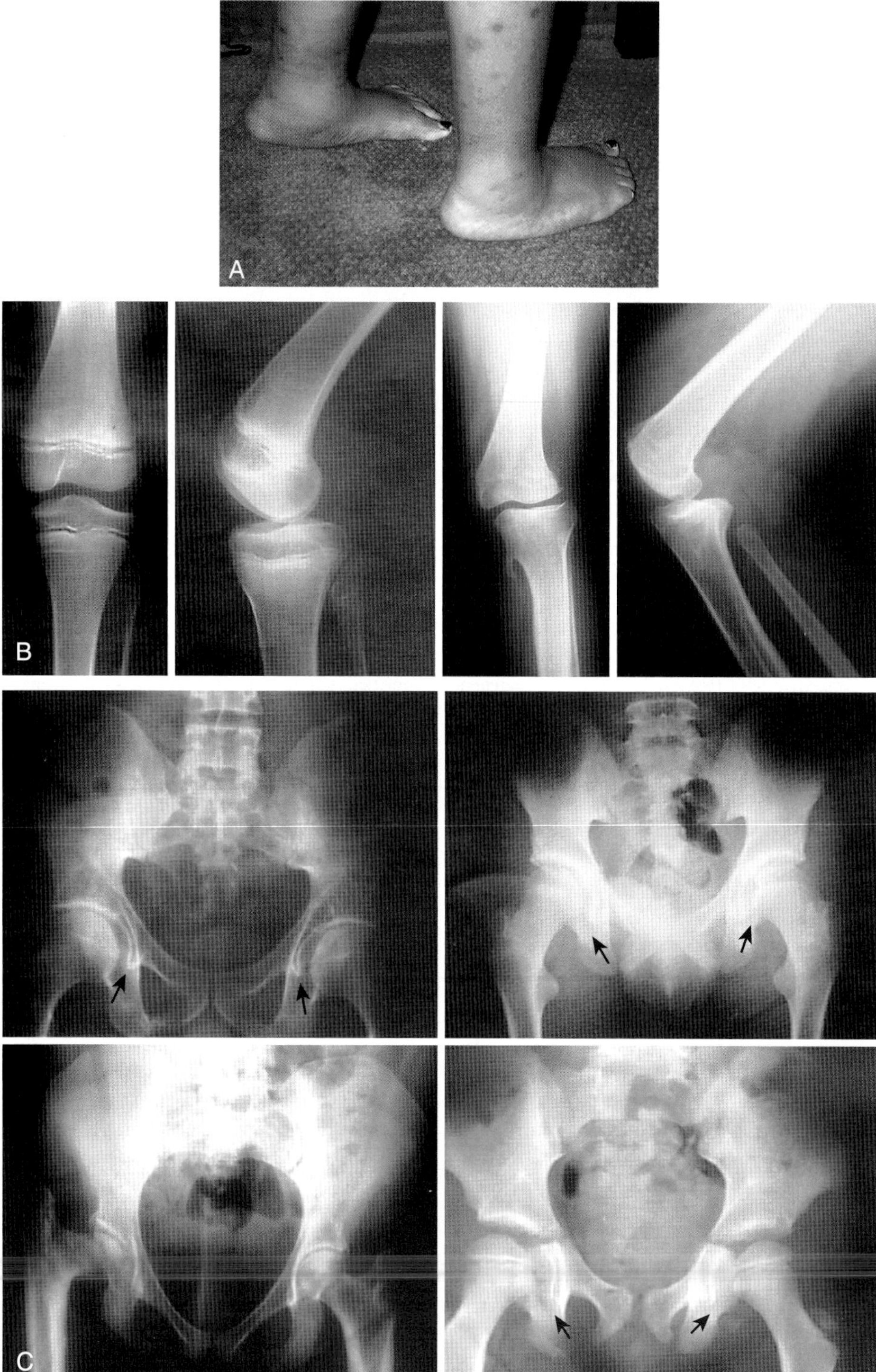

FIGURE 7.2 A, Typical rigid, painful flatfeet in a patient with small patella syndrome and tarsal coalition. B, In small patella syndrome, there is absence or hypoplasia of the patella in the anteroposterior and lateral views of both knees. C, Diagnostic pelvic features consisting of hypoplasia of the descending pubic rami and of the ischiopubic synchondrosis, congenital coxa vara, and so-called ax-cut notching *(arrows)*.

results.[11] Subtalar arthroereisis combined with soft tissue procedures can effectively correct flexible flatfoot in children and it is an important method for severe forefoot abduction reconstruction.[12–15]

Pediatric flatfeet range from the painless flexible normal variant of growth to stiff or painful manifestations of tarsal coalition, collagen abnormalities, neurologic disease, or other underlying condition. Most children with flexible flatfeet do not have symptoms and do not require treatment. In symptomatic children, orthotics, osteotomies, or fusions may be considered.

DIFFERENTIAL DIAGNOSIS

Flexible flatfoot can also occur with tight heel cords in various neurologic disorders, such as muscular dystrophy or mild cerebral palsy. It is unusual for a flatfoot to be stiff and painful, and in such cases trauma, occult infection, a foreign body, bone tumors, osteochondrosis of the tarsal navicular bone, or tarsal coalition should be considered. In these circumstances, radiographic studies using standard and oblique views of the foot and ankle with orthopedic evaluation are merited.

Tarsal coalition can be part of a broader pattern of skeletal dysplasia, such as small patella syndrome (Fig. 7.2), an autosomal dominant condition caused by mutations in *TBX4*.[16] This condition combines absence or hypoplasia of the patella with diagnostic pelvic features (hypoplasia of the descending pubic rami and hypoplasia of the ischiopubic synchondrosis, with congenital coxa vara). Patients with tarsal coalition manifest a familial tendency and may not present until they approach skeletal maturity, when they experience pain in the midtarsal region with activity. Talocalcaneal coalitions are rarely diagnosed on plain radiographs but are easily demonstrated using computed tomography. As opposed to flexible flatfeet, treatment usually requires surgical resection of a middle-facet coalition.[3] Foot morphology in most young children with Charcot-Marie-Tooth disease (an inherited progressive neurologic disorder) is initially pes planovalgus, with the minority being pes cavovarus.[17] As the child grows, the foot becomes cavus or cavovarus, with very few remaining planovalgus or planus. Unexplained regional pain may suggest this diagnosis in children, whereas adolescents and adults present with cavovarus feet, thin calves, or a high-stepping gait. Such patients should be referred to a pediatric neurologist for definitive diagnosis and management.

References

1. Pfeiffer M, Kotz R, Ledl T, et al. Prevalence of flat foot in preschool-aged children. *Pediatrics*. 2006;118:634–639.
2. Evans AM, Rome K. A Cochrane review of the evidence for non-surgical interventions for flexible pediatric flat feet. *Eur J Phys Rehabil Med*. 2011;47:69–89.
3. Sullivan JA. Pediatric flatfoot: evaluation and management. *J Am Acad Orthop Surg*. 1999;7:44–53.
4. Rao UB, Joseph B. The influence of footwear on the prevalence of flat foot: a survey of 2300 children. *J Bone Joint Surg Br*. 1992;74:525–527.
5. Hell AK, Döderlein L, Eberhardt O, et al. S2-leitlinie: der kindliche knick-senk-Fuß [S2-guideline: pediatric flat foot]. *Z Orthop Unfall*. 2018;156(3):306–315.
6. MacKenzie AJ, Rome K, Evans AM. The efficacy of non-surgical interventions for pediatric flexible flat foot: a critical review. *J Pediatr Orthop*. 2012;32:830–834.
7. Dare DM, Dodwell ER. Pediatric flatfoot: cause, epidemiology, assessment, and treatment. *Curr Opin Pediatr*. 2014;26:93–100.
8. Turner C, Gardiner MD, Midgley A, Stefanis A. A guide to the management of paediatric pes planus. *Aust J Gen Pract*. 2020;49(5):245–249.
9. Dars S, Uden H, Banwell HA, Kumar S. The effectiveness of non-surgical intervention (Foot Orthoses) for paediatric flexible pes planus: a systematic review: Update. *PLoS One*. 2018;13(2):e0193060.
10. Evans AM, Rome K, Carroll M, Hawke F. Foot orthoses for treating paediatric flat feet. *Cochrane Database Syst Rev*. 2022;1(1):CD006311.
11. Choi JY, Hong WH, Suh JS, Han JH, Lee DJ, Lee YJ. The long-term structural effect of orthoses for pediatric flexible flat foot: a systematic review. *Foot Ankle Surg*. 2020;26(2):181–188.
12. Smolle MA, Svehlik M, Regvar K, Leithner A, Kraus T. Long-term clinical and radiological outcomes following surgical treatment for symptomatic pediatric flexible flat feet: a systematic review. *Acta Orthop*. 2022;93:367–374.
13. Li B, He W, Yu G, et al. Treatment for flexible flatfoot in children with subtalar arthroereisis and soft tissue procedures. *Front Pediatr*. 2021;9:656178.
14. Elmarghany M, Abd El-Ghaffar TM, Elgeushy A, Elzahed E, Hasanin Y, Knörr J. Is subtalar extra articular screw arthroereisis (SESA) reducing pain and restoring medial longitudinal arch in children with flexible flat foot? *J Orthop*. 2020;20:147–153.
15. García Bistolfi M, Avanzi R, Buljubasich M, Bosio S, Puigdevall M. Subtalar arthroereisis in pediatric flexible flat foot: functional and radiographic results with 5 years of average follow-up. *Foot (Edinb)*. 2022;52:101920.
16. Bongers EM, Duijf PH, van Beersum SE, et al. Mutations in the human *TBX4* gene cause small patella syndrome. *Am J Hum Genet*. 2004;74:1239–1248.
17. Hoellwarth JS, Mahan ST, Spencer SA. Painful pes planovalgus: an uncommon pediatric orthopedic presentation of Charcot-Marie-Tooth disease. *J Pediatr Orthop B*. 2012;21:428–433.

Section III
Other Lower Extremity Deformations

CHAPTER 8

Tibial Torsion

KEY POINTS

- Rotational abnormalities of the lower extremities (in-toeing and out-toeing) are common in young children, and abnormal rotation is termed *torsion*.
- In-toeing is caused by one of three types of deformities: metatarsus adductus (during the first year), internal tibial torsion (in toddlers), and increased femoral anteversion (in early childhood).
- Tibial torsion is especially likely with fetal constraint of the legs in a folded and flexed position, and it is frequently associated with positional equinovarus deformity and metatarsus adductus, which each derives from similar types of mechanical constraints.
- Because spontaneous resolution occurs in 95% of cases by 7 to 8 years of age, management is seldom required.
- Surgery is usually only contemplated in skeletally mature individuals with insufficient spontaneous correction. In such cases, an underlying disorder such as cerebral palsy, hip dysplasia, or skeletal dysplasia should be evaluated.
- Angular deformities, such as genu varum (bowlegs) and genu valgum (knock-knees), need to be distinguished from rotational abnormalities.

GENESIS

Rotation refers to the twist of the tibia along its long axis. Normal rotation in direction and magnitude is termed *version*, and normal values are determined according to age. Abnormal rotation is termed *torsion*, and the degree of rotation is determined by the angle between the transmalleolar axis at the ankle and the bicondylar axis of the proximal tibia at the knee. Rotational abnormalities of the lower extremities (in-toeing and out-toeing) are common in young children. These abnormalities vary by site with advancing age and usually respond to conservative treatment. In-toeing is caused by one of three types of deformities: metatarsus adductus (during the first year), internal tibial torsion (in toddlers), and increased femoral anteversion (in early childhood). Internal tibial torsion may occur in combination with metatarsus adductus, and it can be accentuated by postures such as prone sleeping with the toes turned in (see Fig. 4.2 C) or sitting in a W position.

Torsion of the tibia is sufficiently common in the normal newborn to be considered a normal variant; however, more severe variations are seen in about 3% of infants. Tibial torsion is especially likely with fetal constraint of the legs in a folded and flexed position, and it is frequently associated with positional equinovarus deformity and metatarsus adductus, each of which derives from similar types of mechanical constraints.[1-4] During the seventh week of gestation, the lower limb buds rotate internally, bringing the great toe to the midline from its initial lateral position.[5] During fetal life, the legs are molded so that the femurs rotate externally and the tibiae rotate internally. Internal tibial torsion averaging 4 degrees is normal at birth, after which the tibiae rotate externally to an average of 23 degrees in adulthood (as measured by the transmalleolar axis). In support of the concept that tibial torsion occurs late in gestation because of fetal constraint, this deformation is not encountered in premature infants born before 30 weeks of gestation.[6]

FEATURES

In fetal life the hips are positioned in flexion and lateral rotation, whereas the feet are in medial rotation, resulting in lateral hip rotation that is greater than medial hip rotation and causing internal tibial torsion, most of which corrects by the second year of life.[1-6] The tibia is medially rotated on its long axis at birth, with the most acute incurving occurring distally (Fig. 8.1).

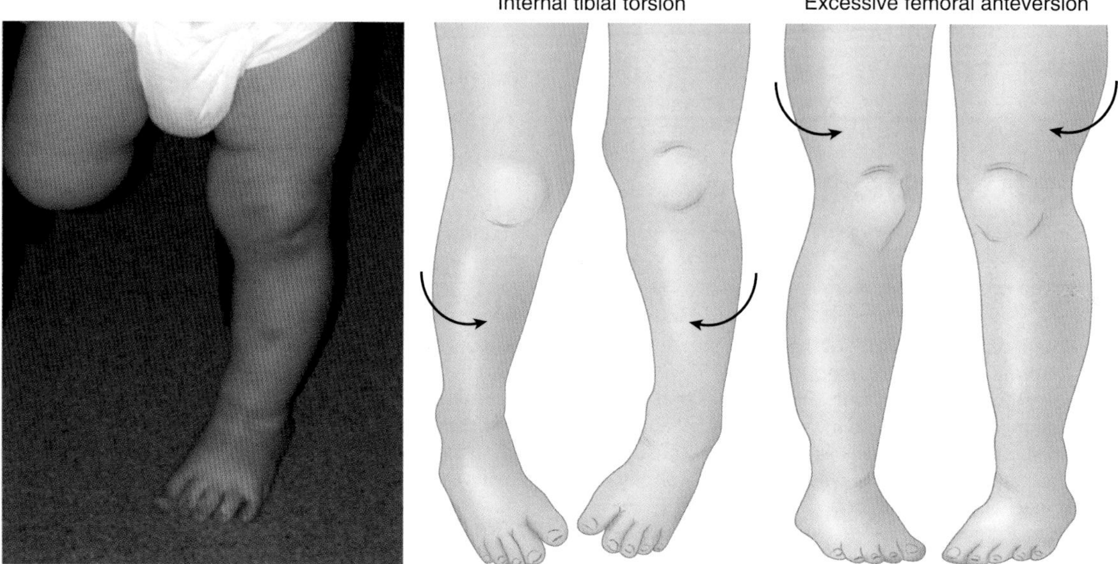

FIGURE 8.1 Internal tibial torsion usually presents as in-toeing during the second year of life, and with persistent tibial torsion, the patellae point forward with walking or standing while the feet point inward. The diagrams compare the patellae and feet in tibial torsion and femoral anteversion. With excessive femoral anteversion, both the patellae and the feet point inward with walking. (Courtesy of Robert M. Bernstein, Cedar Sinai Medical Center, Los Angeles.)

Internal tibial torsion usually presents as in-toeing during the second year of life, and thus it may not be noticed until the child begins to walk. Tibial torsion tends to resolve spontaneously unless accentuated by sleeping in a prone, in-toed position; hence this deformation and metatarsus adductus have decreased in frequency with the adoption of a supine sleeping position. In-toeing in an infant is usually caused by metatarsus adductus, and after 3 years of age, in-toeing is usually caused by excessive femoral anteversion, but a combination of causes is often present.

With persistent tibial torsion, the patellae point forward with walking or standing while the feet point inward (see Fig. 8.1). With excessive femoral anteversion, both the patellae and the feet point inward with walking. Tibial torsion tends to angle the plantar surfaces of the feet toward each other; hence there may also be mild to moderate metatarsus adductus in association with tibial torsion.[1-3] Tibial torsion is usually bilateral, but the degree of tibial torsion varies widely (mean tibial torsion 27.5 ± 8.3 degrees; range −3 to 47.5 degrees), and individual side-to-side differences are common (mean difference, 5 to 6 degrees with the right tibia more externally rotated than the left).[7,8]

Rotational problems can be evaluated by determining the rotational profile. In-toeing is quantified by estimating and following the foot-progression angle, which is the angular difference between the long axis of the foot and the line of progression with ambulation (Fig. 8.2). In-toeing is denoted by a minus (−) sign and out-toeing by a plus (+) sign. The normal foot-progression angle is +10 degrees, with a range of −3 to +20 degrees. Hip rotation in femoral anteversion is measured by having the child lie prone on the examination table with the knees flexed 90 degrees and allowing the legs to fall inward and outward by gravity alone. The amount of internal and external rotation of the hip should be similar, inscribing a total arc of about 90 degrees; medial rotation in excess of 70 degrees suggests excessive femoral anteversion. Tibial rotation is determined by measuring the thigh-foot angle, which is the angular difference between the axis of the foot and the axis of the thigh when the patient is in the prone position with the knees flexed 90 degrees and the foot in neutral position (see Fig. 8.2). A negative value means the tibia is rotated internally (internal tibial torsion), and a positive value means the tibia is rotated externally (external tibial torsion). An infant normally has a negative thigh-foot angle that becomes progressively positive with age, resulting in a mean thigh-foot angle during childhood of +10 to +15 degrees (normal range, −5 to +30 degrees). Quantification of rotational abnormalities can be done by the rotational profile on physical examination,

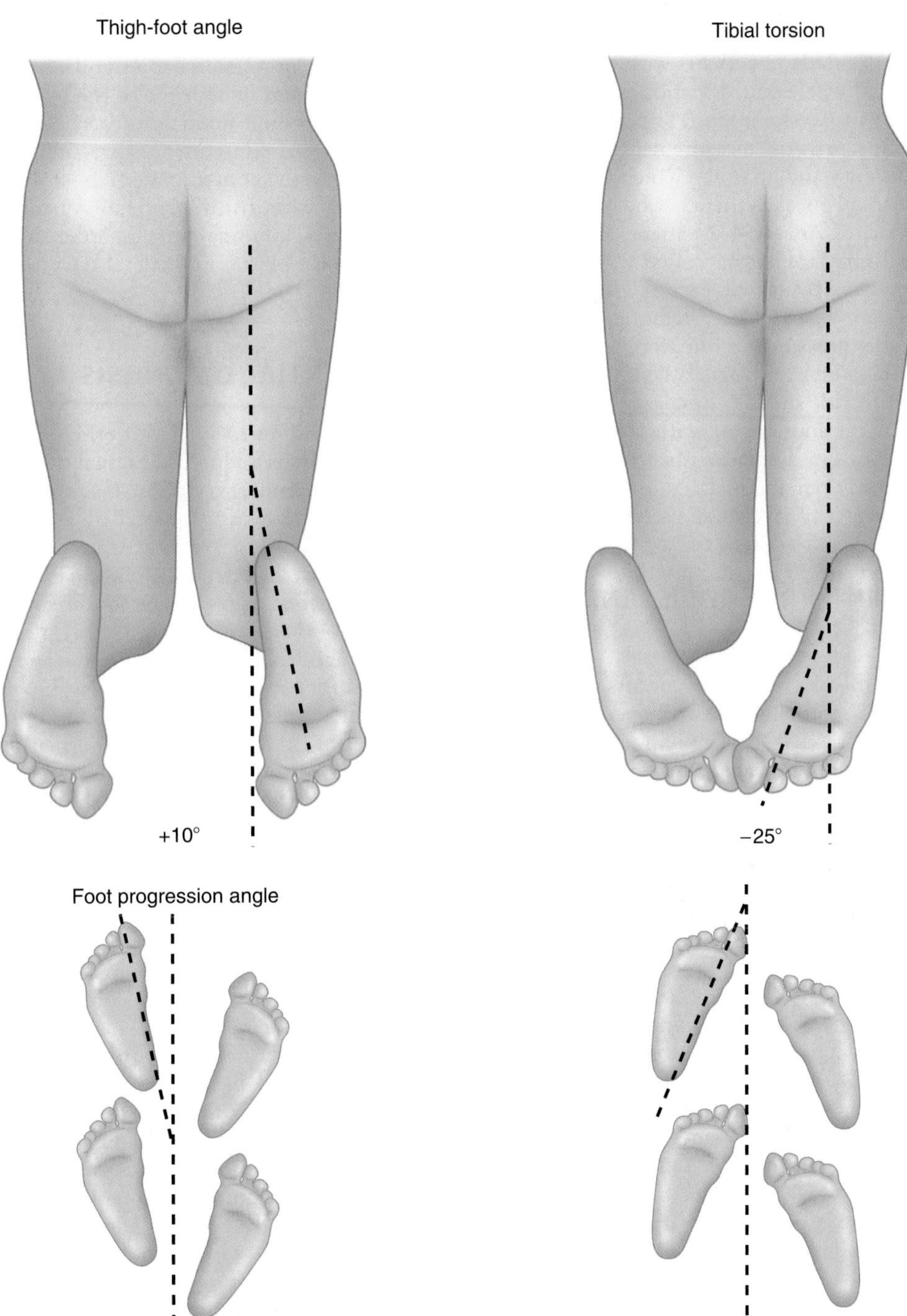

FIGURE 8.2 Diagrams demonstrating normal and abnormal thigh-foot angles and foot-progression angles. The normal foot-progression angle is +10 degrees, with a range from −3 to +20 degrees. Tibial rotation is determined by measuring the thigh-foot angle, which is the angular difference between the axis of the foot and the axis of the thigh when the patient is in prone position with the knees flexed 90 degrees and the foot in neutral position. A negative (−) value means the tibia is rotated internally (internal tibial torsion), and a positive (+) value means the tibia is rotated externally (external tibial torsion). An infant normally has a negative thigh-foot angle that becomes progressively positive with age, resulting in a mean thigh-foot angle during childhood of +10 to +15 degrees (normal range, −5 to +30 degrees).

a computed tomography tortional study and/or gait analysis,[9-11] particularly in patients with cerebral palsy (spastic diplegia) where gait deviation and associated tortional problems are common.[12] The use of software to automatically perform measurements on imaging ensures consistency and accuracy, which may not possible with manual measurements, which depend on assessor experience. Among 472 patients with cerebral palsy, external tibial torsion increased with age, while femoral anteversion decreased. Factors affecting external tibial torsion were increased femoral anteversion, older age, higher gross motor function, and involved/uninvolved limbs of hemiplegia.[12] Pelvic radiographs may be taken to rule out hip dysplasia as a cause of tibial and femoral anteversion, with femoral torsion present in 62% of hip dysplasia, tibial torsion present in 42%, combined torsional malalignment in 21%, and normal femoral and tibial torsion present in 42%.[13,14]

MANAGEMENT, PROGNOSIS, AND COUNSEL

Because spontaneous resolution occurs in 95% of cases by 7 to 8 years of age, management is seldom required. The use of shoe modifications or night splints is not indicated, and parents should be informed that after release from the constraining intrauterine position, progressive straightening of the legs tends to occur.[1-6] However, certain sleeping postures may tend to foster persistence of the tibial torsion, and the same preventive measures for adverse sleeping postures as mentioned for metatarsus adductus may be used. Following the torsional profile over time, with regular examinations and measurements to confirm improvement, can be extremely reassuring to parents. The rotational profile of the lower limb was analyzed in 1319 healthy children.[15] There was no difference between males and females, no significant difference between the right side and the left side, and tibial torsion changed from 34 degrees at 3 years to 36 degrees at 10 years. Tibial torsion persisting after 8 years of age, especially with a family history of rotational anomalies that persist into adulthood, is less likely to resolve spontaneously. The only effective treatment for residual internal tibial torsion is tibial osteotomy, which is usually not performed until after 8 to 10 years of age. Correction of the internal tibial torsion by tibial rotation osteotomy improves, but does not normalize, all gait deviations associated with an in-toeing gait. The decision to perform a derotational osteotomy is usually based on the degree of functional impairment, and neither tibial torsion nor femoral anteversion has a significant influence on the development of arthritis of the hip or knee. Thus parents of asymptomatic children can be reassured that long-term consequences are unlikely.[16] Surgery is usually only contemplated in skeletally mature individuals with insufficient spontaneous correction. In such cases, an underlying disorder such as cerebral palsy, hip dysplasia, or skeletal dysplasia should be evaluated.

DIFFERENTIAL DIAGNOSIS

Three causes of in-toeing affect otherwise normal children: metatarsus adductus, internal tibial torsion, and excessive femoral anteversion resulting from medial rotation of the femur. Internal tibial torsion is at its peak in children 1 to 3 years of age and resolves spontaneously by late adolescence. Rotational anomalies, even if severe, are not painful; therefore any history of pain should prompt a search for another cause. Sometimes a rotational problem is a manifestation of an underlying disorder such as cerebral palsy, hip dysplasia, or a skeletal dysplasia such as pseudoachondroplasia.[17] Any clinical findings such as abnormal muscle tone, gait abnormality, limited hip abduction, leg length discrepancy, or disproportionate short stature should prompt a more intensive evaluation. A child with mild cerebral palsy may walk with mild equinus and in-toeing, whereas hip dysplasia is suggested by a leg length discrepancy and a Trendelenburg gait (i.e., the pelvis tilts toward the normal hip when the affected side bears weight because of weak hip abductors).

Out-toeing is much less common than in-toeing. Femoral retroversion can be caused by external rotation contracture of the hip. It is common in early infancy and becomes apparent before walking when the infant stands with feet turned out nearly 90 degrees in a "Charlie Chaplin" stance. It occurs more commonly in obese children, and when unilateral it is more commonly right-sided. Another cause of out-toeing in the obese child is a slipped capital femoral epiphysis, which requires hip radiographs if suspected. If femoral retroversion persists beyond 2 to 3 years of age, referral to an orthopedist is indicated. External tibial torsion is seen between 4 and 7 years of age. External tibial torsion may be unilateral (more commonly right-sided), causing patellofemoral instability and pain. Tibial torsion may require surgical osteotomy if it persists beyond 10 years of age. Flexible flatfeet may also result in out-toeing.

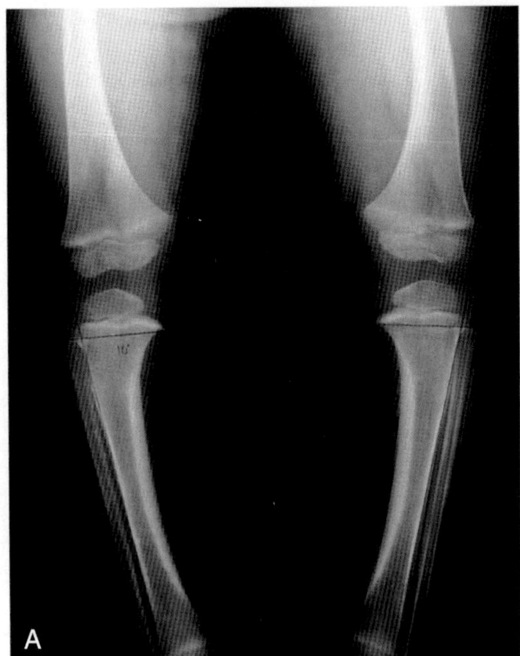

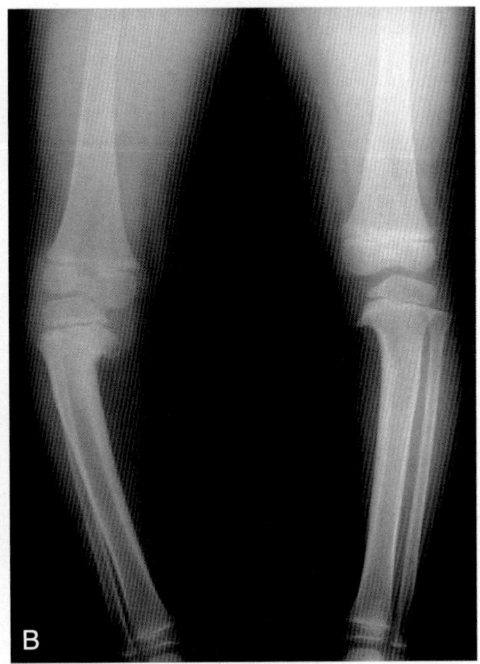

FIGURE 8.3 A, Physiologic bowing in an otherwise normal child. **B,** Tibia vara (Blount disease) results from disordered growth of the proximal medial metaphyses, and a medial metaphyseal lesion is evident on these radiographs in the proximal tibias. Blount disease may be associated with obesity and it must be distinguished from physiologic bowing (**A**). (Courtesy Saul Bernstein, Cedar Sinai Medical Center, Los Angeles.)

The lower legs may be more bowed than usual because of a variety of generalized neuromuscular or skeletal disorders, many which require surgical management. Physiologic bowing confined to the tibia occurs during the first year and usually resolves (Fig. 8.3A). When it occurs during the second year and involves both the tibia and the distal femur, it is often associated with medial tibial torsion. Physiologic bowing usually resolves spontaneously, and bracing does not affect the natural history.

Tibial vara, or Blount disease, results from abnormal proximal tibial metaphyseal growth, often in association with medial tibial torsion (Fig. 8.3B). It is often associated with obesity and is caused by osteochondrosis resulting from mechanical stress, with a medial metaphyseal lesion evident on radiographs in the proximal tibia. In its early stages this disorder is treated with corrective osteotomy.

Angular deformities, such as genu varum (bowlegs) and genu valgum (knock-knees), need to be distinguished from rotational abnormalities (Fig. 8.4).[18] Genu varum is seen from birth to 2 years of age, whereas genu valgum peaks between 2 and 4 years of age. Measurements of the intercondylar and intermalleolar distance taken over time will confirm gradual spontaneous resolution in some cases.[18] Failure to resolve, particularly when there is associated short stature, may suggest the presence of a skeletal dysplasia or metabolic bone disease such as metaphyseal chondrodysplasia, hypophosphatemic rickets, multiple epiphyseal dysplasia, or pseudoachondroplasia.[18]

Limited hip abduction or leg length discrepancy should prompt a search for developmental dysplasia of the hip. An abnormal neurologic examination result should prompt consideration of mild cerebral palsy, spinal dysraphism, hydrocephalus, or hereditary motor-sensory neuropathies. Anterior bowing with a cystic, narrowed, or sclerotic medullary canal may progress to pseudarthrosis in neurofibromatosis or fibrous dysplasia; therefore it is very important to search for café-au-lait spots that might suggest the presence of such an underlying generalized disorder (Fig. 8.5). Various problems in bone formation may also result in malleable or fragile bones, such as those that occur with hypophosphatasia or osteogenesis imperfecta; these bones can lead to bowing. Fibular hemimelia is associated with anterior bowing, dimpling of the skin at the apex of the curve,

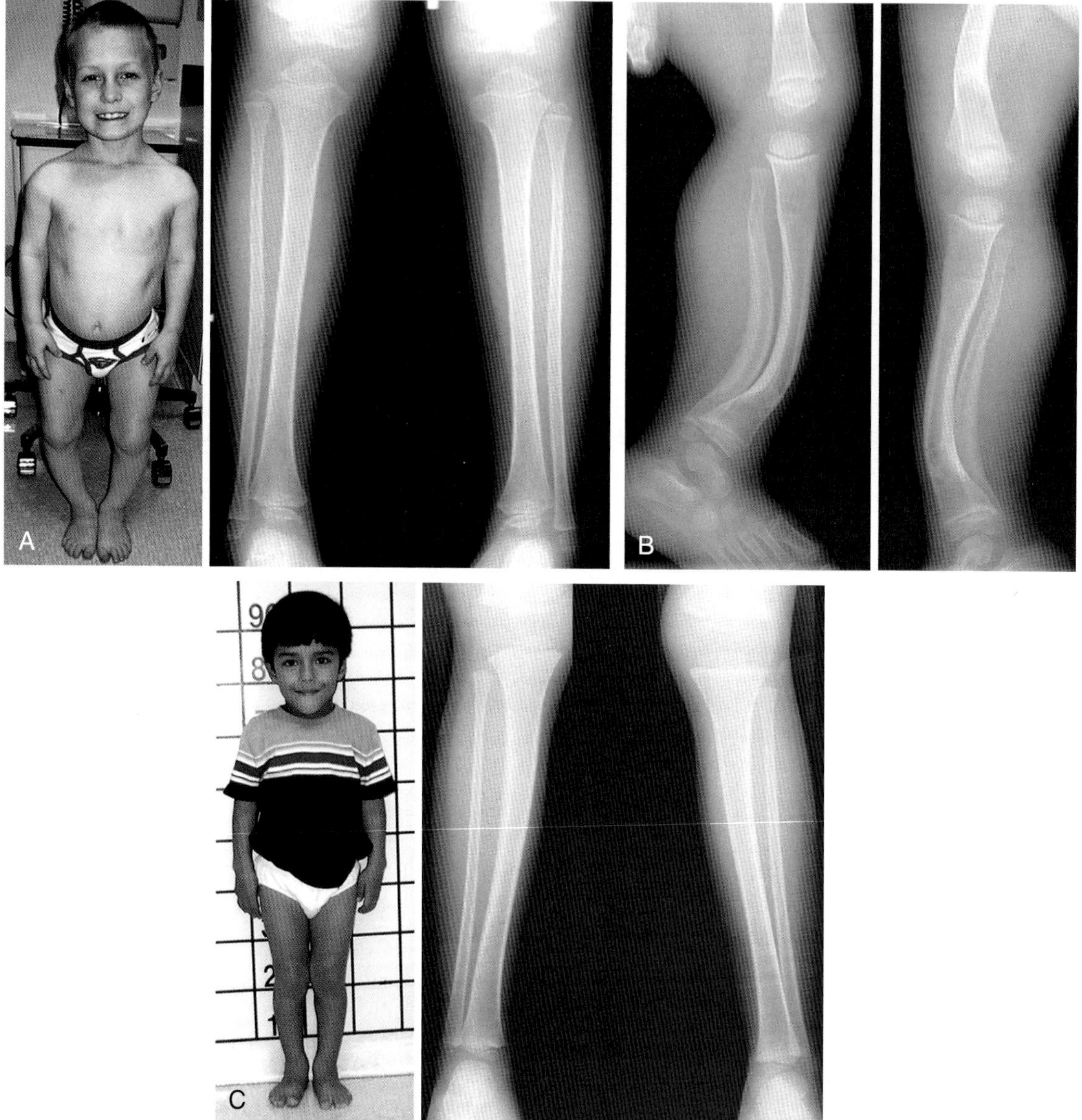

FIGURE 8.4 A, Persistent genu varum (bowlegs) can result from skeletal dysplasias, such as pseudoachondroplasia, presumably as a result of excessive ligamentous laxity. Pseudoachondroplasia can be caused by mutations in cartilage oligomeric matrix protein (COMP). **B,** Persistent genu varum can also result from hypophosphatemic rickets. **C,** Pseudoachondroplasia can also result in genu valgum (knock-knees) caused by ligamentous laxity.

ipsilateral shortening of the long bones (especially the fibula), and an equinovalgus foot position. The tibial cortex is thickened on the concave side of the deformity, and the medullary canal may be partly obliterated. In certain skeletal dysplasias, there is characteristic bowing of the long bones (e.g., camptomelic dysplasia, achondroplasia, or thanatophoric dysplasia), and a complete skeletal survey can help distinguish among these skeletal dysplasias. Osteotomies to correct bowing in skeletal dysplasias (e.g., achondroplasia) are usually not done until 8 to 10 years of age.

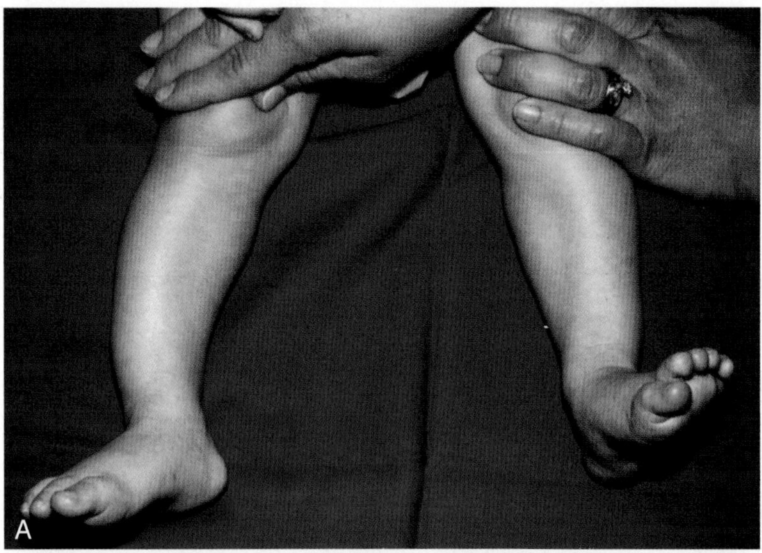

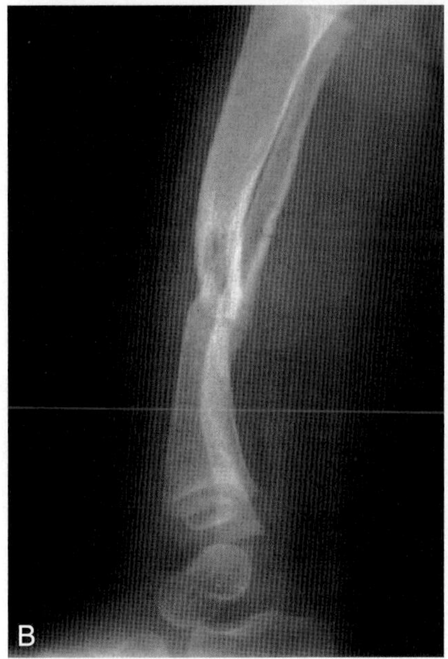

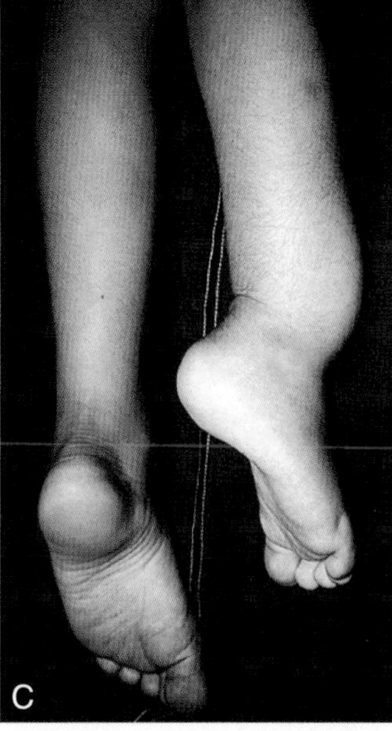

FIGURE 8.5 Anterolateral bowing is a dangerous form of bowing that is usually associated with pseudarthrosis of the tibia. **A,** Pseudarthrosis is often associated with type 1 neurofibromatosis. Radiographs may show a radiolucent lesion at the apex of the bow, but usually only narrowing and sclerosis are seen. Fracture can lead to pseudarthrosis, resulting in nonunion of the fracture and requiring eventual amputation. Thus bracing is often attempted to prevent such a fracture. When fracture occurs (**B** and **C**), the ends of the bone are tapered and sclerotic, with the presence of disorganized bone impairing bone strength. (Courtesy Saul Bernstein, Cedar Sinai Medical Center, Los Angeles.)

References

1. Staheli LT, Corbett M, Wyss C, et al. Lower extremity rotational problems in children. *J Bone Joint Surg Am.* 1985;67:39–47.
2. Staheli LT. Rotational problems in children. *J Bone Joint Surg Am.* 1993;75:939–949.
3. Heirich SD, Sharps CH. Lower extremity torsional deformities in children: a prospective comparison of two treatment modalities. *Orthopedics.* 1991;14: 655–659.
4. Bruce Jr. RW. Torsional and angular deformities. *Pediatr Clin North Am.* 1996;43:867–881.
5. Guidera KJ, Ganey TM, Keneally CR, et al. The embryology of lower-extremity torsion. *Clin Orthoped Relat Res.* 1994;302:17–21.
6. Li YH, Leong JCY. Intoeing gait in children. *Hong Kong Med J.* 1999;5:360–366.
7. Gallo MC, Tucker DW, Reddy A, Pannell WC, Heckmann N, Marecek GS. Large individual bilateral differences in tibial torsion impact accurate contralateral templating

and the evaluation of rotational malalignment. *J Orthop Trauma*. 2021;35(8):e277–e282.

8. Volkmar AJ, Stinner DJ, Pennings J, Mitchell PM. Prevalence of individual differences in tibial torsion: a CT-based study. *J Am Acad Orthop Surg*. 2022;30(2):e199–e203.
9. Borish CN, Mueske NM, Wren TAL. A comparison of three methods of measuring tibial torsion in children with myelomeningocele and normally developing children. *Clin Anat*. 2017;30(8):1043–1048.
10. Stephen JM, Teitge RA, Williams A, Calder JDF, El Daou H. A validated, automated, 3-dimensional method to reliably measure tibial torsion. *Am J Sports Med*. 2021;49(3):747–756.
11. Waelti S, Fischer T, Griessinger J, et al. Ultra-low-dose computed tomography for torsion measurements of the lower extremities in children and adolescents. *Insights Imaging*. 2022;13(1):118.
12. Min JJ, Kwon SS, Kim KT, et al. Evaluation of factors affecting external tibial torsion in patients with cerebral palsy. *BMC Musculoskelet Disord*. 2021;22(1):684.
13. Lerch TD, Liechti EF, Todorski IAS, et al. Prevalence of combined abnormalities of tibial and femoral torsion in patients with symptomatic hip dysplasia and femoroacetabular impingement. *Bone Joint J*. 2020;102-B(12):1636–1645.
14. Cho KJ, Park KS, Shin YR, Yang HY, Yoon TR. Relationship between femoral anteversion and tibial torsion: CT evaluation of 38 unilateral developmental dysplasia of the hip patients. *Hip Int*. 2018;28(5):548–553.
15. Jacquemier M, Glard Y, Pomero V, et al. Rotational profile of the lower limb in 1319 healthy children. *Gait Posture*. 2008;28:187–193.
16. Weinberg DS, Park PJ, Morris WZ, Liu RW. Femoral version and tibial torsion are not associated with hip or knee arthritis in a large osteological collection. *J Pediatr Orthop*. 2017;37(2):e120–e128.
17. Gaebe G, Kruse R, Rogers K, Mackenzie WG, Holmes Jr. L. dynamic lower extremity deformity in children with pseudoachondroplasia. *J Pediatr Orthop*. 2018;38(3):157–162.
18. Greene WB. Genu varum and genu valgum in children: differential diagnosis and guidelines for evaluation. *Compr Ther*. 1996;22:22–29.

CHAPTER 9

Femoral Anteversion

KEY POINTS

- Excessive femoral anteversion results from medial rotation of the femur after birth.
- Surgery consisting of femoral derotation osteotomy is usually only contemplated in children older than 8 years with insufficient spontaneous correction, particularly children with diplegic cerebral palsy.
- Excessive femoral anteversion usually presents as a cause of in-toeing at 3 to 4 years of age, increases in magnitude through 5 to 6 years of age, and then gradually decreases thereafter.
- Management is seldom required, and spontaneous resolution occurs by late childhood in more than 80% of cases.
- Children with cerebral palsy, limbs with anteversion, and significant internal hip rotation during gait analysis may benefit from surgery.

GENESIS

Femoral rotation describes the normal twist present in the femur, and excessive femoral anteversion results from medial rotation of the femur after birth. Normal rotation in direction and magnitude is termed *version*, with normal values determined according to age.[1-6] Abnormal rotation is termed *torsion*, and the rotation of a given bone is determined by the angle between the axis of the head and neck of the femur and the axis of the distal condyles at the most posterior points. If the angle between the proximal and distal axes is positive (+), the femur is considered "anteverted," and if it is negative (−), the femur is "retroverted." Excessive femoral anteversion is the most common cause of in-toeing that develops after age 3 years, and it usually resolves spontaneously by late adolescence.[1-6] Femoral anteversion can be familial, is more common in females, and is usually symmetric. Use of special shoes or bracing does not hasten resolution, but continuation of adverse sleeping or sitting positions may slow or prevent progress. Surgery consisting of femoral derotation osteotomy is usually only contemplated in children older than 8 years with insufficient spontaneous correction, particularly diplegic children with cerebral palsy.[7-9] The rotational profile of the lower limb was analyzed in 1319 healthy children, and femoral anteversion was higher in females and markedly correlated with age in both genders (1% in 6-year-old females and 8.5% in 9-year-old females).[10] Among 950 children studied for spontaneous regression of femoral neck anteversion, these children were divided into three groups: (1) children with normal gait, (2) children with in-toeing gait, and (3) children with an out-toeing gait. On the third examination at 14 years of age, children with an in-toeing gait decreased from 12.8% to 1%, while the number of children with an out-toeing gait did not change significantly during the examination period.[11]

Excessive in-toeing during the second year is usually caused by tibial torsion, and severe in-toeing may be the result of a combination of causes. Out-toeing is much less common than in-toeing. Femoral retroversion can be caused by external rotation contracture of the hip. It becomes apparent before walking when the infant stands with feet turned out nearly 90 degrees in a "Charlie Chaplin" stance. It occurs more commonly in obese children, and when unilateral, it is more commonly right-sided. Another cause of out-toeing in the obese child is a slipped capital femoral epiphysis, which requires hip radiographs if suspected.[7] If femoral retroversion persists beyond 2–3 years of age, referral to an orthopedist is indicated.

FEATURES

Normal femoral anteversion decreases from about 30 to 40 degrees at birth to 10 to 15 degrees by early adolescence, with most of this improvement occurring before 8 years of age.[1-11] Internal tibial torsion is normal at birth, after which the tibiae rotate externally to about 15 degrees in adolescence. Excessive femoral anteversion usually presents as a cause of in-toeing at 3 to 4 years of age, increases in magnitude through 5 to 6 years of age, and then gradually decreases thereafter.[7] With excessive femoral anteversion, both the patellae and the feet point inward with walking, whereas with persistent tibial torsion the patella points forward with walking or standing and the foot points inward. The child with femoral anteversion may trip and fall easily because of crossing over of the feet, and affected children may prefer to sit in the W or reversed tailor position (Fig. 9.1).

Rotational problems should be evaluated by determining the rotational profile. In-toeing is quantified by estimating and following the foot progression angle, which is the angular difference between the long axis of the foot and the line of progression with ambulation. In-toeing is denoted by a minus (−) sign and out-toeing by a plus (+) sign. The normal angle is +10 degrees, with a range of −3 to +20 degrees. Hip rotation is measured by having the child lie prone on the examination table with knees flexed 90 degrees and allowing the legs to fall inward and outward by gravity alone (see Fig. 9.1). The amount of internal and external rotation of the hip should be similar, inscribing a total arc of about 90 degrees. Internal rotation more than 70 degrees suggests excessive femoral anteversion. With mildly excessive femoral anteversion, there are 70 to 80 degrees of internal rotation and 10 to 20 degrees of external rotation. With severe problems, there is no external rotation and internal rotation is greater than 90 degrees. Tibial rotation is determined by measuring the thigh-foot angle, which is the angular difference between the axis of the foot and the axis of the thigh when the patient is in the prone position with the knees flexed 90 degrees and the foot is in neutral position. A negative value means the tibia is rotated internally (internal tibial torsion), and a positive value means the tibia is rotated externally (external tibial torsion). An infant normally has a negative thigh-foot angle that becomes progressively positive with age, resulting in a mean thigh-foot angle during childhood of +10 to +15 degrees (normal range, −5 to +30 degrees). As the child with excessive femoral anteversion ages, compensatory external rotation of the tibia may develop, giving rise to a torsional malalignment syndrome that leads to patellofemoral joint instability and anterior knee pain. Quantification of rotational abnormalities is usually done by physical examination, and imaging via ultrasound or computed tomography is also used.[5,6]

MANAGEMENT, PROGNOSIS, AND COUNSEL

Management is seldom required, and spontaneous resolution occurs by late childhood in more than 80% of cases. After release from the constraining intrauterine position, progressive straightening of the legs tends to occur. The same preventive measures for sleeping posture as were mentioned for metatarsus adductus and tibial torsion may be used. In a patient with a family history of rotational anomalies that persist into adulthood, it is less likely that such rotational anomalies will resolve spontaneously. Treatment for femoral anteversion is controversial, with no effective nonsurgical treatment identified and some risks for complications associated with derotational osteotomies. Children with cerebral palsy have an increased incidence of excessive femoral anteversion, which seldom improves with time. In children with hemiplegia, there is increased femoral anteversion on the hemiplegic side. Physical therapy can be helpful in treating excessive femoral anteversion in children with cerebral palsy, but frequently surgery is necessary.[7-9] An analysis of results from femoral derotational osteotomy in 1088 limbs of children with cerebral palsy revealed that limbs with anteversion and significant internal hip rotation during gait analysis benefited from surgery, but limbs with excessive anteversion and only mild internal hip rotation were at risk of developing an excessive external foot progression angle.[7] There is no evidence that in-toeing causes osteoarthritis or back pain, and the use of shoe modifications or night splints is not indicated.

DIFFERENTIAL DIAGNOSIS

Three causes of in-toeing affect otherwise normal children: metatarsus adductus, internal tibial torsion, and excessive femoral anteversion. Rotational anomalies, even if severe, are not painful; therefore any history of pain should prompt a search for another cause. Surgery is usually only contemplated in skeletally mature individuals with insufficient spontaneous correction. Tibial torsion occurs because the tibia is medially rotated on its long axis at birth, but this may not be noticed until the child begins to walk. The lower legs

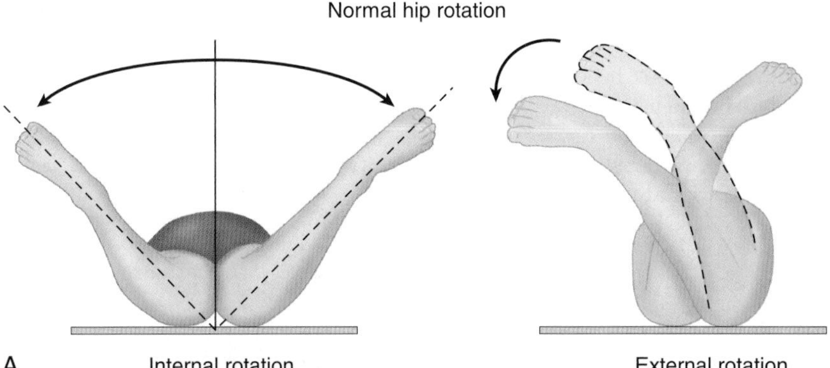

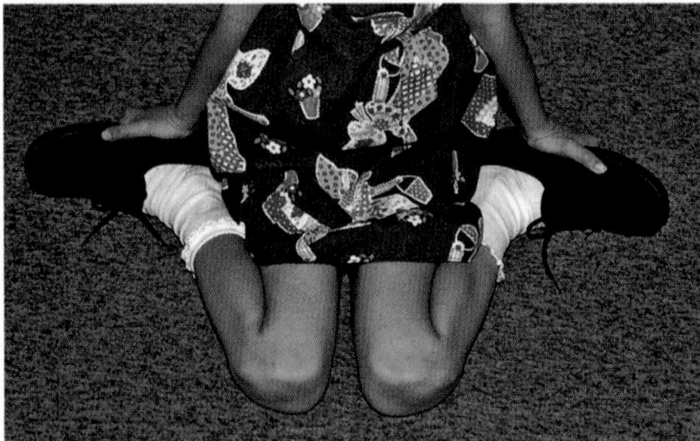

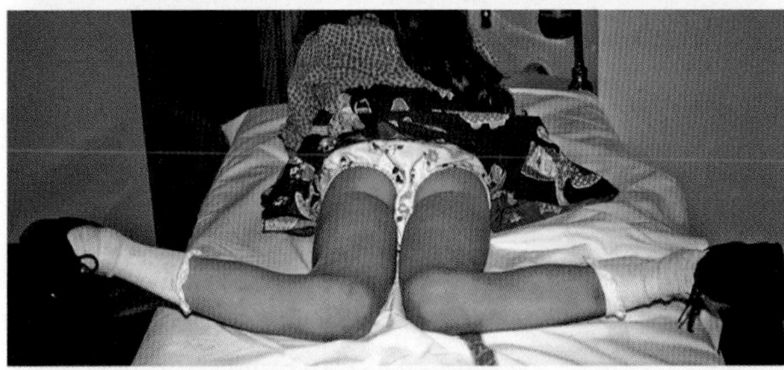

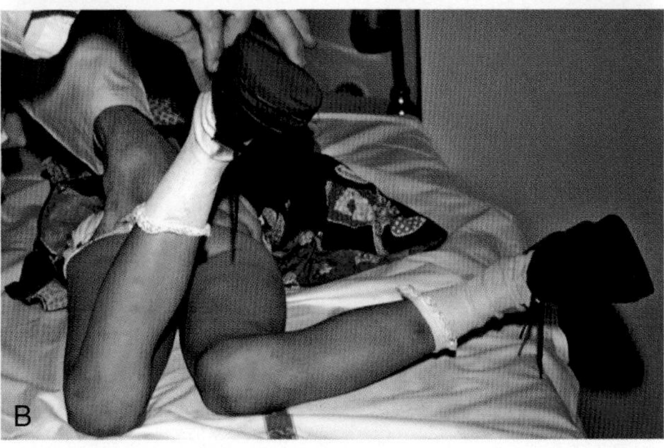

FIGURE 9.1 A, Normal internal and external hip rotation. **B,** Due to excessive femoral anteversion, this moderately affected child prefers to sit in the W or reversed tailor position; femoral torsion can make it difficult or uncomfortable to sit on the floor in a crisscross position. Hip rotation is measured by having the child lie prone on the examination table with the knees flexed 90 degrees and allowing the legs to fall inward and outward by gravity alone. The amount of internal and external rotation of the hip should be similar, inscribing a total arc of about 90 degrees. Internal rotation more than 70 degrees suggests excessive femoral anteversion. With mildly excessive femoral anteversion, there are 70 to 80 degrees of internal rotation and 10 to 20 degrees of external rotation. With severe femoral anteversion, there is no external rotation and internal rotation is greater than 90 degrees. (Courtesy Saul Bernstein, Cedar Sinai Medical Center, Los Angeles.)

may be more bowed than usual because of a variety of generalized neuromuscular or skeletal disorders, many of which require surgical management. Associated short stature may suggest the presence of a skeletal dysplasia or metabolic bone disease. An abnormal neurologic examination should prompt consideration of mild cerebral palsy, spinal dysraphism, hydrocephalus, or hereditary motor-sensory neuropathies.

References

1. Staheli LT, Corbett M, Wyss G, et al. Lower extremity rotational problems in children. *J Bone Joint Surg Am.* 1985;67:39–47.
2. Staheli LT. Rotational problems in children. *J Bone Joint Surg Am.* 1993;75:939–949.
3. Guidera KJ, Ganey TM, Keneally CR, et al. The embryology of lower-extremity torsion. *Clin Orthoped Relat Res.* 1994;302:17–21.
4. Li YH, Leong JCY. Intoeing gait in children. *Hong Kong Med J.* 1999;5:360–366.
5. Scorcelletti M, Reeves ND, Rittweger J, Ireland A. Femoral anteversion: significance and measurement. *J Anat.* 2020;237(5):811–826.
6. Cai Z, Piao C, Zhang T, Li L, Xiang L. Accuracy of CT for measuring femoral neck anteversion in children with developmental dislocation of the hip verified using 3D printing technology. *J Orthop Surg Res.* 2021;16(1):256.
7. Schwartz MH, Rozumalski A, Novacheck TF. Femoral derotational osteotomy: surgical indications and outcomes in children with cerebral palsy. *Gait Posture.* 2014;39:778–783.
8. Desailly E, Badina A, Khouri N. Kinematics after unilateral femoral derotation osteotomy in children with diplegic cerebral palsy. *Orthop Traumatol Surg Res.* 2020;106(7):1325–1331.
9. Vermuyten L, Desloovere K, Molenaers G, Van Campenhout A. Proximal femoral derotation osteotomy in children with CP: long term outcome and the role of age at time of surgery. *Acta Orthop Belg.* 2021;87(1):167–173.
10. Jacquemier M, Glard Y, Pomero V, et al. Rotational profile of the lower limb in 1319 healthy children. *Gait Posture.* 2008;28:187–193.
11. Novais EN, Nunally KD, Ferrer MG, Miller PE, Wylie JD, Dodgen WT. Asymmetrically increased femoral version with high prevalence of moderate and severe femoral anteversion in unilateral Legg-Calvé-Perthes disease. *J Child Orthop.* 2021;15(5):503–509.

Section IV
Joint Dislocations

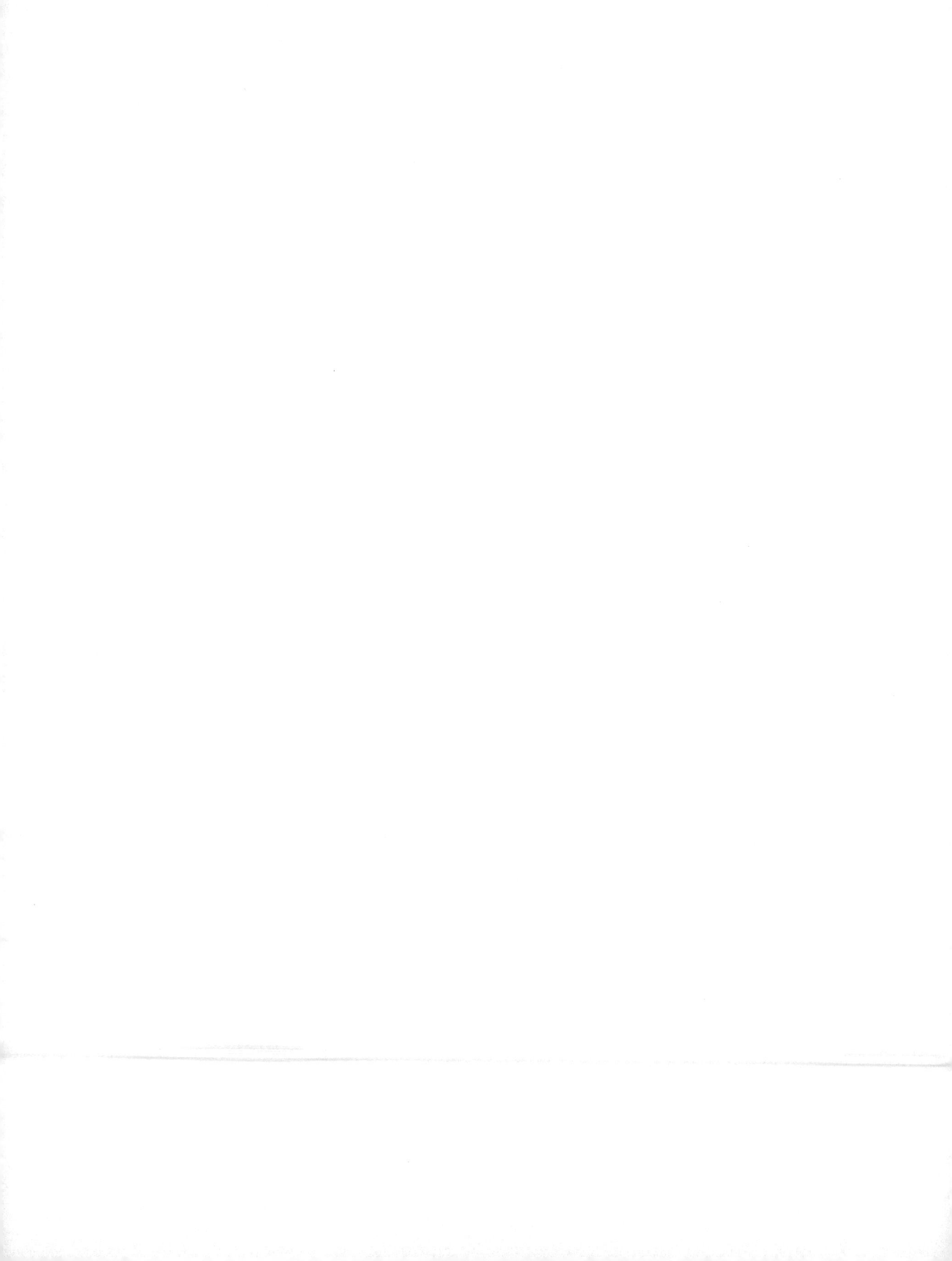

CHAPTER 10

Joint Dislocation

KEY POINTS

- Once a joint has been dislocated, the joint capsule becomes stretched into an unusual form, and ligamentous attachments become elongated and deformed.
- The joint that is most liable to dislocation is the hip joint because of the major forces that may be brought to bear on it by such situations as breech presentation in later fetal life and because of the sloping angulation of the acetabulum.
- When multiple joint dislocations are present, it usually suggests the presence of a genetic malformation syndrome or a genetic connective tissue dysplasia.

GENERAL

Joints normally develop secondarily within the condensed mesenchyme that will form the bones (Fig. 10.1). Hence, a dislocated joint represents a displacement of the bone from the original site of the joint. Once a joint has been dislocated, the joint capsule becomes stretched into an unusual form, and ligamentous attachments become elongated and deformed. If the dislocation is of sufficient duration, the aberrant forces will alter the form of the original joint socket. The occurrence of dislocation is dependent on at least three factors:

1. Biomechanical forces affecting the alignment of bones within the joint
2. Laxity of ligaments that hold the joint together
3. Mesenchymal boney precursors within the joint itself (Fig. 10.2)

The joint that is most liable to dislocation is the hip joint because of the major forces that may be brought to bear on it by such situations as breech presentation in later fetal life and because of the sloping angulation of the acetabulum. The second most common dislocation is of the proximal head of the radius, and the third most common dislocation is at the knee, yielding a genu recurvatum. Because of the relative importance and frequency of dislocation of the hip, it will be given more extensive coverage in this text.

When multiple joint dislocations are present, it usually suggests the presence of a genetic malformation syndrome, such as Larsen syndrome, or a genetic connective tissue dysplasia, such as one of the many different types of Ehlers-Danlos syndrome that are associated with ligamentous laxity. Larsen syndrome results in multiple joint dislocations because of joint malformation.[2] This syndrome is caused by autosomal dominant mutations in filamin B (*FLNB*), a cytoplasmic protein expressed in growth plate chondrocytes and vertebral bodies that serves to regulate the structure and activity of the cytoskeleton by cross-linking actin into three-dimensional networks.[2] Ehlers-Danlos syndrome is a heritable group of connective tissue disorders characterized by joint hypermobility, skin extensibility, and tissue fragility.[1,3-5] Skin extensibility is evaluated on the volar surface of the forearm by pulling the skin until resistance is felt. (This is difficult in young children because of subcutaneous fat.) Joint hypermobility is confirmed by a score of 5 or more points out of 9 on the Beighton scale:

1. Dorsiflexion of the fifth finger of more than 90 degrees (1 point for each hand)
2. Apposition of the thumb to flexor aspect of the forearm (1 point for each hand)
3. Hyperextension of the elbow beyond 10 degrees (1 point for each elbow)
4. Hyperextension of the knee beyond 10 degrees (1 point for each knee)
5. Forward flexion of the trunk with knees extended so that the palms lie flat on the floor (1 point)

Tissue fragility manifests as easy bruising with spontaneous recurrent ecchymoses, causing brownish discoloration and dystrophic scars with a thin,

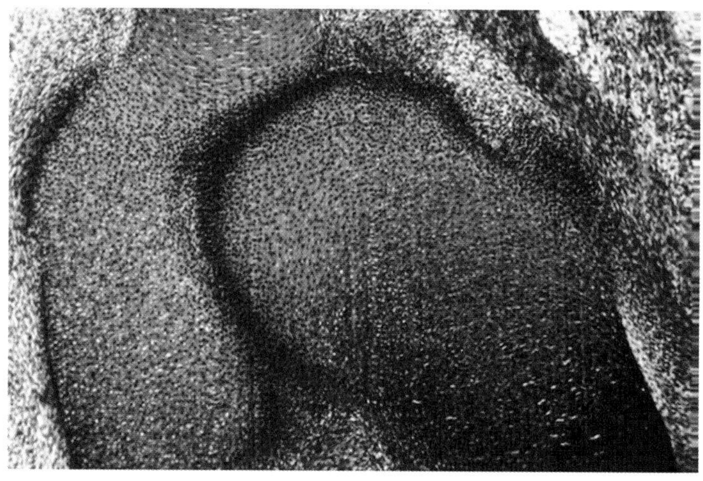

FIGURE 10.1 Normal fetal hip joint developing secondarily within the condensed mesenchyme, which will form the head of the femur and pelvic acetabulum.

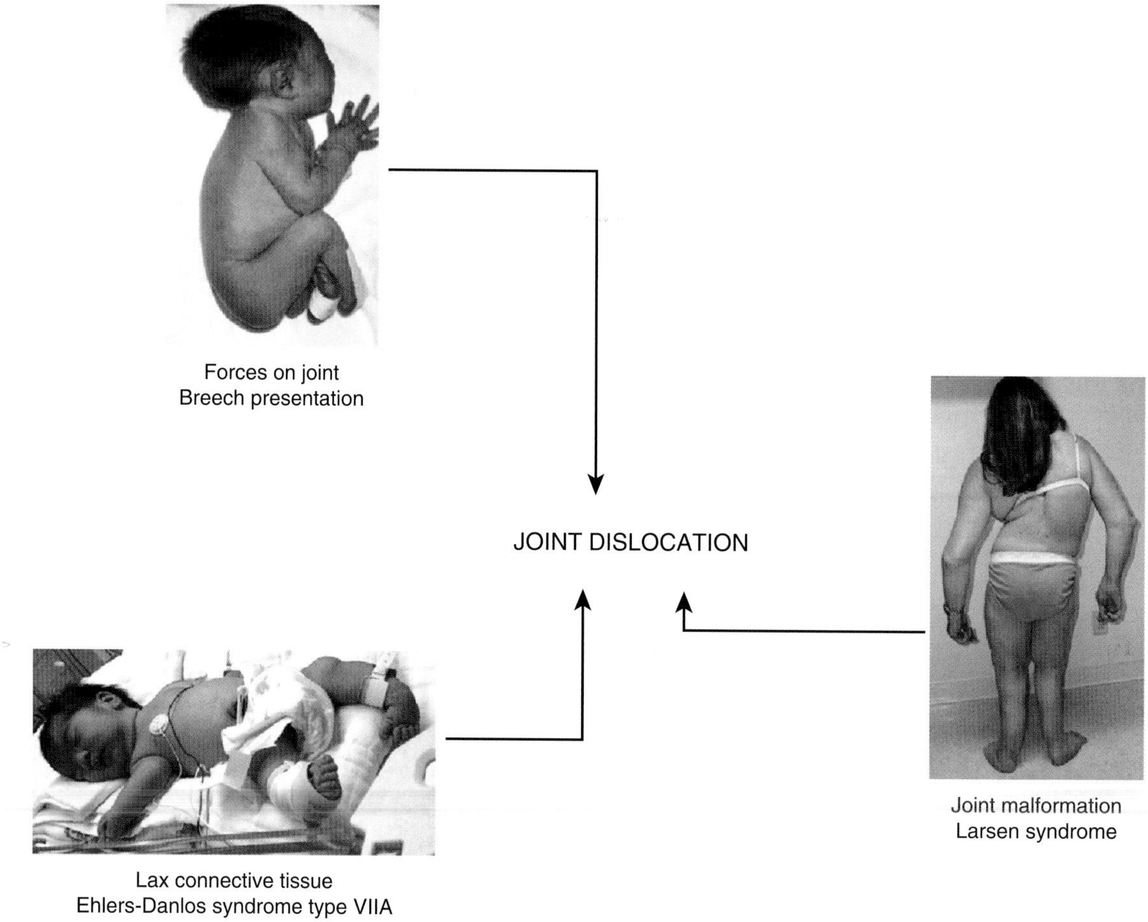

Forces on joint
Breech presentation

JOINT DISLOCATION

Joint malformation
Larsen syndrome

Lax connective tissue
Ehlers-Danlos syndrome type VIIA

FIGURE 10.2 Factors that interact in the genesis of joint dislocation, with examples relating to altered forces resulting from extrinsic deformation (e.g., breech deformation sequence), ligamentous laxity (e.g., Ehlers-Danlos syndrome type VIIA, owing to an autosomal dominant alteration in protease cleavage site from skipping of exon 6 in *COL1A1*),[1] and joint malformation (e.g., Larsen syndrome owing to an autosomal dominant mutation in *FLNB*). In the latter two examples, the presence of multiple joint dislocations suggests a genetic disorder involving connective tissue or skeletal development.

atrophic papyraceous appearance, occurring mostly over pressure points.[3] In addition to the Ehlers-Danlos syndromes and Larsen syndrome, numerous other syndromes result in multiple joint dislocations, such as pseudodiastrophic dysplasia (autosomal recessive), Desbuquois dysplasia (autosomal recessive), and various types of arthrogryposes.

References

1. Ritelli M, Colombi M. Molecular genetics and pathogenesis of Ehlers-Danlos syndrome and related connective tissue disorders. *Genes (Basel)*. 2020;11(5):547.
2. Krakow D, Robertson SP, King LM, et al. Mutations in the gene encoding filamin B disrupt vertebral segmentation, joint formation and skeletogenesis. *Nat Genet*. 2004;36:405–410.
3. Malfait F, Francomano C, Byers P, et al. The 2017 international classification of the Ehlers-Danlos syndromes. *Am J Med Genet C Semin Med Genet.*. 2017;175(1):8–26.
4. Klaassens M, Reinstein E, Hilhorst-Hofstee Y, et al. Ehlers-Danlos syndrome arthrochalasia type (VIIA-B)—expanding the phenotype: from prenatal life through adulthood. *Clin Genet*. 2012;82:121–130.
5. Adham S., Legrand A., Bruno R.M., et al. Assessment of arterial damage in vascular Ehlers-Danlos syndrome: a retrospective multicentric cohort. *Front Cardiovasc Med.* 20223;9:953894.

CHAPTER 11

Developmental Dysplasia of the Hip (Congenital Dislocation of the Hip)

KEY POINTS

- Certain risk factors warrant close surveillance for congenital hip dislocation: positive family history, breech presentation, firstborn children, female gender, accompanying postural deformations, and certain postnatal positioning.
- All gradations of dislocation, from a partially stretched, dislocatable hip to a fully dislocated hip, occur with an overall frequency of about 1%–3%.
- In newborns, positive Ortolani and Barlow tests continue to be effective clinical screening tests for unstable hips.
- The Ortolani and Barlow maneuvers are only indicated during the first 4 months of life, and continued surveillance throughout the first 12 months is merited.
- If either the Ortolani sign or Barlow test is positive during the first few months of life, referral to a pediatric orthopedist is indicated, and in addition, ultrasound or radiographs revealing abnormal findings in the hip should also prompt a referral.
- Splint treatment should ideally begin by 6 weeks of age, and treatment with a Pavlik harness is successful in up to 90% of patients.
- Failed splintage or late presentation usually necessitates surgical intervention depending on the patient's age and the severity of the hip dysplasia and displacement.

GENESIS

The definition of developmental dysplasia of the hip (DDH), formerly termed *congenital dislocation of the hip*, remains complex and controversial, making precise determination of incidence figures difficult. Fig. 10.2 depicts some of the interacting factors that relate to the genesis of DDH. When hip dislocation develops because of a genetic connective tissue dysplasia, such as Marfan syndrome, Ehlers-Danlos syndrome, Larsen syndrome, or osteogenesis imperfecta, it may not become evident until after birth and special treatment considerations may apply.[1] Under such circumstances, use of the term *congenital hip dislocation* is inappropriate. Laxity of connective tissue is an important factor, and the 4:1 to 5:1 female-to-male predilection toward the occurrence of DDH is considered a consequence of the female fetus being laxer than the male. This might be because of a lack of testosterone effect in the female fetus.[1,2] Testosterone in the male fetus may result in tighter muscles and tougher connective tissue, as has been demonstrated in the hip capsule of young rodents.[3] Pelvic ligaments are also more relaxed in infant girls, possibly because of differential receptor responses to relaxing hormones in late gestation. Dunn[4] has shown the excess of dislocation of the hip in the female to be as high as 13:1 when it is an isolated deformation; however when there is breech presentation and/or the presence of multiple deformations, the sex ratio is closer to equal. Carter and Wilkinson[5] noted laxity of three or more joints in 7% of individuals in the general population compared with an incidence of 22% among first-degree relatives with sporadic cases of dislocation of the hip. This suggests a possible heritable tendency toward increased joint laxity in association with congenital hip dislocation. When there were multiple cases of dislocation of the hip in a family, 65% of first-degree relatives had undue joint laxity.[5]

The same forces that tend to thrust the head of the femur out of the acetabulum also cause stretching of the joint capsule and ligamentum teres (Fig. 11.1). These forces are most commonly the result of constraint in late fetal life and thus are more likely to affect firstborn offspring. Certain presentations during late gestation are particularly

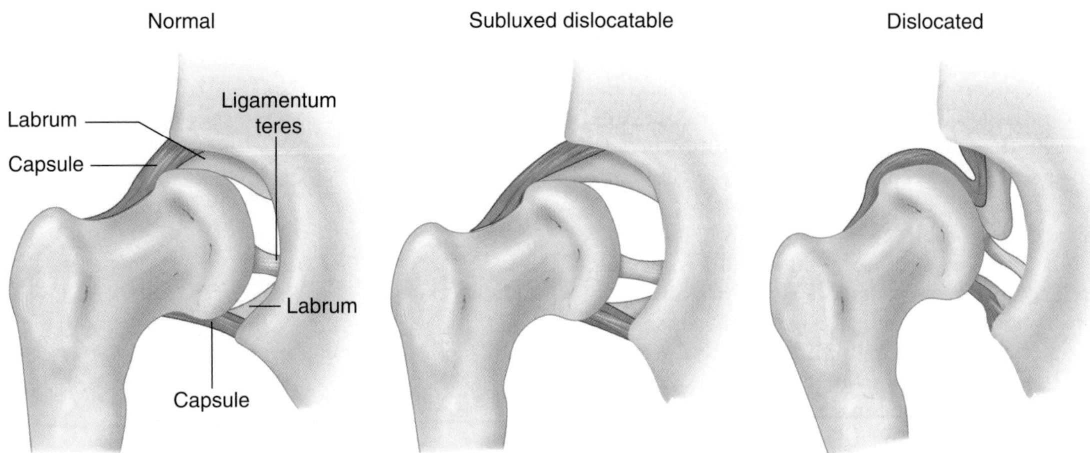

FIGURE 11.1 The normal hip, the moderately stretched capsule, and ligaments of the dislocatable hip, and the overstretched capsule and ligaments of the dislocated hip. (From Clarren S, Smith DW. Congenital deformities. *Pediatr Clin North Am.* 1977;24:665-677.)

likely to cause dislocation of the hip, and breech presentation is notorious in this respect, with about 50% of patients with hip dislocation having been in breech presentation at birth.[4] Among breech term births (about 3.5% of all births), the frequency of dislocation of the hip is 17%, and for breech births with extended legs in utero (frank breech), the incidence is 25%.[4] When 224 term breech singleton infants were compared with 3107 term vertex singleton infants, DDH occurred 15 times more frequently among the infants in breech presentation (0.9%) compared with infants in vertex presentation (0.06%).[6] Breech presentation, with the fetal buttocks located in the maternal pelvis and the hips tightly flexed against the abdomen, tends to displace the femoral heads out of the acetabulum, especially when the legs are extended and "caught" between the fetal abdomen and the maternal uterine wall.

The fact that the fetus more commonly lies with the left side toward the mother's spine may explain why the left hip is more commonly dislocated than the right.[4] Left-sided hip dislocation is noted four times more frequently than right-sided hip dislocation. Constraint of the fetus because of oligohydramnios deformation sequence is associated with an increased frequency of hip dislocation, partly because of the increased frequency of breech presentation with oligohydramnios. Dunn noted that hip dysplasia is more common when other postural deformations are present, particularly congenital muscular torticollis, talipes equinovarus, metatarsus adductus, and hyperextension or dislocation of the knee (usually all resulting from the same deforming posture in late gestation).[4]

The position of the infant after birth is also important in the genesis of DDH. The hip joint may be lax at birth and usually becomes tighter after birth; hence hips rarely become dislocated after birth unless some type of DDH is present. Undue leg extension in early infancy, at a time when the femoral head is not yet perfectly round, can be a factor in the postnatal genesis of DDH.[5] Thus the hip that has been flexed, with a relatively contracted psoas muscle in utero, is more likely to be thrust out of its socket by forced extension of the leg. The increased frequency of DDH among Mongolian infants has been attributed to their practice of swaddling young infants with their legs extended.[7] On the other hand, the relatively low incidence of hip dislocation among the Hong Kong Chinese population has been attributed to the custom of carrying the infant on the mother's lower back, with the infant's hips flexed and partially abducted (which mechanically favors maintenance of the femoral head in the acetabulum).[8] The majority of mothers in the sub-Saharan African country of Malawi back-carry their infants during the first 2–24 months of life in a position similar to that of the Pavlik harness, which results in a very low incidence of DDH in this country where no infant presented with or underwent surgical intervention for symptomatic DDH between 2002 and 2012 in a large hospital where 9842 children underwent other surgical procedures.[9] In addition, there is established evidence indicating that swaddling, the opposite position to back-carrying, causes an increase in the incidence of DDH.[7,9] In dogs, canine hip dysplasia is the most common developmental defect and the risk in very large-sized breeds is 20–50 times greater, respectively, than that in small and medium breeds, with no apparent difference evident between genders.[10]

Therefore certain risk factors warrant close surveillance for congenital hip dislocation: family history of DDH, breech presentation, firstborn children, female gender, accompanying postural deformations (particularly congenital muscular torticollis, which also manifests a left-sided predominance), and certain postnatal positioning practices (papoose swaddling or swaddling with the hips fully extended).[4–7] All gradations of dislocation, from a partially stretched dislocatable hip to a fully dislocated hip, occur with an overall frequency of about 1%–3%.[1,4] Considering the full spectrum, Barlow[11] observed that 60% of these dislocatable hips are stable in the normal location by 1 week of age and 88% are stable by 2 months of age. The remaining 12% represent frank dislocation of the hip that was evident at birth or during early infancy, suggesting a frequency of 1.2 per 1000.

Additional controversy regarding the incidence of DDH results from differences in criteria for defining a genuinely pathologic neonatal hip. Before the introduction of routine clinical screening programs for neonatal detection of DDH (c. 1920–1950), diagnostic criteria were so varied that incidence figures ranged from 0 to 200 per 1000 children.[11] After routine clinical neonatal screening was introduced (c. 1950–1980), data on the incidence of DDH were based mainly on clinical findings that denoted neonatal hip instability, leading to some overdiagnosis and overtreatment, with an incidence of 0.41–168.6 per 1000.[12] After ultrasonography began to be used in neonatal screening for DDH, higher sensitivity resulted in higher incidence figures (71.5–518.5 per 1000), but sonographic diagnoses did not always correlate with clinical diagnoses.[12] In an effort to correlate these data with Barlow's clinical findings (which suggested that 88% of unstable hips eventually become normal without treatment), Bialik and coworkers[12] tried to correlate neonatal ultrasound screening with clinical findings and treatment to determine the true incidence of DDH. They screened 9030 neonates at 1–3 days of life; any infants found to have sonographic abnormalities were reexamined at 2–6 weeks, depending on the severity of their findings. Only hips that had not improved or had deteriorated were treated; all others were examined periodically until 12 months of age. Sonographically abnormal hips had an incidence of 55.1 per 1000 hips, whereas the true incidence of DDH requiring treatment was 5 per 1000 hips, with all others evolving into normal hips and no new instances of DDH at 12 months.[12]

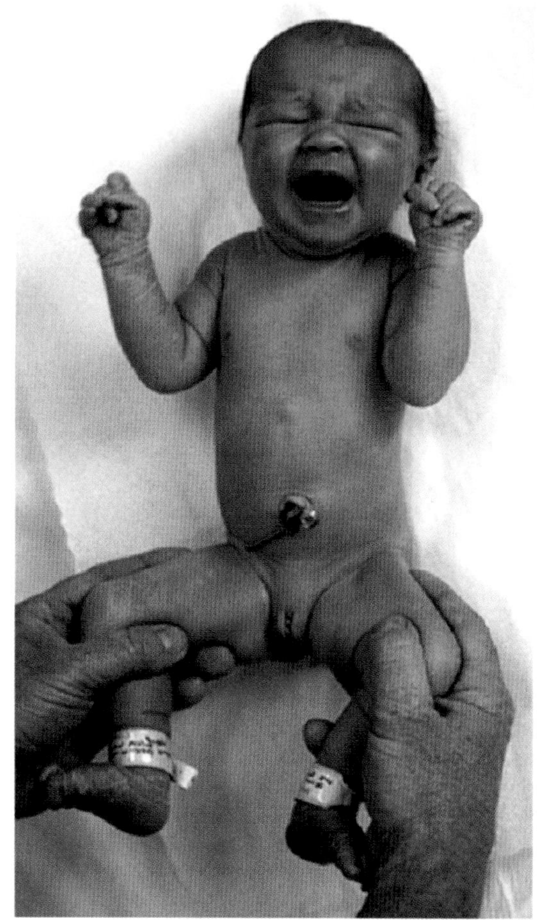

FIGURE 11.2 The usual position of an infant for neonatal hip examination.

FEATURES

The usual direction for hip dislocation is posterior. The major problem with DDH is that it is seldom readily evident on gross inspection of the newborn and may not become apparent until early postnatal life. Thus diagnosis of congenital hip dislocation involves a directed physical examination (Figs. 11.2–11.4 and Video 11.1) searching for signs of the whole dislocation spectrum, from the lax dislocatable hip to the dislocated hip that can still be relocated into the acetabulum, to the dislocated hip that cannot be

relocated. The following hip examinations are warranted for all infants. In newborns, positive Ortolani and Barlow tests (see Figs. 11.3 and 11.4) continue to be effective clinical screening tests for unstable hips. From these tests the examiner should be able to determine whether the hip is dislocated or subluxable.

It is of utmost importance that the infant is relaxed during the hip examination, and use of a pacifier or bottle may be of value in this regard. For the Ortolani test, the infant is placed in the supine position with the hips and knees flexed to 90 degrees and mildly abducted. The examiner, who is facing the baby's buttocks, grasps each thigh. The thumb of each hand is placed on the medial part of the upper thigh, and the index and third fingers are placed over the lateral aspect of the upper thigh at the level of the greater trochanter. The first maneuver is to lift up and out quite gently on the thigh and, at the same time, push the upper thigh toward the groin with the third finger. If the hip is dislocated posteriorly (the usual direction for dislocation) and can be relocated into the acetabulum, the examiner will feel a noticeable "clunk" as the femoral head slips over the acetabular shelf and into the acetabular socket. This is considered a positive Ortolani sign (see Fig. 11.3). If the result of this test is negative, then a Barlow test is performed by pulling out gently on the thigh while at the same time pushing the upper thigh away from the groin with the thumb. Barlow's test (see Fig. 11.4) is a provocative test to determine whether the hip is dislocatable, implying a shallow socket with hip instability. If Barlow's test results in a noticeable (palpable) "clunk" as the femoral head is forced over the acetabular rim into a posteriorly dislocated position, the hip may be referred to as *dislocatable* or *unstable*. Minor clicks may be noted in about one third of

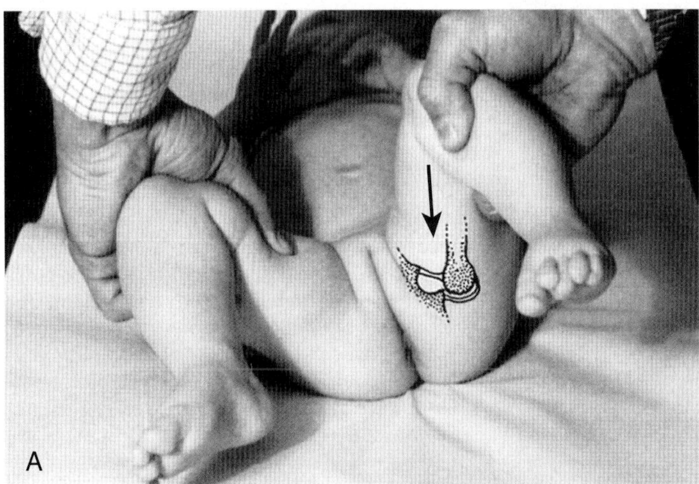

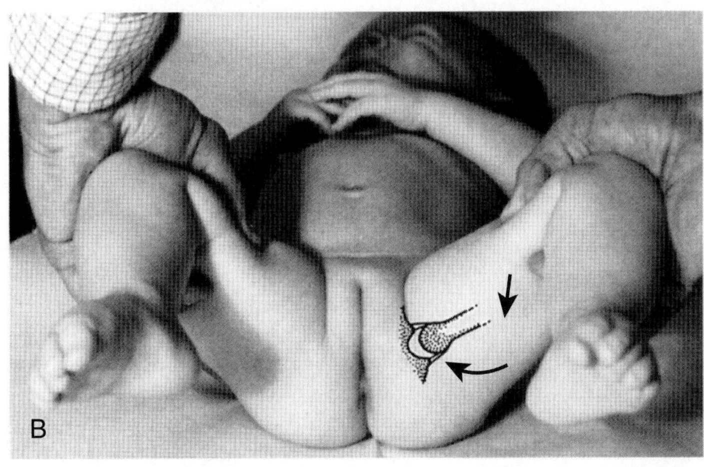

FIGURE 11.3 Technique for the Ortolani maneuver, which assists in the detection of the dislocated hip that can be repositioned into the acetabulum. A, Downward pressure further dislocates the hip. B, Inward rotation of the hip will force the femoral head over the acetabular rim, leading to a noticeable "clunk." (Courtesy Lynn Staheli, Dept. of Pediatric Orthopedics, Children's Orthopedic Hospital, Seattle.)

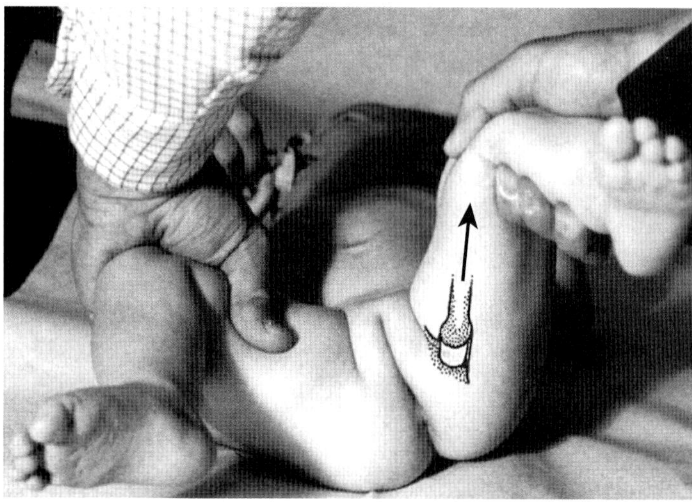

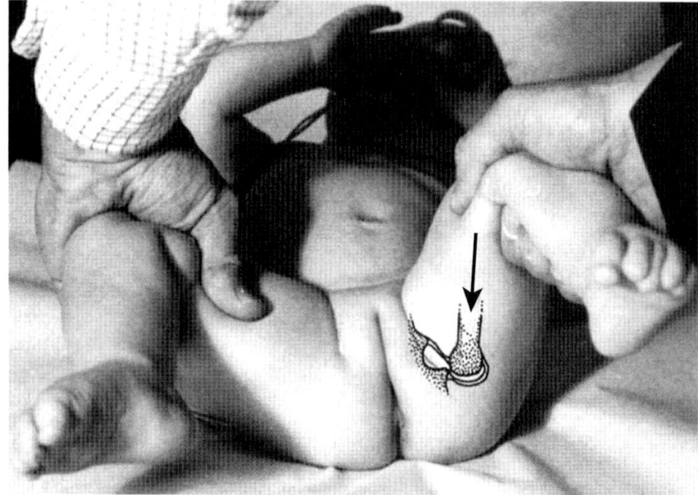

FIGURE 11.4 Technique for the Barlow maneuver, which assists in detecting the unstable dislocatable hip that is in the acetabulum. The leg is forcibly pulled up during the maneuver. Passage over the rim usually yields a noticeable "clunk." (Courtesy Lynn Staheli, Dept. of Pediatric Orthopedics, Children's Orthopedic Hospital, Seattle.)

examinations and do not appear to be of any consequence. Rather it is the palpable "clunk" or "thunk" that is relevant. If either test is positive, referral to a pediatric orthopedist is indicated within the first 2 weeks of life; if equivocal, clinical reevaluation is indicated in 2 weeks. If suspicion still exists after 4 weeks, then hip ultrasonography and referral to an orthopedist are indicated. Ultrasound is the appropriate imaging modality for infants from birth to 4–6 months of age; radiography is used after the femoral heads begin to ossify.

It is important to understand that neither maneuver will be positive in an older infant whose hip is dislocated and cannot be manually relocated; thus the Barlow and Ortolani maneuvers are reserved for infants younger than 3 or 4 months. In older infants with DDH, the hip will usually show a limitation in abduction, the greater trochanter may be felt to be posteriorly and superiorly displaced, and the upper leg may appear relatively short (Fig. 11.5A). When the dislocation is unilateral or asymmetric in degree, then the relative length of the legs may be asymmetric, although the lower legs and feet will be the same length. Thus when the infant is placed in a supine position with the hips and knees flexed and the feet flat on the examination table, if one knee is noticeably lower than the other knee (Galeazzi's sign), DDH is suggested (Fig. 11.5B). An obvious discrepancy may also be observed in the creases of the thigh folds between the two sides (Fig. 11.5C).

Thus the Ortolani and Barlow maneuvers are only indicated during the first 4 months of life. After this

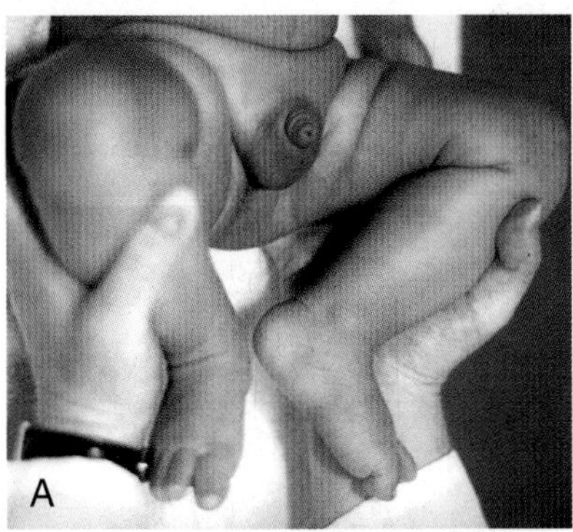

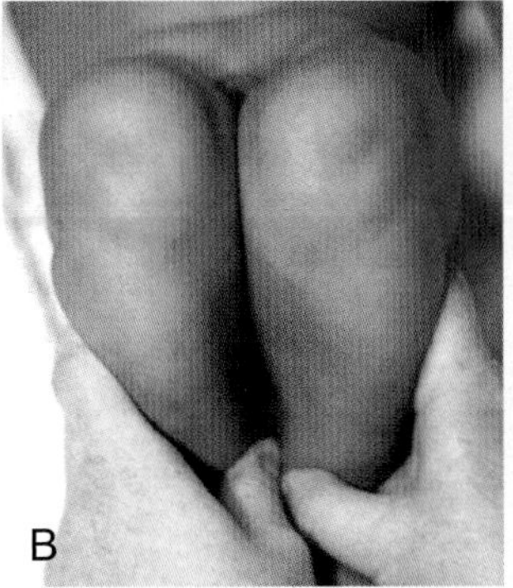

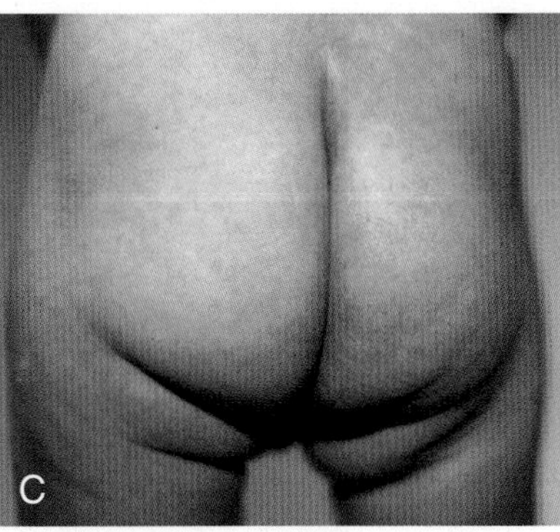

FIGURE 11.5 Developmental dysplasia of the hip in an older infant with rigid spine myopathy. Aberrantly increased muscular forces resulted in postnatal hip dislocation, evident as tight hips with limited abduction (A), upper leg length discrepancy with uneven knee height (B), and asymmetric thigh creases (C). He developed progressive scoliosis and severe lethal respiratory insufficiency. This condition usually results from homozygous or compound heterozygous mutation in the *SEPN1* gene, which encodes a protein that plays a key role in the physiology of skeletal muscles, such as the diaphragm, by maintaining the homeostasis of myocytes and protecting against oxidative stress.

time, the soft tissues around the hip joint tighten and the dislocated hip cannot be replaced within the hip socket. As a result, the adductor muscles appear relatively tight on the involved side, resulting in limited abduction. It is paramount to understand that not all dislocation of the hip can be detected in the newborn nursery, and continued surveillance throughout the first 12 months is merited. To check for DDH in infants older than 4 months, flex both hips and both knees to 90 degrees with the infant lying supine on the exam table, bringing each knee toward the chest, and checking for limited abduction by moving each leg sideways back toward the exam table. Older children with DDH or neuromuscular disease may have a positive Trendelenburg sign, which is tested by having the child stand on one foot and then the other. Normally the hip opposite the weight-bearing leg elevates because the hip on the weight-bearing side abducts. With a positive Trendelenburg sign, the opposite hip drops because the weight-bearing hip does not abduct. This also affects the gait, resulting in a Trendelenburg gait (also called an *abductor lurch*) because of weakness of the abductor muscles. The child with this gait leans the upper trunk over the affected side to maintain his or her center of gravity while walking.

Radiography is of little value in the newborn because of incomplete ossification of the acetabulum and lack of ossification in the femoral head, but it becomes more valuable after 6 months of age. To detect evidence of dislocation when such a problem is clinically suspected, a plain anteroposterior radiograph of the pelvis in the frog leg position is useful. Ultrasonography should be used before this time and in the immediate neonatal period, particularly when the other risk factors mentioned previously are present. Several associated aberrations in morphogenesis may occur secondary to dislocation of the hip (Fig. 11.6), depending on the age of development and the duration and extent of the dislocation. These aberrations include deformation of the femoral head; imperfect articular cartilage; adherence between the articular surface of the femoral head and the capsular tissues; short psoas, adductor, and hamstring muscles; anteversion of the hip; development of a false acetabulum; and elongation of the ligamentum teres with a stretched joint capsule. When such changes are profound, it may be difficult or even impossible to accomplish a closed reduction of the femoral head into its original acetabulum.

MANAGEMENT, PROGNOSIS, AND COUNSEL

If either the Ortolani sign or Barlow test is positive during the first few months of life, referral to a pediatric orthopedist is indicated. Likewise, limited abduction, leg length discrepancy, or asymmetry of skinfolds on the leg in addition to ultrasound or radiographs revealing abnormal findings in the hip should also prompt a referral. Early, simple, conservative management of DDH will usually result in a normal hip by the age of walking. If DDH is discovered after 1

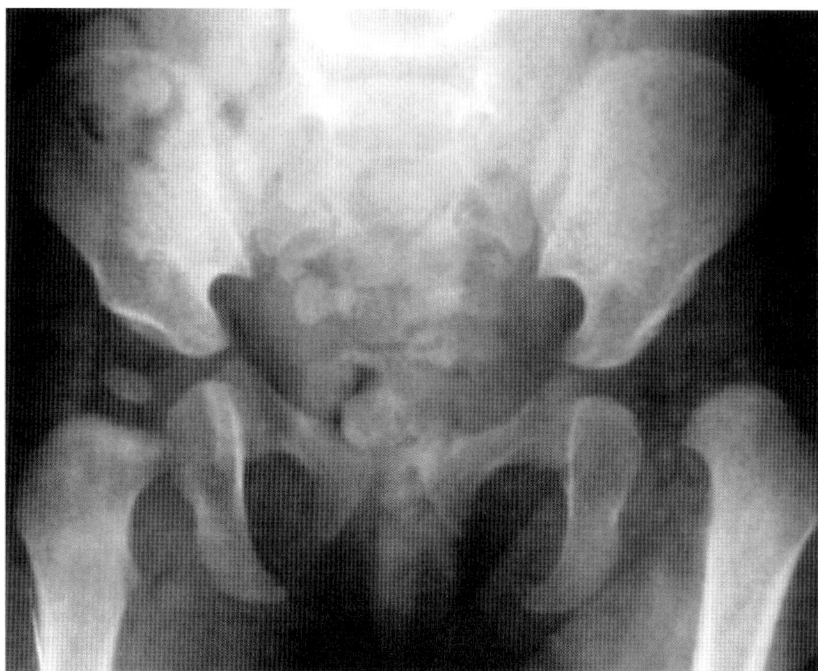

FIGURE 11.6 Secondary changes in the acetabulum and neck of the femur, as well as the unseen hourglass elongation of the hip capsule, elongated ligamentum teres, and foreshortened muscle attachments relating to long-term dislocation of the hip. (Courtesy Lynn Staheli, Dept. of Pediatric Orthopedics, Children's Orthopedic Hospital, Seattle.)

year of age, the condition usually requires prolonged, complicated management and may result in varying degrees of lifelong disability (Fig. 11.7). Hence, early diagnosis, as emphasized previously, is essential to successful management. DDH represents a spectrum of disease ranging from transient neonatal instability to established dislocation. It is accepted that female gender, breech presentation, and family history are risk factors for the disease. Early diagnosis by clinical examination or ultrasound imaging is emphasized, with splint treatment ideally commencing by 6 weeks of age. Treatment using the Pavlik harness is successful in up to 90% of patients. Ultrasound imaging is the gold standard for monitoring a patient during harness wear. Failed splintage or late presentation usually necessitates surgical intervention depending on the patient's age and the severity of the hip dysplasia and displacement. A child aged 6–18 months who requires surgical reduction can be treated by formal anterior open reduction, and additional bony procedures are usually not required in these young patients. Older children, or children with genetic connective tissue problems, may require formal open reduction plus an associated bony osteotomy (acetabular, proximal femoral, or, in some cases, both types of osteotomies) to stabilize the hip.[1,13,14] The addition of a proximal femoral derotational shortening osteotomy for open reduction is commonly used in children as young as 2 years to decrease the forces on the reduced hip and minimize the chances for redislocation and osteonecrosis, with postoperative computed tomography used to accurately confirm the reduction of dislocated hips following surgical reduction because this positioning is critical to the success of the procedure and to the prevention of avascular necrosis.

The most common hip diagnosis at birth is the dislocatable or unstable hip. In a study of 1,059,479 newborns born between 1970 and 1988 in Norway, the overall prevalence of clinically detected neonatal hip instability at birth was 0.9% (0.6% in males and 1.4% in females).[15] With breech presentation, the rate was 4.4% compared with 0.9% with vertex presentation; the incidence was also higher in firstborns. In female infants, the rate of neonatal hip instability increased with the duration of pregnancy, particularly with breech presentation, but this was not seen in males.[15] Family history was important, with the risk of DDH in males increasing from 4.1 per 1000 to 9.4 per 1000

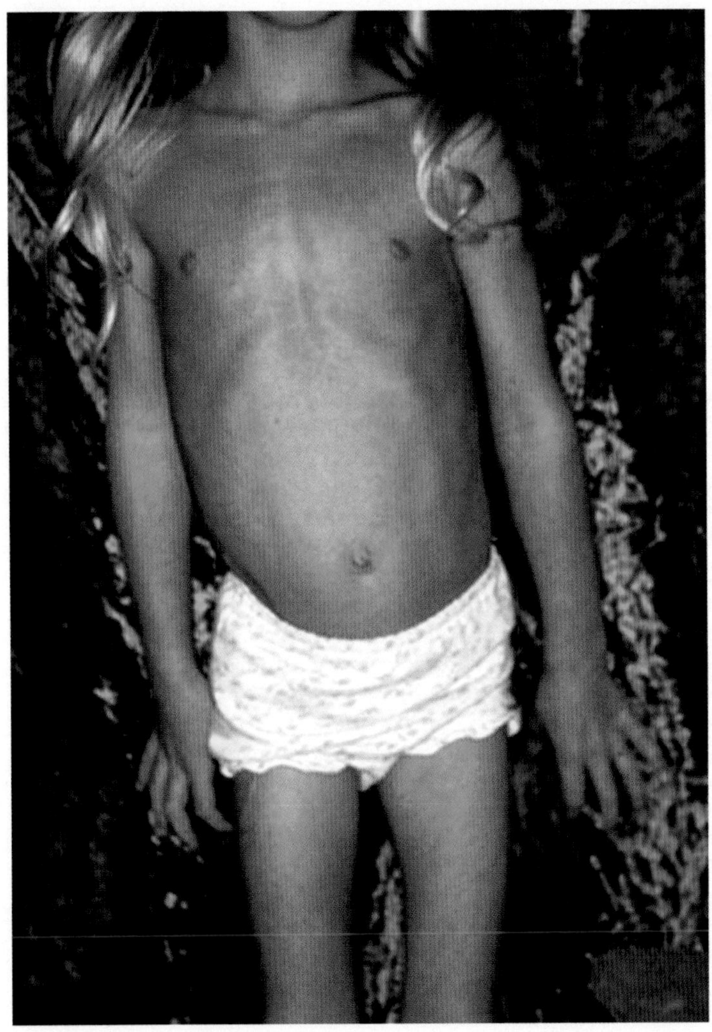

FIGURE 11.7 This girl was born with hip dislocation in breech presentation from a maternal bicornuate uterus. Late diagnosis and treatment resulted in an uneven pelvis and altered gait.

with a positive family history. Risks were even greater in females, increasing from 19 per 1000 to 44 per 1000 with a positive family history. These data support the hypothesis that mechanical factors in combination with familial and hormonal factors (primarily relaxing female hormones) play an important role in causing neonatal hip instability.

Despite the introduction of clinical screening for early detection of DDH in Norway and many other Western countries, the incidence of late DDH appeared to increase, so in 1987 one hospital compared ultrasound and clinical examination prospectively and noted a low incidence of late DDH during the 9-month study period (0.9 per 1000 vs. 3.5 per 1000 with clinical screening from 1982–1985).[16] This same group subsequently showed that the major impact of general ultrasound screening (a combination of clinical screening plus ultrasound screening of all infants) versus clinical screening alone was a higher treatment rate of early DDH using a Frejka pillow splint (3.4% vs. 1.8%) and a lower rate of late DDH, usually requiring hospitalization and surgery (0.3 per 1000 vs. 1.3 per 1000).[17] Selective screening (clinical screening plus ultrasound screening of all female infants and those male infants with known risk factors for DDH) resulted in intermediate figures.[16]

When overall costs for these programs were compared, they were similar for all three groups, but the costs of late treatment accounted for only 22% of the general screening group versus 65% in the other two groups.[18] In 2018, The International Hip Dysplasia Institute conducted a multicenter, international prospective study on infants with hips dislocated at rest. They concluded that there was insufficient evidence to support universal ultrasound screening; instead, selective screening should be performed by 6–8 weeks of age on infants with risk factors of breech presentation, family history, or history of clinical hip instability. Follow-up of infants with risk factors and normal initial screening should be considered to at least 6 months of age.[19] On the other hand, a 2021 study of early universal hip screening by ultrasound compared with clinical examination found that 50.9% of 70/3272 (2.14%) hips positive on the first ultrasound within the first 3 days of life had neither any positive physical signs nor any risk factors, except being a female, resulting in a 20% sensitivity and 98% specificity for physical examination.[20] Another 2021 study of 4000 hips noted that 1.2% of hips were positive on ultrasound, while 2.4% were positive on clinical examination. Analysis of risk factors revealed a significant association between female sex, breech presentation, and family history with pathological ultrasound findings, and the authors concluded that there was inadequate training for DDH during medical school. They concluded that universal ultrasound screening allowed identification of DDH in several children with normal clinical examination and no risk factors.[21]

If the hips are unstable even though the femoral head is in a normal position at birth, it is considered best to provide prophylactic splinting of the dislocatable hip to prevent the very real possibility of insidious hip dislocation during early infancy. Such splinting is continued until the hip is held firmly in place by the baby's own connective tissues, which may have become stretched before birth. The aim of splinting is to maintain the femoral head in the acetabulum with reliable but not excessive constraint. The recommended position is with the hips flexed about 90 degrees and abducted about 25–30 degrees. The full frog leg position has been discouraged because the constant and possibly excessive forcing of the femoral head into the acetabulum may occasionally result in avascular necrosis in the head of the immobilized femur. Various types of splints have been used (Fig. 11.8), but the Pavlik splint is generally preferred. For the dislocatable hip, a period of 4–6 weeks of splinting is usually adequate to yield a "tight" hip.

The dislocated hip that can be relocated into the acetabulum should be splinted, with assurance that the femoral head remains in the acetabulum. For this type of dislocated hip, the Pavlik splint (see Fig. 11.8B) may be preferable. Ultrasound has been found to be valuable for assessment and monitoring treatment with the Pavlik harness, which resulted in a success rate of greater than 95% in a study of 370 ultrasonographically abnormal hips in 221 infants detected through ultrasound screening (treatment rate, 5.1 per 1000 live births), with a low (0.4%) rate of avascular necrosis and a low rate of late presentation (0.26 per 1000 live births).[22] The duration of splinting varies with the severity of the problem and the age at diagnosis. When detected at birth to 1 month of age, the mean duration of splinting was 3.6 months, but detection at 1–3 months required 7 months of splinting. If the dislocation was not detected until 3–6 months, the mean duration of splinting was 9.3 months. Use of ultrasound to monitor treatment in the Pavlik harness makes it possible to distinguish between recalcitrant and gradually improving subluxation, and it also appears to lower the rate of avascular necrosis as well as the rate of late or persistent dysplasia. Among 24 patients (26 hips) who presented late (at age 6–24 months) with a dislocated hip treated primarily by Pavlik harness between 1984 and 2004, 46% were successfully reduced with the Pavlik harness after an average treatment of 14 weeks (4–28 weeks). None of the hips that were reduced with the Pavlik harness developed avascular necrosis, and there were few complications in these patients because of progressive and gentle increases of abduction and flexion, with or without temporary use of an abduction splint, but these authors felt that treatment should be abandoned if the hips did not reduce after 6 weeks because of the risk of avascular necrosis.[23] Others have advocated very early Pavlik harness therapy (mean age at treatment initiation was 5 days, ranging from 1 to 15 days, and mean treatment duration was 34 days, ranging from 15 to 75 days) to ensure rapid hip reduction and stabilization, and optimize the potential of the acetabulum for spontaneous remodeling.[24] The hip was reduced and held in its proper position long enough to allow sufficient capsule and ligament tightening to stabilize the hip so that the acetabular dysplasia underwent self-correction that was not related to treatment duration. In a study of unique ultrasonographic markers in hips with a positive Ortolani sign that were associated with Pavlik harness failure, a retrospective review was done on 85 patients (115 hips) less than 6 months old

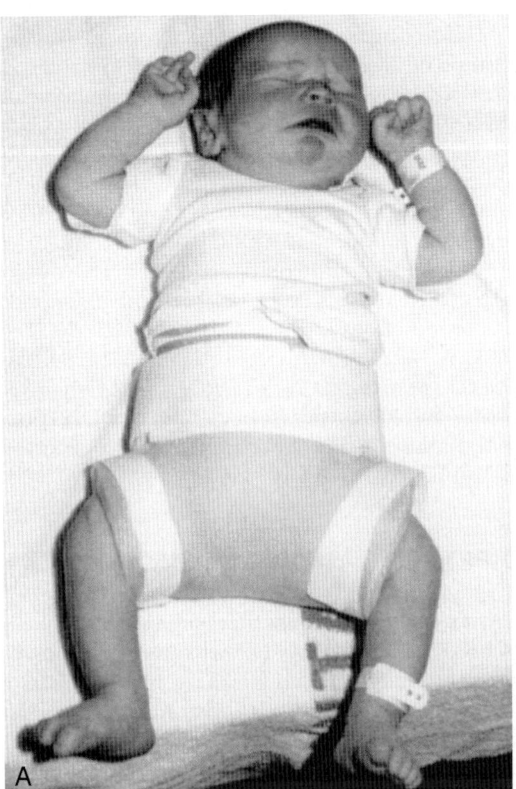
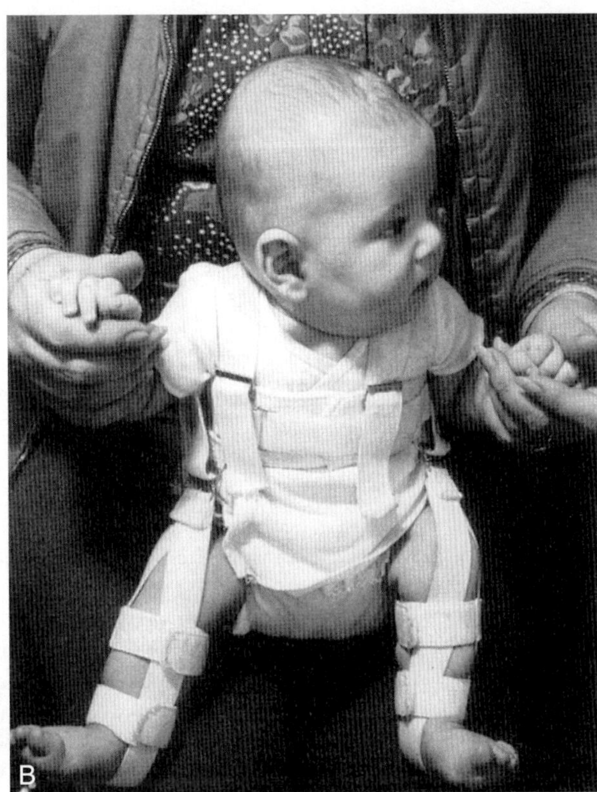

FIGURE 11.8 A, Plastazote splint used for the dislocatable hip in early infancy. B, Pavlik splint used for maintaining the repositioned dislocated hip in early infancy.

who were treated for DDH with a Pavlik harness from 1991 to 2005.[25] Pavlik harness treatment was successful in 72 hips (63%) and failed in 43 hips (37%). A femoral head positioned below the labrum was strongly associated with Pavlik harness treatment success, whereas a hip with a femoral head that was located substantially superior and lateral to the labrum was associated with Pavlik harness treatment failure. Thus the presence of a deficient cartilaginous anlage and an inverted labrum may provide a pathoanatomic explanation for Pavlik harness treatment failure.[23] Another study of children who failed Pavlik harness treatment for DDH compared their rates of avascular necrosis with a group of children who presented late and hence were treated surgically. Among 37 hips in the failed Pavlik group and 86 hips in the no Pavlik group, 10 hips in the failed Pavlik group developed avascular necrosis (27%), whereas this occurred in only seven hips (8%) in the surgical group, with a positive correlation noted with age at presentation and severity of avascular necrosis, so these authors advised close monitoring of hips in the Pavlik harness with discontinuance of its use if the hips did not reduce within 3 weeks.[26]

A prospective study of DDH in the United Kingdom over the period of 1998 to 2008 (36,960 live births) was performed to determine treatment complexity and associated costs of disease detection and hospital treatment, related to age at presentation and treatment modality. Following universal clinical screening of all infants and selective ultrasound screening of at-risk infants, 179 infants (4.8/1000) were identified with hip dysplasia: 34 infants presented late (greater than 3 months of age) and required closed or open reduction, and 145 infants presented at less than 3 months of age, 14 of whom failed early Pavlik harness treatment. Cost analysis revealed 131 early presenters with successful management in a Pavlik harness at a cost of £601 ($1017) per child; 34 late presenters who required surgery (36 hips, 19 closed/17 open reductions, one revision procedure) at a cost of £4352 ($7364) per child; and 14 early presenters with failed management in a Pavlik harness requiring more protracted surgery (18 hips, four closed/14 open reductions, seven revision procedures) at a cost of £7052 ($11,933) per child. Late detection resulted in increased treatment complexity and a sevenfold increase in the short-term costs of treatment compared with early detection and successful management in a Pavlik harness.[27]

If it is not possible to manually reduce the dislocation, leg traction may be used to lengthen the contracted muscles and (ideally) allow for a closed reduction. If this is not possible, then surgical correction merits consideration. Surgery may include lengthening or detachment of contracted muscles and reconstruction of the distorted joint capsule. Surgery is often postponed until the infant is about 1 year old because of the risk of ischemic necrosis following hip surgery at an earlier age. The likelihood of successful closed reduction of a dislocated hip that failed Pavlik harness treatment was 52% with a clinically significant avascular necrosis rate of 7%.[28] As such, these authors advocated closed reduction under general anesthetic for a hip that has failed Pavlik harness treatment. Uncorrected dislocation of the hip will adversely affect walking (see Fig. 11.7), resulting in the development of a limp and osteoarthritis during late adulthood. Although a dislocated hip will usually not become painful until after 40 years of age, a subluxated hip (acetabular dysplasia) becomes painful in late adolescence. In children with untreated DDH who are older than 3 years, it is unclear whether preoperative traction lowers the rate of avascular necrosis, and some surgeons believe that femoral shortening is preferable to traction for the late reduction of DDH.[29] Among 71 adults (90 hips) with late-detected hip dislocation treated between 1958 and 1962, the mean age of patients at the time of the long-term radiographic examination was 51.6 years (range, 44–55 years).[29] Stable reduction was achieved in 83 hips, with a mean age at reduction of 1.7 years (range, 0.3 to 5.4 years). Traction failed in 6 patients (seven hips or 8%), for whom an open reduction was necessary, and 26 patients (30 hips) underwent late surgical procedures because of residual hip dysplasia. A good long-term clinical outcome was assessed for 52 (63%) of the hips, and a satisfactory radiographic outcome (no osteoarthritis) was found for 56 (67%) of the hips. Osteoarthritis had developed in 27 (33%) of the hips, of which 19 had undergone total hip replacement, performed at a mean patient age of 43.7 years (range, 31–54 years). The most important independent risk factors for a poor long-term outcome were an age of 18 months or older at the time of reduction, residual subluxation, and osteonecrosis.[29]

The recurrence risk of the more common type of dislocation of the hip is in the range of 3%–6% and is higher when a male is affected.[5] If both the parent and child are affected, the recurrence risk may be as high as 30%. No specific genes for isolated DDH have reached major significance, but candidate genes associated with the formation of connective tissue (*COL1A1*), osteogenesis (*PAPPA2*, *GDF5*), chondrogenesis (*UQCC1*, *ASPN*), and cell growth, proliferation, and differentiation (*TGFB1*) have been suggested.[30] There is also suggestive evidence of an inducing role of mutations in the *CX3CR1*, *TENM3*, *BMS1*, *FRZB*, *HOXB9*, *HOXD9*, *IL-6*, *TBX4*, *WISP3*, *ATP2B4*, *BMP2K*, *HSPG2*, *MMP24*, *PCNT*, *PDRG1*, *SEMA4D*, *TXNDC3*, *UFSP2*, and *VDR* genes (see Fig. 11.9) in DDH etiopathogenesis, but no firm correlation between genotype and DDH phenotype currently exists.[31,32]

DIFFERENTIAL DIAGNOSIS

Certain malformations that enhance the likelihood of breech positioning, such as spina bifida, and genitourinary malformations leading to oligohydramnios (thereby resulting in both constraint and breech positioning) are associated with an increased frequency of dislocation of the hip secondary to these more primary malformation problems. Several neurologic disorders may lead to dislocation of the hip, presumably based on diminished muscle strength while holding the femoral head in the acetabulum and/or muscular imbalance. Thus dislocation of the hip may be secondary to meningomyelocele and may occur in certain types of cerebral palsy or neuromuscular diseases, especially when there is flexion and/or adduction spasm at the hip. In some forms of arthrogryposis (multiple joint contractures), especially amyoplasia congenita, the hip may be dislocated. Additionally, dislocation of the hip occurs as a frequent or occasional defect in several syndromes. One of the most striking examples is Larsen syndrome, in which there tend to be multiple joint dislocations, an unusually low nasal bridge, and spatulate thumbs. Treatment of these dislocations is not the same as for DDH in an otherwise normal child because this type of joint dislocation is caused by malformation of the joints themselves (see Fig. 10.2).[1] Finally, any syndrome associated with excessive connective tissue laxity is likely to be associated with an increased risk for congenital hip dislocation.[1]

One other entity that warrants mention is voluntary habitual hip dislocation in a child.[33,34] This rare condition is six times more frequent in females than in males and is not associated with underlying joint

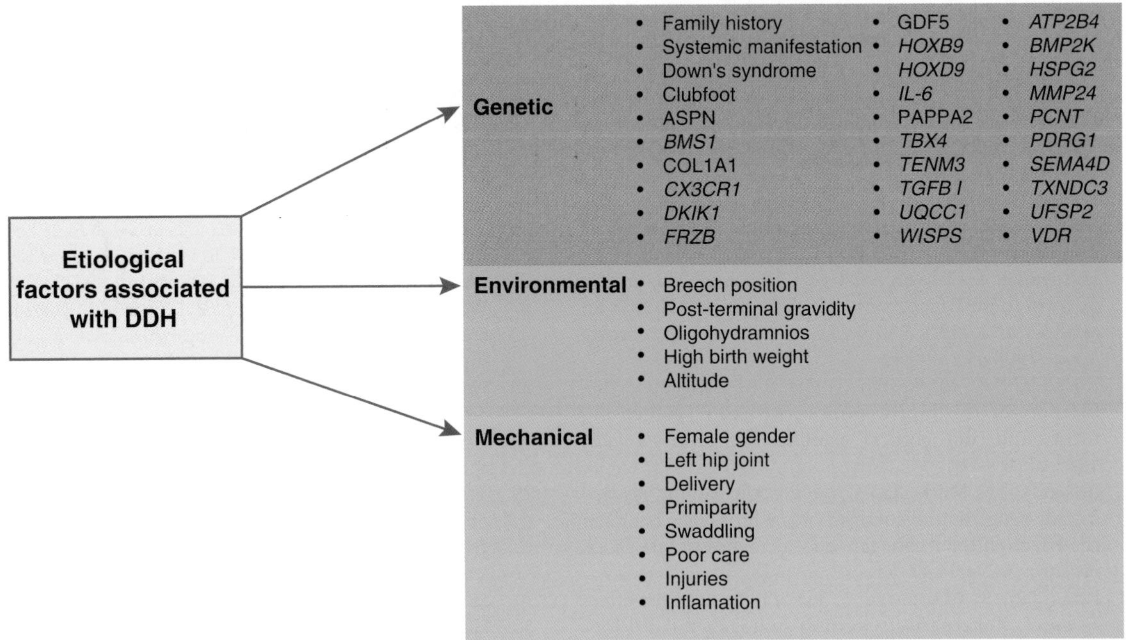

FIGURE 11.9 Genetic, environmental, and mechanical factors associated with developmental dysplasia of the hip. *DDH*, Developmental dysplasia of the hip. (From Harsanyi S, Zamborsky R, Kokavec M, Danisovic L. Genetics of developmental dysplasia of the hip. *Eur J Med Genet*. 2020;63(9):103990.)

laxity or a history of trauma. It consists of voluntary recurrent popping of one hip (more commonly the right hip) with no associated pain, with visualization of a radiographic or sonographic vacuum phenomenon within the hip capsule. Surgery is not needed, and behavioral management halts the behavior with no long-term sequelae.[33,34] A hip click on examination of the newborn hip can occur in stable hips, and it is thought to be benign due to ligaments and myofascial structures around the hips.

Some studies have suggested a link between hip clicks and DDH, and in a study of 90 otherwise normal newborns with a hip click, further evaluation via ultrasound at an average age of 6.6 weeks revealed a 17.8% prevalence of hip abnormalities. Affected infants underwent treatment with a Pavlik harness, and all had normal hips on follow-up.[35]

References

1. Kerrigan A, Ayeni OR, Kishta W. Developmental dysplasia of the hip in patients with connective-tissue disorders. *JBJS Rev*. 2019;7(4):e5.
2. Fernando J, Arena P, Smith DW. Sex liability to single structural defects. *Am J Dis Child*. 1978;132:970–972.
3. Hama H, Yamamuro T, Titkeda T. Experimental studies on connective tissue of the capsular ligament. *Acta Orthop Scand*. 1976;47:473–479.
4. Dunn PM. Perinatal observations on the etiology of congenital dislocation of the hip. *Clin Orthop*. 1976;119:11–22.
5. Carter CO, Wilkinson JA. Genetic and environmental factors in the etiology of congenital dislocation of the hip. *Clin Orthop Rel Res*. 1964;33:119–128.
6. Hsieh Y-Y, Tsai F-J, Lin C-C, et al. Breech deformation complex in neonates. *J Reprod Med*. 2000;45:933–935.
7. Ulziibat M, Munkhuu B, Bataa AE, Schmid R, Baumann T, Essig S. Traditional Mongolian swaddling, and developmental dysplasia of the hip: a randomized controlled trial. *BMC Pediatr*. 2021;21(1):450.
8. Chan A, McCaul KA, Cundy PJ, et al. Perinatal risk factors for developmental dysplasia of the hip. *Arch Dis Child Fetal Neonatal Ed*. 1997;76:94F–100F.
9. Graham SM, Manara J, Chokotho L, Harrison WJ. Back-carrying infants to prevent developmental hip dysplasia and its sequelae: is a new public health initiative needed? *J Pediatr Orthop*. 2015;35(1):57–61.
10. Priester WA, Mulvihill JJ. Canine hip dysplasia: relative risk by sex, size, and breed, and comparative aspects. *J Am Vet Assoc*. 1972;160:735–739.
11. Barlow TG. Early diagnosis and treatment of congenital dislocation of the hip. *J Bone Joint Surg*. 1962;44B:292–301.

12. Bialik V, Bialik G, Blazer S, et al. Developmental dysplasia of the hip: a new approach to incidence. *Pediatrics*. 1999;103:93–99.
13. Swarup I, Penny CL, Dodwell ER. Developmental dysplasia of the hip: an update on diagnosis and management from birth to 6 months. *Curr Opin Pediatr*. 2018;30(1):84–92.
14. Young JR, Anderson MJ, O'Connor CM, Kazley JM, Mantica AL, Dutt V. Team approach: developmental dysplasia of the hip. *JBJS Rev*. 2020;8(9):e20.00030.
15. Hinderaker T, Daltveit AK, Irgens LM, et al. The impact of intra-uterine factors on neonatal hip instability: an analysis of 1,059,479 children in Norway. *Acta Orthop Scand*. 1994;65:239–242.
16. Rosendahl K, Markestad T, Lie RT. Congenital dislocation of the hip: a prospective study comparing ultrasound and clinical examination. *Acta Paediatr*. 1992;81:177–181.
17. Rosendahl K, Markestad T, Lie RT. Ultrasound screening for congenital dislocation of the hip in the neonate: the effect on treatment rate and incidence of late cases. *Pediatrics*. 1994;94:47–52.
18. Rosendahl K, Markestad T, Lie RT, et al. Cost-effectiveness of alternative screening strategies for developmental dysplasia of the hip. *Arch Pediatr Adolesc Med*. 1995;149:643–648.
19. Schaeffer EK, Study Group I, Mulpuri K. Developmental dysplasia of the hip: addressing evidence gaps with a multicentre prospective international study. *Med J Aust*. 2018;208(8):359–364.
20. Gyurkovits Z, Sohár G, Baricsa A, Németh G, Orvos H, Dubs B. Early detection of developmental dysplasia of hip by ultrasound. *Hip Int*. 2021;31(3):424–429.
21. Buonsenso D, Curatola A, Lazzareschi I, et al. Developmental dysplasia of the hip: real world data from a retrospective analysis to evaluate the effectiveness of universal screening. *J Ultrasound*. 2021;24(4):403–410.
22. Taylor GR, Clarke NMP. Monitoring the treatment of developmental dysplasia of the hip with the Pavlik harness: the role of ultrasound. *J Bone Joint Surg Br*. 1997;79B:719–723.
23. Pollet V, Pruijs H, Sakkers R, et al. Results of Pavlik harness treatment in children with dislocated hips between the age of six and twenty-four months. *J Pediatr Orthop*. 2010;30:437–442.
24. Bin K, Laville JM, Salmeron F. Developmental dysplasia of the hip in neonates: evolution of acetabular dysplasia after hip stabilization by brief Pavlik harness treatment. *Orthop Traumatol Surg Res*. 2014;100:357–361.
25. White KK, Sucato DJ, Agrawal S, et al. Ultrasonographic findings in hips with a positive Ortolani sign and their relationship to Pavlik harness failure. *J Bone Joint Surg Am*. 2010;92:113–120.
26. Tiruveedhula M, Reading IC, Clarke NM. Failed Pavlik harness treatment for DDH as a risk factor for avascular necrosis. *J Pediatr Orthop*. 2015;35(2):140–143.
27. Woodacre T, Dhadwal A, Ball T, Edwards C, Cox PJ. The costs of late detection of developmental dysplasia of the hip. *J Child Orthop*. 2014;8(4):325–332.
28. Arneill M, Cosgrove A, Robinson E. Should closed reduction of the dislocated hip be attempted after failed Pavlik harness treatment in developmental dysplasia of the hip? *Bone Jt Open*. 2021;2(8):584–588. 2021 Aug.
29. Terjesen T, Horn J, Gunderson RB. Fifty-year follow-up of late-detected hip dislocation: clinical and radiographic outcomes for seventy-one patients treated with traction to obtain gradual closed reduction. *J Bone Joint Surg Am*. 2014;96:e28.
30. Harsanyi S, Zamborsky R, Krajciova L, Kokavec M, Danisovic L. Developmental dysplasia of the hip: a review of etiopathogenesis, risk factors, and genetic aspects. *Medicina (Kaunas)*. 2020;56(4):153.
31. Kenanidis E, Gkekas NK, Karasmani A, Anagnostis P, Christofilopoulos P, Tsiridis E. Genetic predisposition to developmental dysplasia of the hip. *J Arthroplasty*. 2020;35(1):291–300. e1.
32. Harsanyi S, Zamborsky R, Kokavec M, Danisovic L. Genetics of developmental dysplasia of the hip. *Eur J Med Genet*. 2020;63(9):103990 2020 Sep.
33. Walker J, Rang M. Habitual hip dislocation in a child. *Clin Pediatr*. 1992;31:562–563.
34. Chan YL, Cheng JCY, Tang APY. Voluntary habitual dislocation of the hip: sonographic diagnosis. *Pediatr Radiol*. 1993;23:147–148.
35. Gaffney JT, Spellman J. Prevalence of hip ultrasound abnormalities in newborns with a hip click. *Clin Pediatr*. 2020;59(8):773–777.

CHAPTER 12

Knee Dislocation (Genu Recurvatum)

KEY POINTS

- Hyperextension of the leg with dislocation at the knee may result from the legs being in an extended posture with breech presentation, oligohydramnios, or other unusual late gestational constraint, and it can also occur in various genetic connective tissue disorders.
- If the tibia is displaced anterior to the long axis of the femur, the knee is considered *dislocated,* but if longitudinal contact is at least partially maintained, it is *subluxed.*
- Treatment depends on the severity of the knee dislocation and the age when treatment begins, with early conservative treatment consisting of serial casting and traction.
- Because congenital hip dislocation is often associated with congenital knee dislocation, it is important to evaluate the hips sonographically, because the dislocated knee needs to be reduced before the hip dislocation is treated.

GENESIS

Hyperextension of the leg with dislocation at the knee may result from the legs being in an extended posture with breech presentation, oligohydramnios, or other unusual late gestational constraint caused by uterine myomas or structural defects. It can also occur in various genetic connective tissue disorders, such as Ehlers-Danlos syndrome, Larsen syndrome, and related *FLNB* disorders, or certain neurological disorders such as arthrogryposis or *PIK3CA*-related overgrowth spectrum. Dislocation of the hips is frequently associated with congenital knee dislocation, and this combination is much more common in females, especially when there is no associated syndrome.[1] It is frequently associated with other musculoskeletal problems, especially dislocation of the hip and clubfoot, so it is prudent to search for an underlying disorder, such as Larsen syndrome or arthrogryposis.[2–5] In a fetus at 22 weeks with bilateral clubfoot, fixed extension of the lower limbs, and internal knee rotation, it can be difficult to distinguish congenital knee dislocation from arthrogryposis.[6,7]

FEATURES

Curvature of the knee is "backward" with an unstable and sometimes dislocated knee (Fig. 12.1). Subclassification (Fig. 12.2) depends on the radiographic relationship between the tibia and the femur: (1) simple hyperextension (or severe genu recurvatum), (2) anterior subluxation, or (3) anterior dislocation. If the tibia is displaced anterior to the long axis of the femur, the knee is considered *dislocated*, but if longitudinal contact is at least partially maintained, it is *subluxed*.[2] Another classification is based on the reduction and stability of the knee: (I) easily reducible, with reduction snap when the femoral condyles pass in flexion, remaining stable in flexion; (II) "recalcitrant" dislocation, reducible by posteroanterior "piston" but unstable, with iterative dislocation once posteroanterior pressure on the condyles is relaxed; and (III) irreducible.[8] In a study by Rampal et al., physical therapy with splinting achieved stable reduction in all type I knees. Five type II knees (31%) required traction, none of which needed surgery. Four type III knees (57%) required surgery. The outcome was good or excellent in 82% of type I knees, good in 68% of type II, and poor in all type III knees.[9] Simple hyperextension exists when there is no displacement of the joint surfaces.[2,10–12] The quadriceps muscle tends to be short, and the distal quadriceps may be relatively fibrotic. These findings were noted as early as 19.5 weeks' gestation in a fetus with bilateral, congenitally dislocated knees, and when compared with age-matched controls, there was also absence of a suprapatellar pouch and incomplete patellofemoral joint cavitation.[13,14] Neither altered muscle/joint pathology nor intrauterine

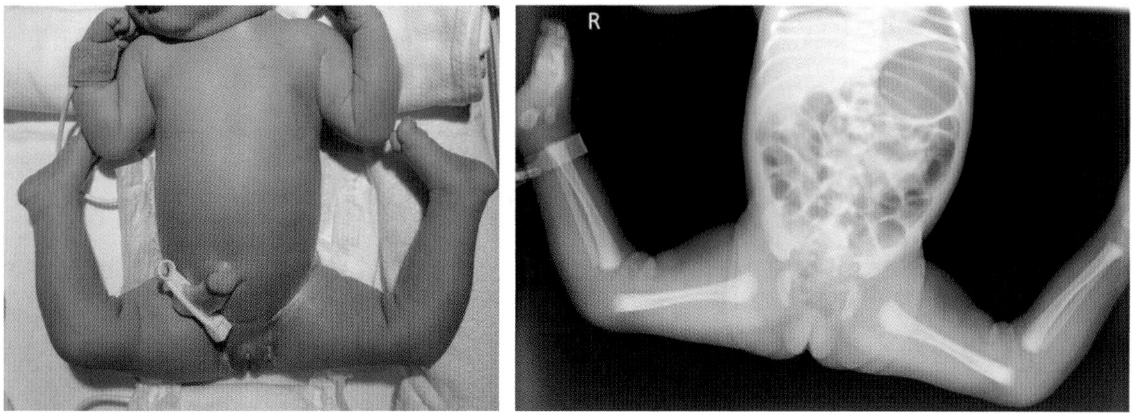

FIGURE 12.1 Hyperextension of the knee joints bilaterally with radiograph showing posterior dislocation of the femurs on the tibias in an otherwise normal female neonate. (From Hirade T, Katsube K, Kato F. Bilateral congenital dislocation of the knee. *J Pediatr.* 2021;229:299-300.)

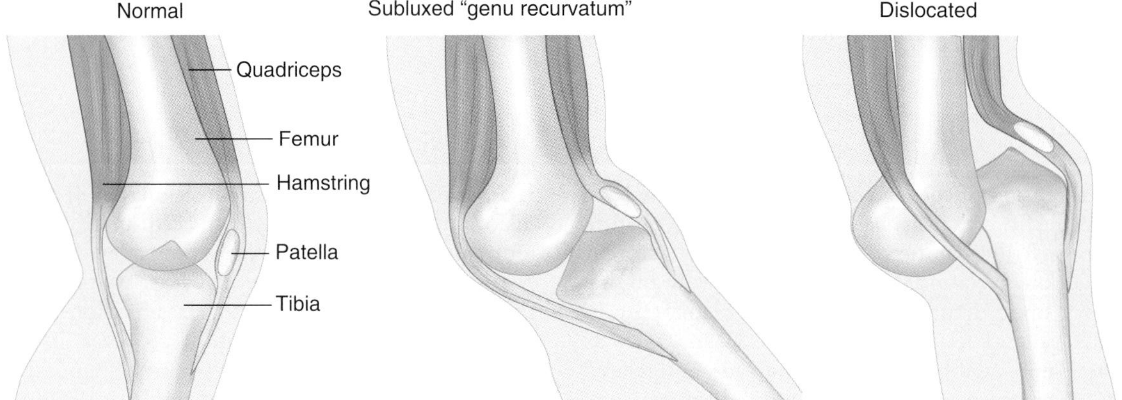

FIGURE 12.2 Normal knee with tissues stretched to the point of being subluxed, also termed *genu recurvatum* (most commonly occurring in prolonged frank breech presentation), and with a dislocated knee. The patella develops as a sesamoid bone in the tendon of the quadriceps muscle. With less tension, the sesamoid bone may be small to absent. (From Clarren SK, Smith DW. Congenital deformities. *Pediatr Clin North Am.* 1977;24:665-677.)

factors explain all cases, and this condition appears to be associated with many different causes. The patella, a sesamoid bone that normally forms in the quadriceps tendon in response to stress, may be small or absent, possibly because of the lack of tension on the quadriceps tendon. Knee dislocation is relatively rare, occurring 1 in 100,000 live births.[15]

MANAGEMENT, PROGNOSIS, AND COUNSEL

Treatment depends on the severity of the knee dislocation and the age when treatment begins, with most authors recommending early conservative treatment consisting of serial casting, leaving surgical treatment for cases in which passive flexion was not achieved above 30 degrees or the conservative treatment failed. In one study, conservative treatment was initiated in all cases, and of the 11 knees treated less than half (36%) required surgery, with good long-term functional results, few complications, and no recurrences.[16] Early traction, manipulation, splinting, and/or serial casting in a corrected position to increase knee flexion may bring about a correction by 8 weeks of age in about 50% of cases, but prompt early treatment is often critical to the success of these measures. For patients with no associated syndrome who are seen within the first 2 days after birth (when high levels of maternal relaxing hormones are still circulating in the neonate and softening the connective tissues), reduction may sometimes be achieved with gentle traction to align the tibia and femur, followed by serial splinting or casting every 2 weeks for 6–8 weeks. After the first 2 days, passive stretching of the quadriceps and anterior knee capsule, combined with serial splinting and casting, may still be successful.[2,15] If these initial measures are not successful, then traction in the prone position for 1–2 weeks may permit closed reduction with or without anesthesia; however, recalcitrant cases usually require quadriceps lengthening with surgical correction of the stretched knee joint capsule and its attachments, with the goal of achieving 90 degrees of flexion intraoperatively.[2,15]

Among 19 neonates with congenital dislocation of the knee, in 6 cases (all females with no associated anomalies) spontaneous reduction was achieved with the application of a simple posterior splint with a fixed degree of knee flexion for a short duration. In four of these patients there were either associated deformations (hip dislocation, foot deformation, or elbow contracture) or fetal constraint resulting from oligohydramnios, uterine myomas, or coiling of the umbilical cord around the affected limb.[1] Cases associated with clubfoot, arthrogryposis, or Larsen syndrome were resistant to such conservative treatment and sometimes required surgery for persistent knee instability. Among 17 patients seen and treated conservatively over a 7-year period, in 5 cases there was immediate reduction within 20 hours of birth; 7 patients seen within 2 days of birth responded to passive stretching of the quadriceps and anterior knee capsule followed by splinting and/or casting; and 5 patients required traction for as long as 26 days, with or without anesthesia, to achieve reduction.[2] The pathoanatomies of congenital knee and hip dislocation are very similar, with soft-tissue contractures becoming more severe if the dislocation is not reduced early; therefore the subluxed or dislocated knee should be treated as early as possible.

Cases with signs of late gestational constraint that reduce spontaneously or with minimal treatment may represent a type of congenital postural deformity produced by abnormal intrauterine posture in late gestation.[1] Because congenital hip dislocation is frequently associated with congenital knee dislocation in more than 50% of cases, it is important to evaluate the hips sonographically, because the dislocated knee needs to be reduced before the hip dislocation is treated.[17] Concurrent treatment of both the knee and hip dislocations with a Pavlik harness has also been successful.[2] Long leg casting has been used to treat concurrent knee and foot deformation after the knee has been reduced. When progressive genu valgus deformity occurs with global instability of the knee resulting from an underlying genetic connective tissue disorder, reconstruction of the medial knee structures with prolonged bracing can provide good results.[2] Recurrence risk is related to whether there is an underlying genetic disorder. Most cases occur sporadically with no prior family history. Because cervical spine instability and/or kyphosis in Larsen syndrome can result in quadriplegia with traction during vaginal delivery, it is recommended that fetuses who are diagnosed prenatally with congenital knee dislocation be delivered by cesarean section.

DIFFERENTIAL DIAGNOSIS

The differential diagnosis is similar to that for dislocation of the hip, but knee dislocation is less likely to occur with neurologic disorders and is especially common in certain genetic connective tissue disorders. The differential diagnosis of associated disorders includes Ellis-van Creveld syndrome, atelosteogenesis (Fig. 12.3), Larsen syndrome (Figs. 12.4 and 12.5),[3,4] Ehlers-Danlos syndrome (Fig. 12.6),[18] *PIK3CA*-related overgrowth syndrome (Fig. 12.7), or arthrogryposis.[6] Ellis-van Creveld is an autosomal recessive form of acromelic-micromelic dwarfism characterized by ectodermal dysplasia, postaxial polydactyly of the hands, and congenital heart disease with significant cardiopulmonary complications. The most significant orthopedic finding is severe and relentlessly progressive valgus deformity of the knees, which is caused by a combination of primary genetic dysplasia of the lateral portion of the tibial plateau combined with severe soft-tissue contractures that tether the tibia into valgus deformations.[19] This progressive valgus deformity is treated by extensive soft-tissue releases, bony osteotomies, and patellar realignment.[20] Knee involvement is very common in patients with arthrogryposis (especially patients with amyoplasia), ranging from soft-tissue contractures (in flexion or hyperextension) to subluxation and dislocation. Flexion contractures are common and disabling, with significant resistance to treatment and increased rates of recurrence. Surgical procedures vary with severity of the contractures and the patient's age, and include soft-tissue

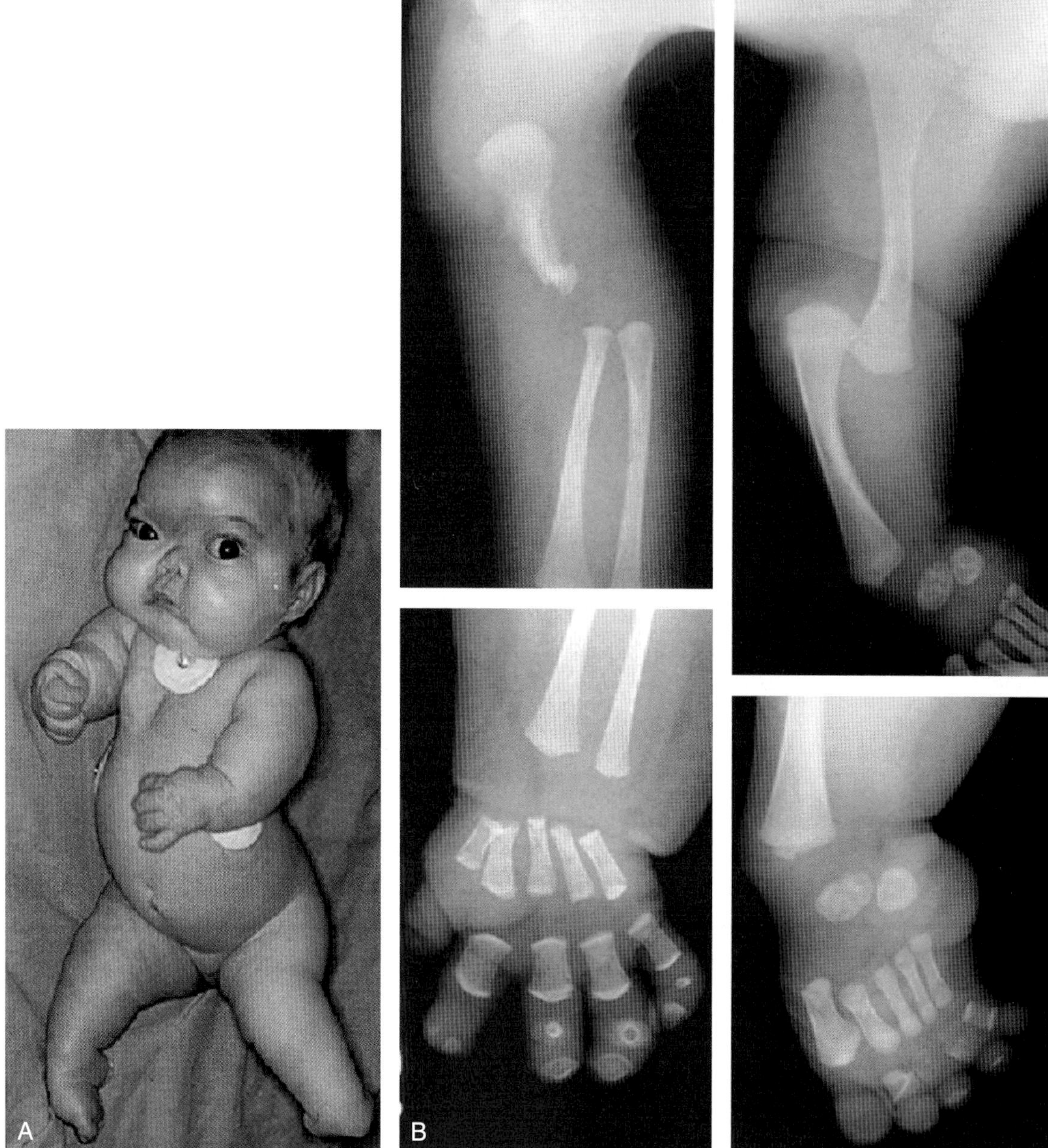

FIGURE 12.3 A, Dislocated knees and elbows in an infant with atelosteogenesis type 3 and a mutation in the *FLNB* gene. B, Radiographs demonstrating dislocations with tapered distal humeri and characteristic hand and foot changes.

releases, femoral shortening-extension osteotomy, and gradual correction with femoral anterior epiphysiodesis. Hyperextension deformities (recurvatum, anterior subluxation, and dislocation) have a better prognosis for walking ability, and surgical options include percutaneous (or mini-open) quadriceps tenotomy, open quadricepsplasty, and femoral shortening osteotomy with limited arthrotomy. Knee dislocations associated with arthrogryposis usually require surgery and should be reduced early.[21] Atraumatic, painful,

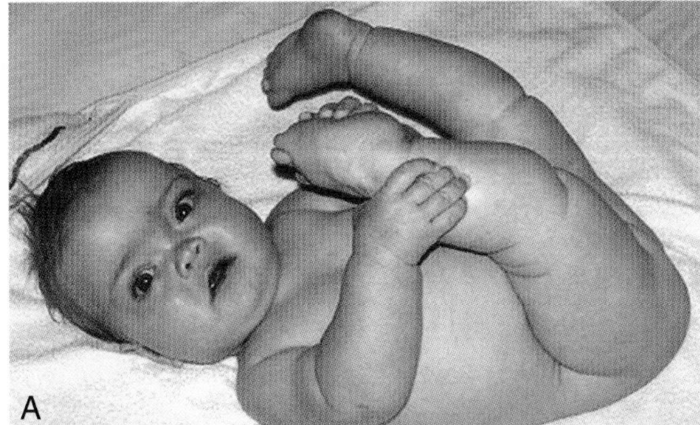

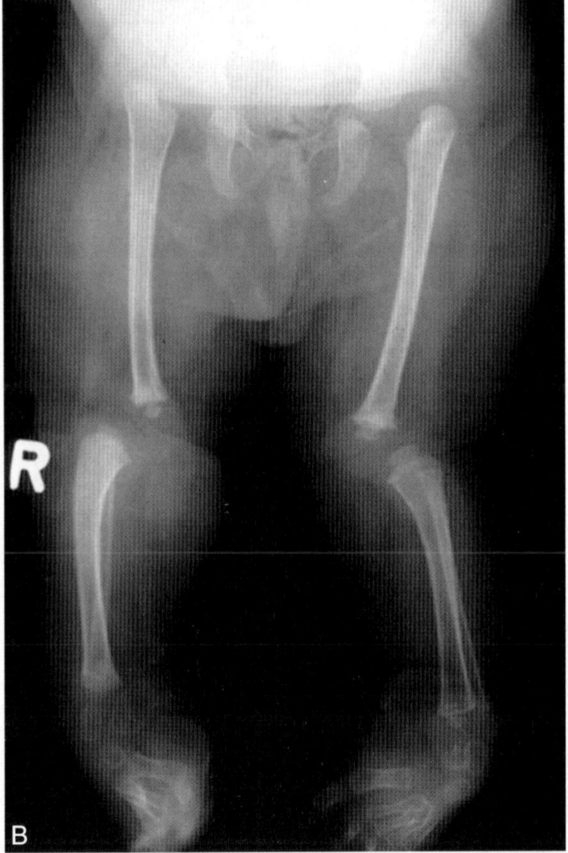

FIGURE 12.4 A-B Multiple joint dislocations in a patient with Larsen syndrome and a mutation in *FLNB*.

recurrent bilateral knee dislocations in an 8-year-old boy were found to be associated with bilateral congenital agenesis of the anterior cruciate ligament (ACL). These were treated with bilateral physeal-sparing ACL reconstructions with an autograft iliotibial band, with no subsequent dislocations during the 14-month follow-up. This appears to be the only reported case of atraumatic spontaneous bilateral knee dislocations in a patient with bilateral congenital absence of the ACL, illustrating a novel indication for physeal-sparing ACL reconstruction in a rare clinical entity.[22]

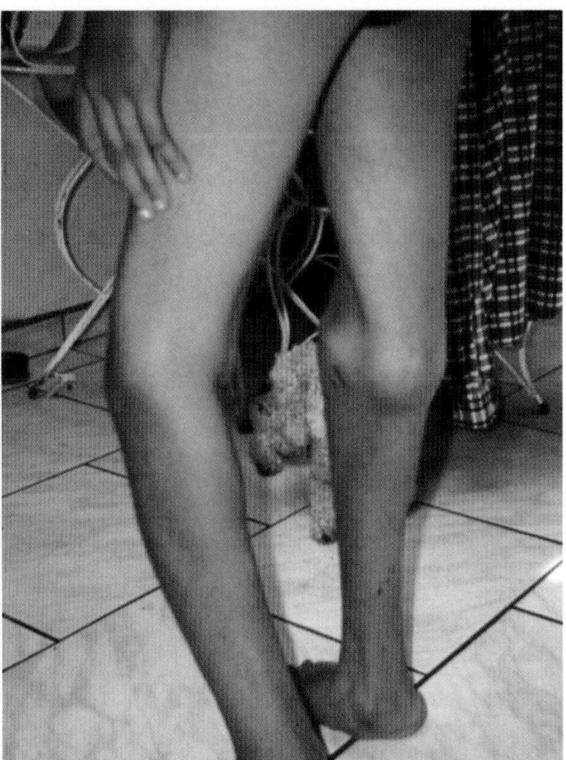

FIGURE 12.5 Genu recurvatum in an older patient with Larsen syndrome.

References

1. Haga N, Nakamura S, Sakaguchi R, et al. Congenital dislocation of the knee reduced spontaneously or with minimal treatment. *J Pediatr Orthop*. 1997;17:59–62.
2. Ko J-Y, Shih C-H, Wenger DR. Congenital dislocation of the knee. *J Pediatr Orthop*. 1999;19:252–259.
3. Matar HE, Garg NK. Management of joint dislocations of the lower limb in Larsen syndrome: practical approach. *Ann R Coll Surg Engl*. 2017;99(1):e8–e10.
4. Hickey SE, Koboldt DC, Mosher TM, et al. Novel in-frame FLNB deletion causes Larsen syndrome in a three-generation pedigree. *Cold Spring Harb Mol Case Stud*. 2019;5(6):a004176.
5. Sehrawat S, Sural S, Sugumar PAA, Khan S, Kar S, Jeyaraman M. Freeman-Sheldon syndrome with stiff knee gait: a case report. *J Orthop Case Rep*. 2021;11(11):64–68.
6. Barreto Mota R, Rodrigues Santos N, Martins R, Soares H. Congenital dislocation of the knee: idiopathic or arthrogryposis? *Cureus*. 2022;14(1):e21684.

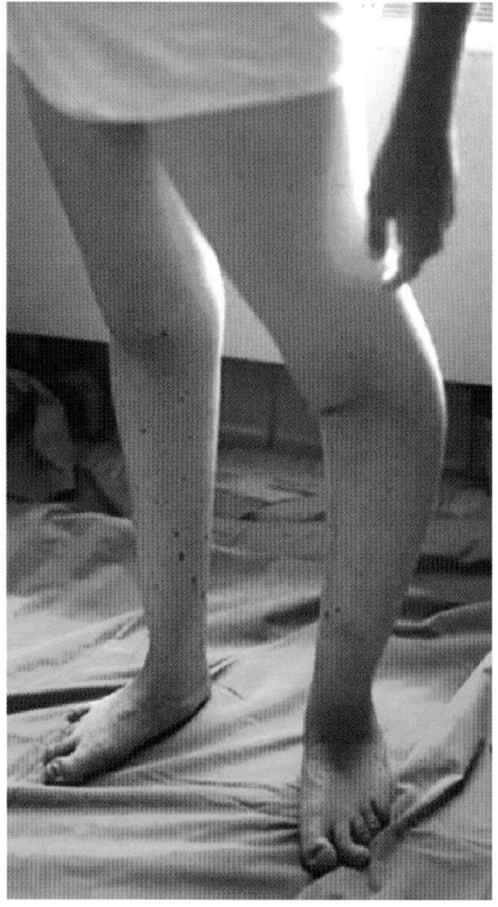

FIGURE 12.6 Genu recurvatum in a patient with Ehlers-Danlos syndrome.

7. Morales-Roselló J, Loscalzo G, Hueso-Villanueva M, Buongiorno S, Jakaitė V, Perales-Marín A. Congenital knee dislocation, case report and review of the literature. *J Matern Fetal Neonatal Med*. 2022;35(4):809–811.
8. Mehrafshan M, Wicart P, Ramanoudjame M, Seringe R, Glorion C, Rampal V. Congenital dislocation of the knee at birth – part I: clinical signs and classification. Orthop Traumatol Surg Res. 2016;102(5):631–633.. *Orthop Traumatol Surg Res*. 2016;102(5):631–633.
9. Rampal V, Mehrafshan M, Ramanoudjame M, Seringe R, Glorion C, Wicart P. Congenital dislocation of the knee at birth – part 2: impact of a new classification on treatment strategies, results and prognostic factors. *Orthop Traumatol Surg Res*. 2016;102(5):635–638.
10. Dasarathy J, Adedipe A, Hawke A. Hyperextension of the bilateral knees in a 1-day-old neonate: no knee fractures or dislocation on x-ray: Dx? *J Fam Pract*. 2019;68(4):E10–E13.
11. Ford B, Burke B, Ainsworth T. Newborn with a hyperextended knee. *Am Fam Physician*. 2018;98(8):535–536.
12. Biswas D, Akter FA, Roy A, Aolad FR, Khan SA. Congenital hyperextension with subluxation of the knees: report of 2 cases. *Mymensingh Med J*. 2014;23(4):811-113.
13. Uthoff HK, Ogata S. Early intrauterine presence of congenital dislocation of the knee *J Pediatr Orthoped*. 141994254–257.
14. Elchalal U, Itzhak IB, Ben-Meir G, et al. Antenatal diagnosis of congenital dislocation of the knee: a case report. *Am J Perinatol*. 1993;10:194–196.
15. Cheng CC, Ko JY. Early reduction for congenital dislocation of the knee within twenty-four hours of birth. *Chang Gung Med J*. 2010;33:266–273.
16. Salvador Marín J, Miranda Gorozarri C, Egea-Gámez RM, Alonso Hernández J, Martínez Álvarez S, Palazón Quevedo Á. Congenital knee dislocation: therapeutic

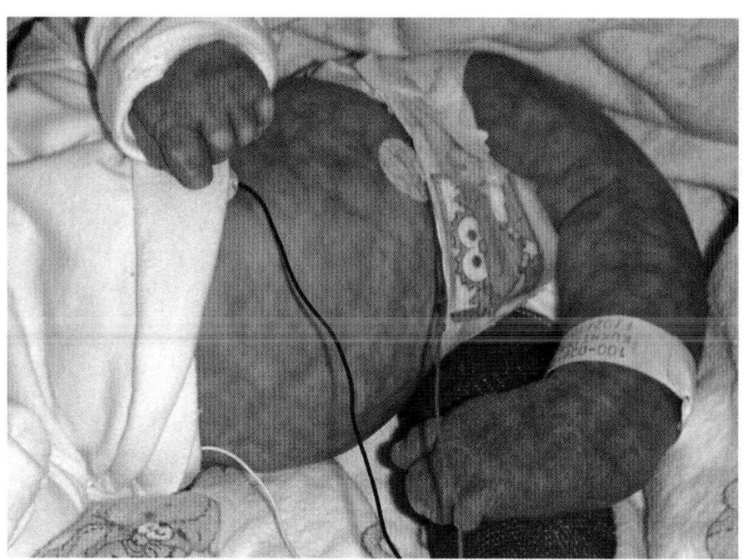

FIGURE 12.7 Genu recurvatum in a patient with postzygotic *PIK3CA* mosaicism and typical extensive cutis marmorata telangiectasia congenita, thick doughy connective tissue, joint laxity, and syndactyly of the second, third, and fourth toes.

protocol and long-term functional results. *Rev Esp Cir Ortop Traumatol (Engl Ed)*. 2021;65(3):172–179.

17. B K AR, Singh KA, Shah H. Surgical management of the congenital dislocation of the knee and hip in children presented after six months of age. *Int Orthop*. 2020;44(12):2635–2644.
18. Homere A, Bolia IK, Juhan T, Weber AE, Hatch GF. Surgical management of shoulder and knee instability in patients with Ehlers-Danlos syndrome: joint hypermobility syndrome. *Clin Orthop Surg*. 2020;12(3):279–285.
19. Weiner DS, Jonah D, Leighley B, et al. Orthopaedic manifestations of chondroectodermal dysplasia: the Ellis-van Creveld syndrome. *J Child Orthop*. 2013;7:465–476.
20. Weiner DS, Tank JC, Jonah D, et al. An operative approach to address severe genu valgum deformity in the Ellis-van Creveld syndrome. *J Child Orthop*. 2014;8:61–69.
21. Lampasi M, Antonioli D, Donzelli O. Management of knee deformities in children with arthrogryposis. *Musculoskelet Surg*. 2012;96:161–169.
22. Moreland CM, Flanagan JC, Christino MA. Bilateral recurrent, atraumatic anterior knee dislocations in a pediatric patient with congenital absence of the anterior cruciate ligament. *J Am Acad Orthop Surg Glob Res Rev*. 2020;4(11):e20 00078.

CHAPTER 13

Dislocation of the Radial Head

KEY POINTS

- Dislocation of the radial head is the most common congenital anomaly of the elbow.
- The direction of bowing of the ulna depends on the type of dislocation of the radial head, and if an abnormal position is initiated by one of the bones of the forearm, the other bone will bend accordingly as it grows.
- Most patients are asymptomatic and treated with observation and monitoring as needed for symptoms.

GENESIS

Dislocation of the radial head is the most common congenital anomaly of the elbow, but it is relatively rare, accounting for 0.15–0.2% of outpatient orthopedic visits.[1–3] It can occur as an isolated abnormality or as part of several different syndromes. The presence of associated anomalies and bilateral involvement suggests a congenital joint dislocation syndrome. Some authors believe that many unilateral cases might be attributed to low-energy greenstick fractures of the ulna, which may result in radial head dislocation as the forearm shortens (eponym Monteggia fracture). These can be relatively benign in appearance with transient mild symptoms that are initially unnoticed by parents and clinicians.[4] Acutely, the traumatically dislocated radial head will still look like a cup (concave) while the chronically dislocated radial head will look round (convex). Over time, however, the acute radial head will round the longer it is dislocated, and eventually it becomes more difficult to distinguish radiographically between congenital dislocation and late post-traumatic cases,[5] so the genesis of many isolated cases is seldom understood.

Radial head dislocation can be associated with radioulnar synostosis, antecubital pterygia, distal hand and limb anomalies, congenital hip dislocation, extra X chromosomes, syndromes resulting from collagen abnormalities, abnormal endochondral ossification of the developing growth plate, abnormalities of forearm ossification outside the growth plate, disproportionate growth of the radius and ulna, and altered HOXD expression or activity, as well as arthrogryposis, Larsen syndrome, Ehlers-Danlos syndrome, occipital horn syndrome (X-linked cutis laxa), multiple exostosis, nail-patella syndrome, cleidocranial dysplasia, surviving camptomelic dysplasia, atelosteogenesis, small patella syndrome, and craniofacial dysostosis.[1,3,6–8]

Bilateral congenital posterior dislocation of the radial heads without other anomalies can also be inherited as an autosomal dominant trait.[9] Vertical transmission within a consanguineous family could be caused by autosomal recessive inheritance, but most isolated hereditary cases appear to manifest autosomal dominant inheritance. Acromesomelic dysplasia type Maroteaux is an autosomal recessive disorder characterized by severe short stature, shortened middle and distal segments of the limbs, redundant skin of fingers, radial head subluxation or dislocation, large great toes and cranium, and normal intelligence. This condition is caused by autosomal loss-of-function variants in the natriuretic peptide receptor B (*NPRB* or *NPR2*), which is involved in endochondral ossification and longitudinal growth of limbs and vertebrae.[10] The combination of short stature, congenital dislocation of the hip, carpal coalition, dislocation of the radial head, cavus deformity, scoliosis, hearing loss, eye defects, and vertebral anomalies was first described in 1993 by Steel in 23 children from Puerto Rico. Steel syndrome is caused by autosomal recessive mutations in *COL27A1*.[11] Posterolateral dislocation of the proximal head of the radius results in the inability to fully supinate at the elbow and some limitation in extension (Fig. 13.1). It generally gives rise to little disability and is seldom treated. Anterior and lateral dislocations are less frequent forms of presentation than posterior dislocation; however, this form is the most frequent congenital pathology of the elbow in children.[8]

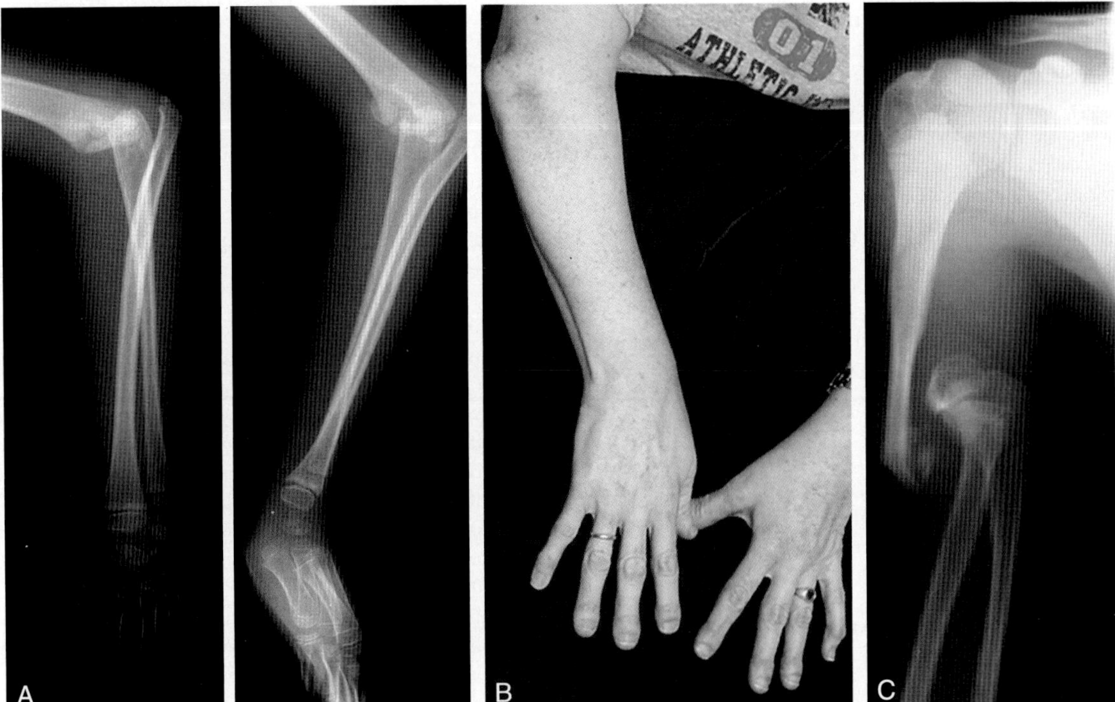

FIGURE 13.1 A, Dislocated radial heads in a child with Larsen syndrome. B and C, Dislocated radial heads in an adult with Larsen syndrome and a mutation in *FLNB*. Note the protrusion of the radial head with long cylindric fingers and broad thumbs.

FEATURES

The family or child will typically observe a bump on the lateral, posterior, or anterior elbow with some limitation to elbow flexion, extension, or supination/pronation movement. Some radial head dislocations result in popping or snapping around the elbow with movement. The direction of bowing of the ulna depends on the type of dislocation of the radial head, and if an abnormal position is initiated by one of the bones of the forearm, the other bone will bend accordingly as it grows (see Fig. 13.1). Therefore in unreduced congenital anterior dislocation of the radial head, the ulna bends forward. In posterior dislocation, it bends backward, and in lateral dislocation, the ulna bends laterally.[5] Radiographic criteria suggesting congenital anterior dislocation includes a hypoplastic or absent capitellum, dome-shaped radial head with a long neck, and a long radius in relation to the ulna.[12] Additional findings that suggest a congenital etiology include bilateral involvement, presence of associated anomalies, familial occurrence, no history of trauma, and dislocation noted at birth.[2] Progression from subluxation to dislocation has been observed, and most patients have no pain and minimal functional limitations during childhood.

MANAGEMENT, PROGNOSIS, AND COUNSEL

Most patients are asymptomatic and treated with observation and monitoring as needed for symptoms. Some untreated patients experience pain, progressive limitation in movement, and prominence of the radial head during adulthood (see Fig. 13.1B–C), in which case radial head excision can alleviate pain and improve appearance but seldom increases movement and risks proximal migration of the radius with interosseous ligament instability and subsequent wrist deformity.[2] In a comparison of 10 patients treated surgically and 6 patients followed without surgery, radial head excision in patients with symptomatic, isolated, congenital radial head dislocations resulted in substantial pain relief and patient satisfaction but modest improvement in forearm rotation and no improvement in elbow flexion-extension; however, more than 25% of the surgically treated limbs developed wrist pain and needed additional surgery. The nonsurgical group did not lose motion, develop pain, or need surgery.[13] Other surgical options are relocation with corrective osteotomies of the ulna[14–16] and salvage one-bone forearm surgeries.[17,18]

Many syndromic cases and those with isolated bilateral involvement are inherited in an autosomal dominant fashion. When radial head dislocation occurs in association with congenital hip dislocation, marked joint hypermobility, and lax redundant skin in a male, the diagnosis of X-linked cutis laxa (occipital horn syndrome) should be considered. When radial head dislocation occurs with patellar hypoplasia and decreased pubic ossification, surviving camptomelic dysplasia or small patella syndrome should be considered. When there are multiple joint dislocations at birth in addition to a flat midface, cleft palate, and broad thumbs with cylindrical fingers, Larsen syndrome should be considered (see Fig. 13.1).[19]

DIFFERENTIAL DIAGNOSIS

Radial head dislocation, which is associated with congenital synostosis of the upper end of the radius, should be considered part of radioulnar synostosis and not a true dislocation. Congenital radioulnar synostosis is caused by defective longitudinal segmentation that results in persistent interzonal mesenchyme between the proximal radius and ulna, which later becomes ossified, resulting in marked limitation of pronation, supination, and extension. Some cases of Erb's palsy result in subluxation of the radial head because of muscle imbalance, but this is not true dislocation.[20]

References

1. Almquist EE, Gordon LH, Blue AI. Congenital dislocation of the head of the radius. *J Bone Joint Surg Am.* 1969;51:1118–1127.
2. Mardam-Bey T, Ger E. Congenital radial head dislocation. *J Hand Surg.* 1979;4:316–320.
3. Agnew DK, Davis RJ. Congenital unilateral dislocation of the radial head. *J Pediatr Orthoped.* 1993;13:526–528.
4. Lloyd-Roberts GC, Bucknill TM. Anterior dislocation of the radial head in children. *J Bone Joint Surg Br.* 1977;59:402–407.
5. Caravias DE. Some observations on congenital dislocation of the head of the radius. *J Bone Joint Surg Br.* 1957;39:86–90.
6. Bongers EM, Van Bokhoven H, Van Thienen MN, et al. The small patella syndrome: description of five cases from three families and examination of possible allelism with familial patella aplasia-hypoplasia and nail-patella syndrome. *J Med Genet.* 2001;38:209–213.
7. Mansour S, Offiah AC, McDowall S, et al. The phenotype of survivors of camptomelic dysplasia. *J Med Genet.* 2002;39:597–602.
8. Al-Qattan MM, Abou Al-Shaar H, Alkattan WM. The pathogenesis of congenital radial head dislocation/subluxation. *Gene.* 2016;586(1):69–76.
9. Reichenbach H, Hörmann D, Theile H. Hereditary congenital posterior dislocation of radial heads. *Am J Med Genet.* 1995;55:101–104.
10. Simsek-Kiper PO, Urel-Demir G, Taskiran EZ, et al. Further defining the clinical and molecular spectrum of acromesomelic dysplasia type Maroteaux: a Turkish tertiary center experience. *J Hum Genet.* 2021;66(6):585–596.
11. Pölsler L, Schatz UA, Simma B, Zschocke J, Rudnik-Schöneborn S. A Syrian patient with Steel syndrome due to compound heterozygous *COL27A1* mutations with colobomata of the eye. *Am J Med Genet A.* 2020;182(4):730–734.
12. Abe M, Kumano H, Kinoshita A, Yokota A, Ohno K. Idiopathic anterior dislocation of the radial head: symptoms, radiographic findings, and management of 8 patients. *J Shoulder Elbow Surg.* 2019;28(8):1468–1475.
13. Bengard MJ, Calfee RP, Steffen JA, et al. Intermediate-term to long-term outcome of surgically and nonsurgically treated congenital, isolated radial head dislocation. *J Hand Surg Am.* 2012;37:2495–2501.
14. Liu R, Miao W, Mu M, Wu G, Qu J, Wu Y. Ulnar rotation osteotomy for congenital radial head dislocation. *J Hand Surg Am.* 2015;40(9):1769–1775.
15. Jie Q, Liang X, Wang X, Wu Y, Wu G, Wang B. Double ulnar osteomy for the treatment of congenital radial head dislocation. *Acta Orthop Traumatol Turc.* 2019;53(6):442–447.
16. Tsumura T, Matsumoto T, Matsushita M, Kishimoto K, Murase T, Shiode H. A three-step method for the treatment of radioulnar synostosis with posterior radial head dislocation. *J Hand Surg Asian Pac.* 2021;26(1):118–125.
17. Gogoi P, Dutta A, Sipani AK, Daolagupu AK. Congenital deficiency of distal ulna and dislocation of the radial head treated by single bone forearm procedure. *Case Rep Orthop.* 2014:526719 2014, Article ID.
18. Wang KK, Vuillermin CB, Waters PM. Single-bone forearm as a salvage procedure in recalcitrant pediatric forearm pathologies. *J Hand Surg Am.* 2020;45(10):947–956.
19. Krakow D, Robertson SP, King LM, et al. Mutations in the gene encoding filamin B disrupt vertebral segmentation, joint formation and skeletogenesis. *Nature Genetics.* 2004;36(4):405–410.
20. McFarland B. Congenital dislocation of the head of the radius. *Br J Surg.* 1936;24:41–49.

Section V
Neurapraxias (Palsies)

CHAPTER 14

Facial Palsy

KEY POINTS

- Traumatic facial nerve palsy has been associated with birth weight greater than 3500 g, forceps-assisted deliveries, and prematurity.
- When facial nerve paralysis is of developmental origin, it may be part of a broader pattern of altered morphogenesis.
- Facial paralysis with associated distal limb deficiency has been seen after early chorion villus sampling, failed dilation and curettage, maternal use of either thalidomide or misoprostol after the first trimester, and maternal hyperthermia during the first trimester, suggesting it may be a manifestation of brainstem disturbances during the first trimester.
- Facial nerve palsy is usually unilateral, and decreased movement on the side of the palsy occurs with facial animation.
- The surgical treatment of facial paralysis consists of staged techniques using autologous muscle or tendon transplantation to the paralyzed side of the face or reanimation procedures using regional muscle transfers and nerve crossovers.

GENESIS

Prolonged compression or stretching of a peripheral nerve may lead to compression palsy, apparently because of neural ischemia. Developmental congenital unilateral facial palsy has an estimated incidence of 2.1 per 1000.[1] The mechanism of injury is usually either direct trauma from delivery or compression of the side of the face and nerve against the sacral promontory, with the side of the injured facial nerve usually corresponding with the side of the fetal face that was lying against the maternal sacrum during delivery. The facial nerve exits the skull through the stylomastoid foramen behind the ear, where it is protected by the mastoid bone, and then travels to the parotid gland, where it divides and sends branches to all the muscles of the face. Direct compression may occur behind the ear or over the parotid region, although both the maternal sacral promontory and fetal shoulder can also cause intrauterine nerve compression. Traumatic cases are usually unilateral and present with weakness of the frontalis, orbicularis oculi, buccinator, orbicularis oris, and platysma. There may be a history of prolonged or difficult labor or forceps delivery, or evidence of periauricular ecchymoses or hemotympanum. Traumatic facial nerve palsy has been associated with birth weight greater than 3500 g, forceps-assisted deliveries, and prematurity.[2,3]

Congenital facial nerve paralysis is generally considered to be of either developmental or traumatic origin. When facial nerve paralysis is of developmental origin, it may be part of a broader pattern of altered morphogenesis, such as Möbius sequence (Fig. 14.1), oculoauriculovertebral sequence (hemifacial microsomia) (Fig. 14.2), or CHARGE syndrome (coloboma, heart disease, atresia choanae, retarded growth and development, and/or central nervous system anomalies, genital hypoplasia, and ear anomalies and/or deafness) (Fig. 14.3).[4,5] In oculoauriculovertebral sequence there is unilateral microtia with conductive deafness and varying degrees of jaw hypoplasia, ocular dermoids, and cervical vertebral abnormalities.[4] CHARGE syndrome can be associated with other cranial nerve deficits, ocular colobomata, choanal atresia, dysplastic ears with sensorineural deafness, hypoplasia of the cochlea and semicircular canals, heart defects, and hypogonadotropic hypogonadism.[5] Of importance to surgeons doing free functional muscle transfers to reanimate the face, facial vessel agenesis is more common in syndromic congenital facial palsy than in those with isolated congenital facial palsy.[6]

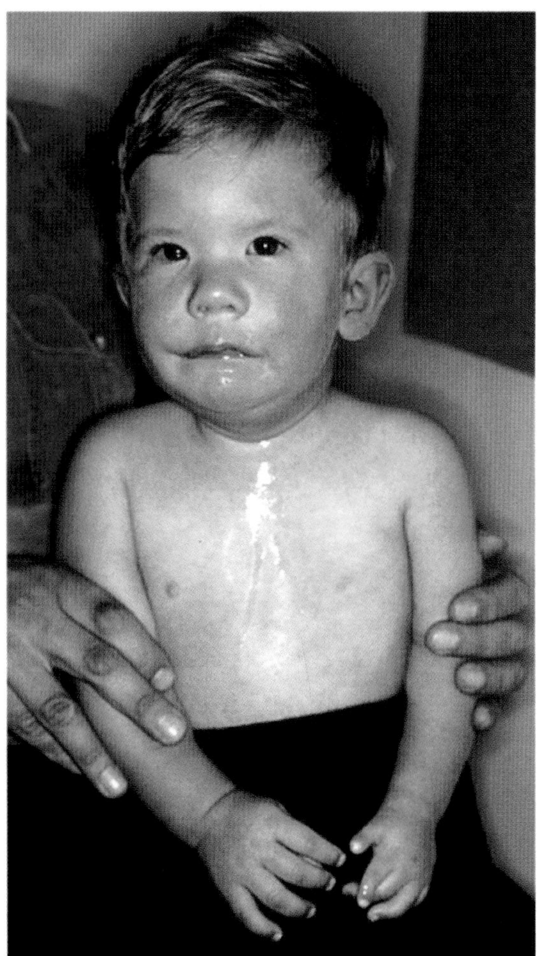

FIGURE 14.1 Möbius sequence with associated absent left pectoralis muscle and hypoplastic left hand (Poland sequence) in a child whose mother had a prolonged high fever toward the end of the first trimester.

Facial paralysis with associated distal limb deficiency has been seen after early chorion villus sampling, failed dilation and curettage, maternal use of either thalidomide or misoprostol after the first trimester, and maternal hyperthermia during the first trimester, suggesting it may be a manifestation of brainstem disturbances during the first trimester.[7-9] Congenital facial paralysis of traumatic etiology in otherwise normal children accounts for 8–25% of all facial nerve palsies occurring in the pediatric population, and it requires a systematic evaluation to exclude other syndromic associated anomalies, particularly those affecting vision and hearing. Among 118 cases of aural atresia (see Fig. 14.2), facial nerve anomalies were present in 13%, and inner ear anomalies were present in 22%.[10]

FEATURES

Facial nerve palsy is usually unilateral, and decreased movement on the side of the palsy occurs with facial animation (Fig. 14.4). At rest, the affected side has decreased forehead wrinkling, increased eye opening (resulting in the inability to close the eye, with resultant corneal drying and irritation), a decreased nasolabial fold, and flattening of the corner of the mouth. With motion, unilateral facial palsy results in an asymmetrical crying face or an asymmetrical smile. Congenital facial palsy may be caused by external/environmental factors present before birth or due to a developmental syndrome or genetic defect. The most common external factor is birth trauma or prenatal compression. Congenital facial palsy caused by birth trauma is mostly transient and usually resolves within 2 years. Facial palsy caused by a developmental defect has a less favorable prognosis. Other external causal factors are prenatal infections, vascular injury, or exposure to teratogens. Associated features in congenital facial palsy can include vessel agenesis and facial nerve agenesis/hypogenesis on the affected side detected by vascular studies, magnetic resonance imaging, and electrodiagnostic studies.[1,6] In central facial palsy, the lesion is located along the corticobulbar tract affecting the upper and lower motor neurons, thereby leaving the dorsal division of the lower motor neurons intact. This causes contralateral facial muscle weakness of the lower part of the face while preserving forehead muscle function. Peripheral facial palsy results from a lesion in the brainstem or more distally along the course of the facial nerve in the middle ear or face, resulting in ipsilateral muscle weakness of both the upper and lower part of the face. There may be a variable clinical picture resulting in facial asymmetry, lagophthalmos, hyperacusis, change in taste (first two-thirds of the tongue), or increased tear production.

Facial nerve palsy has an age-dependent incidence of 2.7 per 100,000 in children under the age of 10 years, and 10.1 per 100,000 in children over age 10 years.[11] The causes of facial nerve palsy can broadly be classified into congenital or acquired, and etiology is unknown in 50–80% of cases (idiopathic facial nerve palsy is known as Bell's palsy).[12] Bilateral facial nerve paralysis is present in Moebius syndrome, with

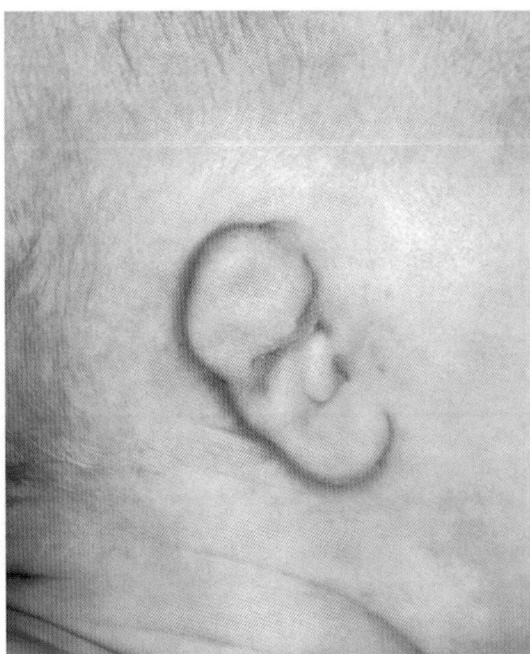

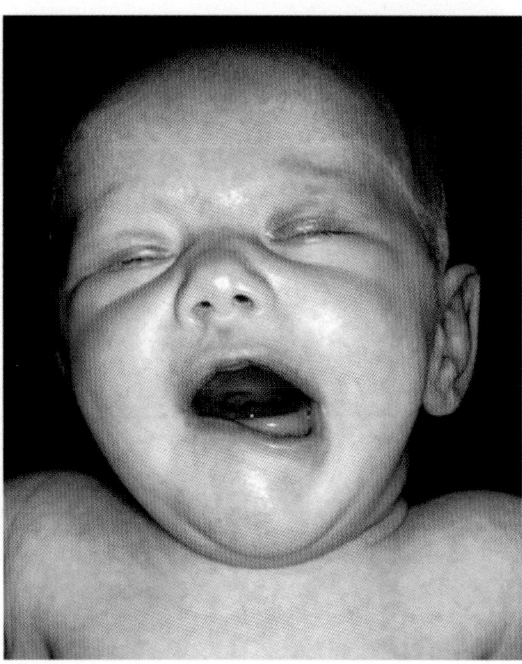

FIGURE 14.2 Right facial nerve palsy in a child with oculoauriculovertebral sequence.

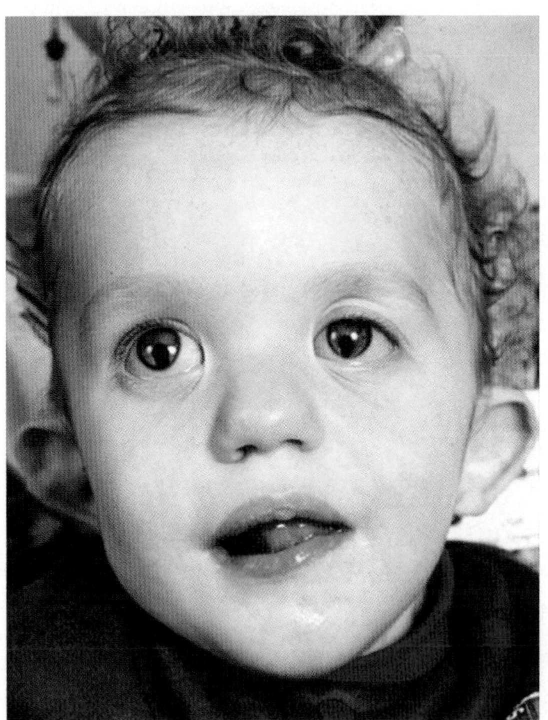

FIGURE 14.3 Child with CHARGE syndrome with right facial weakness, dysplastic ears, and bilateral iris colobomata. This condition is caused by mutations in*CHD7*.

associated palsies of the 6th, 9th, 10th, and 12th cranial nerves. The prevalence of this condition is 1 in 150,000 live births, and the cause remains unknown.[11] One report described a missense mutation in *LMX1A* in a patient with Moebius syndrome.[13]

MANAGEMENT AND PROGNOSIS

Immediate management of facial palsy is usually not necessary, although a careful clinical evaluation should be performed to search for other anomalies.[12] Periauricular bruising or lacerations should heighten the suspicion of facial nerve trauma. Electrophysiologic testing (electroneuronography), whereby the facial nerve is stimulated transdermally near the stylomastoid foramen, can help provide objective assessment of facial nerve function and differentiate Moebius syndrome and other congenital facial weakness disorders.[14] The quantity of nerve deficit parallels the muscle deficit in developmental paralysis, whereas in traumatic cases the nerve may be injured although the muscle is spared. Hereditary congenital facial palsy without ocular muscle weakness has been reported as an autosomal dominant trait in two large Dutch families with defined loci (HCPF1 on 3q21.2-q22.1 and HCFP2 on 10q21.3-q22.1).[15] A third type of hereditary

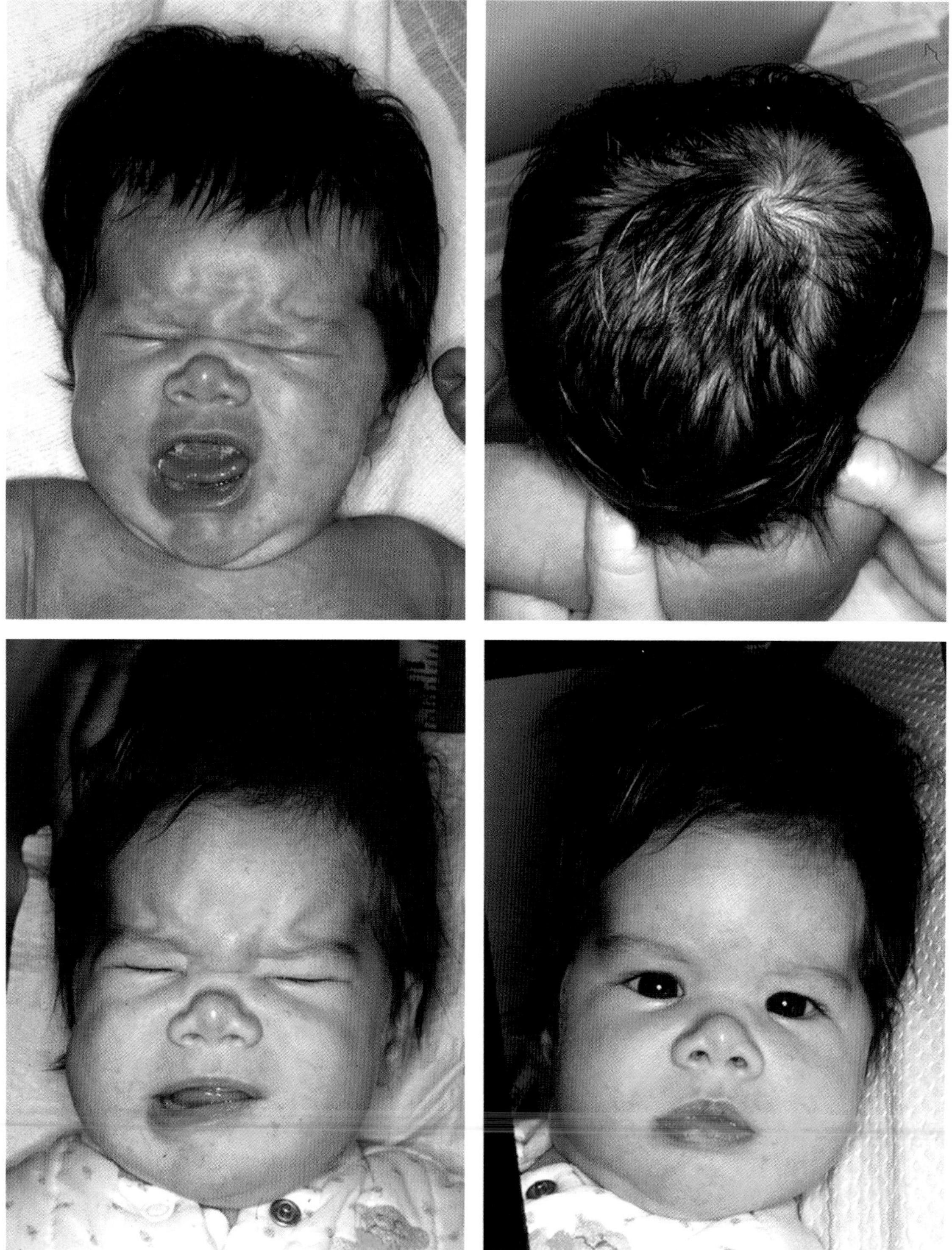

FIGURE 14.4 Child with right lower facial nerve palsy with right facial droop and associated traumatic right parietal cephalohematoma.

congenital facial palsy has been associated with autosomal recessive homozygous mutations in *HOXB1* on 7q21.[16,17] An autosomal dominant syndrome associated with congenital facial palsy, ptosis, and velopharyngeal dysfunction is caused by heterozygous mutations of *TUBB6* on 18p11.[18] Individuals with a specific heterozygous mutation in *TUBB3* (R262H) have a syndrome that includes congenital fibrosis of the extraocular muscles type 3 (CFEOM3), facial palsy, joint contractures, and early-onset peripheral neuropathy.[19]

Congenital unilateral lower lip palsy (also termed asymmetric crying facies) is a congenital facial asymmetry in which one corner of the mouth does not dip downward symmetrically. Electrophysiologic findings in 20 patients suggested that each of the facial nerve branches, including the marginal mandibular branch, functioned normally.[20] This condition results from unilateral agenesis or hypoplasia of the depressor anguli oris muscle, which originates from the mandible and extends to the angle of the mouth. It is mainly innervated by two facial nerve branches, the buccal and the mandibular branch, and it depresses the lower corner of the mouth and pulls it laterally. In cases of hypoplasia/agenesis of the depressor angularis oris muscle, no mouth/lip movement is seen on the hypoplasia side, while the corner of the mouth is pulled downward on the normal side. This diagnosis should be considered in a baby with an asymmetric crying face if the face is completely normal at rest with deviation of the angle of the mouth on crying which disappears on rest.[21,22] Some cases associated with heart defects, bifid uvula, and developmental delay have 22q11.2 deletion syndrome.

When associated limb reduction defects are present, a teratogenic etiology seems more likely than a genetic defect. In developmental cases, temporal bone computed tomography and brainstem auditory evoked-response testing can evaluate the middle ear, inner ear, and semicircular canals for associated anatomic and functional problems, particularly in the case of CHARGE syndrome caused by mutations in *CHD7*, or oculoauriculovertebral sequence. When facial nerve compression has occurred in late gestation or during delivery, there is usually a full return of function within a matter of days to weeks because the injury does not usually disrupt the axon. Spontaneous recovery occurs within 4 weeks in 90% of traumatic congenital facial paralysis cases.[23] Adequate eye care to prevent exposure keratitis is important and consists of taping the eyelid shut and frequently applying artificial tears until the nerve recovers. With developmental facial palsy, the eyelid may need to be partially closed surgically. The surgical treatment of facial paralysis consists of staged techniques using autologous muscle or tendon transplantation to the paralyzed side of the face or reanimation procedures using regional muscle transfers and nerve crossovers (Figs. 14.5 and 14.6).[24,25] These operations are generally not done until early school age, when the child can actively participate in and understand the necessary postoperative physical therapy exercises.

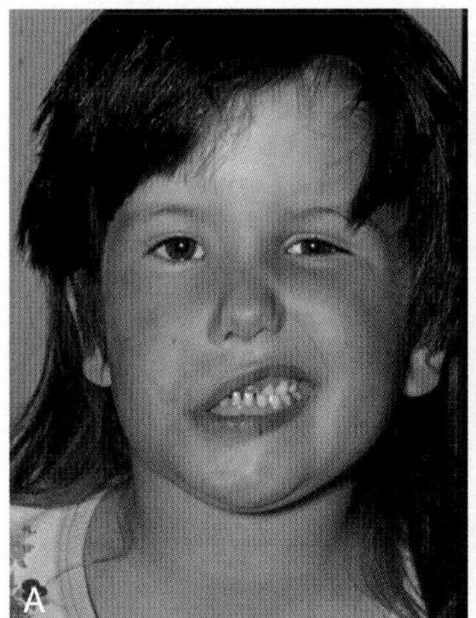

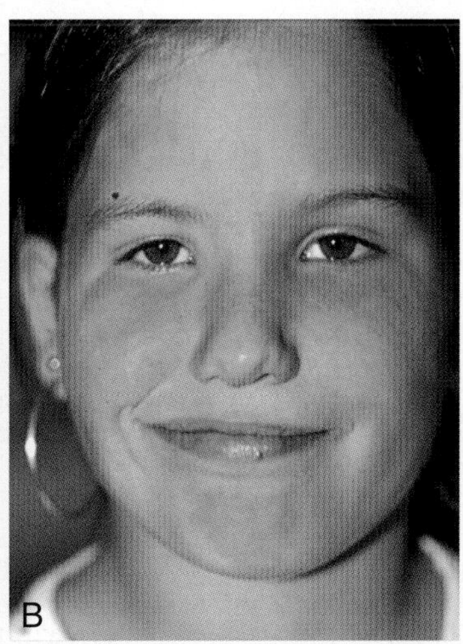

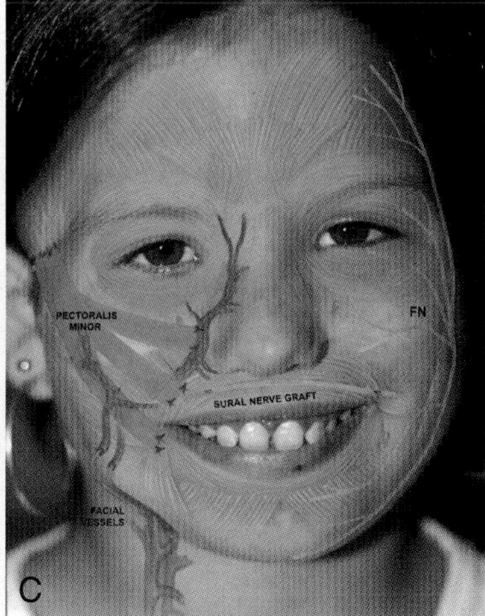

FIGURE 14.5 **A,** Preoperative view of a 10-year-old girl with paralysis of the cervicofacial branch of the facial nerve. **B,** Five months post-op: two-stage reconstruction with craniofacial nerve graft, followed by a free pectoralis minor muscle transfer. **C,** 24 months post-op: smiling. (From Gasteratos K, Azzawi SA, Vlachopoulos N, Lese I, Spyropoulou GA, Grobbelaar AO. Workhorse free functional muscle transfer techniques for smile reanimation in children with congenital facial palsy: case report and systematic review of the literature. *J Plast Reconstr Aesthet Surg*. 2021;74:1423-1435; photograph edited by Manolis Babatsikos.)

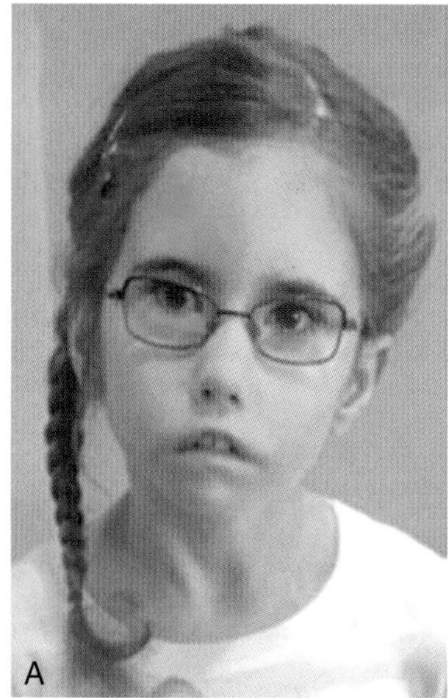

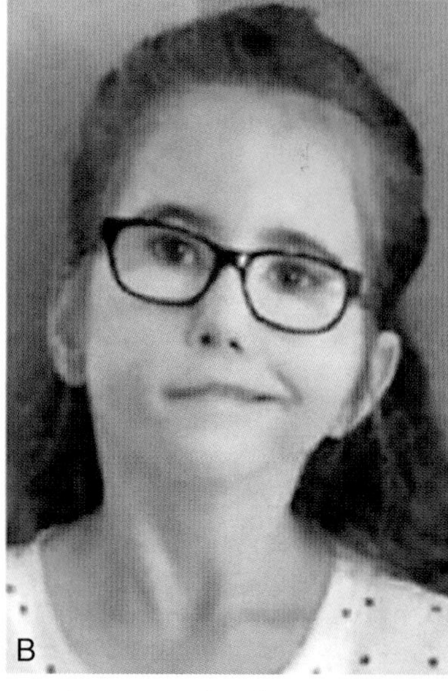

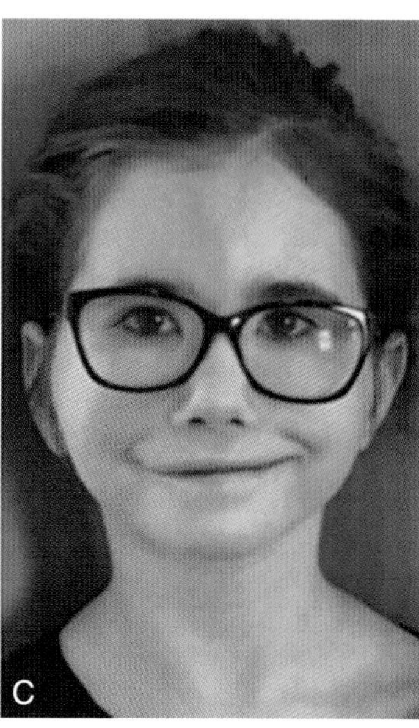

FIGURE 14.6 **A,** Patient with Möbius syndrome in attempted smile preoperatively, **B,** after first-stage left gracilis transfer to the masseteric nerve, and **C,** after second-stage right gracilis transfer to the masseteric nerve. (From Domeshek LF, Zuker RM, Borschel GH. Management of bilateral facial palsy. *Otolaryngol Clin North Am*. 2018;51(6):1213-1226.)

References

1. Decraene L, Boudewyns A, Venstermans C, Ceulemans B. Developmental unilateral facial palsy in a newborn: six cases and literature review. *Eur J Pediatr*. 2020;179(3):367–375.
2. Falco NA, Ericksson E. Facial nerve palsy in the newborn: incidence and outcome. *Plast Reconstr Surg*. 1986;85:1–4.
3. Towner D, Castro MA, Eby-Wilkens E, et al. Effect of mode of delivery in nulliparous women on neonatal intracranial injury. *N Engl J Med*. 1999;341:1709–1714.
4. Carvalho GJ, Song CS, Vargervik K, et al. Auditory and facial nerve dysfunction in patients with hemifacial microsomia. *Arch Otolaryngol Head Neck Surg*. 1999;125:209–212.
5. Graham Jr JM. A recognizable syndrome within CHARGE association: Hall-Hittner syndrome [editorial comment]. *Am J Med Genet*. 2001;99:120–123.
6. Butler DP, Henry FP, Leckenby JI, Grobbelaar AO. The incidence of facial vessel agenesis in patients with syndromic congenital facial palsy. *Plast Reconstr Surg*. 2014;134(6):955e–958e.
7. Pastuszak AL, Schuler L, Speck-Martins CE, et al. Use of misoprostol during pregnancy and Möbius syndrome in infants. *N Engl J Med*. 1998;338:1881–1885.
8. Grundfast KM, Guarisco JL, Thornsen JR, et al. Diverse etiologies of facial paralysis in children. *Int J Pediatr Otorhinolaryngol*. 1990;19:223–229.
9. Graham Jr JM, Edwards MJ, Edwards MJ. Teratogen update: gestational effects of maternal hyperthermia due to febrile illnesses and resultant patterns of defects in humans. *Teratology*. 1998;58:209–221.
10. Dhandayutham S, Damam NK, Gomez TH, Sasidharan M, Sathees C. Facial nerve anomalies as an obscure co-occurrence with external ear malformations: a case report. *Cureus*. 2022;14(7):e26907.
11. Malik M, Cubitt JJ. Paediatric facial paralysis: an overview and insights into management. *J Paediatr Child Health*. 2021;57(6):786–790.
12. Yılmaz U, Cubukçu D, Yılmaz TS, Akıncı G, Ozcan M, Güzel O. Peripheral facial palsy in children. *J Child Neurol*. 2014 Nov;29(11):1473–1478.
13. Alnefaie GO. A Missense mutation in *LMX1A* in a patient with moebius syndrome: a case report. *Cureus*. 2022;14(10):e30127.
14. Lehky T, Joseph R, Toro C, et al. Moebius Syndrome Research Consortium. Differentiating Moebius syndrome and other congenital facial weakness disorders with electrodiagnostic studies. *Muscle Nerve*. 2021;63(4):516–524.
15. Michielse CB, Bhat M, Brady A, et al. Refinement of the locus for hereditary congenital facial palsy on chromosome 3q21 in two unrelated families and screening of positional candidate genes. *Eur J Hum Genet*. 2006;14(12):1306–1312.
16. Vogel M, Velleuer E, Schmidt-Jiménez LF, et al. Homozygous *HOXB1* loss-of-function mutation in a large family with hereditary congenital facial paresis. *Am J Med Genet A*. 2016;170(7):1813–1819.
17. Vahidi Mehrjardi MY, Maroofian R, Kalantar SM, Jaafarinia M, Chilton J, Dehghani M. A novel loss-of-function

mutation in *HOXB1* associated with autosomal recessive hereditary congenital facial palsy in a large Iranian family. *Mol Syndromol.* 2017;8(5):261–265.
18. Fazeli W, Herkenrath P, Stiller B, et al. A *TUBB6* mutation is associated with autosomal dominant non-progressive congenital facial palsy, bilateral ptosis and velopharyngeal dysfunction. *Hum Mol Genet.* 2017;26(20):4055–4066.
19. Whitman MC, Barry BJ, Robson CD, et al. *TUBB3* Arg262His causes a recognizable syndrome including CFEOM3, facial palsy, joint contractures, and early-onset peripheral neuropathy. *Hum Genet.* 2021 Dec;140(12):1709–1731.
20. Baba S, Kondo K, Yamasoba T. Electrophysiological evaluation of the facial muscles in congenital unilateral lower lip palsy. *Otol Neurotol.* 2018;39(1):106–110.
21. Saylam E, Arya K. *Congenital unilateral lower lip palsy*. In: *StatPearls [Internet]*. Treasure Island (FL): StatPearls Publishing; 2022 Jan.PMID: 32809530.
22. Kamal NM, Omair MM, Attar R, et al. Facial asymmetry in a newly born baby: diagnostic challenge! *Clin Med Insights Case Rep.* 2022;1511795476221088487.
23. Smith JD, Crumley RL, Lee AH. Facial paralysis in the newborn. *Otolaryngol Head Neck Surg.* 1981;89:1021–1024.
24. Gasteratos K, Azzawi SA, Vlachopoulos N, Lese I, Spyropoulou GA, Grobbelaar AO. Workhorse free functional muscle transfer techniques for smile reanimation in children with congenital facial palsy: case report and systematic review of the literature. *J Plast Reconstr Aesthet Surg.* 2021;74(7):1423–1435.
25. Domeshek LF, Zuker RM, Borschel GH. Management of bilateral facial palsy. *Otolaryngol Clin North Am.* 2018;51(6):1213–1226.

CHAPTER 15

Brachial Plexus Palsy

Erb Palsy, Klumpke Palsy, Obstetric Palsy, and Birth-Related Brachial Plexus Palsy

KEY POINTS

- The frequency of brachial plexus palsy has been decreasing with improved obstetric management.
- Lesions that affect the upper segments (C5–C7) result in Erb palsy, whereas lesions that affect the lower spinal segments (C7–T1) result in Klumpke palsy.
- Traction to the plexus, especially the upper plexus, occurs during delivery when the angle between the neck and shoulder is suddenly and forcibly increased, with the arms in an adducted position.
- The advent of microsurgical techniques and neuroelectrodiagnostic techniques has fostered the development of new neurosurgical techniques to repair brachial plexus injuries, although most infants recover spontaneously by 4 months of age.
- The absence of biceps clinical recovery in the sixth month of life and the presence of nerve root rupture signs are indications for surgery.
- Brachial plexus palsy can progress to significant sequelae, such as muscle contractures and glenohumeral dysplasia.
- Recovery usually begins distally, with all cases of complete recovery evident by 5 months of age.
- Surgery is rarely performed before 3 months of age but almost always performed before 9 months of age.

GENESIS

The frequency of brachial plexus palsy has been decreasing with improved obstetric management from 1 per 1000 births before 2000, to 0.5 per 1000 births after 2000.[1] Supraclavicular traction or stretching of the brachial plexus during delivery can injure nerve fibers; hence this injury is sometimes termed *obstetric palsy*. Historically risk factors have included shoulder dystocia, fetal macrosomia, labor abnormalities, forceps or vacuum delivery, and prior neonatal brachial plexus palsy, but these risk factors have not been shown to be reliable predictors. Other factors include familial congenital brachial plexus palsy, maternal uterine malformation, congenital varicella syndrome, osteomyelitis involving the proximal head of the humerus or cervical vertebral bodies, exostosis of the first rib, tumors and hemangioma in the region of the brachial plexus, and intrauterine maladaptation, but Kaiser Wilhelm syndrome (neonatal brachial plexus palsy due to placental insufficiency) is no longer considered to be a cause of brachial plexus palsy.[2] Most cases occur in infants weighing less than 4500 g, whose mothers are not diabetic with no other identifiable risk factors, and cesarean section reduces but does not completely eliminate the risk for neonatal brachial plexus palsy.[3] In a summary of 63 publications covering 17 million births, the likelihood of *not* having concomitant shoulder dystocia was 76% overall.[1] In studies from the United States, the rate of permanent neonatal brachial plexus palsy is 1.1–2.2 per 10,000 births and 2.9–3.7 per 10,000 births in other countries.[1]

The brachial plexus is formed by joining the anterior branches of the roots of C5, C6, C7, C8, and T1, and it emerges between the anterior and middle scalene muscles. In some cases, it receives a contribution from C4 (termed *prefixed*), while the contribution from T2 is termed *postfixed*. The brachial plexus is usually injured by excessive traction during labor, which can occur in up to 15% of newborns with shoulder dystocia. In most cases the lesion resolves within 6–12 months, but severe cases may require surgery, with risk of permanent damage in up to 10% of occurrences.[4] The fibers that originate from the 5th and 6th cervical segments, which innervate the supraspinatus and infraspinatus muscles, are usually the most commonly (90% of cases) and severely affected. Occasionally fibers from C7, C8, and T1 also can be affected. Lesions that affect the upper segments (C5–C7) result in Erb palsy, whereas lesions that affect the lower spinal segments (C7–T1) result in Klumpke palsy. There is also total (mixed) palsy, which results in both motor and sensory palsy of the entire affected limb due to injury to all of the brachial plexus. There may be associated injuries suggesting a difficult delivery, such as fracture of the clavicle or humerus (9–21% of cases), diaphragmatic paralysis (5–9%), or facial palsy (5–14%).[5,6] The position at delivery is related to the risk of brachial plexus injury, and infants delivered vaginally from an occipitoposterior position have a higher incidence of Erb palsy and facial palsy than those delivered from the occipitoanterior position.[7]

Traction to the plexus, especially the upper plexus, occurs during delivery when the angle between the neck and shoulder is suddenly and forcibly increased, with the arms in an adducted position. This can occur during vertex deliveries when traction is placed on the head to deliver the after-coming shoulder, particularly when the shoulders are caught against the pelvic brim in shoulder dystocia, as forceful contractions push the head and trunk forward. Brachial plexus palsy also can occur during breech deliveries when the adducted arm is pulled forcefully downward to free the after-coming head (accounting for 24% of brachial plexus palsies) or during other malpresentations when the head is rotated to achieve an occipitoanterior presentation.[3] The lower plexus is most susceptible to injury when traction is exerted on an abducted arm, such as occurs in vertex deliveries when traction is applied to an abducted prolapsed arm, or during breech deliveries when traction is applied to the trunk or legs while the after-coming arm is fixed in abduction.[3] Spinal nerves are attached to the vertebral transverse process distal to the intervertebral foramen, encased in funnel-shaped dural sleeves, and enmeshed in a network of rami, cords, and trunks to form the brachial plexus; these factors serve to protect the plexus from traction injury. When traction is excessively rapid and forceful, then diffuse multifocal injury occurs, including avulsion of the roots from the cord in the most severe injuries. Previous risk factors (before 2000) have included technically difficult (57%) or breech (9%) deliveries, fetal macrosomia (weight greater than 4 kg) (55%), shoulder dystocia, multiparous mothers, prolonged labor, or fetal hypotonia leading to loss of the normal cushioning effect of intact muscle tone.[3–5] Among 751 cases of neonatal brachial plexus palsy, 248 patients were born following routine deliveries and 503 patients were born following difficult deliveries. The routine delivery infants were more likely to have upper Erb palsy, whereas the difficult delivery group of infants were significantly more likely to develop total palsy. Poor functional recovery was more common in the difficult delivery group regarding shoulder, wrist, and hand function, suggesting that higher peak forces applied by the clinician in difficult deliveries affect the extent of neonatal brachial plexus palsy.[6] There are also reports of prenatal-onset brachial plexus injuries in which denervation was demonstrated by electromyography (EMG) shortly after birth.[4] One child demonstrated left brachial plexus injury, left Horner syndrome, left phrenic nerve injury, and hypoplasia of the left hand in addition to distortion of the first four ribs because of pressure on the left side of the neck and shoulder from the septum of a bicornuate uterus.[8] In a retrospective study of the predictive value of prenatal ultrasound in 152 deliveries (2004–2012) complicated by shoulder dystocia, birthweight (odds ratio 12.1 for greater than or equal to 4000 g; 95% CI, 4.18–35.0) and vacuum extraction (odds ratio 3.98; 95% CI, 1.25–12.7) were the most significant clinical risk factors. Among cases with shoulder dystocia, the incidence of brachial plexus palsies was high (40%) and the impact of diabetes as a risk factor for shoulder dystocia decreased, reflecting improved screening and treatment.[9]

The advent of microsurgical techniques and neuroelectrodiagnostic techniques has fostered the development of new neurosurgical techniques to repair brachial plexus injuries, although most infants recover spontaneously by 4 months of age. Severe lateral flexion of the infant's neck at delivery makes avulsion of the lower brachial plexus nerve roots more likely than avulsion of the upper plexus. Among 91 infants observed through 2 years of age who sustained a brachial plexus birth injury and were treated with only physical and occupational therapy, 63 children with an upper or middle plexus injury recovered good to excellent shoulder and hand function.[10] Of the remaining 28 infants, 12 sustained global injury, resulting in a useless arm, and 16 infants showed inadequate recovery of deltoid and biceps function by 6 months of age. These authors concluded that children with global injury would clearly benefit from early nerve reconstruction, and careful examination by age 6 months, in the sitting position, could confirm the potential for almost full recovery in most infants. Recovery of motor and sensory nerve function is attributed to axonal regeneration with re-innervations of original target muscle tissue, and functional improvement, which may continue for 5 years or longer. This longer period of recovery mirrors adaptational mechanisms at the spinal and supraspinal levels, which overcome initial motor neuron loss.[10] According to the literature, hand functions are conserved in upper-root brachial plexus injury, and there is no need to evaluate them, but there can be activity restrictions related to hand functions involving forearm rotation. In children with total plexus injury, grasp was absent and thumb function was deficient.[11] After perinatal upper brachial plexus injury to spinal roots C5 and C6, spinal root C7 contributes to biceps and deltoid innervations, but this does not occur in the adult.[12] The absence of biceps clinical recovery in the 6th month of life and the presence of nerve root rupture signs are indications for surgery.[13] Magnetic resonance imaging is the most sensitive and specific technique for identifying preganglionic nerve injuries such as rootlet avulsion, which has the poorest prognosis and may dictate the need for surgical intervention.[14] Brachial plexus palsy can progress to significant sequelae, such as muscle contractures and glenohumeral dysplasia. Timely characterization of these entities based on different imaging modalities is a high priority for optimal patient outcomes.

FEATURES

Lesions that affect the upper segments (C5, C6, and sometimes C7) result in Erb palsy, paralyzing the abductors, external rotators, and extensors of the shoulder as well as injuring the flexors and supinators of the forearm (Fig. 15.1). The infant's arm tends to hang limply adducted and internally rotated at the shoulder, with pronation and extension at the elbow, absent biceps and brachioradialis tendon jerks, and absent Moro response on the side of the lesion.[3,4] If C7 is also involved, then a wrist drop will be noted, with the hand flexed in a "waiter's tip" position and with an absent triceps jerk. Upper plexus injuries (Erb palsy) may be present without lower plexus injuries; however, lower plexus injury is usually accompanied by some degree of upper plexus damage. Lesions that affect only lower spinal segments (C7, C8, and T2) are much less common, and loss of C7 results in paralysis of the elbow, wrist, and finger extensors, causing wrist drop. Loss of C8 and T1 causes loss of wrist and finger flexors, as well as intrinsic hand muscles, causing extension of the metacarpal-phalangeal joints and flexion at the proximal and distal interphalangeal joints (Klumpke palsy).[3,4] The infant manifests a flexed arm with the shoulder in a normal position with flexed wrist and fingers, absent grasp reflex, sensory loss, and loss of sweating on the arm and hand. Injury to T1 at the root level can affect sympathetic fibers to the face, resulting in ipsilateral Horner syndrome (ptosis, miosis, anhydrosis, facial flushing, and failure of iris pigmentation). Among 220 infants with extended Erb palsy, 209 infants were without Horner syndrome and 11 had concurrent Horner syndrome. The rate of spontaneous recovery of elbow flexion in the former group was 59% versus 27% in the latter group, with 61% spontaneous recovery of wrist extension in the former group versus 0% in the latter group. Thus concurrent Horner syndrome in infants with extended Erb palsy is a poor prognostic sign for recovery of the 6th and 7th cervical roots.[15] Lesions that affect C5 and C6 are most common and account for 58–72% of brachial plexus palsies, followed by those affecting C5, C6, and C7 (18%) and those affecting the entire brachial plexus (C5–T1) (10%). Most cases are unilateral (56% right-sided, 41% left-sided), with only 3% affecting both arms.[3-5]

MANAGEMENT AND PROGNOSIS

Diagnosis is based on clinical features of lower motor neuron weakness. Additional studies may help determine prognosis, such as motor conduction velocities in the median and ulnar nerves; assessment of sensory action potentials in the median, ulnar, and radial nerves; EMG of affected muscles; radiographs; and magnetic resonance imaging or myelography with contrast when avulsion of roots is suspected. Although the mainstay of treatment is physical therapy with range-of-motion exercises, no treatment is advised during the first 7–10 days after birth because traumatic neuritis makes arm movement painful.[3] Physical therapy should then be promptly initiated because contractures can develop quickly in this condition. For upper plexus injuries, range-of-motion exercises should be initiated for the shoulder and elbow, along with abduction of the arm with the scapula fixed by one hand

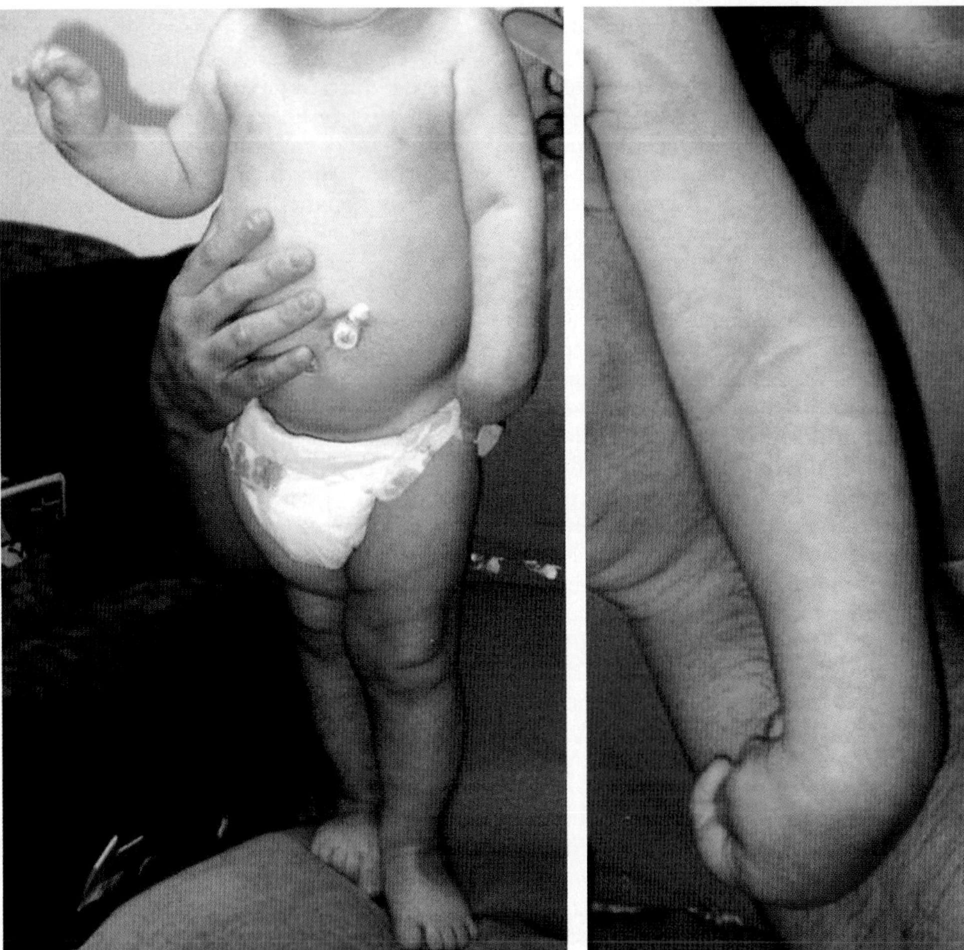

FIGURE 15.1 This large-for-gestational-age infant experienced shoulder dystocia, resulting in a left brachial plexus palsy affecting C5, C6, and C7 and resulting in Erb palsy, with paralyzed abductors, external rotators, and extensors of his left shoulder and deficient flexors and supinators of his forearm. His arm hangs limply adducted and internally rotated at the shoulder, with pronation and extension at the elbow, absent biceps, and brachioradialis tendon jerks, and absent Moro response on the side of the lesion. Because of involvement of C7, he manifests wrist drop, with the hand flexed in a "waiter's tip" position and with an absent triceps jerk.

to prevent the development of scapulohumeral adhesions.[3] For middle and lower plexus injuries, the paralyzed hand and wrist require range-of-motion exercises as well as a long opponens splint to maintain the hand and wrist in a position of function, with the wrist slightly extended and the phalanges slightly flexed.[3]

Complete recovery occurs in 70–92% of cases; in most of the remaining cases, recovery is partial. Recovery usually begins distally, with all cases of complete recovery evident by 5 months of age. Although some improvement may continue through 18 months of age, no improvement has been noted after 24 months of age. Children with residual deficits usually manifest shoulder muscle weakness (especially in the external rotators), with associated muscular atrophy and contractures. Infants with lower plexus injuries are less likely to make a complete recovery than those with upper plexus injuries. Associated elevation of the hemidiaphragm on chest radiograph, Horner syndrome, inability to retract or shrug the shoulders, or scapular winging may indicate damage to nerve fibers that originate from spinal roots close to the cord, thereby signifying avulsion, which is an irreversible injury. The most useful prognostic indicator is recovery that begins within 2 weeks after delivery.[3] The "towel test" has been advocated as a clinical tool to assess shoulder and elbow flexion/extension, biceps contraction, and finger flexion/extension because absence of biceps recovery by 3 months of age is an indication to consider surgical reconstruction.[16] The infant's face is covered with a towel, and the infant is then observed to see if they can remove the towel with either arm. Among 21 infants with brachial plexus palsy, none of the infants could remove the towel with either arm at 2–3 months; at 6 and 9 months, all infants could remove the towel with the normal arm, but 11 of 21 could not remove it with the affected arm.[16]

Management of neonatal brachial plexus palsy requires close follow-up of the baby up to 3–6 months, and if there are no signs of recovery, microsurgical repair is indicated. Surgery is rarely performed before 3 months of age but almost always performed before 9 months of age.[17] Serial physical examinations, supplemented by a thorough maternal and perinatal history, are critical to the formulation of the treatment plan that relies upon occupational/physical therapy and rehabilitation management but may include nerve reconstruction and secondary musculoskeletal surgeries. Adjunctive imaging and electrodiagnostic studies provide additional information to guide prognosis and treatment. Infants with severe lesions can be identified at 1 month of age by testing elbow extension, elbow flexion, and recording motor unit potentials in the biceps muscle, and children without active elbow extension at 1 month are usually referred to a specialized center. When there is active elbow extension but no active elbow flexion, an EMG may be needed. EMG at 1 month can identify severe cases of flexion paralysis for early surgical referral, whereas EMG of the biceps at 3 months can be misleading because of abnormal axonal branching and aberrant central motor control.[18] Neuromas involving ruptured nerve roots of C5 and C6 are the most common lesions (found in 95% of plexi explored). If EMG conduction post-neuroma decreases by more than 50% compared with pre-neuroma, the lesion is excised with grafting of the proximal and distal nerve roots, which usually involves interpositional sural nerve grafts to guide the proximal sprouting neural bulb to the severed ends. Pseudomeningoceles resulting from nerve root avulsions are thought to be predictive of significant injury to the brachial plexus and can be visualized by magnetic resonance imaging.[14]

After diagnosing the severity of brachial plexus palsy, early intensive and complex therapy should be started. After approximately a week or 10 days following birth, the mildest form (neurapraxia) normalizes without any intervention, and signs of recovery can be detected around this period. Therapy includes unipolar nerve point electro-stimulation and regular stimulation of elementary sensorimotor patterns, which activate both extremities simultaneously.[19] Full recovery can be achieved in 50% of patients, and even in the most severe cases (nerve root lesion). Palliative secondary procedures are used to further improve the overall function of the upper extremity in patients who present late or fail to improve after primary management. These secondary procedures include transfers of free vascularized and neurotized muscles.[20–23] Older children with brachial plexus injuries (more than 3 years after injury) require tendon and muscle transfers to achieve functional improvement. Recovery of function can occur up to 4–5 years after nerve reconstruction. Some children in whom complete neurologic recovery is apparent may develop a shoulder contracture or subluxation during growth; therefore ongoing monitoring and intervention are recommended to minimize functional problems. Glenoid dysplasia and posterior shoulder subluxation with resultant shoulder stiffness is a well-recognized complication in infants with neonatal brachial plexus palsy.[24] It is attributed to slowly progressive glenohumeral deformation resulting from muscle imbalance and/or physeal trauma. Clinical signs include asymmetric axillary skinfolds, asymmetric humeral shortening, asymmetric fullness in the posterior shoulder region, and/or a palpable click during shoulder manipulation (thereby resembling the clinical signs of congenital hip dislocation). Long considered as the ultimate surgery for limb salvage in cases of brachial plexus palsy, shoulder fusion has reduced indications with the development of new microsurgical and multiple tendon transfers. This option remains relevant because of its impact on pain and function, but this demanding surgery can have complications, and the position of the fusion remains difficult to determine.[25]

DIFFERENTIAL DIAGNOSIS

Amyoplasia involving the upper limbs (Fig. 15.2) and neonatal muscular dystrophy should be easily distinguished by the presence of joint stiffness or ankylosis and the absence of associated features suggesting birth

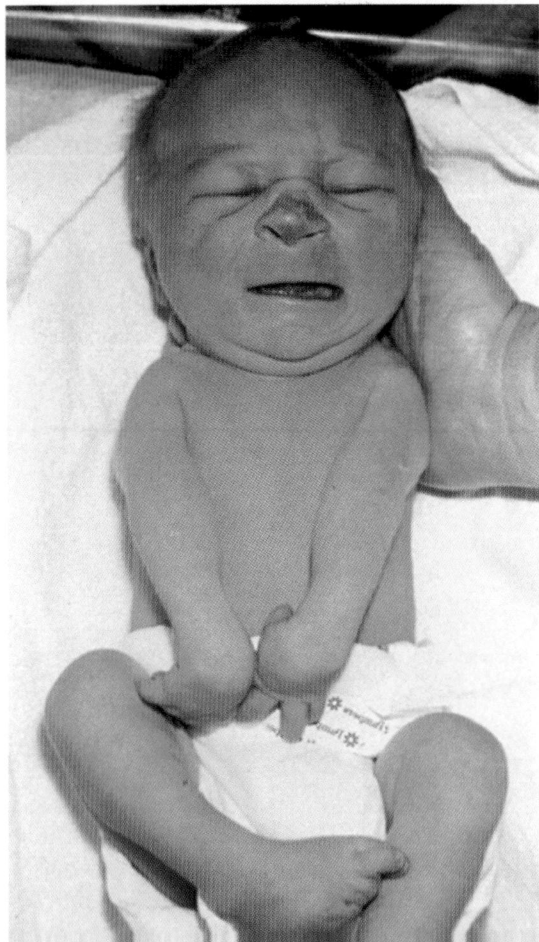

FIGURE 15.2 This infant was born with upper limb amyoplasia, which required multiple orthopedic corrective surgeries. His fixed upper limb contractures at birth, along with distal digital amputation defects in toes 3–5 suggesting prenatal vascular disruption, easily distinguish him from a child with neonatal brachial plexus palsy.

trauma. The limb is flaccid at birth in Erb palsy compared to amyoplasia, where significant contractures are present at birth. Of interest, the fifth and sixth spinal nerves are commonly injured during birth in individuals with Erb palsy, and this area of the cervical spinal cord is also likely to be involved when amyoplasia involves the upper limbs.[26] Sometimes pseudoparalysis can occur after a humeral fracture.

References

1. Chauhan SP, Blackwell SB, Ananth CV. Neonatal brachial plexus palsy: incidence, prevalence, and temporal trends. *Semin Perinatol.* 2014;38:210–218.
2. Alfonso DT. Causes of neonatal brachial plexus palsy. *Bull NYU Hosp Jt Dis.* 2011;69(1):11–16.
3. Ozounian JG. Risk factors for neonatal brachial plexus palsy. *Semin Perinatol.* 2014;38:219–221.
4. Galbiatti JA, Cardoso FL, Galbiatti MGP. Obstetric paralysis: who is to blame? A systematic literature review. *Rev Bras Ortop (Sao Paulo).* 2020;55(2):139–146.
5. Painter MJ, Bergman I. Obstetrical trauma to the neonatal central and peripheral nervous system. *Semin Perinatol.* 1982;6:89–104.
6. El-Sayed AA. Obstetric brachial plexus palsy following routine versus difficult deliveries. *J Child Neurol.* 2014;29(7):920–923.
7. Pearl ML, Roberts JM, Laros RK, et al. Vaginal delivery from the persistent occiput posterior position: influence on maternal and neonatal morbidity. *J Reprod Med.* 1993;38:955–961.
8. Dunn DW, Engle WA. Brachial plexus palsy: intrauterine onset. *Pediatr Neurol.* 1985;1:367–369.
9. Parantainen J, Palomäki O, Talola N, et al. Clinical and sonographic risk factors and complications of shoulder dystocia—a case-control study with parity and gestational age matched controls. *Eur J Obstet Gynecol Reprod Biol.* 2014;177:110–114.
10. DiTaranto P, Campagna L, Price AE, et al. Outcome following nonoperative treatment of brachial plexus injuries. *J Child Neurol.* 2004;19:87–90.
11. Delioğlu K, Uzumcugil A, Kerem Gunel M. Activity-based hand-function profile in preschool children with obstetric brachial plexus palsy. *Hand Surg Rehabil.* 2022;41(4):487–493.
12. Vredeveld JW, Blaauw G, Slooff BA, et al. The findings in paediatric obstetric brachial palsy differ from those in older patients: a suggested explanation. *Dev Med Child Neurol.* 2000;42:158–161.
13. Barsaoui M, Safi H, Said W, Nessib MN. Nerve surgery in obstetric brachial plexus palsy, report of 68 cases. *Tunis Med.* 2017;95(3):196–200.
14. Girard AO, Suresh V, Lopez CD, et al. Radiographic imaging modalities for perinatal brachial plexus palsy: a systematic review. *Childs Nerv Syst.* 2022;38(7):1241–1258.
15. El-Sayed AA. The prognostic value of concurrent Horner syndrome in extended Erb obstetric brachial plexus palsy. *J Child Neurol.* 2014;29(10):1356–1359.
16. Bertelli JA, Ghizoni MF. The towel test: a useful technique for the clinical and electromyographic evaluation of obstetric brachial plexus palsy. *J Hand Surg Br.* 2004;29:155–158.
17. Yang LJ. Neonatal brachial plexus palsy: management and prognostic factors. *Semin Perinatol.* 2014;38:222–234.
18. Van Dijk JG, Pondaag W, Buitenhuis SM, et al. Needle electromyography at 1 month predicts paralysis of elbow flexion at 3 months in obstetric brachial plexus lesions. *Dev Med Child Neurol.* 2012;54:753–758.
19. Berényi M, Szeredai M, Cseh Á. Neonatal brachial plexus palsy: early diagnosis and treatment. *Ideggyogy Sz.* 2022;75(7-08):247–252.

20. El-Gammal TA, El-Sayed A, Kotb MM, et al. Traumatic brachial plexus palsy in children: long-term outcome and strategy of reconstruction. *J Reconstr Microsurg.* 2021;37(8):704–712.
21. Ellabban MA, Sadek AF, Galhom A, Hafez AE, Ramadan A. Comparison between long and lower medial head triceps branches in dual neurotization for shoulder function restoration in upper brachial plexus palsy. *Microsurgery.* 2021 Feb;41(2):124–132.
22. Krauss EM, Noland SS, Hill EJR, Jain NS, Kahn LC, Mackinnon SE. Outcome analysis of medial triceps motor nerve transfer to axillary nerve in isolated and brachial plexus-associated axillary nerve palsy. *Plast Reconstr Surg.* 2022 Jun 1;149(6):1380–1390.
23. Abzug JM, Miller E, Case AL, Hogarth DA, Zlotolow DA, Kozin SH. Single versus double tendon transfer to improve shoulder external rotation during the treatment of brachial plexus birth palsy. *Hand (N Y).* 2022 Jan;17(1):55–59.
24. González-Mantilla P, Abril A, Bedoya MA. Brachial plexus birth palsy: practical concepts for radiologists. *Semin Musculoskelet Radiol.* 2022;26(2):182–193.
25. Clavert P, Antoni M. Shoulder arthrodesis in brachial plexus palsy. *Hand Surg Rehabil.* 2022;41S:S54–S57.
26. Hall JG. Amyoplasia involving only the upper limbs or only involving the lower limbs with review of the relevant differential diagnoses. *Am J Med Genet Part A.* 2014;164A:859–873.

CHAPTER 16

Diaphragmatic Paralysis

Diaphragmatic Eventration

KEY POINTS

- Eventration of the diaphragm is defined as abnormal elevation of the diaphragm, which can originate from a congenital defect or be acquired.
- Acquired eventration caused by injury to the phrenic nerve with resultant paralysis and elevation of the entire diaphragm can be secondary to an injury sustained during cardiothoracic surgery, or due to birth trauma.
- Brachial plexus palsy is the most common comorbidity with phrenic nerve injury, although 66–92% of these brachial plexus palsies resolve by 2 months of age.
- Neonates are less able to tolerate diaphragmatic paralysis than older children or adults; hence they often require prolonged ventilatory support with supplemental oxygen.
- If early recovery of diaphragmatic function is going to occur, it will do so during the first 2 weeks after birth, and after that time, diaphragmatic plication may be indicated in infants with persistent paralysis.

GENESIS

Eventration of the diaphragm is defined as abnormal elevation of the diaphragm. It may originate from a congenital defect or be acquired. Congenital eventration is a rare developmental abnormality characterized by muscular aplasia or hypoplasia of the diaphragm. The diaphragm is the main inspiratory muscle of the respiratory system, and it is innervated by the left and right phrenic nerves, which are branches of the cervical plexus arising at C3–C5. Acquired eventration is caused by injury to the phrenic nerve with resultant paralysis and elevation of the entire diaphragm. The paralysis may be secondary to an injury sustained during cardiothoracic surgery (1.2–5.5%), or due to birth trauma (1 per 15,000–30,000 live births).[1–3] Because the cervical plexus arises near the brachial plexus (C5–T1), in a study by Rizeq et al., 2% of 5832 newborns with birth-related brachial plexus palsies also had diaphragmatic paralysis, which was usually ipsilateral. Of these 122 infants, 32% were born to diabetic mothers, 65% required mechanical ventilation, and 27% required surgical diaphragmatic plication at a median age of 36 days.[4] Traction to the phrenic nerve during difficult deliveries or vaginal breech deliveries has been reported, and brachial plexus palsy is the most common comorbidity with phrenic nerve injury, although 66%–92% of these brachial plexus palsies resolve by 2 months of age.[5] Thoracic surgery for cardiovascular or tracheoesophageal fistula repair may also injure the phrenic nerve and result in diaphragmatic paralysis. Tetralogy of Fallot correction was the most associated cardiothoracic surgery, followed by arterial switch operation, Fontan procedure, and Blalock-Tausig shunt surgery.[2,3]

FEATURES

Symptoms of diaphragmatic paralysis are relatively nonspecific and can include respiratory distress (tachypnea, paradoxical breathing, cyanosis, shortness of breath, or increased work of breathing) and recurrent atelectasis and/or pneumonia, and asymmetric chest excursions, with chest radiographs demonstrating elevation of the diaphragm on one side as the infant is breathing spontaneously (Fig. 16.1). A careful examination for associated ipsilateral birth-related brachial plexus palsy is merited. If bilateral paralysis is present or if the infant is being ventilated, chest radiographs may not be diagnostic, and chest fluoroscopy or bedside ultrasonography to demonstrate an immobile diaphragm or one with paradoxical motion (i.e.,

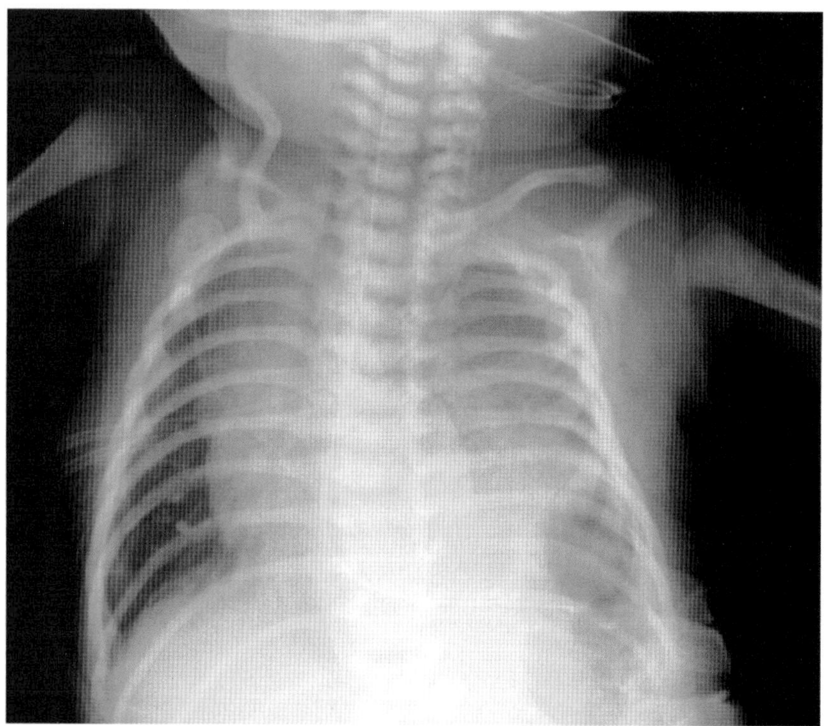

FIGURE 16.1 This infant was delivered from an obese mother and had shoulder dystocia, left Erb palsy and a left diaphragmatic paralysis that resulted in respiratory distress during the first 3 weeks, which then resolved. Note the elevated left hemidiaphragm and stomach bubble. This hemidiaphragm did not move on fluoroscopy.

elevation during inspiration) may be required.[3] Several recent electrophysiological tools have become available in some centers, such as phrenic nerve transcutaneous stimulation and diaphragm electromyogram, and compound diaphragmatic action potentials through transcutaneous stimulation of the phrenic nerves can be used to determine if functional diaphragmatic recovery might be expected.[3]

MANAGEMENT AND PROGNOSIS

Neonates are less able to tolerate diaphragmatic paralysis than are older children or adults; hence they often require prolonged ventilatory support with supplemental oxygen. Most authors state that if early recovery of diaphragmatic function is going to occur, it will do so during the first 2 weeks after birth, during which time ventilatory support is usually necessary. After that time, diaphragmatic plication may be indicated in infants with persistent paralysis. Plication prevents inspiratory shifting of abdominal contents into the ipsilateral thoracic cavity, thereby allowing for greater lung expansion. In a study by Denamur et al., eventual recovery of diaphragmatic function occurred in 63% of 51 infants with diaphragmatic paralysis following cardiac surgery, while 37% required diaphragmatic plication.[6] Another study of 88 children with diaphragmatic paralysis (59 related to cardiac surgery and 29 other causes) noted that 31% required plication.[7] Treatment depends on the degree of respiratory compromise, with mild cases requiring little more than close monitoring, chest physical therapy, and the use of antibiotics for any associated pneumonia. Advancements in endoscopic technology and technique have resulted in minimally invasive methods (video-assisted thoracoscopic plication of the diaphragm) for repair of this defect with modest benefits when compared with the open thoracotomy.[8] Among eight patients who underwent thoracoscopic plication, one patient underwent conversion to an open procedure because the operative field was too small. The mean operative time was 60.5 minutes, and chest drainage was placed in six patients. There were two recurrences, and at follow-up all patients were asymptomatic with a normal level for the diaphragm, suggesting thoracoscopic plication is feasible and safe, but certain modifications may be necessary to reduce the potential risk of recurrence.[9]

DIFFERENTIAL DIAGNOSIS

A congenital pulmonary malformation, such as pulmonary sequestration or congenital cystic adenomatoid malformation, should be suspected in infants with recurrent lower respiratory symptoms or unifocal infiltrations. The possibility of congenital pulmonary malformation associated with additional abnormalities, such as diaphragmatic hernia, is relatively high and can lead to misdiagnosis of diaphragmatic eventration.[10] Diaphragmatic paralysis has been reported in four infants with congenital Zika virus infection and associated arthrogryposis.[11] Various genetic neuromuscular conditions have been reported with diaphragmatic weakness or paralysis. These include monoallelic pathogenic variants in *BICD2*, which are associated with autosomal dominant spinal muscular atrophy lower extremity predominant type 2A and 2B (SMALED2A and SMALED2B, respectively) as well as spinal muscular atrophy with respiratory distress type 1 (SMARD1), a very rare autosomal recessive disorder caused by mutations in the immunoglobulin μ-binding protein-2 (*IGHMBP2*) gene.[12-14] Diaphragmatic paralysis has also been reported in *BAG-3* myofibrillar myopathy, Nemalin myopathy, and *CNTNAP1*-associated congenital hypomyelinating neuropathy.[15-17]

References

1. Fraser 3rd CD, Ravekes W, Thibault D, et al. Diaphragm paralysis after pediatric cardiac surgery: an STS congenital heart surgery database study. *Ann Thorac Surg.* 2021;112(1):139–146.
2. Akbariasbagh P, Mirzaghayan MR, Akbariasbagh N, Shariat M, Ebrahim B. Risk factors for post-cardiac surgery diaphragmatic paralysis in children with congenital heart disease. *J Tehran Heart Cent.* 2015;10(3):134–139.
3. Gerard-Castaing N, Perrin T, Ohlmann C, et al. Diaphragmatic paralysis in young children: a literature review. *Pediatr Pulmonol.* 2019;54(9):1367–1373.
4. Rizeq YK, Many BT, Vacek JC, et al. Diaphragmatic paralysis after phrenic nerve injury in newborns. *J Pediatr Surg.* 2020;55(2):240–244. (Elsevier Journal).
5. Reiter AJ, Rizeq YK, Many BT, Vacek JC, Abdullah F, Goldstein SD. A rare case of contralateral diaphragm paralysis following birth injury with brachial plexus palsy: a case report and review of the literature. *Case Rep Pediatr.* 2020;2020:8844029.
6. Denamur S, Chenouard A, Lefort B, et al. Outcome analysis of a conservative approach to diaphragmatic paralysis following congenital cardiac surgery in neonates and infants: a bicentric retrospective study. *Interact Cardiovasc Thorac Surg.* 2021;33(4):597–604.
7. Goldberg L, Krauthammer A, Ashkenazi M, et al. Predictors for plication performance following diaphragmatic paralysis in children. *Pediatr Pulmonol.* 2020;55(2):449–454.
8. Gritsiuta AI, Gordon M, Bakhos CT, Abbas AE, Petrov RV. Minimally invasive diaphragm plication for acquired unilateral diaphragm paralysis: a systematic review. *Innovations (Phila).* 2022;17(3):180–190.
9. Borruto FA, Ferreira CG, Kaselas C, et al. Thoracoscopic treatment of congenital diaphragmatic eventration in children: lessons learned after 15 years of experience. *Eur J Pediatr Surg.* 2014;24(4):328-231.
10. Kuo HC, Chang CY, Leung JH. Pulmonary sequestration and diaphragmatic eventration in a 6-month-old infant. *Pediatr Neonatol.* 2012;53:63–67.
11. Rajapakse NS, Ellsworth K, Liesman RM, et al. Unilateral phrenic nerve palsy in infants with congenital Zika syndrome. *Emerg Infect Dis.* 2018;24(8):1422–1427.
12. Chin HL, Huynh S, Ashkani J, et al. An infant with congenital respiratory insufficiency and diaphragmatic paralysis: a novel *BICD2* phenotype? *Am J Med Genet A.* 2022;188(3):926–930.
13. Pekuz S, Güzin Y, Sarıtaş S, Kırbıyık Ö, Ünalp A, Yılmaz Ü. Spinal muscular atrophy with respiratory distress type 1 (SMARD1): a rare cause of hypotonia, diaphragmatic weakness, and respiratory failure in infants. *Turk J Pediatr.* 2022;64(2):364–374.
14. Chiu ATG, Chan SHS, Wu SP, et al. Spinal muscular atrophy with respiratory distress type 1-A child with atypical presentation. *Child Neurol Open.* 2018;52329048X18769811.
15. Zhan L, Lv L, Chen X, Xu X, Ni J. Ultrasound evaluation of diaphragm motion in BAG-3 myofibrillar myopathy: a case report. *Medicine (Baltimore).* 2022;101(1):e28484.
16. Wen Q, Chang X, Guo J. A childhood-onset nemaline myopathy caused by novel heterozygote variants in the nebulin gene with literature review. *Acta Neurol Belg.* 2020;120(6):1351–1360.
17. Lesmana H, Vawter Lee M, Hosseini SA, et al. *CNTNAP1*-related congenital hypomyelinating neuropathy. *Pediatr Neurol.* 2019;93:43–49.

CHAPTER 17

Other Peripheral Nerve Palsies

KEY POINTS

- Radial nerve compression along the humerus from fetal crowding in late gestation may lead to wrist drop as a function of radial nerve palsy.
- Sciatic nerve compression may cause weakness in one or both legs.
- Prolonged extreme abduction, flexion, and external rotation of the leg at the hip can result in traction on the obturator nerve, and obturator palsy in the newborn results in limitation of active internal rotation and adduction of the thigh, as well as limitation of knee extension.
- Although the mainstay of treatment is physical therapy with range-of-motion exercises, no treatment is advised for the first 7–10 days of life because traumatic neuritis makes limb movement painful.
- Complete recovery is usually evident by 5 months of age, and significant improvement may continue for another 12 months, but no improvement has been noted in any series after 24 months of age.

GENESIS AND FEATURES

Radial nerve compression along the humerus resulting from fetal crowding in late gestation may lead to wrist drop (Fig. 17.1) as a function of radial nerve palsy.[1–5] Among 953 infants evaluated for upper extremity weakness, 25 (2.6%) had isolated radial nerve palsy with good shoulder function and intact flexion of the elbow, and 17 affected infants (68%) had a subcutaneous nodule representing fat necrosis in the inferior posterolateral portion of the affected arm. Full recovery occurred in all patients within a range of 1 week to 6 months, and 72% of the patients (18/25) had fully recovered by the time they were 2 months old.[2] The pathophysiology of isolated radial nerve palsy in the newborn is thought to be secondary to prolonged pressure on the inferior upper arm from the pelvic brim either in utero or during prolonged or difficult delivery. Neonatal radial nerve palsy should be suspected in newborns presenting with absent wrist and digital extension but intact deltoid, biceps, and triceps function with wrist and digital flexor function. The presence of ecchymosis and/or fat necrosis along the posterolateral humerus may support the notion that neonatal radial nerve palsy is caused by a compression injury during or before labor (Fig. 17.2).[2–5] Wrist drop may also result from compression of the posterior interosseous nerve when prolonged intrauterine palmar flexion results in traction on the posterior interosseous nerve over a fixed point at the origin of the nerve in the supinator muscle. Among 55 reported cases of congenital radial nerve palsy, all had some form of recovery, with full recovery in most cases by 8–9 weeks of age, regardless of initial severity.[2–5] Constricting amniotic bands can also lead to distal nerve dysfunction (Fig. 17.3).[6,7]

Initial examination should delineate which nerves are not functioning and confirm that no humeral fracture is present.[7] Humeral fracture is an unlikely cause of radial palsy, and it is commonly caused by birth trauma in neonates.[8] It may be difficult to separate a brachial plexus palsy from a radial palsy. Lack of a grasp reflex and a weak hand grip can be seen in brachial plexus palsy but not radial palsy. Shoulder and elbow functions are normal in radial nerve palsies but may not be in brachial plexus palsy (Video 17.1).[3] Moro reflex should elicit shoulder abduction and elbow extension with radial nerve palsy, but this may be impaired with brachial plexus palsy. With radial nerve palsy, the asymmetric tonic neck reflex is normal (flexion of the upper and lower extremities on one side, with extension of the arm and leg on the contralateral side). Skin findings at the mid-humeral level on the affected side (bruising and subcutaneous nodules suggesting the presence of fat necrosis due to compression) indicate radial nerve palsy (see Fig. 17.2). Treatment includes observation, physical therapy (passive range-of-motion exercises), and nighttime

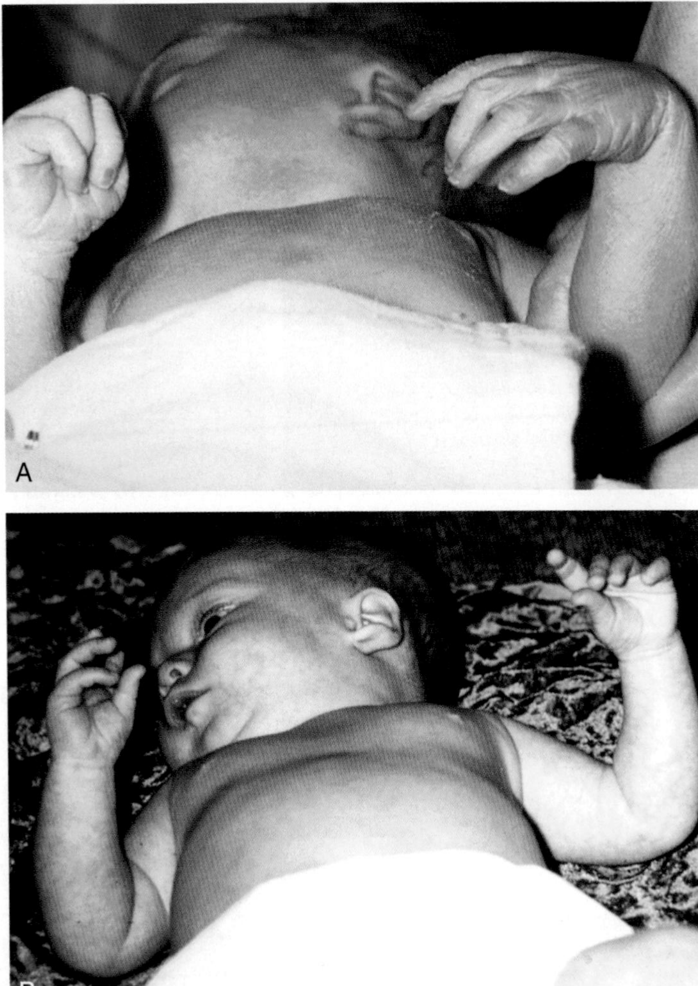

FIGURE 17.1 Unilateral radial palsy from compression at birth (**A**) and 12 weeks later (**B**), by which time wrist function was normal. The compression in this case was caused by prolonged engagement in a restricted birth canal for 5 weeks before delivery.

wrist splints, but recovery can occur in the absence of any treatment.[3]

Peripheral nerve palsies affect the upper extremities much more often than the lower extremities, and in a newborn they are usually attributable to mechanical factors operating in utero. Sciatic compression may cause weakness in one or both legs. In infants with prolonged breech presentation and extended legs, traction on the sciatic nerve may exert a selective effect on the peroneal nerve because of relative fixation of the nerve at the neck of the fibula. This results in foot drop caused by weakness of ankle dorsiflexion.[9] The peroneal nerve is a division of the sciatic nerve, which splits above the popliteal fossa to form the tibial and common peroneal nerves. The latter nerve extends anterolaterally around the neck of the fibula, where it is exposed to potential injury.[9] Prolonged extreme abduction, flexion, and external rotation of the leg at the hip can result in traction on the obturator nerve, as it is stretched between fixation points at the pubic ramus and knee joint. Obturator palsy in the newborn results in limitation of active internal rotation and adduction of the thigh and limitation of knee extension.[10] Among 12 newborn children with sciatic nerve

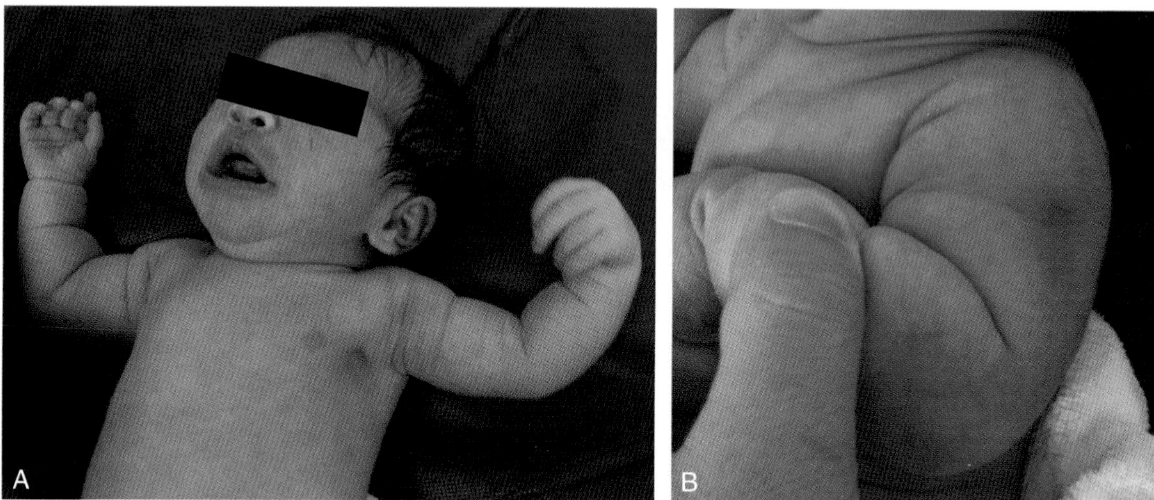

FIGURE 17.2 Left-sided wrist drop in an infant with left congenital radial nerve palsy. Ecchymosis present on the left lateral arm at the mid-humerus level in an infant with a congenital radial nerve palsy. (Image courtesy Joshua M. Abzug, MD, Dept. of Orthopedics, University of Maryland Brachial Plexus Clinic, University of Maryland School of Medicine, Timonium.)

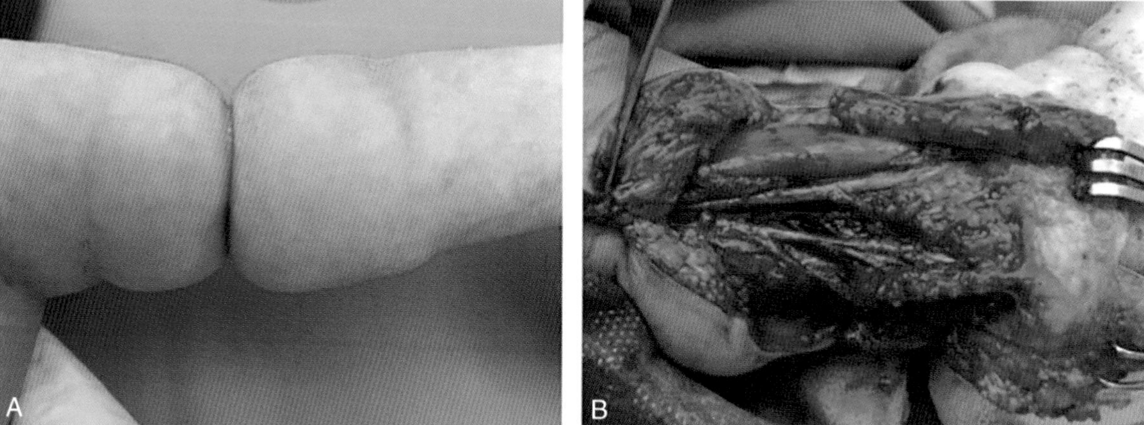

FIGURE 17.3 **A,** A newborn with a deep, circular constriction band in the mid-diaphyseal humerus region. **B,** After circular resection of the constriction band and creation of multiple z-plasties, the neurovascular bundles are released. A flattened median nerve and severely flattened ulnar nerve were found and neurolyzed. (From Gallone G, Di Gennaro GL, Farr S. Peripheral nerve compression syndromes in children. *J Hand Surg Am*. 2020;45(9):857-863.)

paralysis, complete paralysis was present in 6 and partial paralysis in 6 neonates. In all cases of breech delivery, there was a history of prolonged labor and forceful extraction by pulling the leg of the fetus.[11] Recovery was incomplete in most of these cases with total sciatic nerve palsy. Sciatic nerve paralysis is a rare entity in the newborn, and in most cases the sciatic palsy has been observed after misplaced injections into the buttocks. Among 21 newborns with sciatic palsy, no cause was apparent in most cases. Cesarean delivery was associated with incomplete recovery, and time of recovery took 4–14 months (median 8.8 months), with independent ambulation in all cases by 10–24 months.[12]

MANAGEMENT AND PROGNOSIS

Diagnosis is based on clinical features of lower motor neuron weakness. Neonatal radial nerve palsy should be suspected in newborns presenting with wrist drop and absent wrist and digital extension but intact deltoid, biceps, and triceps function with preserved wrist and digital flexor function. The presence of ecchymosis and/or fat necrosis along the posterolateral upper arm above the elbow in the region of the spiral groove (see Fig. 17.2), where the radial nerve is most vulnerable to compression injury, suggests that neonatal radial nerve palsy is caused by a compression injury during or before labor, and there is often a history of failure of progression of labor. There is usually complete spontaneous recovery of radial nerve function if there is no associated infectious or constriction band pathology.[2–5] Electrophysiologic studies such as motor conduction velocities, sensory action potentials, and electromyography of affected muscles may help determine the prognosis. Early electrophysiologic examination of a newborn with peripheral neuropathy may provide valuable information about the time of onset and pathophysiologic features of the nerve lesion.[13] In spite of the early electromyogram findings revealing severe nerve injury, a good prognosis is possible in newborns with a peripheral neuropathy.[13] The evidence for in utero compression includes active denervation of the muscle (as evidenced by fibrillation on electromyography) within the first week after birth, when normally such denervation would be expected to appear a minimum of 10 days after injury to the nerve.[2] Neuromuscular ultrasound has also been used to complement clinical examination and electrodiagnostic evaluation of peripheral neuropathies.[14,15]

Although the mainstay of treatment is physical therapy with range-of-motion exercises, no treatment is advised for the first 7–10 days of life because traumatic neuritis makes limb movement painful.[1] Physical therapy should then be promptly initiated because contractures may develop quickly in this condition. The paralyzed hand and wrist require range-of-motion exercises in addition to splinting to maintain the hand and wrist in a position of function, with the wrist slightly extended and the phalanges slightly flexed.[1] Complete recovery occurs in most cases, and patients who do not completely recover usually show some degree of improvement. Complete recovery is usually evident by 5 months of age, but significant improvement may continue for another 12 months. No improvement has been noted in any series after 24 months of age.[1] The most useful prognostic indicator is recovery that begins within 2 weeks of delivery.[1]

References

1. Painter MJ, Bergman I. Obstetrical trauma to the neonatal central and peripheral nervous system. *Semin Perinatol.* 1982;6:89–104.
2. Alsubhi FS, Althunyan AM, Curtis CG, Clarke HM. Radial nerve palsy in the newborn: a case series. *CMAJ.* 2011;183:1367–1370.
3. Song X, Abzug JM. Congenital radial nerve palsy. *J Hand Surg Am.* 2015;40(1):163–165.
4. Carsi MB, Clarke AM, Clarke NP. Transient neonatal radial nerve palsy: a case series and review of the literature. *J Hand Ther.* 2015;28(2):212–215. (Elsevier Journal).
5. Böhringer E, Weber P. Isolated radial nerve palsy in newborns: case report of a bilateral manifestation and literature review. *Eur J Pediatr.* 2014;173(4):537–539.
6. Weeks PM. Radial, median, and ulnar nerve dysfunction associated with a congenital constricting band of the arm. *Plast Reconst Surg.* 1982;69:333–336.
7. Gallone G, Di Gennaro GL, Farr S. Peripheral nerve compression syndromes in children. *J Hand Surg Am.* 2020;45(9):857–863.
8. Mahapatra SK, Jangira V, Kalra M. Neonatal radial nerve palsy associated with humerus fracture: is the fracture to be blamed? *Orthop Surg.* 2014;6(2):162–164.
9. Hawkes CP, McNamara B, O'Mahony O, et al. Your diagnosis? Congenital foot drop. *Eur J Pediatr.* 2013;172:1145–1147.
10. Craig WS, Clark JM. Obturator palsy in the newly born. *Arch Dis Child.* 1962;37(196):661–662.
11. Sriram K, Sakthivel A. Sciatic nerve palsy in the newborn. *Ann Acad Med Singap.* 1981;10(4):472–475.
12. Ramos-Fernández JM, Oliete-García FM, Roldán-Aparicio S, Kirchschläger E, Barrio-Nicolás A. Parálisis ciática neonatal: etiología y seguimiento a propósito de 21 casos [Neonatal sciatic palsy: etiology and outcome of 21 cases]. *Rev Neurol.* 1998 May;26(153):752–755. Spanish.
13. Yilmaz Y, Oge AE, Yilmaz-Değpirmenci S, et al. Peroneal nerve palsy: the role of early electromyography. *Eur J Paediatr Neurol.* 2000;4:239–242.
14. Baute Penry V, Cartwright MS. Neuromuscular ultrasound for peripheral neuropathies. *Semin Neurol.* 2019;39(5):542–548.
15. Hannaford A, Vucic S, Kiernan MC, Simon NG. Review article "Spotlight on ultrasonography in the diagnosis of peripheral nerve disease: the evidence to date". *Int J Gen Med.* 2021;14:4579–4604.

Section VI
Thoracic Cage and Spinal Deformations

CHAPTER 18

Lung Hypoplasia and Pediatric Thoracic Insufficiency

KEY POINTS

- Lung hypoplasia implies an abnormal reduction in the weight and/or volume of the lung without the absence of any of its lobes.
- Decreased lung weight and volume can result from fewer bronchial branches, reduced numbers of alveoli, decreased alveolar size, or any combination of these phenomena.
- Thoracic insufficiency syndrome is the inability of the thorax to support normal respiration or lung growth, and this condition includes a wide group of constrictive thoracospinal conditions.
- Distension of the lung with lung liquid and fetal lung movements are both needed for normal lung growth.
- The risk for pulmonary hypoplasia diminishes when oligohydramnios occurs after 24 weeks of gestation, and the duration of severe oligohydramnios and gestational age at which oligohydramnios had its onset are independent risk factors.
- Some thoracic insufficiency conditions are lethal in the neonatal period because of a severely restricted thoracic cage, whereas others are compatible with life.
- Vertical expandable prosthetic titanium rib (VEPTR) expansion thoracoplasty has also been used to manage thoracic insufficiency syndrome.
- Severe diaphragmatic hernias have poor outcomes and may be candidates for fetal endoscopic tracheal occlusion.

GENESIS

Lung hypoplasia implies an abnormal reduction in the weight and/or volume of the lung without the absence of any of its lobes; this condition is different from agenesis or aplasia of the lungs. Lung hypoplasia can result from various phenomena. During the fourth week of gestation, the laryngotracheal groove forms in the esophageal portion of the endotracheal tube, and shortly thereafter lung development begins with the evagination of two buds from the ventral surface of this groove. Between 6 and 16 weeks of gestation, these buds invade the thoracic mesenchyme by dichotomous branching so that the conducting airway system is complete by the end of the 16th week. Formation of the acini begins proximally and proceeds distally in the lung, and alveoli appear as early as 32 weeks and continue to develop throughout childhood.[1]

Decreased lung weight and volume can result from a decreased number of bronchial branches, reduced numbers of alveoli, decreased alveolar size, or any combination of these phenomena.[1] Pulmonary hypoplasia can be associated with various types of problems: oligohydramnios, thoracic wall abnormalities, diaphragmatic hernia, central nervous system abnormalities, or a group of miscellaneous conditions, including fetal hydrops, extralobar sequestration, or cloacal dysgenesis.[1,2] Restriction of thoracic cage expansion by a small uterine cavity can also rarely be associated with lung hypoplasia. Certain lethal skeletal dysplasias that result in rib shortening and a small thorax (e.g., thanatophoric dysplasia or asphyxiating thoracic dysplasia [Figs. 18.1 and 18.2]) can have the same impact. Thoracic insufficiency syndrome is the inability of the thorax to support normal respiration or lung growth, and this condition includes a wide group of constrictive thoracospinal conditions (congenital scoliosis, skeletal, neuromuscular, and other structural thoracic disorders) (Figs. 18.3 and 18.4).[3–5] Intervention is primarily via growth-sparing surgery, for which several device options exist, to preserve vertical growth prior to a definitive spinal fusion at skeletal

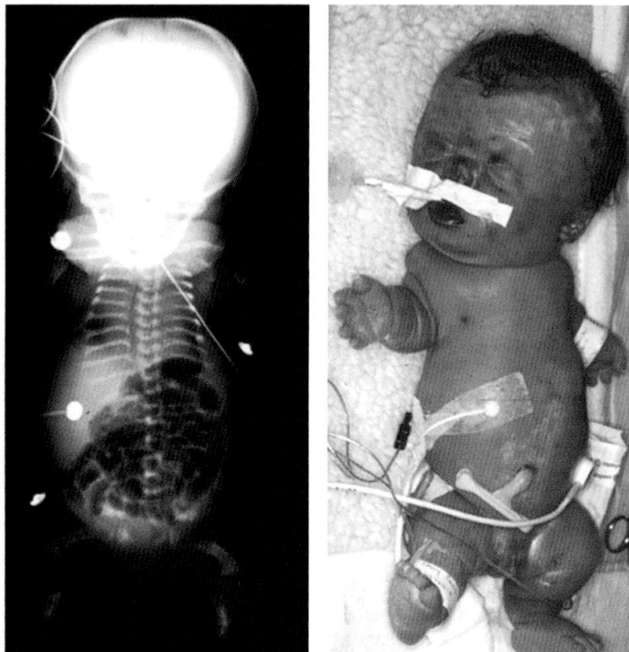

FIGURE 18.1 Thanatophoric dysplasia is caused by mutations in *FGFR3* and results in extremely short limbs with very short ribs, a small thorax, and markedly hypoplastic lungs.

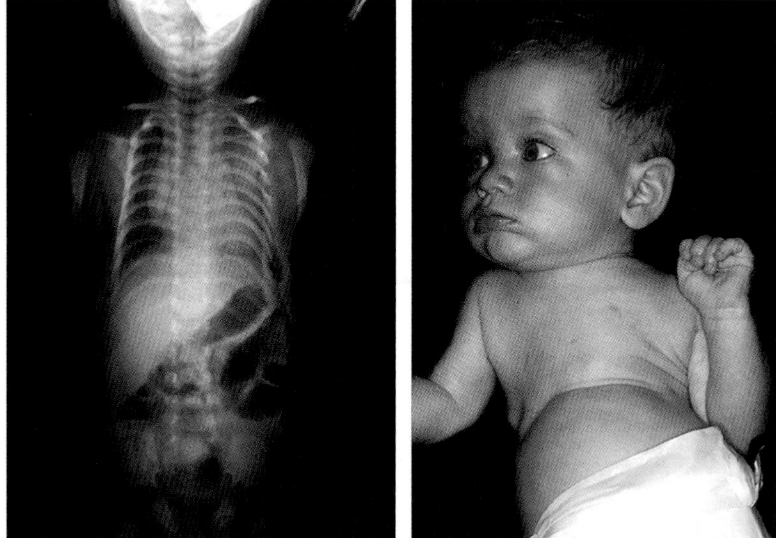

FIGURE 18.2 Radiographic and clinical appearance of a patient with asphyxiating thoracic dystrophy (Jeune syndrome), showing reduced thoracic volume. This condition is an autosomal recessive condition caused by mutations in over 21 different skeletal ciliopathy genes.

maturity (Fig. 18.5; Table 18.1). In a cohort of 42 individuals with thoracic insufficiency syndromes from a pediatric orthopedic clinic that underwent exome sequencing, the identified genes encoded components of the primary cilium, bone, and extracellular matrix. Exome sequencing identified a molecular etiology in 24/42 (57%) of the participants, with short-rib thoracic dysplasia syndromes manifesting the highest

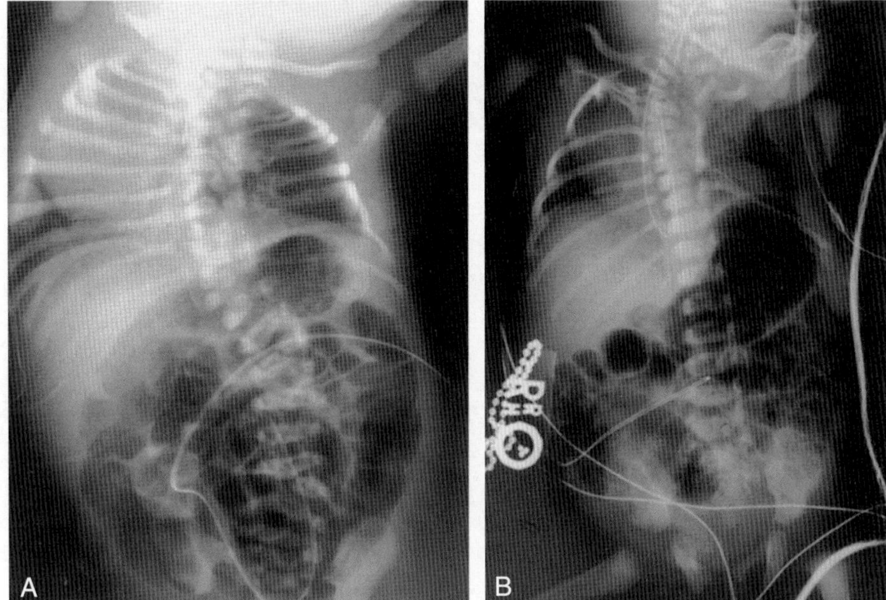

FIGURE 18.3 Radiographs of two different neonates with Jarcho-Levin syndrome. **A,** Spondylothoracic dysplasia; **B,** Spondylocostal dysostosis.

molecular diagnostic rate (81%) and *DYNC2H1* being the most common gene (7/16; 44%).[4]

Congenital diaphragmatic hernia occurs in approximately 2.3–2.8 per 10,000 live births and it can result in high neonatal morbidity and mortality, largely associated with the severity of pulmonary hypoplasia and pulmonary arterial hypertension.[6] Fetal akinesia that results in diaphragmatic paralysis and failure to swallow amniotic fluid is associated with polyhydramnios, and it leads to a lack of lung expansion and pulmonary hypoplasia. Prolonged oligohydramnios resulting from either renal agenesis or prolonged rupture of membranes can lead to pulmonary hypoplasia. Thus distension of the lung with lung liquid and fetal lung movements are both needed for normal lung growth.[7]

Restrained thoracic growth was initially hypothesized to cause the lungs to remain small and underdeveloped in oligohydramnios sequence, but it is the inhibition of breathing movements (essential for lung growth) and/or abnormal fluid dynamics within the lung that result in decreased intraluminal fluid pressures and cause poor lung growth.[8] The gestational age at the time of premature rupture of membranes relates to the histologic development of the lungs, which can be divided into three stages. During the pseudoglandular stage (5–17 weeks of gestation), all major lung elements are formed except those related to gas exchange. During the canalicular stage (16–25 weeks), terminal bronchioles give rise to respiratory bronchioles and then to thin-walled terminal sacs. During the terminal sac stage (24 weeks to birth), the number of terminal sacs rapidly increases, which increases the total gas exchange area. If oligohydramnios is limited to the terminal sac stage, it does not affect lung growth, but when oligohydramnios is induced during the canalicular stage, it results in a cumulative reduction in lung size.[8] Thus the risk for pulmonary hypoplasia diminishes when oligohydramnios occurs after 24 weeks of gestation.[8-11] The duration of severe oligohydramnios and the gestational age at which oligohydramnios had its onset are independent risk factors, and severe oligohydramnios lasting more than 14 days with rupture of membranes before 25 weeks results in a mortality rate greater than 90%.[11]

FEATURES

Lung hypoplasia is best defined by the ratio of lung weight to body weight; hence the pathologist usually defines it during postmortem examination. This ratio is 0.012 for infants older than 28 weeks of

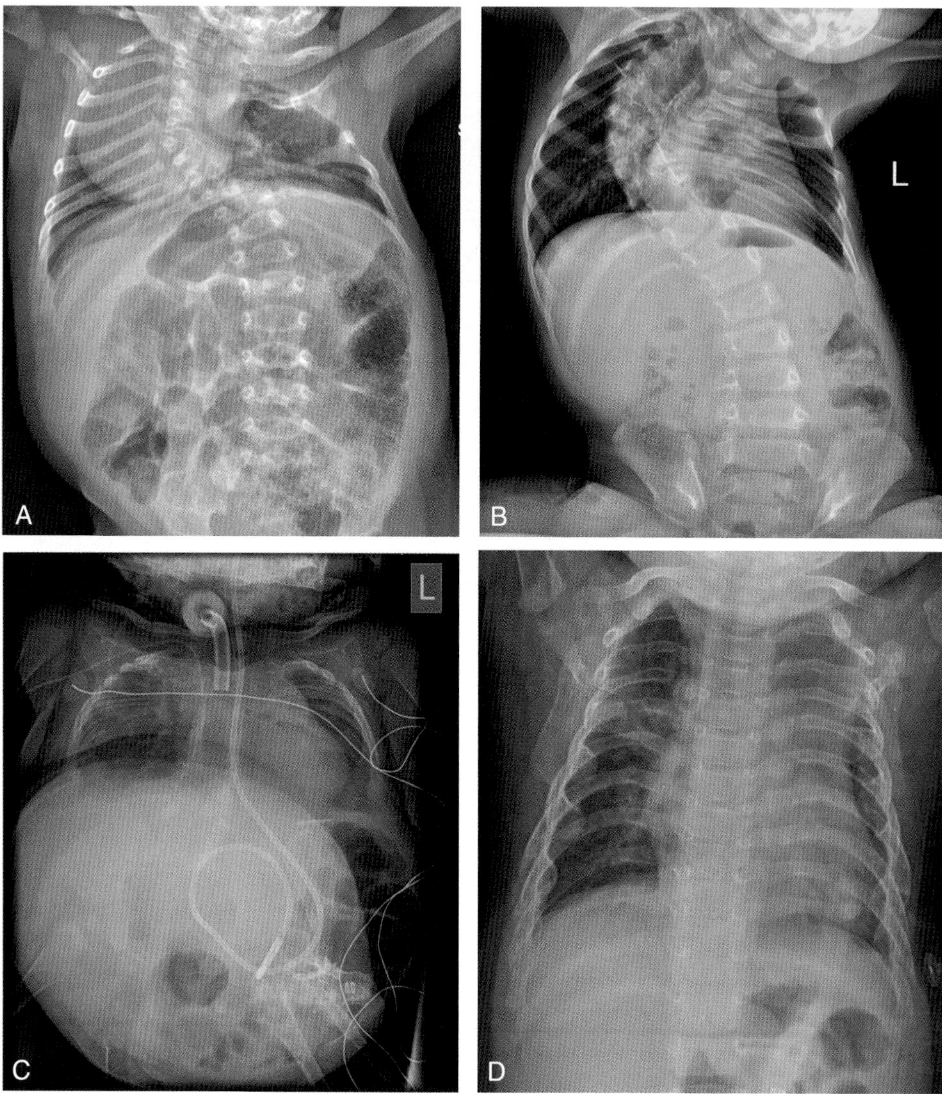

FIGURE 18.4 Types of thoracic volume depletion as classified by Campbell and Smith. **A,** Type I, absent ribs and scoliosis (this patient had agenesis of the left-sided ribs of most of the upper vertebral bodies, as well as rib fusion at T1–T4, and of the 8th, 9th, and 10th ribs proximally); **B,** Type II, fused ribs and scoliosis; **C,** Jarcho-Levin syndrome; **D,** Jeune syndrome, also called asphyxiating thoracic dystrophy. (From Tsukahara K, Mayer OH. Thoracic insufficiency syndrome: approaches to assessment and management. *Paediatr Respir Rev*. 2022;44:78-84; Campbell Jr RM, Smith MD. Thoracic insufficiency syndrome and exotic scoliosis. *J Bone Joint Surg Am*. 2007;89(Suppl 1):108-122.)

gestation and 0.015 for younger fetuses.[12] Another method of detecting lung hypoplasia involves the radial alveolar count, which is the number of alveolar septae traversed by a perpendicular line drawn from the center of a respiratory bronchiole to the nearest connective tissue septum. As the lung matures, bronchioles extend peripherally, so pathologists often take the most peripheral bronchiole in the section and count the number of alveoli to the pleural surface. The radial count is standardized for gestational age. At 18 weeks of gestation the count averages 1.5 alveolar spaces, whereas at term it averages five alveolar spaces.[13] Pulmonary hypoplasia, with limited alveolar development, leads to respiratory insufficiency.

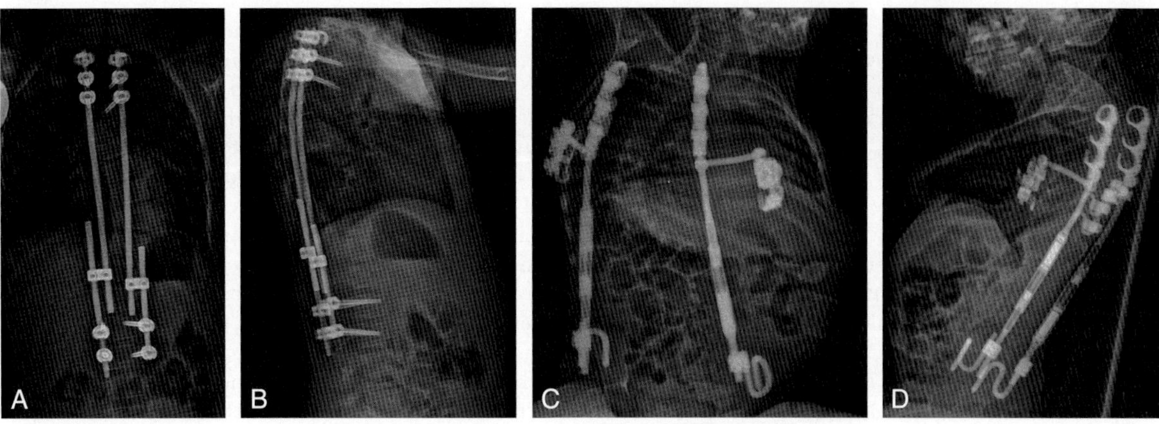

FIGURE 18.5 Examples of growth-friendly surgical intervention. **A, B,** Traditional growing rods. **C, D,** MAGnetic Expansion Control (MAGEC) growing rods with lateral rib supports. (From Tsukahara K, Mayer OH. Thoracic insufficiency syndrome: approaches to assessment and management. *Paediatr Respir Rev*. 2022;44:78-84.)

Table 18.1 COMPARISON OF GROWTH-FRIENDLY SURGICAL IMPLANTS

Device	Fixation Point	Mechanism
Growing rod	Proximal and distal spine	Surgical distraction, typically every 6–8 months
Vertical Expandable Prosthetic Titanium Rib (VEPTR)	Rib, spine, or iliac crest	Surgical distraction, typically every 6–8 months
MAGnetic Expansion Control (MAGEC) rod	Proximal and distal spine	Magnetic expansion mechanism activated externally; can be done in the outpatient office
Shilla	Rods fixed to vertebrae of curve apex	Sliding pedicle screws placed above below curve guide spinal growth and allow the device to self-distract
Vertebral body tether[a]	Consecutive anterior vertebrae along major curve	Polyethylene tether anchored to convex side of spinal curve unilaterally limits spinal growth

[a]Not routinely used for complex scoliosis.

From Samdani AF, Pahys JM, Ames RJ, et al. Prospective follow-up report on anterior vertebral body tethering for idiopathic scoliosis: interim results from an FDA IDE study. *J Bone Joint Surg Am*. 2021;103:1611-1619; Mayer O, Campbell R, Cahill P, Redding R. Thoracic insufficiency syndrome. *Curr Probl Pediatr Adolesc Health Care*. 2016;46:72-97; McCarthy RE, Luhmann S, Lenke L, McCullough FL. The Shilla growth guidance technique for early-onset spinal deformities at 2-year follow-up: a preliminary report. *J Pediatr Orthop*. 2014;34:1-7; Tsukahara K, Mayer OH. Thoracic insufficiency syndrome: approaches to assessment and management. *Paediatr Respir Rev*. 2022;44:78-84.

MANAGEMENT AND PROGNOSIS

Premature rupture of membranes occurs in approximately 10% of all pregnancies, and pulmonary hypoplasia occurs in 13–21% of cases with second-trimester premature rupture of membranes.[13] The duration of severe oligohydramnios (amniotic pocket less than 1 cm and lasting more than 14 days) and gestational age (fetus younger than 25 weeks of gestation) are independent risk factors for lethal pulmonary hypoplasia.[14,15] Lethality usually results in a 25-week fetus with more than 3 days of oligohydramnios, but when chronic leakage of amniotic fluid occurs after 27 weeks of gestation, every measure toward providing adequate oxygenation should be taken in the hope of maintaining survival until lung development can become adequate for normal respiration.

The lungs in thanatophoric dysplasia (see Fig. 18.1) and fetal akinesia sequence are usually too hypoplastic to allow for survival, and extended respiratory support is generally futile. In other conditions, such as short-rib thoracic dysplasia or spondylocostal dysostosis (SCD), the prognosis is extremely variable, which leaves little tolerance for additional insults such as respiratory syncytial virus infection. Short-rib thoracic dysplasia with or without polydactyly refers to a group of autosomal recessive skeletal ciliopathies that are characterized by a constricted thoracic cage, short ribs, shortened tubular bones, and a "trident" appearance of the acetabular roof.[16] This group of disorders includes the perinatal lethal short-rib polydactyly syndromes and the less severe asphyxiating thoracic dystrophy (Jeune syndrome), Ellis-van Creveld syndrome, and cranioectodermal dysplasia (see Figs. 18.2 and 18.3). Polydactyly is variably present, and there is phenotypic overlap in these various conditions, which differ by visceral malformation and metaphyseal appearance. Non-skeletal involvement can include cleft lip/palate as well as anomalies of major organs such as the brain, eye, heart, kidneys, liver, pancreas, intestines, and genitalia. Some conditions are lethal in the neonatal period because of respiratory insufficiency from a severely restricted thoracic cage, whereas others are compatible with life. One-stage thoracic expansion also has been attempted in nine children with Jeune syndrome.[17] There were two deaths within 3 months of surgery resulting from pulmonary causes. At the median follow-up of 11 months, three children had been discharged home, and two had significantly reduced respiratory support. One child remained on noninvasive ventilation and another continued to require ventilatory support with a high oxygen requirement. Among 24 patients with Jeune syndrome treated at a mean age of 23 months with VEPTR dynamic posterolateral expansion thoracoplasty and followed to an average age of 8.4 years, average chest width increased from 121 to 168 mm at follow-up ($P < .001$), total lung volumes increased 484 to 740 mm^3 ($P < .001$), and assisted ventilation rate status tended to improve ($P = .07$).[18] The survival rate with surgery was nearly 70% (compared with 70%–80% mortality without treatment) with less ventilator dependence.

Jarcho-Levin syndrome includes two conditions that result in severe shortening of the chest: SCD and spondylothoracic dysplasia (STD). SCD is usually associated with severe scoliosis and chaotic patterns of absent and/or fused ribs. It can be treated with expansion thoracoplasty using a VEPTR technique.[19,20] STD results in more severe volume restriction of the thorax with mild scoliosis but extreme shortening of the thoracic spine (see Fig. 18.3A), averaging 25% of the normal height with most of the posterior ribs fused in a "crablike" pattern. STD had a very high mortality rate reported in the earlier literature within the first year of life, but recent reports have noted an improved survival rate of 55%–58%, with most deaths occurring in the first year of life from respiratory failure. A VEPTR expansion thoracoplasty technique for the posterior fused rib mass in STD has been developed.[21] Together, SCD and STD are a genetically heterogeneous group of axial skeletal disorders characterized by generalized multiple segmentation defects of the vertebrae, misalignment of the ribs with variable points of intercostal fusion, and often a reduction in rib number, resulting in a small, broadly symmetric chest with compromised thoracic and lung function. SCD occurs in 1 in 40,000 live births and this condition is inherited, predominantly as autosomal recessive traits due to mutations in genes that are involved in the Notch-signaling pathway such as the *DLL3*, *MESP2*, *LFNG*, *HES7*, *TBX6*, *RIPPLY2*, and *DLL1* genes.[22,23] Early mortality resulting from respiratory insufficiency and life-threatening pulmonary hypertension can occur, but surgical enlargement of the chest may lead to improved survival in some cases.

VEPTR expansion thoracoplasty has also been used to manage thoracic insufficiency syndrome in early-onset scoliosis in 21 children.[24] Mean forced vital capacity increased from 0.65 to 0.96 L ($P < .0001$), but this increase in lung volume did not keep up with the growth of the child, and the percentage of the predicted forced vital capacity decreased while chest wall stiffness increased. Coronal correction was maintained, but there was some increase in proximal thoracic kyphosis.

With the advent of prenatal imaging, the prognosis of congenital diaphragmatic hernia can be evaluated by assessing the fetal lung size, the degree of liver herniation, and the fetal pulmonary vasculature. Severe diaphragmatic hernias have poor outcomes and may be candidates for fetal endoscopic tracheal occlusion, which is usually performed between 26 and 30 weeks' gestation. In utero, an endoscope is passed through the fetal mouth and down to the carina; the balloon is deployed just above the carina, and at approximately 34 weeks' gestation, the balloon is deflated and removed.[6,25] Fetal endoscopic tracheal occlusion is thought to improve outcomes by minimizing pulmonary hypoplasia and pulmonary arterial hypertension, but following delivery, neonates still require diaphragm repair. Bilateral renal agenesis leads to complete absence of urine production, termed Potter syndrome, which is associated with extremely hypoplastic lungs (Figs. 18.5–18.7), which is usually lethal.

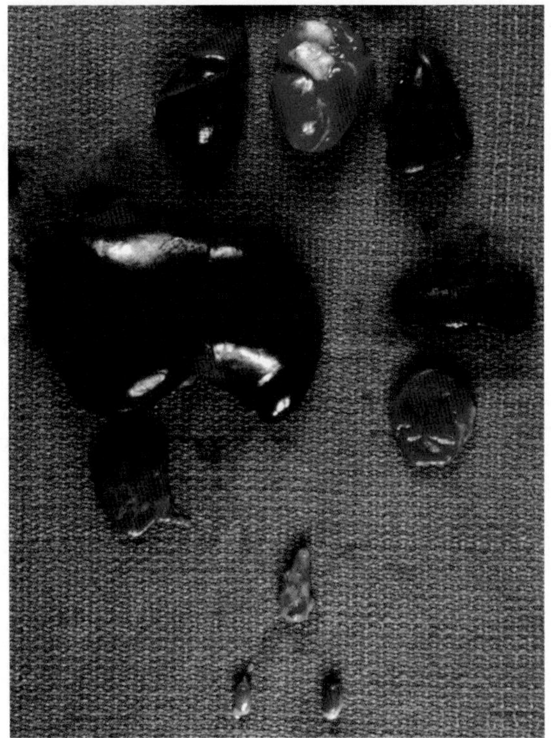

FIGURE 18.6 Relative organ size in an infant with bilateral renal agenesis, resulting in prolonged oligohydramnios due to failure of urine flow. Note the extremely small size of both lungs and the discoid appearance of both adrenal glands when both kidneys are absent.

DIFFERENTIAL DIAGNOSIS

Oligohydramnios may be the result of inadequate urine flow into the amniotic space (e.g., bilateral renal agenesis, polycystic kidney disease, or cystic dysplastic kidneys), in which case the prognosis is usually poor. Instillation of fluid has been used successfully in cases of oligohydramnios, and fetal bladder catheterization has been used in other cases of bladder outlet obstruction. (See Chapter 46 for a more complete discussion of the oligohydramnios deformation sequence.) Diaphragmatic hernia not only limits lung development on the side of the hernia, but also shifts the mediastinal contents toward the opposite side, thereby limiting lung growth on that side as well. Hence, infants with this condition may die from respiratory insufficiency caused by lung hypoplasia unless fetal surgery is attempted to correct the diaphragmatic hernia. Several skeletal dysplasias have a profound impact on thoracic cage growth, thereby resulting in lung hypoplasia and associated respiratory insufficiency. These disorders are extremely heterogeneous from a genetic standpoint and establishing an accurate genetic diagnosis can be extremely useful in providing prenatal diagnosis for future pregnancies.

References

1. Askin F. Respiratory tract disorders in the fetus and neonate. In: Wigglesworth JS, Singer DB, eds. *Textbook of*

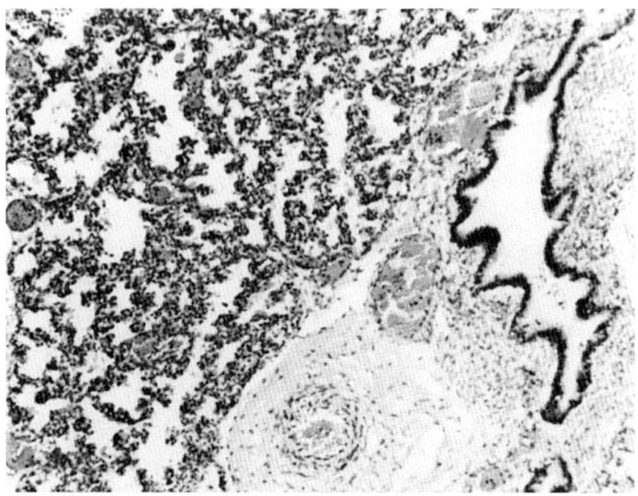

FIGURE 18.7 Histology in hypoplastic lungs caused by prolonged oligohydramnios.

Fetal and Perinatal Pathology. Boston: Blackwell Scientific; 1991:643–688.
2. Gilbert-Barness E. *Potter's pathology of the fetus and infant*. St. Louis: Mosby; 1997:733–734.
3. Tsukahara K, Mayer OH. Thoracic insufficiency syndrome: approaches to assessment and management. *Paediatr Respir Rev*. 2022;44:78–84.
4. Strong A, Behr M, Lott C, et al. Molecular diagnosis and novel genes and phenotypes in a pediatric thoracic insufficiency cohort. *Sci Rep*. 2023;13(1):991.
5. Campbell Jr RM, Smith MD. Thoracic insufficiency syndrome and exotic scoliosis. *J Bone Joint Surg Am*. 2007;89(Suppl 1):108–122.
6. Kirby E, Keijzer R. Congenital diaphragmatic hernia: current management strategies from antenatal diagnosis to long-term follow-up. *Pediatr Surg Int*. 2020;36(4):415–429.
7. Wigglesworth JS, Desai R. Is fetal respiratory function a major determinant of perinatal survival? *Lancet*. 1982;1:264–267.
8. Richards DS. Complications of prolonged PROM and oligohydramnios. *Clin Obstet Gynecol*. 1998;41:817–826.
9. Nimrod C, Varela-Gittins F, Machin G, et al. The effect of very prolonged membrane rupture on fetal development. *Am J Obstet Gynecol*. 1984;148:540–543.
10. Moessinger AC, Collins MH, Blanc WA, et al. Oligohydramnios-induced lung hypoplasia: the influence of timing and duration in gestation. *Pediatr Res*. 1986;20:951–954.
11. Kilbride HW, Yeast J, Thiebault DW. Defining limits of survival: lethal pulmonary hypoplasia after midtrimester premature rupture of membranes. *Am J Obstet Gynecol*. 1996;175:675–681.
12. Wigglesworth JS, Desai R, Guerrini P. Lung hypoplasia: biochemical and structural variations and their possible significance. *Arch Dis Child*. 1981;56:606–615.
13. Cooney TP, Thurlbeck WM. The radial alveolar count method of Emery and Mithal: a reappraisal. 2. Intrauterine and early postnatal lung growth. *Thorax*. 1982;37:580–583.
14. Rotschild A, Ling EW, Poterman ML, et al. Neonatal outcome after prolonged preterm rupture of the membranes. *Am J Obstet Gynecol*. 1990;162:46–52.
15. Suzuki K. Respiratory characteristics of infants with pulmonary hypoplasia syndrome following preterm rupture of membranes: a preliminary study for establishing clinical diagnostic criteria. *Early Hum Dev*. 2004;79:31–40.
16. Zhang W, Taylor SP, Ennis HA, et al. Expanding the genetic architecture and phenotypic spectrum in the skeletal ciliopathies. *Hum Mutat*. 2018;39(1):152–166.
17. Muthialu N, Mussa S, Owens CM, Bulstrode N, Elliott MJ. One-stage sequential bilateral thoracic expansion for asphyxiating thoracic dystrophy (Jeune syndrome). *Eur J Cardiothorac Surg*. 2014;46(4):643–647.
18. O'Brien A, Roth MK, Athreya H, et al. Management of thoracic insufficiency syndrome in patients with Jeune syndrome using the 70 mm radius vertical expandable prosthetic titanium rib. *J Pediatr Orthop*. 2015;35(8):783–797.
19. Ramirez N, Flynn JM, Emans JB, et al. Vertical expandable prosthetic titanium rib as treatment of thoracic insufficiency syndrome in spondylocostal dysplasia. *J Pediatr Orthop*. 2010;30(6):521–526.
20. Karlin JG, Roth MK, Patil V, et al. Management of thoracic insufficiency syndrome in patients with Jarcho-Levin syndrome using VEPTRs (vertical expandable prosthetic titanium ribs). *J Bone Joint Surg Am*. 2014 Nov 5;96(21):e181.
21. Joshi AP, Roth MK, Simmons JW, Shardonofsky F, Campbell Jr. RM. Expansion thoracoplasty for thoracic insufficiency syndrome associated with Jarcho-Levin syndrome. *JBJS Essent Surg Tech*. 2015;5(2):e12.
22. Nóbrega A, Maia-Fernandes AC, Andrade RP. Altered cogs of the clock: insights into the embryonic etiology of spondylocostal dysostosis. *J Dev Biol*. 2021;9(1):5.
23. Umair M, Younus M, Shafiq S, Nayab A, Alfadhel M. Clinical genetics of spondylocostal dysostosis: A mini review. *Front Genet*. 2022;13:996364.
24. Dede O, Motoyama EK, Yang CI, Mutich RL, Walczak SA, Bowles AJ, Deeney VF. Pulmonary and radiographic outcomes of VEPTR (vertical expandable prosthetic titanium rib) treatment in early-onset scoliosis. *J Bone Joint Surg Am*. 2014;96(15):1295–1302.
25. Ruano R, Ali RA, Patel P, et al. Fetal endoscopic tracheal occlusion for congenital diaphragmatic hernia: indications, outcomes, and future directions. *Obstet Gynecol Surv*. 2014;69:147–158.

CHAPTER 19

Pectus Excavatum and Pectus Carinatum

KEY POINTS

- Pectus excavatum and pectus carinatum are the most common abnormalities of the thorax. The incidence of pectus excavatum is between 1 and 8 per 1000 persons, and pectus carinatum is two to four times less frequent than pectus excavatum.
- Pectus excavatum is thought to result from overgrowth of costal cartilages, which becomes more apparent during the period of rapid skeletal growth in early adolescence.
- Pectus carinatum is thought to be caused by abnormal growth of costal cartilages with precocious fusion of sternal growth plates.
- Severe pectus excavatum is usually repaired during adolescence because this deformity tends to worsen during the adolescent growth spurt.
- For younger pediatric patients with pectus carinatum, noninvasive orthotic bracing treatment should be considered first.
- Sternal depression surgery may be the preferred treatment for patients over 15 years of age with severe pectus carinatum.

GENESIS

Pectus excavatum and pectus carinatum are the most common abnormalities of the thorax. The incidence of pectus excavatum is between 1 and 8 per 1000 persons, and pectus carinatum is two to four times less frequent than pectus excavatum, with a significant male-to-female excess for both pectus carinatum and pectus excavatum.[1] If no features of an underlying disorder are detected, then the pectus abnormality is considered to be an isolated abnormality. Although cases of nonsyndromal pectus excavatum or carinatum with a positive family history fitting mendelian inheritance have been described, no single gene has been identified as a causative factor for either deformity, and the recurrence risk for a nonfamilial isolated pectus deformity appears to be low.[1] If other features are present, then appropriate further diagnostic studies are indicated because pectus excavatum or carinatum can be part of many syndromes.[1] The most frequently observed monogenic syndromes with pectus abnormalities are Marfan syndrome (Fig. 19.1) and Noonan syndrome (Fig. 19.2A).

Pectus excavatum or carinatum can be present at birth, but both disorders are usually not recognized until early childhood, when the deformity progresses (Fig. 19.2B). The cause of each condition is not known with certainty, but pectus excavatum is thought to result from an inward overgrowth of costal cartilages, which becomes more apparent during the period of rapid skeletal growth in early adolescence. Pectus carinatum is thought to be caused by abnormal outward growth of costal cartilages with precocious fusion of sternal growth plates, resulting in anterior bowing of the superior costal cartilages and consequent protrusion of the superior portion of the sternum. Most recent studies agree that the primordial defect leading to deformation of the anterior chest wall is related to the costal hyaline cartilage structure and function, and the origin of pectus deformities may be found in the ultrastructure of the costal cartilage.[2] A positive family history is observed in 43% of pectus excavatum cases and 25% of pectus carinatum cases,[3] and the mean prevalence of adolescent idiopathic scoliosis in patients with pectus deformity is 13.1%.[4] This association may represent the occurrence of a common underlying condition, and abnormal skeletal growth in a variety of skeletal dysplasias and genetic connective tissue disorders can result in pectus deformities, which are especially frequent in patients with Marfan syndrome.

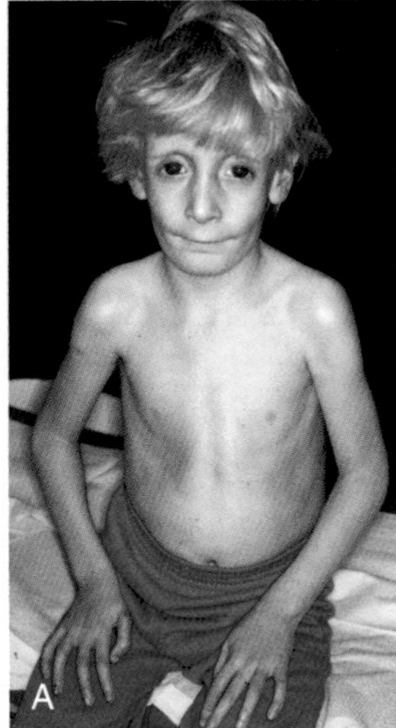
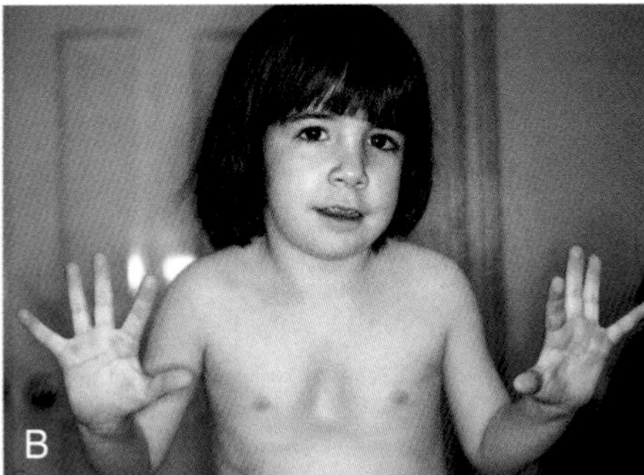
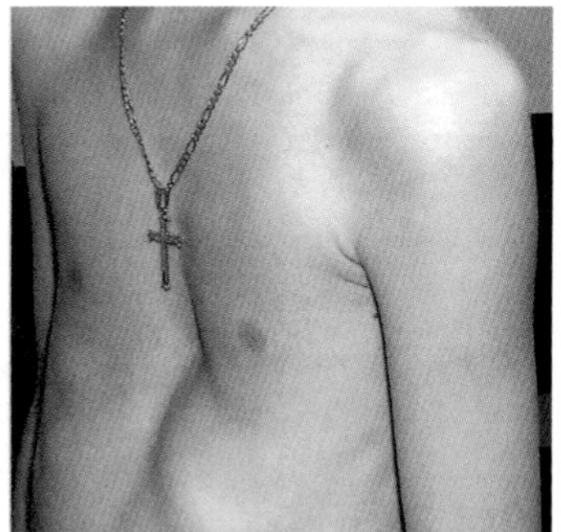

FIGURE 19.1 A, Pectus carinatum and **B,** pectus excavatum in unrelated children with Marfan syndrome, an autosomal dominant connective tissue disorder that results in laxity of connective tissues because of mutations in *FBN1*.

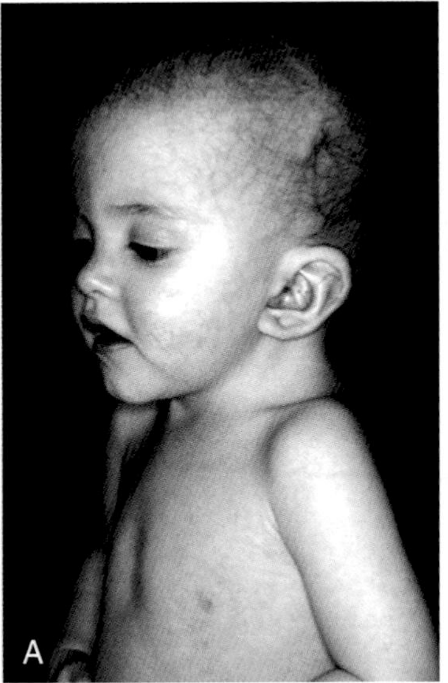
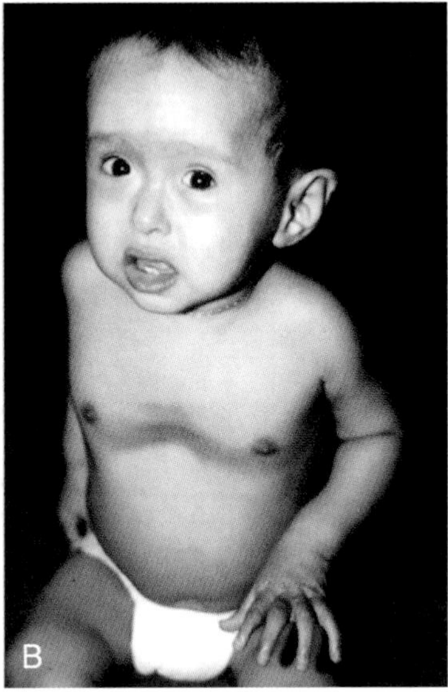
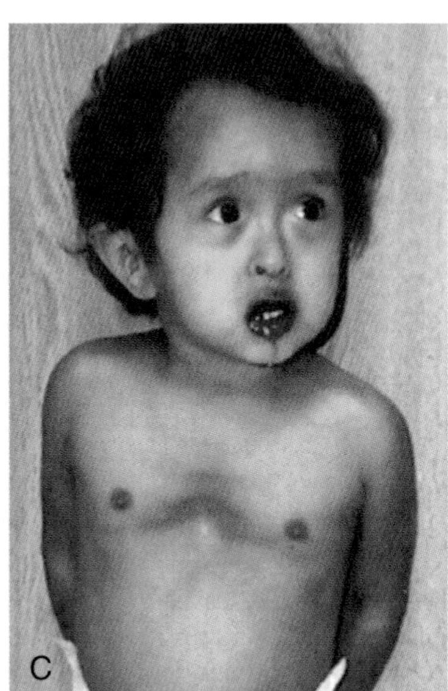

FIGURE 19.2 A, Early pectus excavatum in a 10-month-old girl with Noonan syndrome, and **B, C** progression of pectus excavatum between 2 and 4 years of age in a boy with Van Den Ende-Gupta syndrome.

Pectus deformities affect a significant proportion of the general population (0.8%) and an even greater proportion of patients with Marfan syndrome (up to 70%).[5] Pectus excavatum can be a clue to the early diagnosis of Morquio syndrome,[6] a rare autosomal recessive type of mucopolysaccharidosis that can take several years (mean 2.6 years) from initial presentation to definitive diagnosis (mean age 4.7–4.9 years). Since enzyme replacement is available, late diagnosis complicates disease management. These authors reported a case of Morquio A syndrome in which definitive diagnosis was made within 2 months of initial presentation.[6]

Chest wall deformities can be divided into two main categories, congenital and acquired. Congenital chest wall deformities may present any time between birth and early adolescence. Acquired chest wall deformities typically follow prior chest surgery or a posterolateral diaphragmatic hernia repair (Bochdalek). Open thoracotomy for repair of cardiovascular defects during early childhood sometimes affects the growth of costal cartilages, leading to pectus deformities with secondary associated scoliosis. Large congenital diaphragmatic hernias can be repaired with either a muscle flap or prosthetic patch. Prospectively, 75% of flap patients and 67% of patch patients had pectus, and 13% of flap patients and 33% of patch patients had scoliosis. The operative technique did not appear to affect the incidence of subsequent skeletal deformity.[7]

FEATURES

Pectus excavatum results in a central anterior chest depression (inward sternum), whereas pectus carinatum results in sternal protrusion (prominent sternum). Both may be symmetric, but they are usually asymmetric. Frequently the sternum faces to the right in pectus excavatum, and the deepest depression is usually near the xiphoid. Deep inspiration commonly accentuates the pectus depression, and the heart is often displaced into the left chest, interfering with right atrial filling and limiting pulmonary expansion on inspiration. Respiration during exercise often requires deeper diaphragmatic excursions to compensate for diminished chest wall expansion and younger adolescents may become easily fatigued during exercise, with decreased stamina and endurance.[1] Some patients experience exercise-induced asthma and/or low anterior chest pain as well as bronchiectasis. Spontaneous regression of pectus excavatum or pectus carinatum rarely occurs. Echocardiography and static and exercise pulmonary function testing are recommended before surgical reconstruction for pectus excavatum, and for pectus carinatum, only static and exercise pulmonary function assessments are recommended unless a genetic disorder of connective tissue or syndrome is suspected (e.g., Marfan syndrome or Noonan syndrome).[1] About 20–25% of patients with pectus excavatum have associated mild to moderate scoliosis, particularly with genetic connective tissue disorders, and body-building resulting in hypertrophy of chest muscles can accentuate sternal depression. Severe pectus excavatum is usually repaired during adolescence because this deformity tends to worsen during the adolescent growth spurt. With improved surgical techniques, surgery yields improvements in respiratory symptoms and exercise tolerance, with excellent cosmetic results and short hospital stays.

MANAGEMENT AND PROGNOSIS

In mild cases no management is necessary, but because most cases progress with growth, surgical intervention merits early consideration. The primary goal of surgical repair is to correct the chest deformity, which improves self-acceptance and may improve the patient's breathing, posture, and cardiac function. In 1949, Ravitch described a repair technique requiring resection of deformed costal cartilages, xiphoid excision, and transverse sternal osteotomy to displace the sternum anteriorly.[8] Traditionally, an open repair (the Ravitch technique) was performed in which the abnormal cartilage was resected and the sternum was fractured and fixed in a corrected position. More recently, beginning in the late 1990s, the Ravitch technique has been supplanted by the significantly less invasive Nuss procedure, in which a curved bar is passed upside down with thoracoscopic assistance and then flipped into position under the sternum, effectively lifting the sternum and chest wall into a corrected position. Routine thoracoscopy and sternal elevation have helped to prevent intraoperative cardiac injuries. The Nuss procedure has gained popularity because it has been shown to have minimal blood loss, a shorter operating time, good postoperative results and satisfaction, and a low rate of complications with no visible scar on the anterior chest. Nuss recommends surgical repair for those with severe symptomatic pectus excavatum at around 13–15 years of age, since the chest wall is still typically flexible and because this allows the bar to be kept in place as the patient progresses through puberty, which may help decrease growth-related recurrences. Current management has moved away from operating on children except in rare symmetric cases. Postoperative management includes pain control via cryoablation of intercostal nerves, deep breathing, and early ambulation. Exercise restriction is mandatory for the first 6 weeks with slow resumption of normal activity after 12 weeks.[9] In a retrospective study of 62 children with pectus excavatum treated with the Nuss procedure, age of surgery was evaluated regarding surgical outcome: group A (3–12 years old) and group B (>12 years old), with 31 cases in each group. The overall response rate to treatment in group A (93.55%) was higher than that of group B (70.97%; $P < .05$), while left ventricular ejection fraction, cardiac index, stroke volume, forced expiratory volume in 1 second, and peak expiratory flow levels were increased compared to before the operation, and the improvement in these indicators of group A was better than in group B (all $P < .05$). Thus a younger age indicates a better effect.[10]

Among 24 physically active pediatric patients aged 9–18 years with severe pectus excavatum, cardiopulmonary exercise testing was performed before and after the Nuss procedure. After the repair, the exercise capacity as measured by maximal oxygen consumption improved significantly, primarily due to increase in oxygen pulse, an indirect measurement of stroke volume.[11] Among 392 patients over 18 years of age who had preoperative cardiopulmonary exercise testing, abnormal oxygen consumption was present in 68% of patients. Consistent improvements in cardiopulmonary function were seen for these adult patients with pectus excavatum after the Nuss procedure for pectus excavatum, supporting the existence of adverse preoperative cardiopulmonary consequences, as well as the benefits of surgical repair.[12] Both lung volume and weight significantly increased in 10 patients averaging 13.8 years after Nuss surgery, suggesting that growth of the lung parenchyma is associated with the correction of chest deformity in younger patients with pectus excavatum.[13] Indications for surgery are driven largely by the presence of symptoms.

Patients with mild to moderate pectus excavatum may be treated with therapeutic deep breathing, posturing, and aerobic exercises, and in appropriately selected patients, vacuum bell therapy may also be offered.[9] This technique creates negative pressure up to 15% below the atmospheric pressure by application on the anterior chest wall. A hand pump is operated by the patient, who learns to place the middle of the device's window above the deepest point of the deformity. There are three different sizes of vacuum bell approved by the United States Food and Drug Administration (16, 19, and 22 cm in diameter, respectively) according to patient age, ventral surface, and self-perception of the deformity, and another model is available for adolescents and adult female patients. A review of 13 studies involving the use of vacuum bell therapy revealed depth-improvement in 37–90%, with 10–40% having an excellent correction to normal.[14] This technique is contraindicated in patients with skeletal disorders (e.g., osteogenesis imperfecta), vasculopathies (e.g., Marfan syndrome, aortic aneurysm, or dilated aortic root), coagulopathies (e.g., hemophilia or thrombocytopenia), and cardiac disorders. Younger patients with good chest pliability are the best candidates for vacuum bell therapy.[15]

Haje et al. reported treating 84 patients with broad pectus excavatum (mean age 13.3 years) and 115 patients with localized pectus excavatum (mean age 12.8 years) with a dynamic orthotic that applied pressure to lower rib projections and prescribed exercises with at least 36 months of follow-up. Evaluation more than a year after treatment ended revealed good results in 70–83% of patients who used the brace and performed the exercises, especially when treatment was started earlier for milder more flexible deformities.[16,17]

Another nonsurgical treatment for pectus excavatum includes the use of a dermal filler such as hyaluronic acid gel, which has previously been used in plastic surgery for volume and contour enhancement. Males over 18 years of age with no functional problems received 50–150-mL injections at the site of their pectus excavatum, and 58% of the gel remained 24 months after treatment. This treatment was well tolerated with good patient satisfaction.[18]

Different minimally invasive surgical techniques have been used for pectus carinatum, such as the anti-Nuss procedure or the Abramson technique, in which a steel bar is placed over the sternum and secured to the ribs. Among 112 patients with a mean age 14.5 years, the operation took 68 minutes on average with a mean length of stay of 3–4 days and good or excellent results in 87.5% of patients.[19] This operation was effective in repairing both symmetric and asymmetric pectus carinatum patients (Fig. 19.3). Satisfactory cosmetic results were reported for 42 patients with pectus excavatum who underwent minimally invasive surgery with the bar left in place for 2 years.[20] Surgical correction does not impair cardiopulmonary function.[21]

In 1992, good results were reported with prolonged use of an orthotic sternal brace for pectus carinatum in 21 children and adolescents (Fig. 19.4).[22] A *dynamic compressor system* orthotic brace was created in Argentina in 2001 as an alternative to surgery, and it has been used worldwide.[23] In a study of 61 patients with pectus carinatum (43 symmetric, 18 asymmetric) who were treated with a dynamic chest compression brace at a mean age of 13.5 years, with a mean use time of 19 hours per day, 47 patients completed this treatment with excellent aesthetic results and 14 patients were improving under active treatment with satisfactory initial results. None of the 61 patients in this study abandoned the treatment, and no complications were reported.[24] Continued bracing until skeletal maturity provides the most complete and

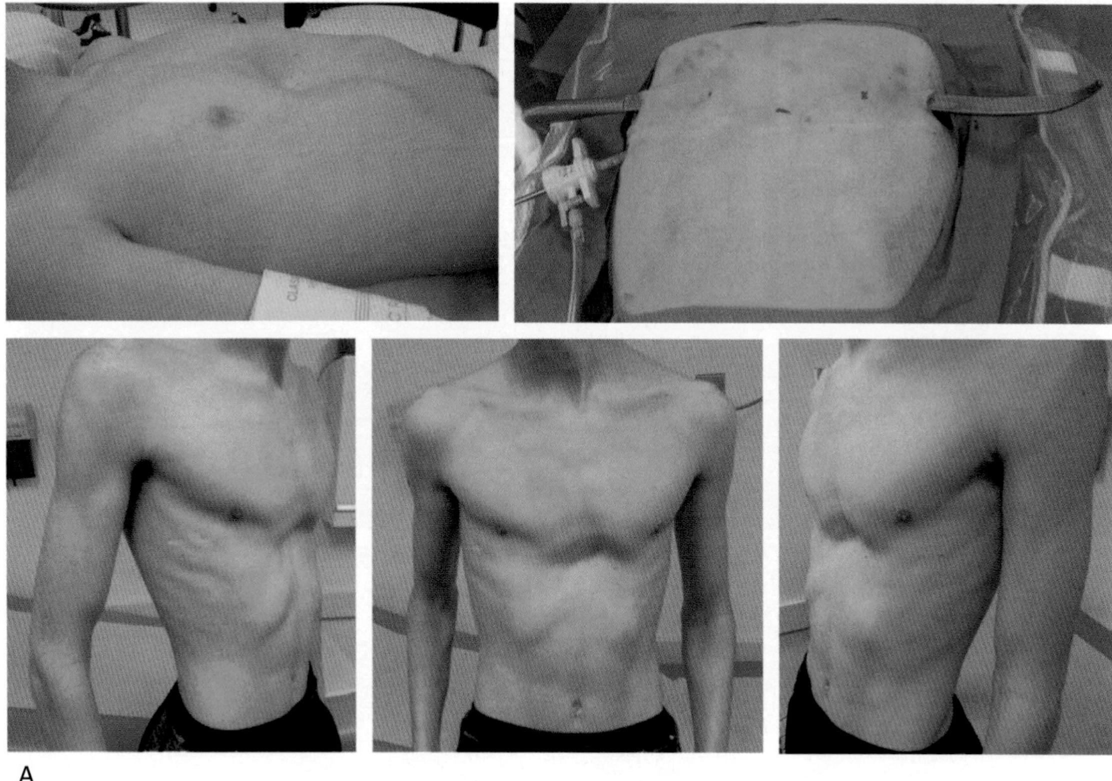

A

FIGURE 19.3 A, Pectus excavatum before and during surgery (insertion of substernal bar) (*top*). Post-operative results 33 months after surgery and removal of substernal bar (*bottom*).

stable correction. Among 61 patients with pectus carinatum who wore orthotic braces that allowed gradual compression, the brace was worn 6 hours per day during the first week and the bracing time was extended an additional hour per week until 16 hours per day was reached. Pulmonary function tests were not affected by brace treatment, and gradual progression of bracing increased the patient's compliance.[25] Between January 2008 and December 2012, 69 pectus carinatum patients were treated with custom-fitted braces. Mean length of therapy was 7 months, and mean duration of brace wearing was 12–15 hours per day. Patients who reported the result "unchanged" had a mean daily brace-wearing time of 8.73 hours, whereas those who judged the result as "good" wore the brace for 14.53 hours and those who judged the result as "excellent" wore the brace for 18.36 hours. Thus daily brace-wearing time should be greater than 14 hours, ideally 24 hours, and the duration of treatment should be around 1 year since treatment results correlate directly with the cooperation of the patients.[26]

Among patients with pectus carinatum evaluated by three-dimensional (3D) whole-body scans, 40 patients underwent compressive orthotic bracing and 10 were observed without treatment. Among 23 patients who were compliant with bracing for more than 12 hours per day, and 17 patients who were noncompliant, compliant patients exhibited an 8.2% improvement versus 1.5% improvement in noncompliant patients and 2.5% improvement in non-brace patients. The change in compliant patients was significantly better compared with non-brace patients and noncompliant patients, indicating that three-dimensional body scans are an effective, radiation-free, and objective means to evaluate patients treated with compressive orthotic bracing.[27] Another study compared pre- and post-treatment radiographs with 3D body surface scanning.[28] Bracing therapy produced favorable outcomes in all 63 patients who underwent compressive orthotic bracing.

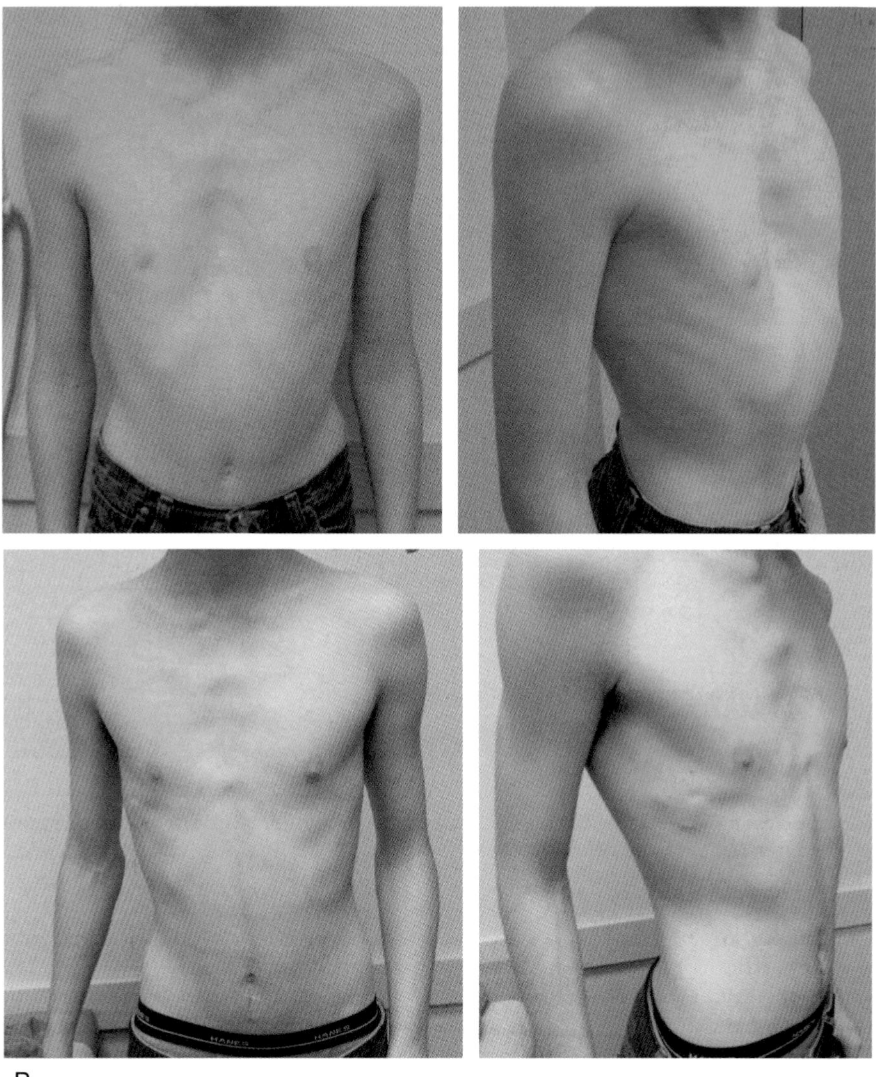

B

FIGURE 19.3, cont'd B, Pectus excavatum in one brother before surgery (*top*) and 41 months after surgery (*bottom*).

Measurements obtained via 3D body surface scanning were strongly correlated with those obtained via chest radiography, thus 3D body surface scanning is an effective, radiation-free method for the evaluation of pectus excavatum treatment. In a metaanalysis of five studies comparing optical imaging versus computed tomography and plain radiography to quantify pectus excavatum in a total of 75 patients, there was high correlation between 3D optical surface scanning and radiological assessment, reducing concerns over ionizing radiation.[29]

Among 137 pectus carinatum patients treated between 2008 and 2011, the median age for 122 bracing patients was 14 years. Five patients (4%) were lost to follow-up and 13 (11%) failed treatment, whereas 37 patients (30%) exhibited flattening of the sternum after 6 months without surgery. After flattening, patients then wore the brace for progressively fewer hours each day as a "retainer" for 5 months. Five patients (4%) experienced recurrence about 5 months after brace treatment was discontinued, and complications were limited to transient skin breakdown in

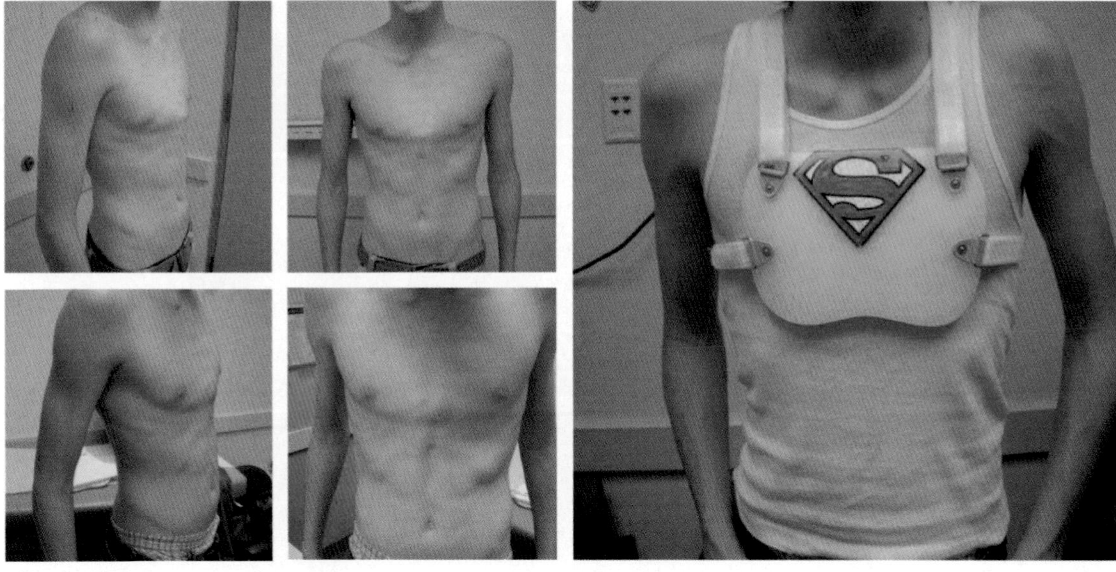

C

FIGURE 19.3, cont'd C, Pectus carinatum in other brother before (*top, left*) and after 12 months of therapy (*bottom, left*) with brace (*right*). Note erythema over sternum from pressure of brace. (Figures courtesy Dr. Eugene Kim, Chief of Pediatric Surgery at Cedars-Sinai Medical Center).

nine patients. Three of the 13 brace failures and 15 other pectus carinatum patients were treated surgically. Thirteen underwent an Abramson minimally invasive operation, whereas five had an open repair, all with good initial correction. In three patients with stiff chests, costal cartilage was resected thoracoscopically during Abramson repair, which measurably improved compliance. Staged treatment of pectus carinatum allowed most teenagers to be managed nonoperatively. For patients who fail bracing or are not compliant with bracing, minimally invasive surgical treatment is a viable option.[30] Among 767 pediatric patients, 644 achieved satisfactory chest appearance through orthotic bracing, for a success rate of 84.0%. Younger pediatric patients had better orthotic outcomes. Among the 123 failure cases, 108 pediatric patients successfully completed minimally invasive surgery with a mean operation time of 113 minutes and an average length of hospital stay after surgery of 7 days.[31] For younger pediatric patients with pectus carinatum, noninvasive orthotic bracing treatment should be considered first. For older pediatric patients, the failure rate for bracing was higher and outcomes were often unsatisfactory, so minimally invasive sternal depression may be the preferred treatment for patients over 15 years of age with pectus carinatum. As the anti-Nuss procedure has been modified in recent years, patients have experienced shorter operative durations and postoperative hospitalizations, with shorter plate removal durations.[32]

DIFFERENTIAL DIAGNOSIS

Pectus deformities may occur concomitantly with abdominal muscle weakness in several neurologic disorders, and they also occur with certain genetic connective tissue disorders and skeletal dysplasias (e.g., Jeune syndrome [see Fig. 18.2]), as well as in many other conditions.[1] About two-thirds of patients with Marfan syndrome have pectus excavatum, which may manifest later in childhood than in other patients, who usually present before 2 years of age. Patients with Marfan syndrome are also much more likely to experience recurrence if sternal support bars are not used postoperatively, and they may benefit from pectus repair performed before aortic replacement is necessary.[33] Pectus excavatum can be inherited without any associated syndrome, with most cases fitting a multifactoral mode of inheritance.[34]

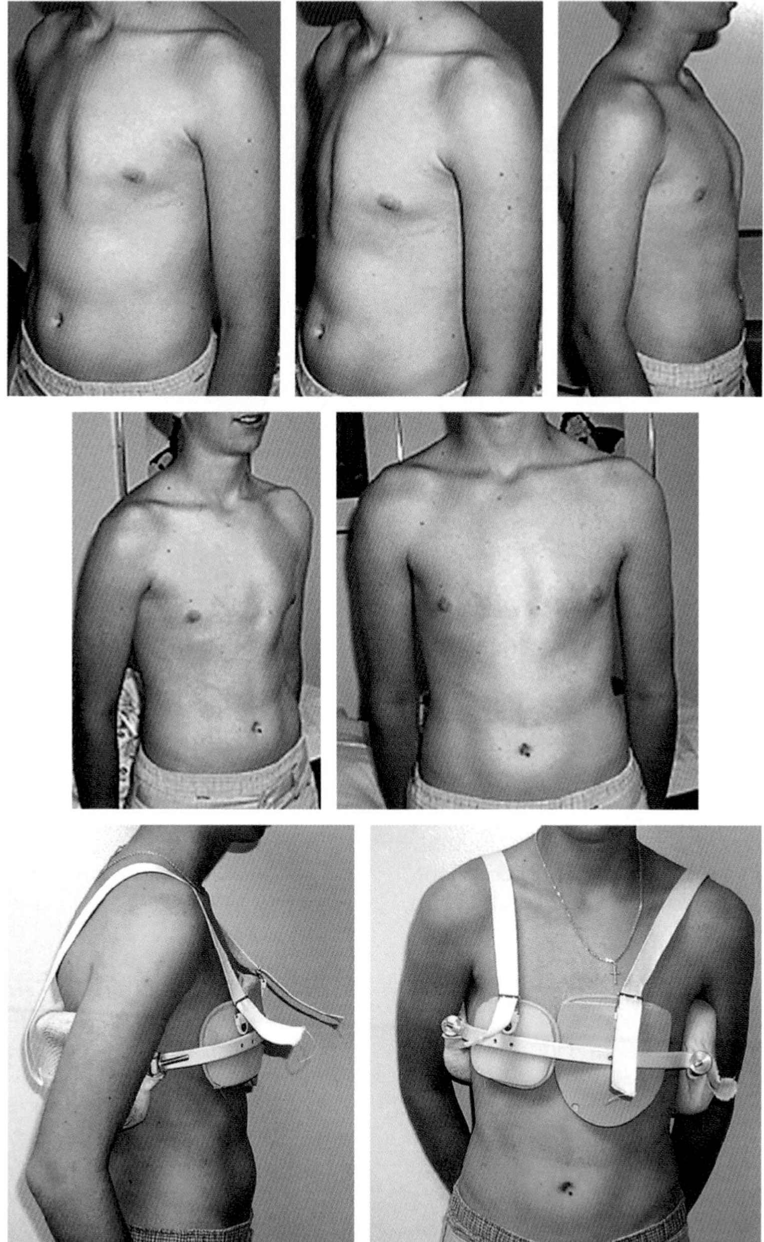

FIGURE 19.4 An otherwise normal adolescent with pectus carinatum. Nonsurgical correction of pectus carinatum was attempted via orthotic bracing.

References

1. Cobben JM, Oostra RJ, van Dijk FS. Pectus excavatum and carinatum. *Eur J Med Genet*. 2014;57:414–417.
2. David VL. Current concepts in the etiology and pathogenesis of pectus excavatum in humans—a systematic review. *J Clin Med*. 2022;11(5):1241.
3. Ramadan S, Wilde J, Tabard-Fougère A, et al. Cardiopulmonary function in adolescent patients with pectus excavatum or carinatum. *BMJ Open Respir Res*. 2021;8(1):e001020.

4. Fraser S, Child A, Hunt I. Pectus updates and special considerations in Marfan syndrome. *Pediatr Rep.* 2018;9(4):7277.
5. van Es LJM, van Royen BJ, Oomen MWN. Clinical significance of concomitant pectus deformity and adolescent idiopathic scoliosis: systematic review with best evidence synthesis. *N Am Spine Soc J.* 2022;11:100140.
6. Yamauchi K, Hirano D, Wada M, Ida H. Pectus carinatum as the key to early diagnosis of Morquio A syndrome: a case report. *J Med Case Rep.* 2021;15(1):150.
7. Russell KW, Barnhart DC, Rollins MD, et al. Musculoskeletal deformities following repair of large congenital diaphragmatic hernias. *J Pediatr Surg.* 2014;49:886–889.
8. Ravitch MM The operative treatment of pectus excavatum. Ann Surg. 1949;129:429.
9. Nuss D, Obermeyer RJ, Kelly Jr. RE. Pectus excavatum from a pediatric surgeon's perspective. *Ann Cardiothorac Surg.* 2016;5(5):493–500.
10. Liu Q, Wang W, Hong C, et al. Effect of minimally invasive repair of pectus excavatum on postoperative chest flatness, cardiopulmonary function, and bone metabolism indexes in children at different ages. *Am J Transl Res.* 2022;14(6):3955–3963.
11. Das BB, Recto MR, Yeh T. Improvement of cardiopulmonary function after minimally invasive surgical repair of pectus excavatum (Nuss procedure) in children. *Ann Pediatr Cardiol.* 2019;12(2):77–82.
12. Jaroszewski DE, Farina JM, Gotway MB, et al. Cardiopulmonary outcomes after the Nuss procedure in pectus excavatum. *J Am Heart Assoc.* 2022;11(7):e022149.
13. Ito Y, Suzuki H, Sasahara Y, Mitsukawa N, Yoshino I. Can surgical repair for pectus excavatum contribute to lung growth? *Interact Cardiovasc Thorac Surg. 22.* 2021;33(6):928–934.
14. Loufopoulos I, Karagiannidis IG, Lampridis S, Mitsos S, Panagiotopoulos N. Vacuum bell: is it a useful innovative device for pectus excavatum correction? *Turk Thorac J.* 2021;22(3):251–256.
15. Yi E, Lee K, Jung Y, et al. Finding suitable candidates for vacuum bell therapy in pectus excavatum patients. *Sci Rep.* 2021;11(1):22787.
16. Haje DP, Haje SA, Volpon JB, da Silva ACO, Lima LFB, Huang W. Broad pectus excavatum treatment: long term results of a Brazilian technique. *Acta Ortop Bras.* 2021;29(4):197–202.
17. Haje DP, Haje SA, Volpon JB, Silva ACOD, Lima LFB, Huang W. Localized pectus excavatum treated with brace and exercise: long term results of a Brazilian technique. *Acta Ortop Bras.* 2021;29(3):143–148.
18. Hedén P, Sinna R. an open, prospective study to evaluate the effectiveness and safety of hyaluronic acid for pectus excavatum treatment. *Aesthet Surg J.* 2019;39(6):NP189–NP201.
19. Zhang X, Hu F, Bi R, Wang L, Jiang L. Minimally invasive repair of pectus carinatum with a new steel bar. *J Thorac Dis.* 2022 Aug;14(8):2781–2790.
20. Ping W, Fu S, Li Y, et al. A new minimally invasive technique for correction of pectus carinatum. *J Cardiothorac Surg.* 2021;16(1):280.
21. Sigl S, Del Frari B, Harasser C, Schwabegger AH. The effect on cardiopulmonary function after thoracoplasty in pectus carinatum: a systematic literature review. *Interact Cardiovasc Thorac Surg.* 2018;26(3):474–479.
22. Haje SA, Bowen RJ. Preliminary results of orthotic treatment of pectus deformities in children and adolescents. *J Pediatr Orthop.* 1992;12:795–800.
23. Martinez-Ferro M, Bellia Munzon G, Fraire C, et al. Non-surgical treatment of pectus carinatum with the FMF® Dynamic Compressor System. *J Vis Surg.* 2016;2:57.
24. Lopez M, Patoir A, Varlet F, et al. Preliminary study of efficacy of dynamic compression system in the correction of typical pectus carinatum. *Eur J Cardiothorac Surg.* 2013;44:e316–e319.
25. Ateş O, Karakuş OZ, Hakgüder G, et al. Pectus carinatum: the effects of orthotic bracing on pulmonary function and gradual compression on patient compliance. *Eur J Cardiothorac Surg.* 2013;44:e228–e232.
26. Loff S, Sauter H, Wirth T, Otte R. Highly efficient conservative treatment of pectus carinatum in compliant patients. *Eur J Pediatr Surg.* 2015;25(5):421–424.
27. Wong KE, Gorton 3rd GE, Tashjian DB, et al. Evaluation of the treatment of pectus carinatum with compressive orthotic bracing using three-dimensional body scans. *J Pediatr Surg.* 2014;49:924–927.
28. Song SH, Kim CH, Moon DH, Lee S. Usefulness of 3-dimensional body surface scanning in the evaluation of patients with pectus carinatum. *Korean J Thorac Cardiovasc Surg.* 2020;53(5):301–305.
29. Daemen JHT, Loonen TGJ, Lozekoot PWJ, et al. Optical imaging versus CT and plain radiography to quantify pectus severity: a systematic review and meta-analysis. *J Thorac Dis.* 2020;12(4):1475–1487.
30. Cohee AS, Lin JR, Frantz FW, et al. Staged management of pectus carinatum. *J Pediatr Surg.* 2013;48: 315–320.
31. Shang Z, Hong C, Duan X, Li X, Si Y. Orthotic bracing or minimally invasive surgery? A summary of 767 pectus carinatum cases for 9 years. *Biomed Res Int.* 2021;2021:6942329.
32. Wang L, Liu J, Shen S, et al. Comparison of outcomes between anti-Nuss operation and modified anti-Nuss operation using a flexible plate for correcting pectus carinatum: a retrospective study. *Front Surg.* 2021;7: 600755.
33. Scherer LR, Arn PH, Dressel DA, et al. Surgical management of children and young adults with Marfan syndrome and pectus excavatum. *J Pediatr Surg.* 1988;23:1169–1172.
34. Creswick HA, Stacey MW, Kelly Jr RE, et al. Family study of the inheritance of pectus excavatum. *J Pediatr Surg.* 2006;41:1699–1703.

CHAPTER 20

Scoliosis

KEY POINTS

- External fetal constraint rarely causes persistent scoliosis but can result in infantile idiopathic scoliosis that responds to physical therapy.
- Congenital scoliosis is caused by a failure of vertebral segmentation, which may lead to progressive spinal deformity with growth.
- Neuromuscular scoliosis is caused by central nervous system dysfunction, peripheral neuromuscular dysfunction, or combined sensory and motor dysfunction.
- Idiopathic scoliosis is divided into infantile (in children from birth up to 3 years of age), juvenile (in children 3–10 years of age), adolescent (in children older than 10 years of age), or adult.
- It is estimated that 20% of scoliosis can be attributed to neuromuscular, syndromic, or congenital disorders, while 80% is idiopathic.
- Recent high-quality evidence has been published on the effect of conservative treatment approaches (braces and exercises) for idiopathic scoliosis.
- A lateral bending of the spine and an associated rotation of vertebral bodies over 5–10 segments of the spine characterize adolescent idiopathic scoliosis.
- Current treatment guidelines recommend observation or physiotherapy for curves below 25 degrees and bracing for curves between 25 and 40 degrees.
- Surgery is indicated when progressive scoliosis exceeds 45 degrees in patients with an immature skeleton or when progression or associated pain occurs after skeletal maturity.

GENESIS

Scoliosis is the most common deformity of the spine, and it is defined as a lateral curvature of the spine that is 10 degrees or greater on a standing coronal radiographic image.[1]

Congenital scoliosis is caused by a failure of vertebral segmentation, which may lead to progressive spinal deformity with growth. Neuromuscular scoliosis is caused by central nervous system dysfunction (e.g., spastic quadriplegia), peripheral neuromuscular dysfunction (e.g., muscular dystrophy and spinal muscular atrophy), or combined sensory and motor dysfunction (e.g., syringomyelia). Scoliosis commonly occurs in patients with neurofibromatosis or genetic connective tissue diseases (e.g., Marfan syndrome or Ehlers-Danlos syndrome). In most patients with scoliosis, however, the cause is unrecognized and termed *idiopathic scoliosis*. Idiopathic scoliosis is divided into infantile (in children from birth up to 3 years of age), juvenile (in children 3–10 years of age), adolescent (in children older than 10 years of age), or adult. In adults, scoliosis may be caused by degenerative disk disease. First-degree relatives of a person with scoliosis have a 10% risk of developing scoliosis, suggesting a genetic basis for this condition, but specific genetic determinants remain unclear.[1]

External fetal constraint rarely causes persistent scoliosis but can result in infantile idiopathic scoliosis that responds to physical therapy (Fig. 20.1). Infantile idiopathic scoliosis has been associated with a history of breech presentation,[2] and Lloyd-Roberts and Pilcher studied the natural history of 100 infants with no associated malformations or radiologic defects who presented with a lateral curve of the thoracic spine that did not disappear on suspension (67% male predilection).[3] Convexity to the left was noted in 85% of cases, with similar sex and sidedness predilections as noted for torticollis. The mean angle of curvature was 15 degrees (range 5–40 degrees), and the affected infants were observed for an average of 3 years until complete resolution (92%)

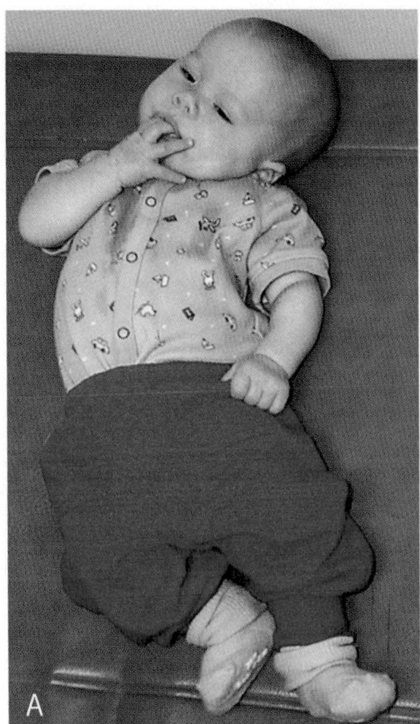

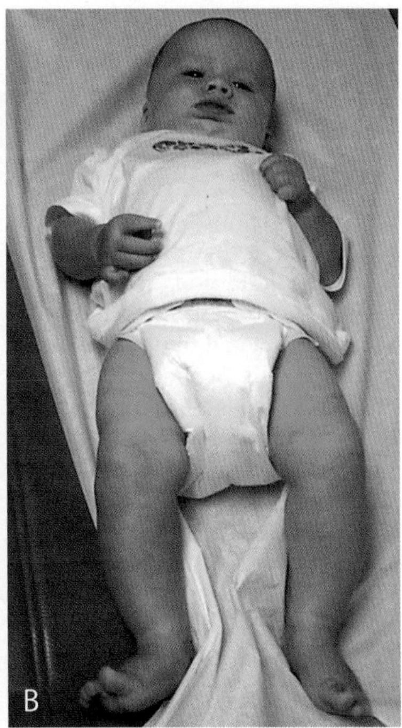

FIGURE 20.1 Infantile scoliosis before (**A**) and after (**B**) physical therapy in an infant with late fetal constraint caused by an abnormal fetal lie. At 3 months of age, he presented with scoliosis and left torticollis-plagiocephaly deformation sequence. His mother wore an elastic maternity girdle during the final 2 weeks of her pregnancy to keep her fetus in vertex presentation after undergoing version for a transverse lie.

or obvious progression (5%), with secondary structural scoliosis (double primary curves) noted in 3%.[2] Because of the high rate of associated torticollis-plagiocephaly deformation sequence (83%), with rib prominence on the convex side (50%) and pelvic tilting that followed the curve of the trunk, these researchers interpreted these defects as being secondary to fetal constraint and used the term *molded baby syndrome*.

Spontaneous resolution during infancy occurred in most cases of infantile idiopathic scoliosis, but curves with an initial rib-vertebra angle difference greater than 20 degrees that failed to improve in 3 months, or those who developed compensatory curves above and/or below the primary curve, tended to relentlessly progress, compromising cardiorespiratory function.[3-5] In a study of causative factors of infantile idiopathic scoliosis, Wynne-Davies noted an excess of males, with most curves convex to the left, as well as postnatal development of forehead flattening on the same side as the convexity and accompanied by contralateral occipital flattening.[5] She noted an excess of breech presentation (17.6%), with only 3% of such infants sleeping in the prone position (which she compared with the markedly reduced incidence of infantile idiopathic scoliosis among prone-sleeping North American infants). Among infants with idiopathic scoliosis, 64% were born between July and December, and they developed curves between October and March, suggesting that limitation to free movement resulting from being heavily wrapped during cold weather played a role.[6] Infantile idiopathic scoliosis differs from adolescent-onset idiopathic scoliosis in that it frequently resolves spontaneously, is more common in males, and shows a marked predilection for left thoracic curves, whereas most adolescent-onset cases progress and occur more commonly in females and on the right side. The occurrence of resolving infantile idiopathic scoliosis in Edinburgh, Scotland, was markedly reduced, from 42% of all patients with idiopathic scoliosis in 1968–1971 to 4% in 1980–1982, when infant sleep positioning changed from supine to prone, and centralized heating became more available.[7] Because the current infant sleeping practice has switched back to supine sleep positioning, the incidence of infantile idiopathic scoliosis may increase once again, but this can easily be treated with physical therapy.[8]

Chest and trunk asymmetry is common in otherwise healthy children and adolescents, and few high school students have completely symmetric posture. Among more than 2000 children assessed in a school screening program, 4.1% had positive screening for scoliosis based on rib prominence while standing and bending forward (the Adams forward-bend test), 1.8% had idiopathic scoliosis of greater than 10 degrees, and 0.4% required active treatment.[1] Idiopathic scoliosis is usually not progressive, but the likelihood of progression is higher in girls and in children with a large curvature and remaining growth. Scoliotic deformity that is less than 30 degrees at the end of growth rarely worsens during adulthood, whereas scoliosis of greater than 50 degrees does tend to worsen during adulthood at a rate of 0.75–1.00 degree per year.[1] Therefore a patient with an immature skeleton and scoliosis of greater than 25–30 degrees is at risk for progression. Lung volume doubles between the age of 10 years and skeletal maturity, and growth of the thoracic spine is necessary to achieve adult chest volume. Adolescents with thoracic scoliosis of greater than 50 degrees are at increased risk for shortness of breath later in life. Lung volumes are diminished when idiopathic scoliosis reaches 70 degrees, and symptomatic restrictive pulmonary disease occurs in patients with curves that exceed 100 degrees.[1]

Several risk factors have been set forth for adolescent idiopathic scoliosis, which is of unknown etiology. It is estimated that 20% of scoliosis can be attributed to neuromuscular, syndromic, or congenital disorders, while 80% is idiopathic.[9] Adolescent idiopathic scoliosis is a complex three-dimentional deformity of the spine and trunk, which has a commonly accepted prevalence of 2–3% in the general population, with higher prevalence and severity in girls than boys. The female-to-male ratio increases from 1.4:1.0 for mild curves (10–20 degrees) to 7.2:1.0 for more severe curves (more than 40 degrees).[9] It is thought that tall, slim spines are more likely to bend than shorter, thicker spines, and girls' spines tend to be more slender with narrower vertebral bodies than boys'.[9] Other factors include joint hypermobility, growth-related factors (height, delayed puberty, and low body mass index), and family history.[9] Using data from the Swedish Twin Registry, the heritability of scoliosis is around 38%.[9]

Progressive scoliosis also has been noted after chest wall resection in children who undergo surgical repair of esophageal atresia, diaphragmatic hernia, or congenital heart defects. The degree of curvature is related to the number of ribs resected, with posterior rib resection leading to scoliosis much more readily than anterior rib resection (which seldom leads to significant scoliosis).[10]

The 22q11.2 deletion syndrome results in a 20–25-fold increased risk for developing scoliosis, with curve progression in 54.2% of cases (mean progression rate of 2.5 degrees/year, similar to idiopathic scoliosis with progression in 49% and 2.2–9.6 degrees/year), and a prevalence of intraspinal anomalies on magnetic resonance imaging of 10.5% in 22q11.2 deletion syndrome (comparable to 11.4% reported for idiopathic scoliosis).[11] Presence of a 22q11.2 deletion, a history of thoracotomy before the age of 12 years, and most severe category of congenital heart disease, but not sex, were significant independent risk factors for scoliosis. The prevalence of scoliosis in those with congenital heart disease, but without a 22q11.2 deletion, was like that of the general population, while among the congenital heart disease population with a 22q11.2 deletion, the prevalence of scoliosis is like that of others with 22q11.2 deletion syndrome, suggesting that this chromosomal deletion is a significant risk factor for both congenital heart disease and scoliosis.[12]

Scoliosis also may result from plural tethering following tumors, irradiation, or empyema. In the past, paralytic scoliosis after poliomyelitis was a cause of scoliosis, and there is progressive neuromuscular scoliosis in spinal muscular atrophy,[13] acute flaccid myelitis with extensive thoracic spinal cord involvement,[14] as well as in Friedrich's ataxia (90%, with more than 50% requiring surgical intervention).[15] Scoliosis is also common in children with cerebral palsy (41%), with strong associations with poor gross motor function and dystonic movement disorders, particularly in nonambulant children.[16] Boys with Duchenne muscular dystrophy often develop scoliosis that progresses, which can by delayed or prevented by using spinal orthosis, thereby improving sitting position and especially pulmonary function.[17] Spine flexibility is a significant influencing factor for the effectiveness of bracing. There is a period of fully reducible curve in muscular dystrophy patients at the initial onset of scoliosis, but as the spinal curve progresses, flexibility decreases over time, so it is crucial to detect the scoliosis when the curve is fully reducible. Therefore patients should be regularly evaluated radiographically over time.[17]

Patients with anterior chest wall deformities manifest associated scoliosis in more than 20% of cases, and 18% and 14% of patients with pectus excavatum and pectus carinatum, respectively, require therapeutic intervention for scoliosis via bracing or surgery.[18]

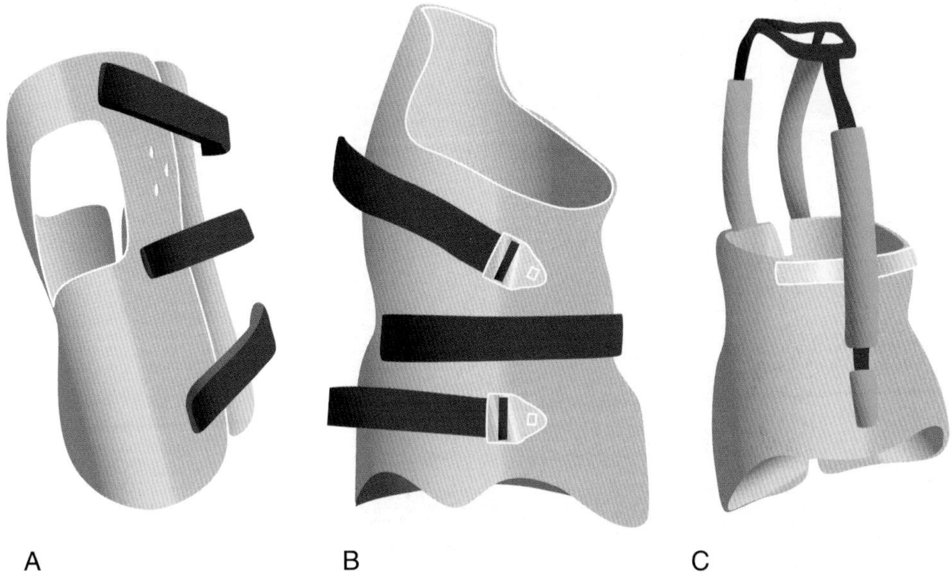

FIGURE 20.2 Common types of braces for scoliosis. **A,** Boston back brace (also called a thoracolumbosacral orthosis, a low-profile brace, or an underarm brace). Typically used for curves in the lumbar (low-back) or thoracolumbar sections of the spine. **B,** Charleston bending brace (also known as a part-time brace). Commonly used for spinal curves of 20–35 degrees, with the apex of the curve below the level of the shoulder blade. **C,** Milwaukee brace (also called cervicothoracolumbosacral orthosis) is used for high thoracic (mid-back) curves. (From DesJardins. *Clinical Manifestations and Assessment of Respiratory Disease*. Philadelphia, PA: Mosby, 2011;323-333.)

FEATURES

Constraint-related infantile scoliosis (see Fig. 20.1) is not associated with vertebral anomalies or underlying neuromuscular disease, and there is usually a history of fetal constraint and/or abnormal fetal lie, supported by an unusual position of comfort shortly after birth (see Fig. 20.1). Recently published high-quality evidence has been made available on the effect of conservative treatment approaches (braces and exercises) for idiopathic scoliosis, particularly in the areas of efficacy of bracing (Fig. 20.2) and physiotherapeutic scoliosis-specific exercises.[19] Congenital scoliosis can be caused by abnormal development of the vertebral bodies during the sixth week of gestation, resulting in unilateral bar, block vertebrae, hemivertebrae, wedge vertebrae (Fig. 20.3), and other complex forms resulting from multiple vertebral anomalies.[20] It is usually progressive, with the degree and rate of progression dependent on the type and location of the spinal defects. Bracing is ineffective, and operative intervention with posterior spinal fusions, with or without instrumentation, combined with anterior and posterior arthrodeses, is necessary in about 50% of such cases to preserve respiratory function and stabilize progressive curvature. Therefore surgery is usually done early, and any associated spinal dysraphism or tethering of the cord must be identified before surgery.[20] As mentioned in Chapter 19, early-onset scoliosis can be treated with a vertical expandable prosthetic titanium rib device, and the speed of proximal anchor failure was greatest in neuromuscular scoliosis compared to idiopathic and congenital scoliosis.[21]

Scoliosis is defined as a three-dimensional spinal deformity consisting of a lateral curvature greater than 10 degrees with rotation of the vertebrae within the curve. It can be classified as congenital, neuromuscular, or idiopathic. Idiopathic scoliosis is further classified by age of onset: infantile (birth to 2 years), juvenile (3–9 years), and adolescent (10 years and older). It is the most common pediatric musculoskeletal disorder that causes a three-dimensional spinal deformity that involves an axial rotation of the vertebrae, not just displacement and rotation in the frontal plane. Adolescent idiopathic scoliosis is the most common form because the spinal deformity evolves during periods of significant physical growth and it is diagnosed when other etiological factors cannot be identified, such as congenital neurological or musculoskeletal anomalies, or inflammatory or demyelinating processes leading to primary or secondary motor neuron damage.[22]

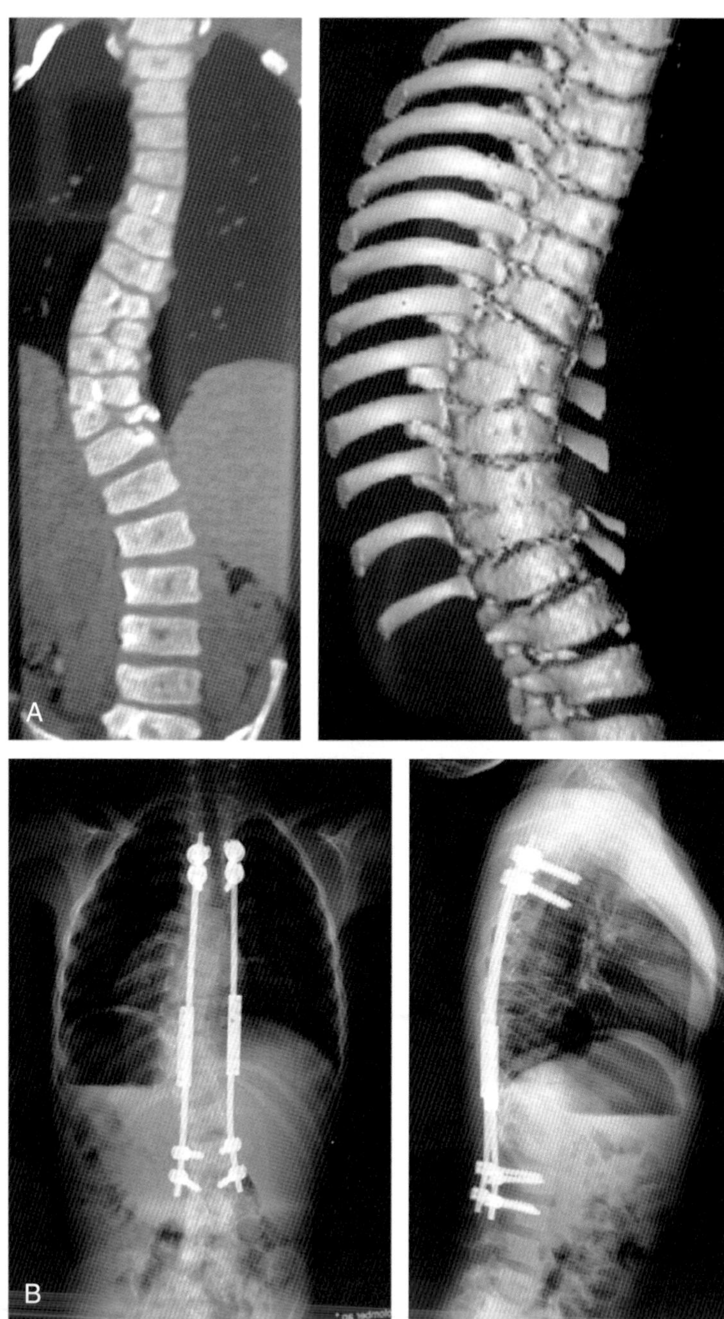

FIGURE 20.3 A, Despite multiple failure of formation anomalies at the lower thoracic region, the curve was significantly flexible. **B,** The patient underwent growing rod insertion to control the curve and to maintain growth. After surgery the deformity improved significantly. (From Salari et al. Growing rods in the treatment of congenital spinal deformity, seminars in spine surgery: evaluation and treatment of congenital spinal deformities. 2010;22(3):131–125, Figure 2, parts B and C.)

A lateral bending of the spine and an associated rotation of vertebral bodies over 5-10 segments of the spine characterize adolescent idiopathic scoliosis. Classic findings of scoliosis on examination are shoulder and scapular asymmetry, rib prominence on forward flexion on the Adams test, and asymmetry of the waist and trunk. Axial rotation of the trunk on the Adams test can be quantified with an inclinometer, and rotation of less than 7 degrees is associated with a 95% probability of a curve that is less than 30 degrees

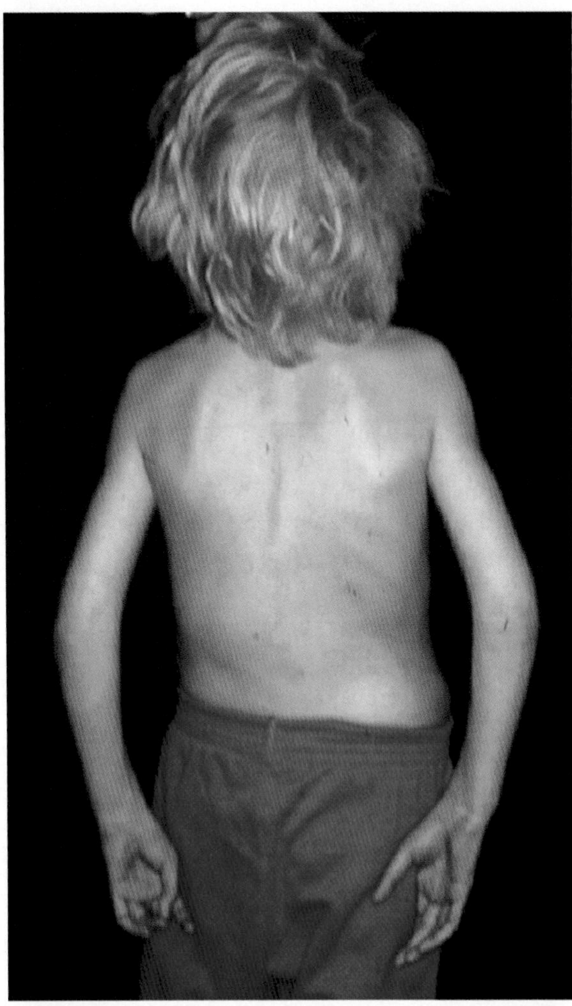

FIGURE 20.4 Scoliosis is associated with laxity of connective tissues in Marfan syndrome, an autosomal dominant genetic connective tissue disorder that results from mutations in the *FBN1* gene.

on radiography. Skin examination is warranted to rule out manifestations of neurofibromatosis (café-au-lait spots, inguinal/axillary freckling, neurofibromas) or occult spinal dysraphism (e.g., midline spinal dimpling, hairy patch, or hemangioma/lipoma) that might suggest a tethered cord. The extremities should be assessed for arachnodactyly or joint laxity, which might suggest a genetic connective tissue disorder such as Marfan syndrome (see Figs. 19.1 and 20.4), as well as for inequality in leg length, which may cause a false positive result on the Adams test. Among patients with Marfan syndrome, development of severe, progressive scoliosis was associated with pathogenic *FBN1* protein-truncating variants within the region associated with neonatal Marfan syndrome (exons 25–33),[23] as illustrated in Figs. 19.1 and 20.4.

Although the etiology of idiopathic scoliosis is unknown, genetic factors appear to play a role because family history is positive in 27–30% of cases.[20] Daughters of mothers with scoliosis have a 1.5-times higher risk for adolescent idiopathic scoliosis, and the sibling recurrence risk is 18%, with positive family history increasing the risk for curves requiring treatment.[9] A systematic scoping review of 40 genetic studies revealed 15 genes with significant association with progressive adolescent idiopathic scoliosis, but none showed sufficient power to sustain clinical applications, while nine studies of epigenetic changes showed promising results regarding reliable markers.[24]

MANAGEMENT AND PROGNOSIS

Physical therapy is merited for infantile scoliosis resulting from fetal constraint, with manipulative stretching exercises performed by caretakers and careful follow-up to determine whether full correction occurs after initiation of physical therapy. Physiotherapy scoliosis-specific exercises are a therapeutic intervention, which can be used alone or in combination with bracing or surgery to stabilize progressive scoliosis curves, produce a significant reduction in the Cobb angle, improve back asymmetry, correct posture, and improve secondary muscle imbalance and related pain.[25-27] Nonoperative treatment consists of observation, physiotherapy, and/or bracing. Current treatment guidelines recommend observation or physiotherapy for curves below 25 degrees and bracing for curves between 25 and 40 degrees.[28] There is sparse evidence regarding the effectiveness of bracing for curves over 40 degrees and in adult degenerative scoliosis, although one systemic literature review suggested that spinal bracing may have a positive short- to medium-term influence on pain and function in adults with either progressive primary degenerative scoliosis or progressive idiopathic scoliosis.[29] Specific exercises should be prescribed in children and adolescents with a Cobb angle in excess of 15 degrees. In progressive curves, they should be used in conjunction with bracing. Similarly, bracing and exercises should be prescribed for patients with kyphosis, particularly when the lumbar spine is involved.[30] Surgery should be considered only when the symptoms cannot be managed conservatively. Initial in-brace correction and compliance seem to be the most important predictive factors for successful treatment outcome. A meta-analysis of 215 patients from the three randomized control trials suggested that the compliance-enhancing intervention group had 2.92 more bracing hours per day than the usual care control group, with sensor monitoring showing the most significant improvement in bracing duration.[31] Moderate evidence suggests that thoracic and double curves, and curves over 30 degrees at an early growth stage, have more risk for failure. High and low body mass index scores are also associated with lower success rates. For a curve at high risk of progression, rigid and daytime braces are significantly more effective than soft or nighttime braces.[28] There is no high-quality evidence demonstrating that surgical treatment is superior to conservative treatment for the management of adolescent idiopathic scoliosis and kyphosis, and surgery is associated with a number of long-term complications.

Consensus guidelines of the American Academy of Pediatrics, Scoliosis Research Society, American Academy of Orthopedic Surgeons, and Pediatric Orthopedic Society of North America recommend screening for scoliosis by means of visual inspection in girls in fifth grade (age 10–11 years) and again in seventh grade, and in boys in eighth grade (age 13–14 years).[1] Most pediatric orthopedists believe that the probability of progression is low if the scoliotic curve is 15 degrees or less and growth is complete. For patients who are skeletally immature with curves between 20 and 25 degrees, observation and follow-up evaluations are indicated. For curves between 25 and 45 degrees with a high probability of progression, treatment usually includes underarm bracing with a thoracolumbosacral orthosis worn under the clothing during the day and at night. Occasionally a nighttime brace is used to hold the spine in an overcorrected position (see Fig. 20.2).

Indications for magnetic resonance imaging in patients with idiopathic scoliosis are onset before 10 years of age, kyphotic apex of the scoliosis, clinically significant pain, a neurologic abnormality, neurofibromatosis, or midline cutaneous anomalies (which are known to occur with occult spinal dysraphism and a tethered cord). The onset of scoliosis before 10 years of age is associated with an occult intraspinal abnormality in approximately 20% of patients, and magnetic resonance imaging of the spine from the craniocervical junction to the sacrum is recommended in this age group if the scoliosis exceeds 20 degrees.[1]

Treatment with the use of a rigid thoracolumbar orthotic brace is currently preferred for children 3 years of age through adolescence who have a curve magnitude of 25–45 degrees and considerable remaining growth to arrest the progression of scoliosis below the cutoff requiring surgical treatment. In a prospective observational study involving girls 10–15 years of age with scoliosis of 25–35 degrees, the rate of success (defined as progression of less than 6 degrees) at 4 years was 74% among those who underwent bracing, compared with 34% in an observation group. Results from bracing appeared to be best when the average daytime brace wear was at least 12 hours; a typical brace prescription is for 18–20 hours per day, because full adherence is rarely achieved.[32] A multicenter, randomized trial compared bracing with watchful waiting, and this study confirmed treatment success was 72% after bracing, compared with 48% after observation. There was a significant positive association between hours of brace wear and rate of treatment success. Bracing significantly decreased the progression of high-risk curves to the threshold for surgery in patients with adolescent idiopathic scoliosis, and the benefit increased with longer hours of brace wear.[33]

Operative treatment is indicated when progressive scoliosis exceeds 45 degrees in patients with an immature skeleton or when progression or associated pain occurs after skeletal maturity.[1] Surgery is also recommended for mature adolescents with curves of 40–50 degrees that are likely to progress during adulthood. Surgery is intended to diminish the scoliotic curve and maintain spinal correction during the next 6 months while fusion and healing occur. At present in children younger than 10 years of age, implants are placed without fusion to allow continued spinal and chest growth. Improvements in surgical techniques and implants have resulted in reduced complications and improved outcomes. Spinal instrumentation prevents the need for postoperative immobilization in a cast or brace, and there are usually few long-term limitations. Because current techniques still involve spinal fusion over the implant, the trade-off for the correction of the curvature is a loss of spinal motion. In the thorax, the restriction of rotation is well tolerated, and many patients return to their usual preoperative activities after surgery. However, spinal fusion extending into the lumbar spine has been associated with reduced activity levels and development of degenerative arthritis. A complication characterized by pain and the loss of lumbar lordosis occurred after the original Harrington distraction technique, and it occurred much less frequently with modern segmental spinal instrumentation, which corrects the scoliosis while maintaining balanced thoracic kyphosis and lumbar lordosis. Most surgeons prefer a dual-rod segmental spinal-fixation system that allows multiple anchor points for attachment to the deformed spine (see Fig. 20.3).[1]

The typical postoperative hospital stay in the United States is 4 or 5 days, and most adolescents return to school 4–6 weeks after the procedure. As with other procedures involving metallic implants, infection is a major concern. Multimodal intraoperative neurologic monitoring with sensory-evoked and motor-evoked potentials is used to detect and prevent neurologic complications during surgery. Ten years after initial surgery for idiopathic scoliosis, 3–10% of patients undergo subsequent surgery. A retrospective case series involving more than 20 years of follow-up of 156 patients who underwent surgery or bracing showed similar general health and extent of disability when successful fusion was achieved, although both groups had a higher frequency of back pain, sick-leave days (see Fig. 20.4), and degenerative disk disease compared with age-matched controls.[1] A recent review of results in 124 patients with adolescent idiopathic scoliosis who underwent posterior instrumentation with pedicle screw fixation (the average number of pedicle screws was 1.96/vertebra) revealed the average curve correction was 48.3% for the proximal thoracic curve, 83.1% for the main thoracic curve, and 80.2% for the thoracolumbar/lumbar curve at final follow-up 5 years after surgery, with no significant loss of correction at final follow-up.[34] A South Korean nationwide population database study of 268,372 patients with idiopathic scoliosis revealed an overall incidence of 0.5%, with the incidence in females 1.44 times higher than that for males, and 0.7% of patients undergoing surgical treatment within 5 years of diagnosis for curves of more than 40 degrees under 15 years of age, or curves of more than 50 degrees at 15 years of age or older, or scoliosis with thoracic lordosis.[35]

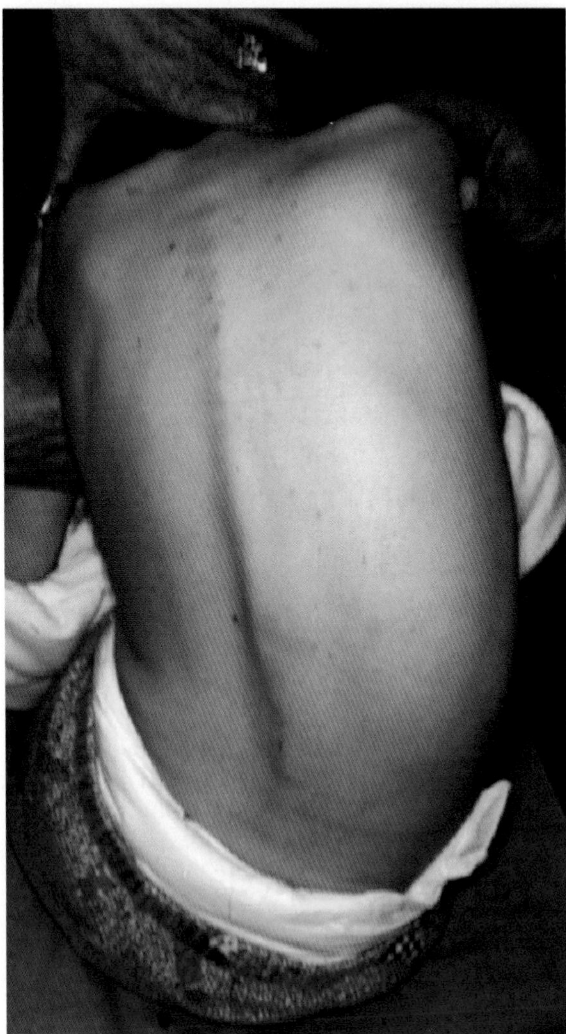

FIGURE 20.5 Neuromuscular scoliosis is associated with increased muscle tone in a young woman with Rett syndrome, an X-linked dominant disorder that is lethal in males and is caused by mutations in *MECP2,* a gene involved in the process of silencing other genes.

DIFFERENTIAL DIAGNOSIS

Vertebral anomalies can result in congenital scoliosis (see Fig. 18.3), as can neurologic problems that alter muscle tone (Fig. 20.5). Among 913 females with classic Rett syndrome, scoliosis frequency and severity increased with age, with severe scoliosis found in 251 patients (27%), and 168 patients (18%) required surgical correction.[36] Some genetic connective tissue disorders such as Marfan syndrome, Loeys-Dietz syndrome, or Ehlers-Danlos syndrome (EDS) (see Figs. 20.4 and 20.6) can lead to scoliosis,[37] as can certain skeletal dysplasias such as camptomelic dysplasia or diastrophic dysplasia (Fig. 20.7). The arthrochalasia type of EDS (caused by specific mutations in *COL1A1* or *COL1A2*), kyphoscoliotic type of EDS (caused by mutations in *PLOD1* or *FKBP14*), and spondylodysplastic type of EDS (caused by mutations in *B4GALT7* or *B3GALT6*) are each associated with kyphoscoliosis.[37] Musculocontractural EDS is caused by mutations in *CHST14*, and posterior spinal fusion has been reported in three cases with progressive kyphoscoliosis; however careful attention is required for massive blood loss due to tissue fragility, which warrants extreme caution.[38] Arterial fragility has also been noted in autosomal recessive kyphoscoliotic EDS due to *PLOD1* mutations.[39] Use of traditional growing rods has also been advocated for the treatment of early-onset scoliosis in

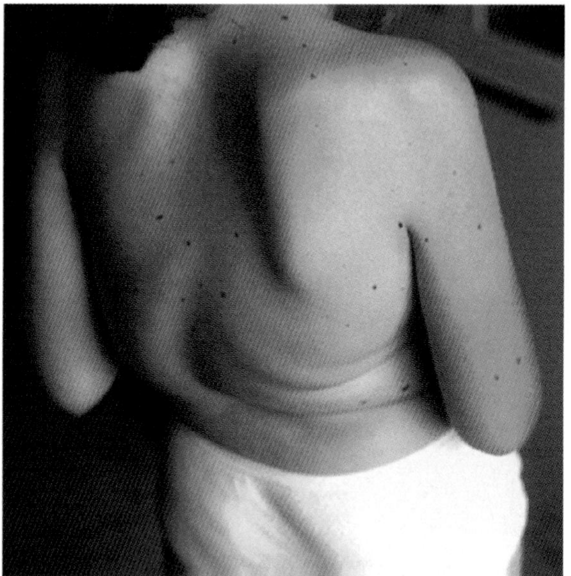

FIGURE 20.6 Progressive kyphoscoliosis in a young woman with Ehlers-Danlos syndrome.

EDS.[40] Diastrophic dysplasia is an autosomal recessive skeletal dysplasia caused by pathogenic variants in *SLC26A2*, which codes for a sulfate transporter protein in the cell membrane and results in abnormal cartilage due to production of under sulfated proteoglycans within cartilage cells. It is characterized by short limbs, a normal head and intelligence, hitchhiker thumbs, scoliosis, exaggerated lumbar lordosis, cervical kyphosis, and contractures of the large joints with early-onset osteoarthritis. Most infants have some degree of cervical kyphosis, with one third of infants and toddlers having clinically significant kyphosis. If the kyphosis is less than 60 degrees, it will often improve with growth.[40] Cervical spine surgery in infancy is restricted to individuals with clinical or neurophysiologic evidence of spinal cord impingement, and postpubertal surgical correction of scoliosis is recommended unless severe spinal deformity is causing respiratory compromise or neurologic signs. The spine frequently develops excessive lumbar lordosis and thoracolumbar kyphoscoliosis. In anteroposterior radiographs of the

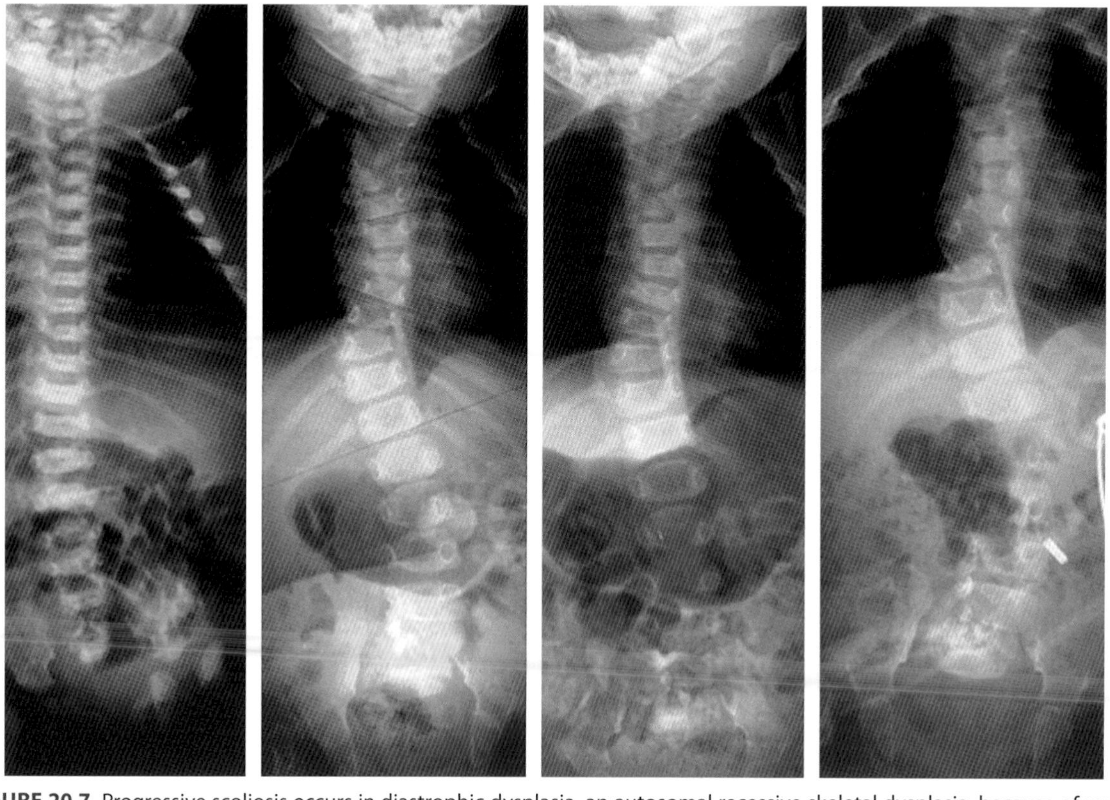

FIGURE 20.7 Progressive scoliosis occurs in diastrophic dysplasia, an autosomal recessive skeletal dysplasia, because of mutations in a sulfate transporter gene (*SLC26A2*). This condition typically results in abnormal connective tissues with fixed equinovarus foot deformities, phalangeal synostosis, and proximally placed thumbs and halluces. The changes in spinal curvature shown in this patient occurred over the course of the first 18 months of her life.

lumbar spine, a decrease of the vertebral interpedicular distance is often noted, but neurologic symptoms are uncommon. Bracing does not prevent progression of the spinal deformity in patients with diastrophic dysplasia, and anteroposterior surgery is indicated in patients with severe spinal deformities, but the risk for major complications is high, especially in patients with marked kyphosis.[41]

References

1. Hresko MT. Idiopathic scoliosis in adolescents. *N Engl J Med.* 2013;368:834–841.
2. Wynne-Davies R, Littlejohn A, Gormley J. Aetiology and relationship of some common skeletal deformities (talipes equinovarus and calcaneovalgus, metatarsus varus, congenital dislocation of the hip, and infantile idiopathic scoliosis). *J Med Genet.* 1982;19:321–328.
3. Lloyd-Roberts GC, Pilcher MF. Structural idiopathic scoliosis in infancy: a study of the natural history of 100 patients. *J Bone Joint Surg Br.* 1965;47:520–523.
4. Ferreira JH, James JIP. Progressive and resolving infantile idiopathic scoliosis. *J Bone Joint Surg Br.* 1972;54:648–655.
5. Thompson SK, Bentley G. Prognosis in infantile idiopathic scoliosis. *J Bone Joint Surg Br.* 1980;62:151–154.
6. Wynne-Davies R. Infantile idiopathic scoliosis: causative factors, particularly in the first six months of life. *J Bone Joint Surg Br.* 1975;57:138–141.
7. McMaster MJ. Infantile idiopathic scoliosis: can it be prevented? *J Bone Joint Surg Br.* 1983;65:612–617.
8. Philippi H, Faldum A, Bergmann H, et al. Idiopathic infantile asymmetry, proposal of a measurement scale. *Early Hum Dev.* 2004;80:79–90.
9. Fadzan M, Bettany-Saltikov J. Etiological theories of adolescent idiopathic scoliosis: past and present. *Open Orthop J.* 2017;11:1466–1489.
10. DeRosa GP. Progressive scoliosis following chest wall resection in children. *Spine.* 1985;10:618–622.
11. de Reuver S, Homans JF, Schlösser TPC, et al. 22q11.2 deletion syndrome as a human model for idiopathic scoliosis. *J Clin Med.* 2021;10(21):4823.
12. Homans JF, de Reuver S, Heung T, et al. The role of 22q11.2 deletion syndrome in the relationship between congenital heart disease and scoliosis. *Spine J.* 2020;20(6):956–963.
13. Rodillo E, Marini ML, Heckmatt JZ, et al. Scoliosis in spinal muscular atrophy: review of 63 cases. *J Child Neurol.* 1989;4:118–123.
14. Suresh KV, Karius A, Wang KY, Sadowsky C, Sponseller PD. Scoliosis in pediatric patients with acute flaccid myelitis. *Top Spinal Cord Inj Rehabil.* 2022;28(1):34–41.
15. Rummey C, Flynn JM, Corben LA, et al. Scoliosis in Friedreich's ataxia: longitudinal characterization in a large heterogeneous cohort. *Ann Clin Transl Neurol.* 2021;8(6):1239–1250.
16. Willoughby KL, Ang SG, Thomason P, et al. Epidemiology of scoliosis in cerebral palsy: a population-based study at skeletal maturity. *J Paediatr Child Health.* 2022;58(2):295–301.
17. Choi YA, Shin HI, Shin HI. Scoliosis in Duchenne muscular dystrophy children is fully reducible in the initial stage, and becomes structural over time. *BMC Musculoskelet Disord.* 2019;20(1):277.
18. Waters P, Welch K, Micheli LJ, et al. Scoliosis in children with pectus excavatum and pectus carinatum. *J Pediatr Orthop.* 1989;9:551–561.
19. Negrini S, Donzelli S, Aulisa AG, et al. 2016 SOSORT guidelines: orthopaedic and rehabilitation treatment of idiopathic scoliosis during growth. *Scoliosis Spinal Disord.* 2018;10(13):3.
20. Lopez-Sosa F, Guille JT, Bowen JR. Rotation of the spine in congenital scoliosis. *J Pediatr Orthop.* 1995;15:528–534.
21. Park HY, Matsumoto H, Feinberg N, et al. The classification for early-onset scoliosis (C-EOS) correlates with the speed of vertical expandable prosthetic titanium rib (VEPTR) proximal anchor failure. *J Pediatr Orthop.* 2017;37(6):381–386.
22. Karpiel I, Ziębiński A, Kluszczyński M, Feige D. A survey of methods and technologies used for diagnosis of scoliosis. *Sensors (Basel).* 2021;21(24):8410.
23. Taniguchi Y, Takeda N, Inuzuka R, et al. Impact of pathogenic *FBN1* variant types on the development of severe scoliosis in patients with Marfan syndrome. *J Med Genet.* 2023;60(1):74–80.
24. Faldini C, Manzetti M, Neri S, et al. Epigenetic and genetic factors related to curve progression in adolescent idiopathic scoliosis: a systematic scoping review of the current literature. *Int J Mol Sci. 25.* 2022;23(11):5914.
25. Berdishevsky H, Lebel VA, Bettany-Saltikov J, et al. Physiotherapy scoliosis-specific exercises: a comprehensive review of seven major schools. *Scoliosis Spinal Disord.* 2016;11:20.
26. Seleviciene V, Cesnaviciute A, Strukcinskiene B, Marcinowicz L, Strazdiene N, Genowska A. Physiotherapeutic scoliosis-specific exercise methodologies used for conservative treatment of adolescent idiopathic scoliosis, and their effectiveness: an extended literature review of current research and practice. *Int J Environ Res Public Health.* 2022 Jul 28;19(15):9240 2022.
27. Liu D, Yang Y, Yu X, et al. Effects of specific exercise therapy on adolescent patients with idiopathic scoliosis: a prospective controlled cohort study. *Spine (Phila Pa 1976).* 2020;45(15):1039–1046.
28. Karavidas N. Bracing in the treatment of adolescent idiopathic scoliosis: evidence to date. *Adolesc Health Med Ther.* 2019;10:153–172.
29. McAviney J, Mee J, Fazalbhoy A, Du Plessis J, Brown BT. A systematic literature review of spinal brace/orthosis treatment for adults with scoliosis between 1967 and 2018: clinical outcomes and harms data. *BMC Musculoskelet Disord.* 2020 Feb 8;21(1):87 2020.
30. Bettany-Saltikov J, Turnbull D, Ng SY, Webb R. Management of spinal deformities and evidence of treatment effectiveness. *Open Orthop J.* 2017;11:1521–1547.

31. Li X, Huo Z, Hu Z, et al. Which interventions may improve bracing compliance in adolescent idiopathic scoliosis? A systematic review and meta-analysis. *PLoS One*. 2022 Jul 20;17(7):e0271612.
32. Morton A, Riddle R, Buchanan R, et al. Accuracy in the prediction and estimation of adherence to brace wear before and during treatment of adolescent idiopathic scoliosis. *J Pediatr Orthop*. 2008;28:336–341.
33. Weinstein SL, Dolan LA, Wright JG, et al. Effects of bracing in adolescents with idiopathic scoliosis. *N Engl J Med*. 2013;369:1512–1521.
34. Hwang CJ, Baik JM, Cho JH, Yoon SJ, Lee DH, Lee CS. posterior correction of adolescent idiopathic scoliosis with high-density pedicle screw-only constructs: 5 years of follow-up. *Yonsei Med J*. 2020;61(4):323–330.
35. Sung S, Chae HW, Lee HS, et al. Incidence and surgery rate of idiopathic scoliosis: a nationwide database study. *Int J Environ Res Public Health*. 2021;18(15):8152.
36. Killian JT, Lane JB, Lee HS, et al. Scoliosis in Rett syndrome: progression, comorbidities, and predictors. *Pediatr Neurol*. 2017;70:20–25.
37. Meester JAN, Verstraeten A, Schepers D, Alaerts M, Van Laer L, Loeys BL. Differences in manifestations of Marfan syndrome, Ehlers-Danlos syndrome, and Loeys-Dietz syndrome. *Ann Cardiothorac Surg*. 2017;6(6):582–594.
38. Uehara M, Oba H, Hatakenaka T, et al. Posterior spinal fusion for severe spinal deformities in musculocontractural Ehlers-Danlos syndrome: detailed observation of a novel case and review of 2 reported cases. *World Neurosurg*. 2020;143:454–461.
39. Henneton P, Legrand A, Giunta C, Frank M. Arterial fragility in kyphoscoliotic Ehlers-Danlos syndrome. *BMJ Case Rep*. 2018bcr2018224423, 2018.
40. Campbell JW. Dysplasias in the Child's Spine. *Neurosurg Clin N Am*. 2022;33(1S):e1–e10.
41. Jalanko T, Remes V, Peltonen J, Poussa M, Helenius I. Treatment of spinal deformities in patients with diastrophic dysplasia: a long-term, population based, retrospective outcome study. *Spine (Phila Pa 1976)*. 2009;34(20):2151–2157.

Section VII
Head and Neck Deformations

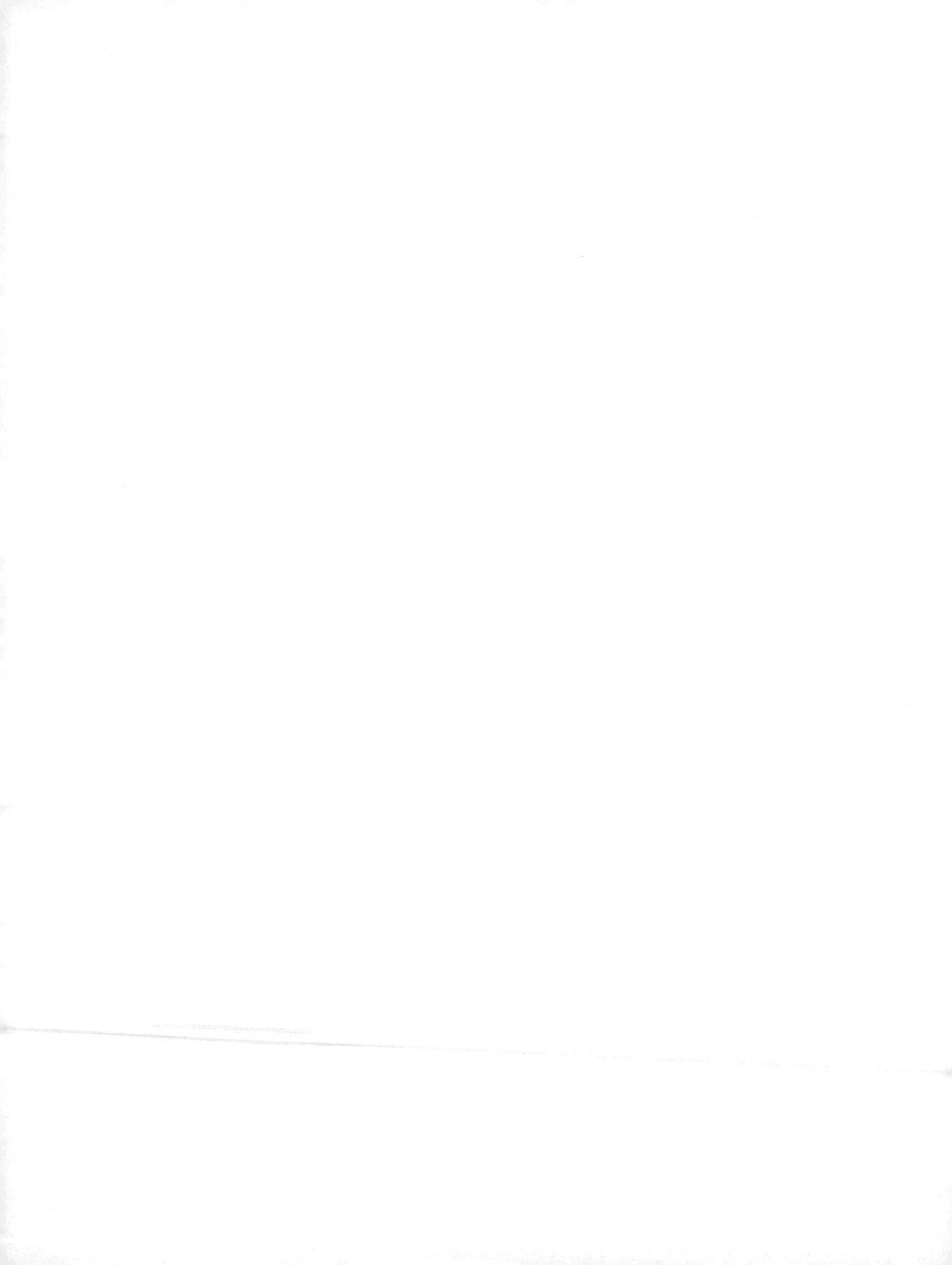

CHAPTER 21

Nasal Deformation

KEY POINTS

- Nasal deformities can result from constraint or a birth-related trauma in newborns.
- Nasal septum deviations must be distinguished from deformities of the whole nose.
- Spontaneous correction of nasal deformities can occur within the first 3 months of life.
- Nasal obstruction in infants may require intervention, especially if it leads to significant respiratory distress and oxygen desaturation.
- Failure to recognize and treat dislocation may lead to permanent deformity.
- Computed tomography (CT) and magnetic resonance (MRI) imaging modalities can complement the physical exam.

GENESIS

A small or short nose may result from constraint-related limitation of nasal growth in a face presentation, transverse lie, or from compression resulting from a small uterine cavity. During delivery the delicate structures of the face are predominantly exposed to external force effects, and hence deformities on the nose can emerge as a birth-related trauma in newborns.[1]

A compressed nose is also a feature of oligohydramnios and severe crowding, such as can occur in a bicornuate uterus (Fig. 21.1). Infants born to mothers with a bicornuate uterus have about a fourfold greater risk of congenital defects, and nasal hypoplasia and limb deficiencies occur more frequently in infants born to mothers with a bicornuate uterus.[2] Nasal deformities consisting of columellar necrosis, flaring of nostrils, and snubbing of the nose have been reported in very low-birth-weight infants after prolonged application of flow-driver nasal prongs for continuous positive airway pressure.[3] Midfacial hypoplasia also has been reported in preterm infants with bronchopulmonary dysplasia who were subjected to prolonged nasotracheal intubation for 68–243 days.[4]

Among 3425 children born between 1980 and 1981, 29 neonates (0.86%) showed a deviation of the bony and cartilaginous nose. After 11–12 years, nine children had a straight nose and five children (36%) showed a deviation of the nasal pyramid to the same side as found at birth.[5] CT images of 105 spontaneously aborted fetuses aged between 12 and 40 weeks of gestation revealed nasal septal deviations in 15 (14.3%) fetuses,[6] and among 4090 consecutive newborns investigated for nasal septal deviations over a 2-year period, there was a 0.93% incidence of anterior nasal septal cartilaginous dislocation.[7] This nasal septal dislocation was treated shortly after birth, and among treated infants followed for a 3-year period, there was no recurring septal deformity. Nasal septal deviations (Fig. 21.2) occur in as many as 17–22% of newborns examined immediately after vaginal delivery, and it is less frequent in infants delivered by cesarean section; therefore nasal septal deviations are thought to be related to passage through the birth canal.[8,9] Among 273 newborns examined at 12-hour intervals, the septum straightened spontaneously during the first 3 days of life.[6] Newborns delivered from a left occipitoanterior presentation were more prone to anterior nasal septal deviations to the right, whereas newborns delivered from a right occipitoanterior presentation had deviations directed to the left. During left occipitoanterior presentation, the head turns in a clockwise direction and the nasal cartilage moves to the right as the nasal tip is directed to the left; the reverse is true for infants delivered from a right occipitoanterior presentation.[8,9] Gray is generally credited with attributing anterior nasal septum deviations to deformation from maxillary pressure during pregnancy or birth, noting a 4% incidence of anterior nasal cartilage deformity among 2380 neonates.[10] More severe deviation of the nasal septum can result in frank nasal septum dislocation. About 2–4% of neonates

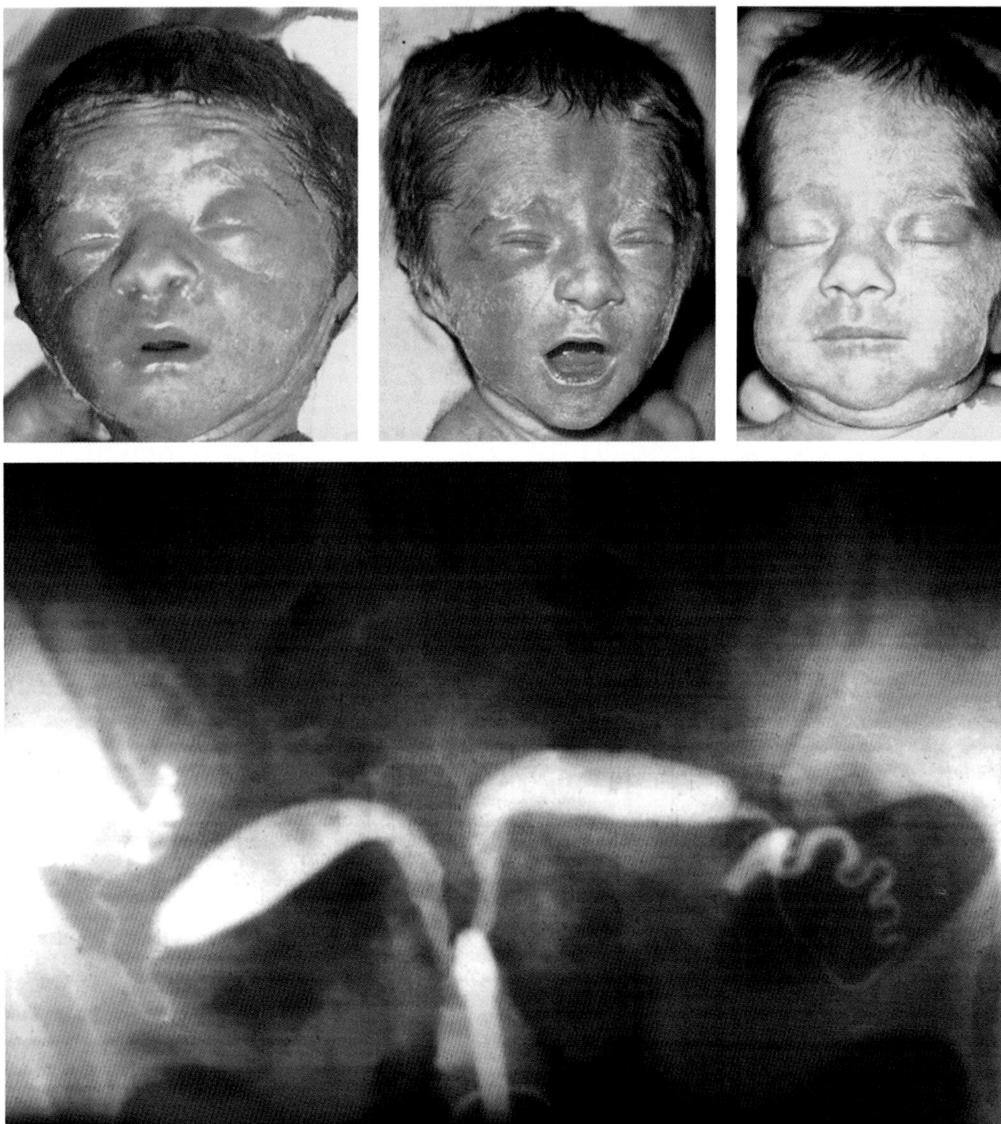

FIGURE 21.1 Nasal compression can occur with severe crowding resulting from a maternal bicornuate uterus, with gradual recovery over the first few weeks of postnatal life, as shown.

have an anterior dislocation of the nasal septum, and about 17–22% of neonates have some type of septum deformation.[11]

FEATURES

A deviated nose is not rare and appears to be secondary to mechanical force during normal vaginal delivery. The lower edge of the nasal cartilage may be dislocated from its usual placement on the vomerine ridge, which results in an asymmetric nose with slanting of the columella and a smaller nasal aperture on the side toward which the cartilaginous septum is dislocated (see Fig. 21.2). Deviations of the nasal septum must be distinguished from deformities that comprise the whole nose, in particular with involvement of the entire cartilaginous nasal frame (the nasal septum and adjacent cartilaginous parts), as demonstrated by the incidence figures in the preceding figures.[12]

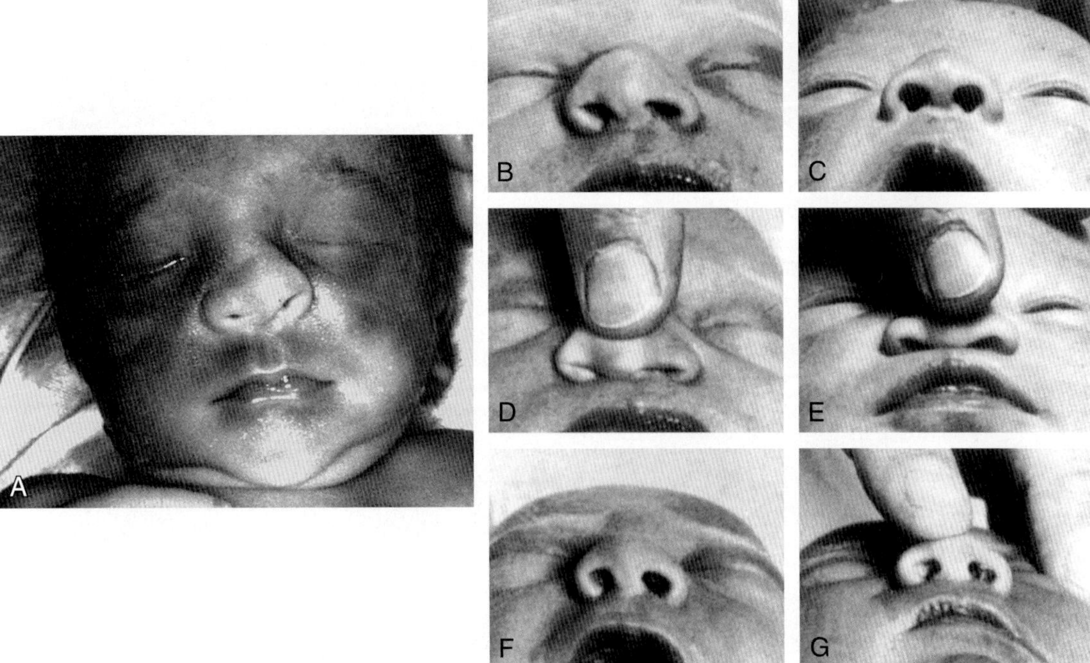

FIGURE 21.2 A, Nasal deviation caused by mechanical pressure during vaginal delivery from a right occiput transverse position. **B** and **C,** Deviated nasal septum (**B**) versus normal (**C**). The compression test is positive when dislocation of the lower edge of the nasal cartilage has occurred (**D**) and the nasal cartilage is unable to return to its former slot in the vomerine ridge (**E**). The normal response to compression is shown on the right. After reduction of the dislocation of the cartilaginous septum, there is still slight asymmetry (**F**), but the compression test (**G**) shows that the cartilage is relocated into its slot in the vomerine ridge. (From Stoksted P, Schønsted-Madsen U. Traumatology of the newborn's nose. *Rhinology.* 1979;17:77–82.)

MANAGEMENT AND PROGNOSIS

Nasal compression and nasal septum deviation generally resolve spontaneously, but most authors believe that nasal septum dislocation should be treated by cautious manual reduction in the newborn nursery (see Figs. 21.2 and 21.3).[7,11–13] If a nasal obstruction in an infant leads to significant respiratory distress and oxygen desaturation, an intervention becomes mandatory because infants are obligate nose breathers. An unresolved dislocated nasal septum should probably be treated by the third day after birth by repositioning the septal cartilage into the anatomic groove in the floor of the nose; however, there are examples in which spontaneous correction has occurred over the first 3 months.[14] The cartilaginous part of the nose should be grasped (with gauze) between the thumb and forefingers and then lifted forward while a probe or elevator is inserted into the nares below the free edge of the dislocated septum, forcing it into its normal location.[11] A slight nasal asymmetry may persist for several weeks after relocation before the normal form is fully reestablished. Failure to recognize and treat dislocation may lead to permanent deformity. Regarding the deformed septum that is not dislocated, there is no known contraindication to manipulation in an effort to restore the nasal septum to a normal alignment.

DIFFERENTIAL DIAGNOSIS

A short nose secondary to an underlying deformation may be a distinguishing feature of a number of disorders such as Stickler syndrome, 22q11.2 deletion syndrome, trichorhinophalangeal syndrome, and CHARGE syndrome, and therefore all children should be examined for associated malformations.[15] A wide variety of congenital nasal lesions can present to clinical attention due to airway obstruction, the presence of a mass, and/or cosmetic deformity, including pyriform aperture stenosis, choanal atresia, nasopharyngeal atresia, arrhinia, congenital germline fusion cysts,

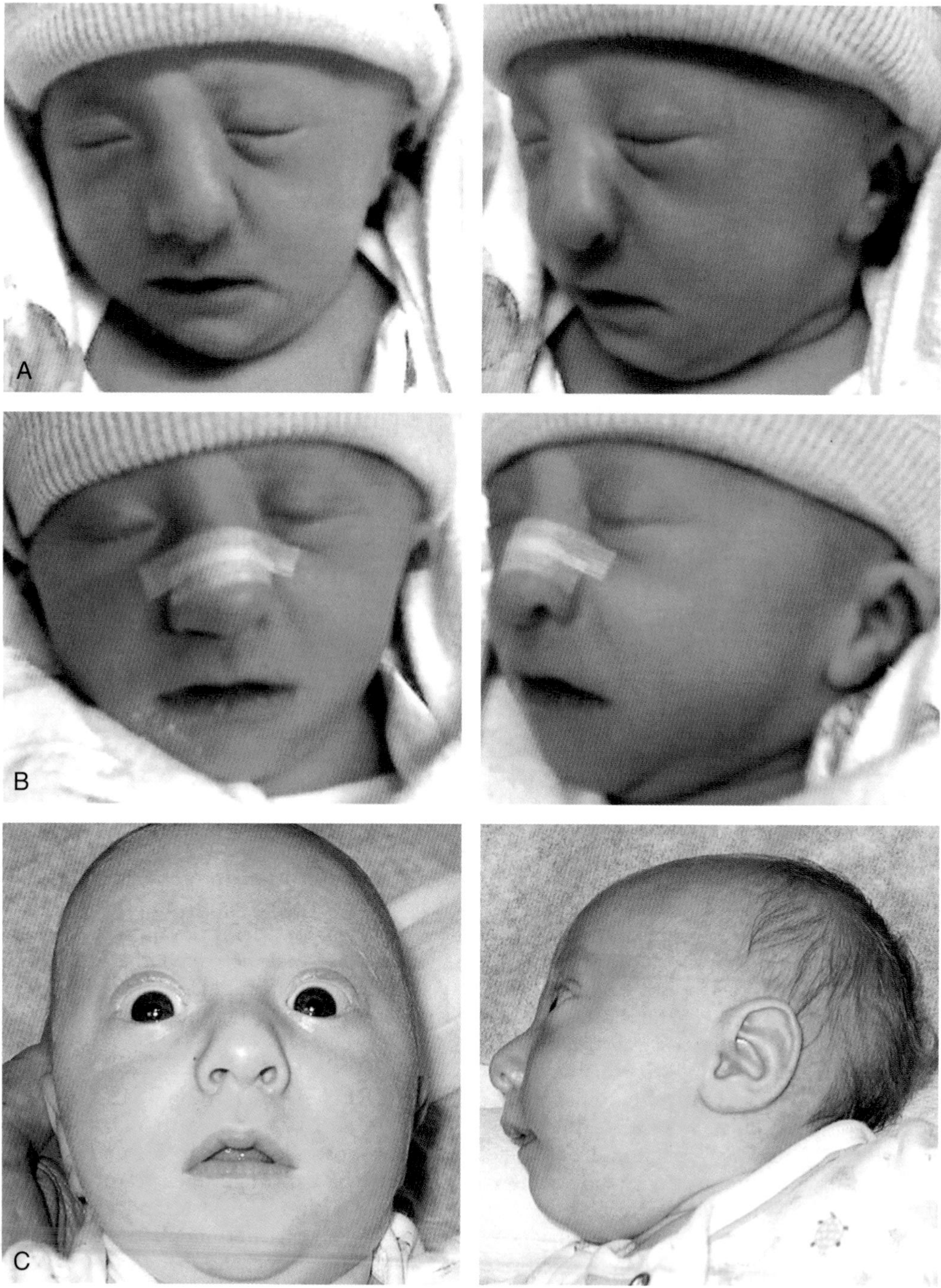

FIGURE 21.3 **A,** This infant was delivered by cesarean section at 37 weeks from a prolonged face presentation with a nasal septum dislocation to the left side. **B,** His nasal septum was relocated shortly after birth, and external taping was used to maintain the correction. **C,** At age 2 months, his nose appeared fully corrected with symmetric nares. (**A** and **B** Courtesy Dr. Gene Liu, Cedar Sinai Medical Center, Los Angeles.)

cephaloceles, neuroglial heterotopia, nasolacrimal duct mucoceles, hamartomas, supernumerary nostril, and bifid nose. A comprehensive classification scheme dedicated to congenital nasal anomalies is reviewed by Losee et al.[16,17] In general, computed tomography is the modality of choice for evaluating lesion-associated airway obstruction, while magnetic resonance imaging is better suited for evaluating nasofrontal mass lesions, although these modalities often serve complementary roles.[18,19]

References

1. Luers JC, Welzing L, Roth B, Streppel M. Traumatic luxation of the nose in a newborn: case report and review of the literature. *Eur Arch Otorhinolaryngol.* 2009 Sep;266(9):1489–1493.
2. Martinez-Frias ML, Bermejo E, Rodriquez-Pinilla E, et al. Congenital anomalies in the offspring of mothers with a bicornuate uterus. *Pediatrics.* 1998;101:e10.
3. Robertson NJ, McCarthy LS, Hamilton PA, et al. Nasal deformities resulting from flow driver continuous positive airway pressure. *Arch Dis Child.* 1996;75:F209–F212.
4. Rotschild A, Dison PJ, Chitayat D, et al. Midfacial hypoplasia associated with long-term intubation for bronchopulmonary dysplasia. *Am J Dis Child.* 1990;144:1302–1306.
5. Pentz S, Pirsig W, Lenders H. Long-term results of neonates with nasal deviation: a prospective study over 12 years. *Int J Pediatr Otorhinolaryngol.* 1994;28:183–191.
6. Teul I, Slawinski G, Lewandowski J, et al. Nasal septum morphology in human fetuses in computed tomography images. *Eur J Med Res.* 2010;15(Suppl 2):202–205.
7. Podoshin L, Gertner R, Fradis M, et al. Incidence and treatment of deviation of nasal septum in newborns. *Ear Nose Throat J.* 1991;70:485–487.
8. Korantzis A, Cardamakis E, Chelidonis E, et al. Nasal septum deformity in the newborn infant during labor. *Eur J Obstet Gynecol Reprod Funct.* 1992;44:41–46.
9. Kawalski H, Spiewak P. How septum deformations in newborns occur. *Int J Pediatr Otorhinolaryngol.* 1998;44:23–30.
10. Gray LP. Deviated nasal septum: incidence and etiology. *Ann Otol Rhinol Laryngol.* 1978;87(Suppl 50):3–20.
11. Stoksted P, Schønsted-Madsen U. Traumatology of the newborn's nose. *Rhinology.* 1979;17:77–82.
12. Tasca I, Compadretti GC. Immediate correction of nasal septum dislocation in newborns: long-term results. *Am J Rhinol.* 2004;18:47–51.
13. Luers JC, Welzing L, Roth B, Streppel M. Traumatic luxation of the nose in a newborn: case report and review of the literature. *Eur Arch Otorhinolaryngol.* 2009;266:1489–1493.
14. Deitmer T, Kiebler A. A self-redressment of neonatal nose-trauma. *Int J Pediatr Otorhinolaryngol.* 2013;77:443–445.
15. Patel VA, Carr MM. Congenital nasal obstruction in infants: a retrospective study and literature review. *Int J Pediatr Otorhinolaryngol.* 2017 Aug;99:78–84.
16. Losee JE, Kirschner RE, Whitaker LA, Bartlett SP. Congenital nasal anomalies: a classification scheme. *Plast Reconstr Surg.* 2004;113(2):676–689.
17. Fijałkowska M, Antoszewski B. Classification of congenital nasal deformities: a proposal to amend the existing classification. *Eur Arch Otorhinolaryngol.* 2017;274(3):1231–1235.
18. Ginat DT, Robson CD. Diagnostic imaging features of congenital nose and nasal cavity lesions. *Clinical Neuroradiology.* 2015;25(1):3–11.
19. Chaturvedi A, Chaturvedi A, Stanescu AL, Blickman JG, Meyers SP. Mechanical birth-related trauma to the neonate: an imaging perspective. *Insights Imaging.* 2018 Feb;9(1):103–118.

CHAPTER 22

External Ears

KEY POINTS

- Congenital ear deformities are common, with an incidence as high as 58% of all newborns.
- Congenital ear anomalies are divided into malformations and deformations.
- Malformations involve chondro-cutaneous defects, while deformations involve mechanically distorted architectural anomalies of the newborn's pinna.
- Crumpled and distorted ears can be secondary to late gestational deformational forces.
- Apparent ear enlargement on the side opposite the muscular torticollis is common.
- Many ear shape abnormalities can be corrected by splinting the ear into a normal shape with custom molds if initiated before the first 3 weeks of life.

GENESIS

Congenital ear anomalies are generally divided into malformations (chondro-cutaneous defects) and deformations (misshaped architectural anomalies of the newborn's pinna, in which normal auricular components are fully developed yet mechanically distorted). Overfolding of the upper helix and/or other parts of the cartilaginous auricle are common constraint-related deformations, as is flattening of the ear against the head (Figs. 22.1 and 22.2). Prolonged constraint of the external ear may also result in asymmetric overgrowth of the ear.[1] Apparent ear enlargement is commonly observed on the side opposite the muscular torticollis in torticollis-plagiocephaly deformation sequence (Fig. 22.3). On the side of the tightened sternocleidomastoid muscle, the ear is usually measurably smaller, with an uplifted lobe caused by pressure from the shoulder. In nonsynostotic deformational posterior plagiocephaly, the position of the ear is also displaced anteriorly on the side toward which the head is turned (as the occiput on that side becomes flattened with persistent supine positioning). Such ear malposition usually corrects with timely and appropriate treatment of the torticollis-plagiocephaly deformation sequence. Similarly, the vertical position of the ear can be lowered with unilateral coronal or lambdoidal craniosynostosis, and it also improves with timely and appropriate surgical correction (Fig. 22.4). Protrusion of the auricles is also common with positional brachycephaly.

The incidence of ear deformation varies with age and the degree of attentiveness of the observer. The incidence of congenital ear deformities has been documented to be as high as 58% of all newborns.[2] Matsuo studied the ears of 1000 neonates over time and noted that more than 50% of the neonates had external ear shape abnormalities, most of which self-corrected during the first few months.[3] Extrinsic and intrinsic ear muscles play a role in shaping ears and may overcome the impact of fetal head constraint in many instances.[3,4] For example, Stahl's ear (third crus) was noted in 47% of neonates but only seen in 7% of the same infants at 1 year of age. On the other hand, protruding ears were only seen in 0.4% of neonates, but 5.5% of the same infants had protruding ears at 1 year of age, usually caused by persistently turning the head toward one side while being maintained in a supine sleeping position.[3] These researchers noted that when constriction was accompanied by a lop ear deformity, it was unlikely to correct spontaneously over time. A lop ear deformity can be defined as a deficient helix and scapha, underdeveloped antihelix, and downfolding of the helix.[4]

Inactivity of the posterior auricular muscles with associated loss of facial nerve function in Möbius syndrome leads to prominent ears, which suggests that some ear deformities result from aberrant neuromuscular function.[5] Maternal relaxing hormones that circulate before parturition can soften the cartilages of the fetus and neonate, making the auricles

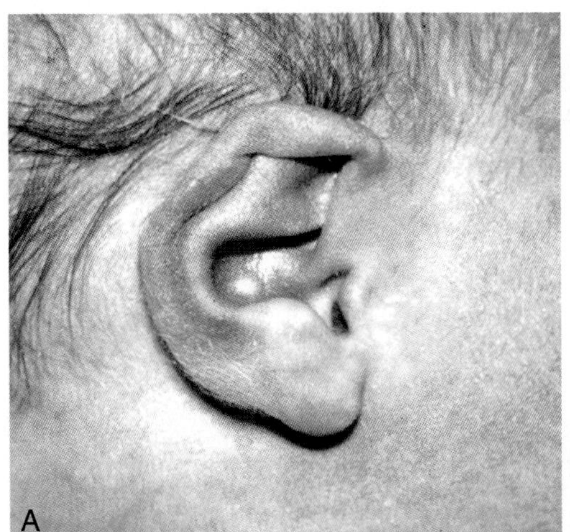

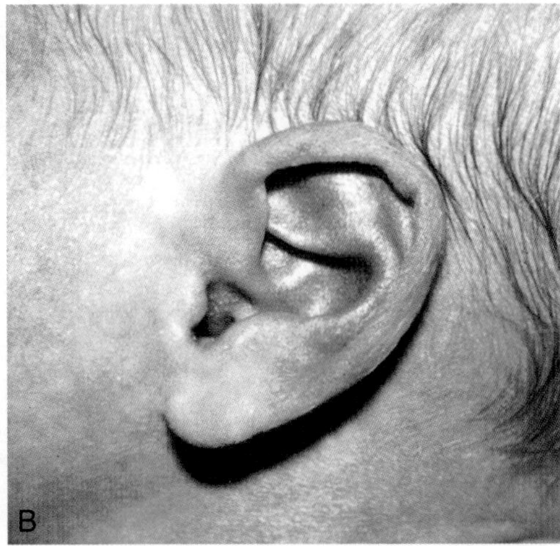

FIGURE 22.1 Constraint-induced overfolding of the scapha helix (**A**) and partial crumpling of the concha (**B**). In a more severe example of abdominal pregnancy with prolonged oligohydramnios, the right ear is markedly enlarged owing to compression, whereas the left ear is markedly crumpled. Respiratory insufficiency associated with oligohydramnios led to death shortly after birth.

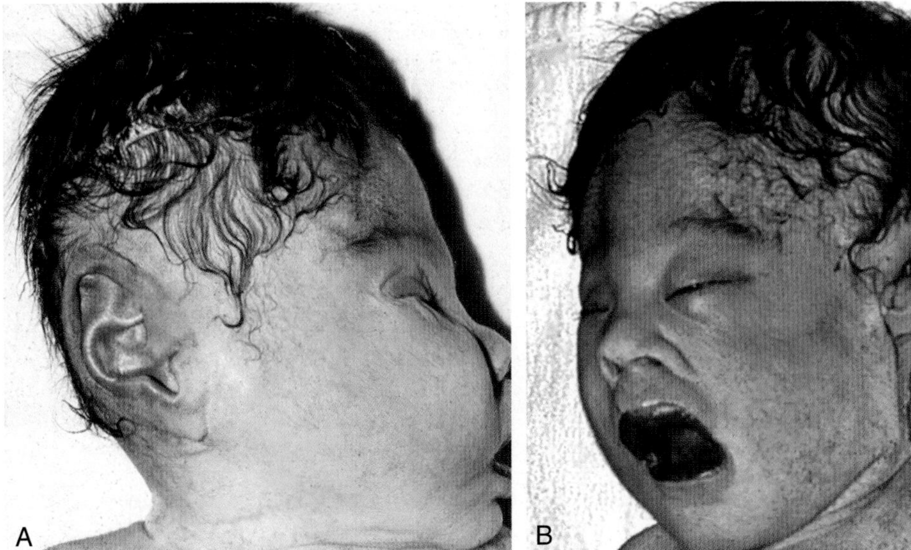

FIGURE 22.2 **A** and **B** Crumpling of the helix as the result of late gestational constraint owing to prolonged oligohydramnios associated with an ectopic abdominal pregnancy. (Courtesy of Will Cochran, Beth Israel Hospital and Harvard Medical School, Boston.)

more susceptible to deforming external forces.[3] Based on this pliability of ear cartilage in the first few days after birth, many ear shape abnormalities can be corrected by splinting the ear into a normal shape with custom molds fashioned from polymer dental compound, thermoplastic materials, or flexible wire splints encased in plastic tubing and taped in place for the first few weeks.[3,6–9] Such splinting is much less effective and generally requires longer treatment periods when initiated in older children.[9] In one study by Chen et al. of 173 individuals (274 ears), the mean treatment duration of participants who started ear molding within 14 days of birth was shorter than that of those who started treatment more than 14 days after birth with the same ear deformation.[10] The elasticity of ear cartilages affects successful treatment more than

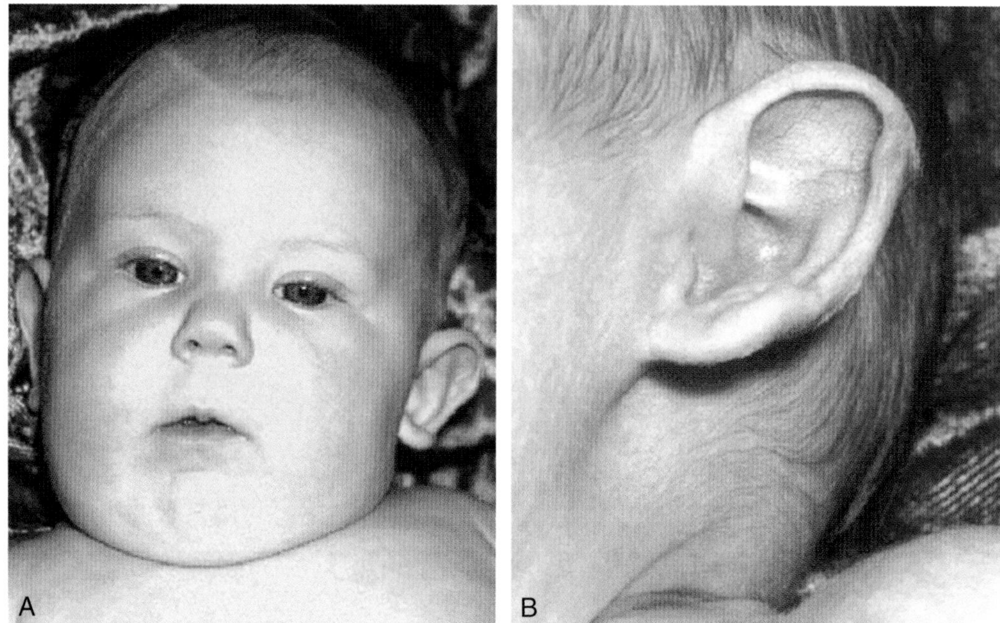

FIGURE 22.3 **A,** Uplifted left ear lobe caused by an oblique skewed head position in utero, with the left auricle between the head and left shoulder and the right ear compressed against the calvarium. **B,** Note the asymmetric overgrowth of the right ear and the prominent sulcus under the left mandible caused by compression against the left shoulder.

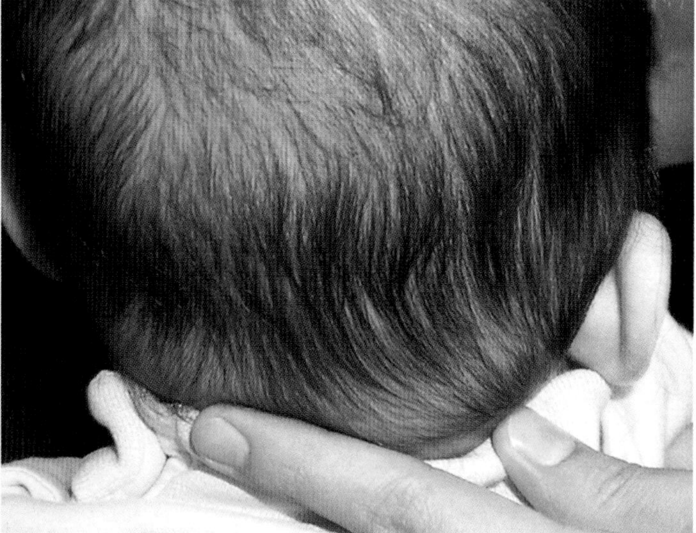

FIGURE 22.4 Posterior bony prominence of the right mastoid region with downward displacement of the right ear owing to right lambdoid synostosis.

does age, and ear cartilages tend to lose elasticity with age. Many types of congenital auricular deformities are caused by abnormalities in intrinsic and extrinsic ear muscles, with shortened muscles increasing the prominence of cartilages. Thus shortened muscles can be corrected by mechanical stretching with a splint, but stretched muscles are more difficult to shorten by splinting.[11]

FEATURES

Ears are often crumpled and distorted by late gestational forces, and their folded forms reflect the impact of these deforming forces. If an ear can be straightened out beneath a plate of clear glass or plastic so that all of its normal cartilaginous landmarks can be identified, this suggests the presence of deformations rather than malformations. Some minor ear shape abnormalities can be inherited in an autosomal dominant pattern, which is readily ascertained by inspection of the parents' ears. Other ear shape anomalies and malformations should prompt a search for other anomalies that might suggest the presence of a recognizable syndrome, such as oculoauriculovertebral spectrum (OAVS), branchiootorenal syndrome, Treacher Collins syndrome, or CHARGE syndrome.[12,13] In a series of 1000 patients with branchial arch malformations resulting in microtia, 36.5% had obvious soft tissue and bony abnormalities suggesting hemifacial microsomia, 15.2% had facial nerve weakness, 2.5% had macrostomia, 4.3% had cleft lip and/or palate, 4% had urogenital defects, 2.5% had cardiovascular abnormalities, and 1.7% had other anomalies such as cervical vertebral abnormalities.[14] Microtia occurs in 1 in 5000 live births and is more frequently right-sided (58.2%) than left-sided (32.4%) or bilateral (9.4%), and it is found more frequently in males (63.1%).[14]

In a retrospective review of 204 patients from The Netherlands referred for microtia reconstruction, 60.8% were male and 91.7% were unilateral (66.3% right-sided). In unilateral patients lobule-type microtia was seen in 59.9%, (small) concha type in 34.4%, and anotia in 5.7%. Atresia of the acoustic meatus (76.0%) was the most commonly associated anomaly, followed by preauricular skin tags (30.5%), hemifacial microsomia (27.5%), facial nerve paralysis (8.3%), and congenital heart disease (2.5%). Familial occurrence of microtia in this cohort was 2.0%.[15]

OAVS is characterized mainly by anomalies of the ear, hemifacial microsomia, epibulbar dermoids, and vertebral anomalies. Among 355 infants diagnosed with OAVS during the 1990–2009 period, 19% were detected prenatally and 70% were diagnosed at birth.[16] The best time to evaluate fetal ears with ultrasonography is at 20–24 weeks of pregnancy. Among infants with OAVS, microtia (89%), hemifacial microsomia (49%), and ear tags (44%) were the most frequent anomalies, followed by atresia/stenosis of the external auditory canal (25%), and diverse vertebral (24%) and eye (24%) anomalies. There was a high rate (69.5%) of associated anomalies in other organ systems, the most common being congenital heart defects in 27.8% of patients. The prevalence of OAVS, defined as microtia/ear anomalies and at least one major characteristic anomaly, was 3.8 per 100,000 births. Twinning, assisted reproductive techniques, and maternal prepregnancy diabetes were confirmed as risk factors.[17]

MANAGEMENT AND PROGNOSIS

A return to normal auricular form within the first few postnatal days tends to confirm the deformational origin of such ear defects, which usually require no management. When the ear is abnormally crumpled into a form that is unlikely to resolve within the first day or so, wax molds or thermoplastic splints can be individually fashioned and taped in place (Figs. 22.5–22.8). This is most effective if done in the first few days of life, while the ear cartilage is still relatively soft and pliable as a consequence of maternal relaxing hormones still circulating in the neonatal bloodstream.[3,6–11] Since 2010, the gold standard for achieving a permanent change in the shape of a newborn ear has been with the use of an infant ear-molding device such as the EarWell® System. The device is typically kept in place for 4–6 weeks and can correct most ear deformities with a high rate of success. When a child's ear was protruded laterally because of torticollis-plagiocephaly deformation sequence, one parent with an engineering background designed a modification for the child's cranial orthotic device that compressed the protruding auricles against the adjacent cranium (Fig. 22.9). Microtia requires surgical correction (Fig. 22.10), which is usually done using a patient's rib cartilages to create an ear framework around 6 years of age before correction of any associated canal atresia or mandibular asymmetry is attempted.[7,14] The alternative method of ear reconstruction is based on a porous polyethylene implant that is covered with fascia and skin as young as 4 years of age. It is extremely important to assess a child with auricular malformations for the possibility of associated hearing loss.[12,13] This can be done safely and effectively in young infants through otoacoustic emission evaluations, which can detect malfunction of cochlear hair cells at hearing thresholds greater than 35 decibels, or by auditory brainstem responses, which can detect neurologic hearing losses at greater than 80 decibels.[17] Early amplification is extremely important for the normal development of speech, and cochlear implantation in early childhood is indicated for children with severe or profound cochlear deafness.[17] Correction of the mandibular asymmetry

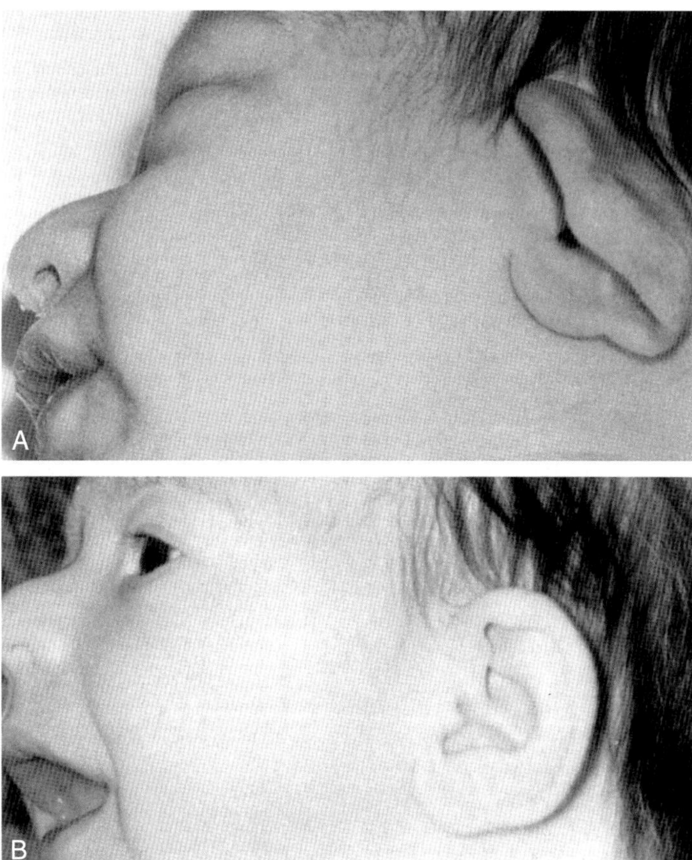

FIGURE 22.5 A, Overfolded auricle secondary to constraint during an asymmetric breech presentation in a septate uterus. **B,** 12 weeks later, the auricle has largely returned to normal form. Taping the ear may accelerate the process of reformation.

is typically delayed until skeletal maturity (approximately 17 years old) unless the patient is symptomatic from the small jaw.

A 2012 systematic review of 20 suitable papers revealed that splinting can be performed in many ways provided that the ear is permanently kept in the desired shape without distorting it.[18] The time needed to splint for permanent correction depends upon the age at the time of starting the treatment. For a newborn, 2 weeks often sufficed, whereas for older children splinting time became more variable—up to 6 months. The results tended to be poor in older children, who required longer splinting. No serious complications occurred and skin irritation was seen sporadically. The antihelical fold was more easily corrected than a deep concha (correction in 69.8% vs. 26.8%). Considering splinting therapy for protruding ears, a reasonable chance of success can only be offered to parents of children up to 6 weeks of age.[18]

A 2020 review of the literature identified 16 articles published in the previous decade that summarized their experience and outcomes.[19] Although some authors initiate treatment at 24 or 72 hours, several recommended waiting 1 week after birth before initiating treatment, to give spontaneous correction the opportunity to occur. Byrd et al. stated that only 50% of molding therapy was effective if initiated after the first 3 weeks of life. The rate of satisfactory improvement seems to be confounded by factors that include compliance, comfort, individual moldability, prolonged treatment for dissatisfactory results, and age at initiation of treatment.

DIFFERENTIAL DIAGNOSIS

Congenital malformational auricular anomalies are characterized by a partial absence of the skin or

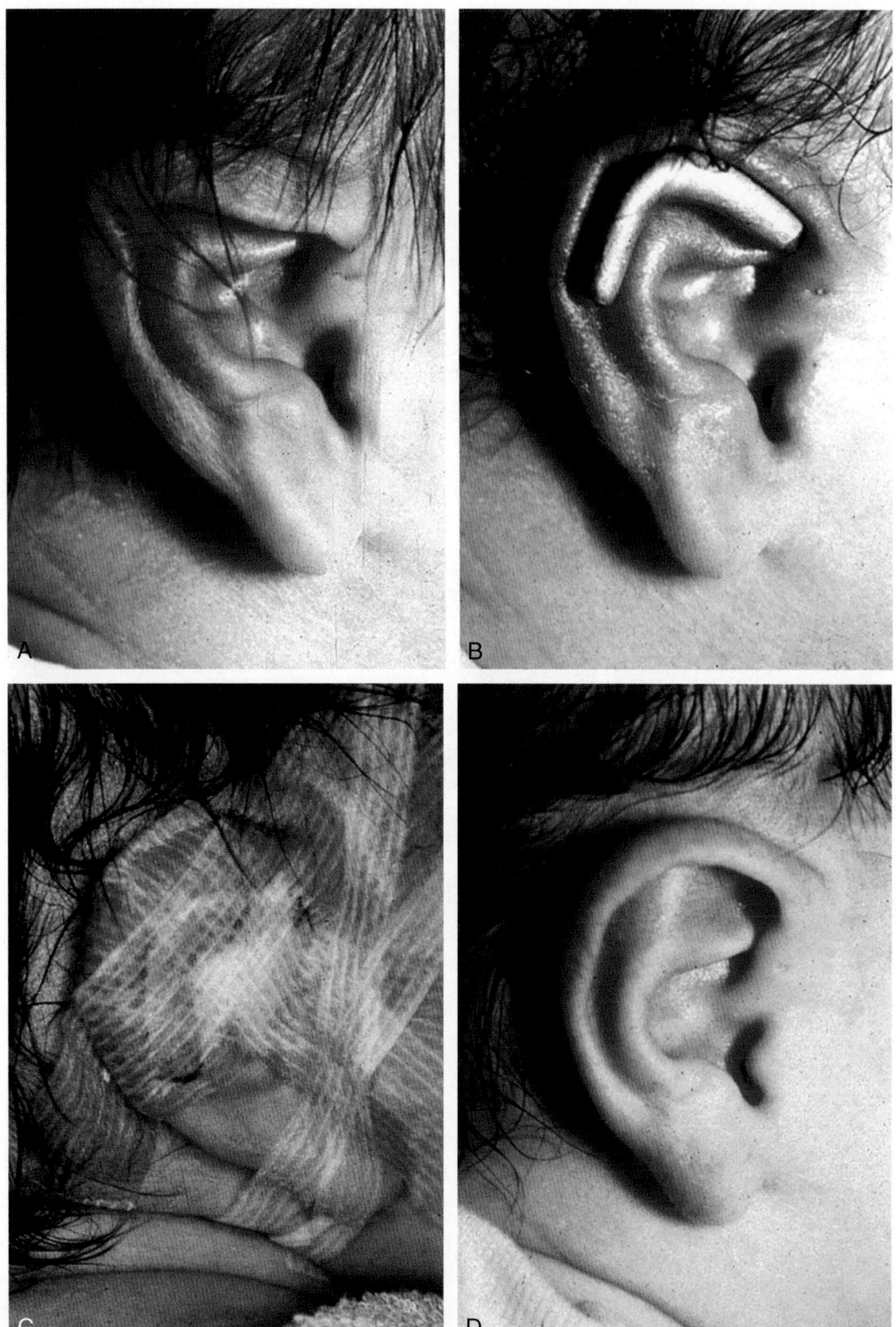

FIGURE 22.6 Crumpled ears can be reformed with the aid of dental wax molds. **A,** Initial Stahl's ear deformity that had also been present in the infant's mother, who required surgical correction. Dental wax molds were applied to reshape the ear (**B**) and were taped securely in place (**C**). **D,** The ear form remained normal after removal of taping and wax molds.

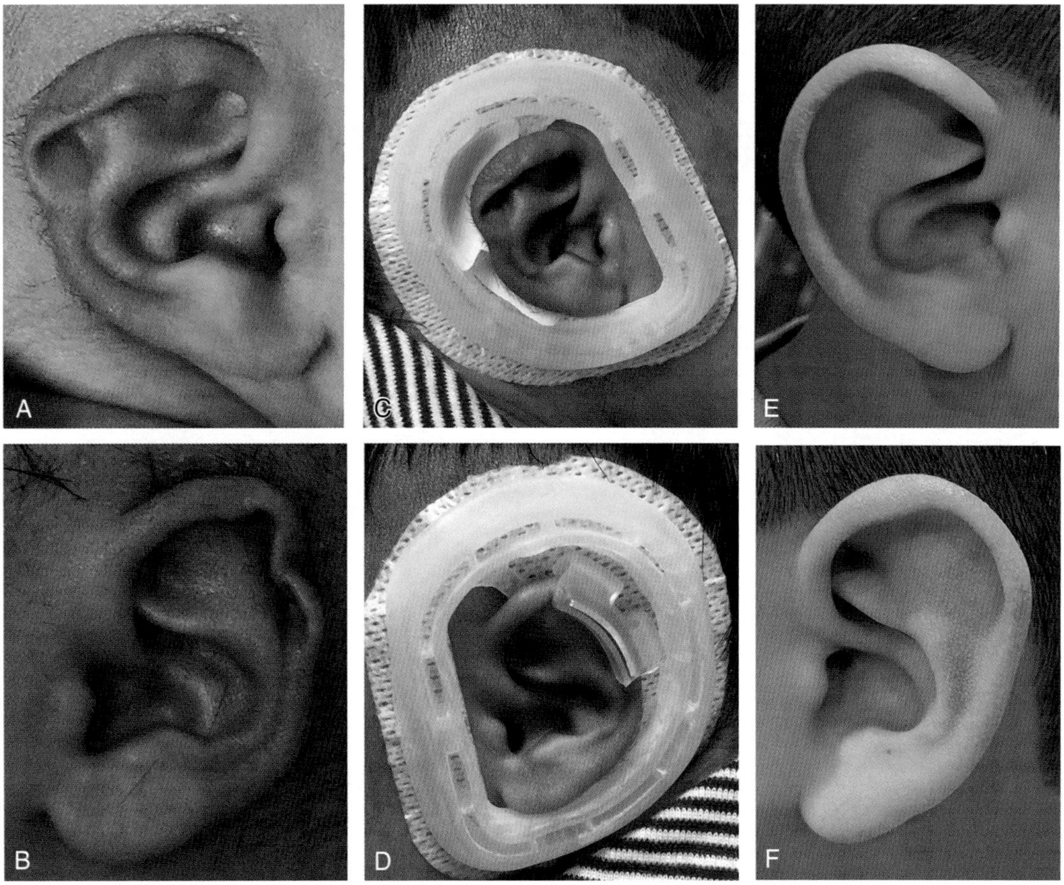

FIGURE 22.7 Bilateral congenital crumpled ears at 2 weeks of age (**A** and **B**), during treatment with an EarWell® infant ear correction system (**C** and **D**). Complete resolution with no residual deformity at 7-year follow-up (**E** and **F**).

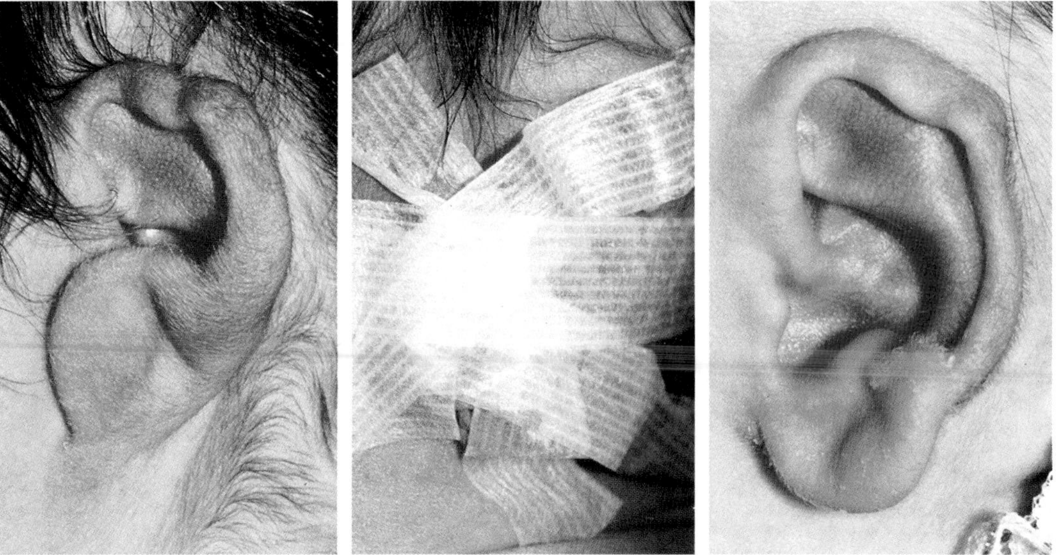

FIGURE 22.8 This crumpled ear in an infant with Turner syndrome was corrected nonsurgically by taping molds in place to correct the abnormally folded ears.

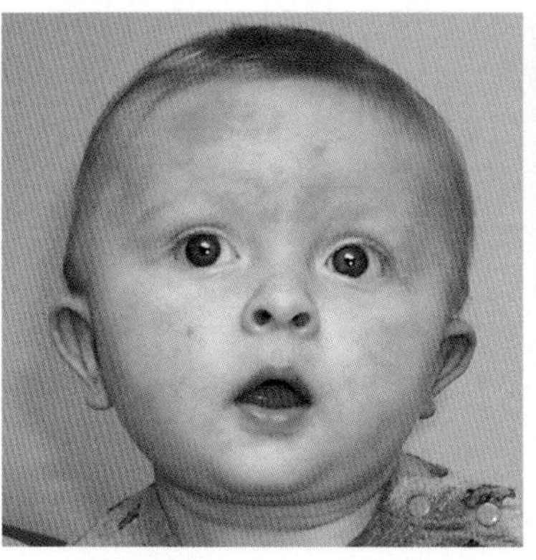
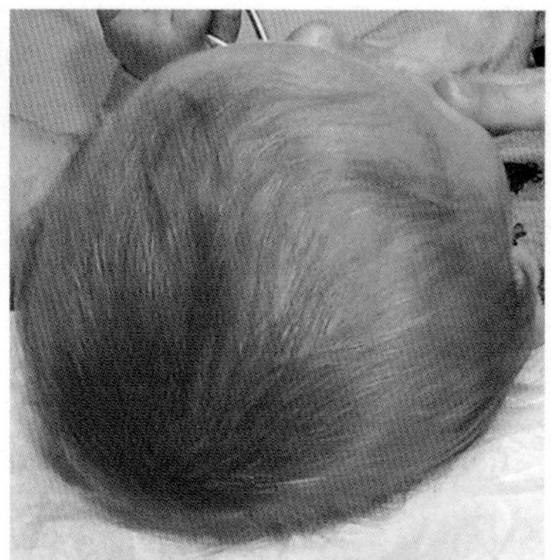
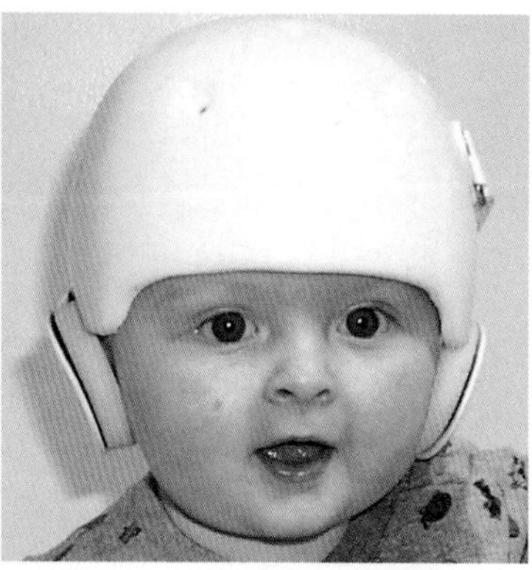

FIGURE 22.9 When this infant's ear protruded laterally because of brachycephaly with a head turn to the right, a parent with an engineering background designed a modification for the cranial orthotic device, which compressed the protruding auricle against the adjacent cranium.

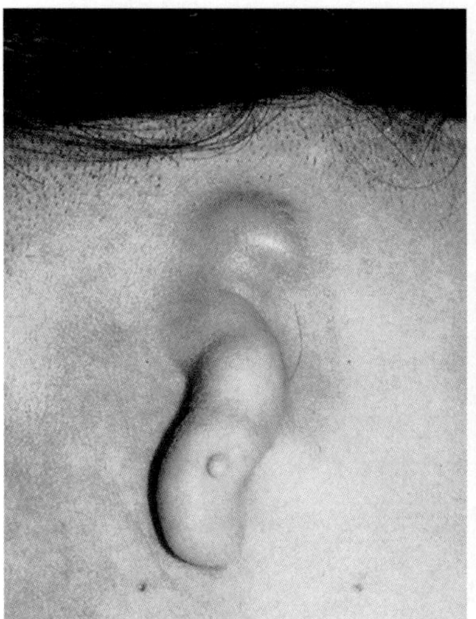
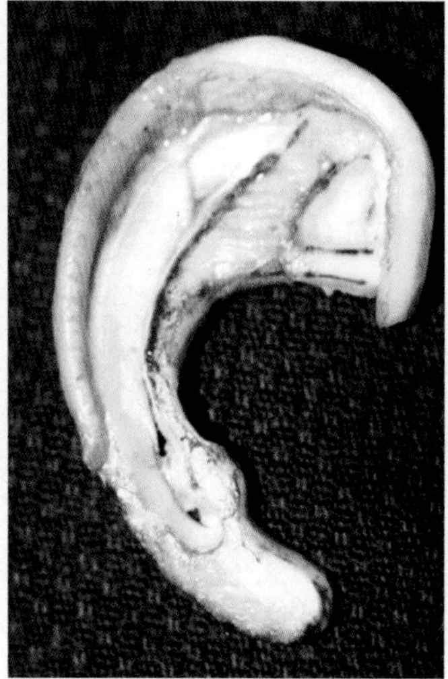
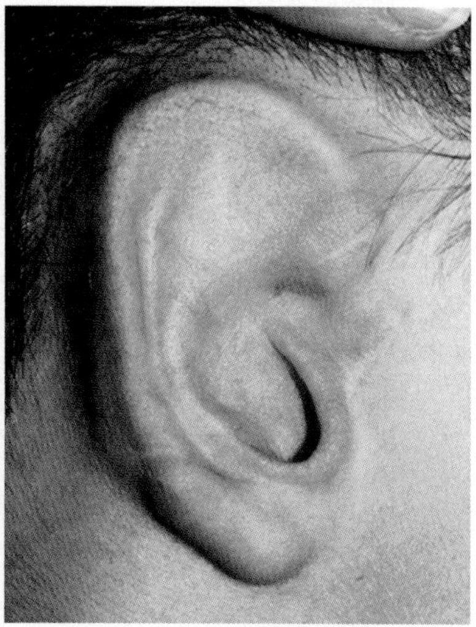

FIGURE 22.10 This microtic ear in a child with hemifacial microsomia was surgically corrected by carving a portion of the child's rib cartilage into a normal auricular form, sliding this form under the skin, and using the ear tag to help form an ear lobe. (Courtesy of Dr. Robert Ruder, Cedar-Sinai Medical Center, Los Angeles.)

cartilage resulting in a constricted or underdeveloped pinna, and they require surgical correction. Malformational auricular anomalies are caused by embryologic maldevelopment that occurs between the 5th and 9th weeks of gestation, resulting in deficient and/or supernumerary auricular components. Deformational auricular anomalies, on the other hand, result from in utero or postnatal deformational forces, including those caused by aberrant insertion of the intrinsic or extrinsic auricular muscles. Deformations are characterized by a misshapen but fully developed pinna and are best treated by auricular molding. Aberrations of ear form caused by defects in the development and/or function of intrinsic or extrinsic auricular ear muscles, such as protruding auricle or lop ear, usually do not improve after birth. Ear malformations that result from deficient cartilaginous support seldom improve and may be associated with a significant risk for hearing loss and renal anomalies.[12,13] A truly low-set ear is a very rare malformation, but vertical or anterior displacement is quite common and usually is a consequence of associated cranial abnormalities such as deformational plagiocephaly, or lambdoidal or multisuture craniosynostosis. Some types of ear deformities spontaneously resolve on their own without treatment, such as the characteristic ear swelling seen in diastrophic dysplasia (Fig. 22.11).

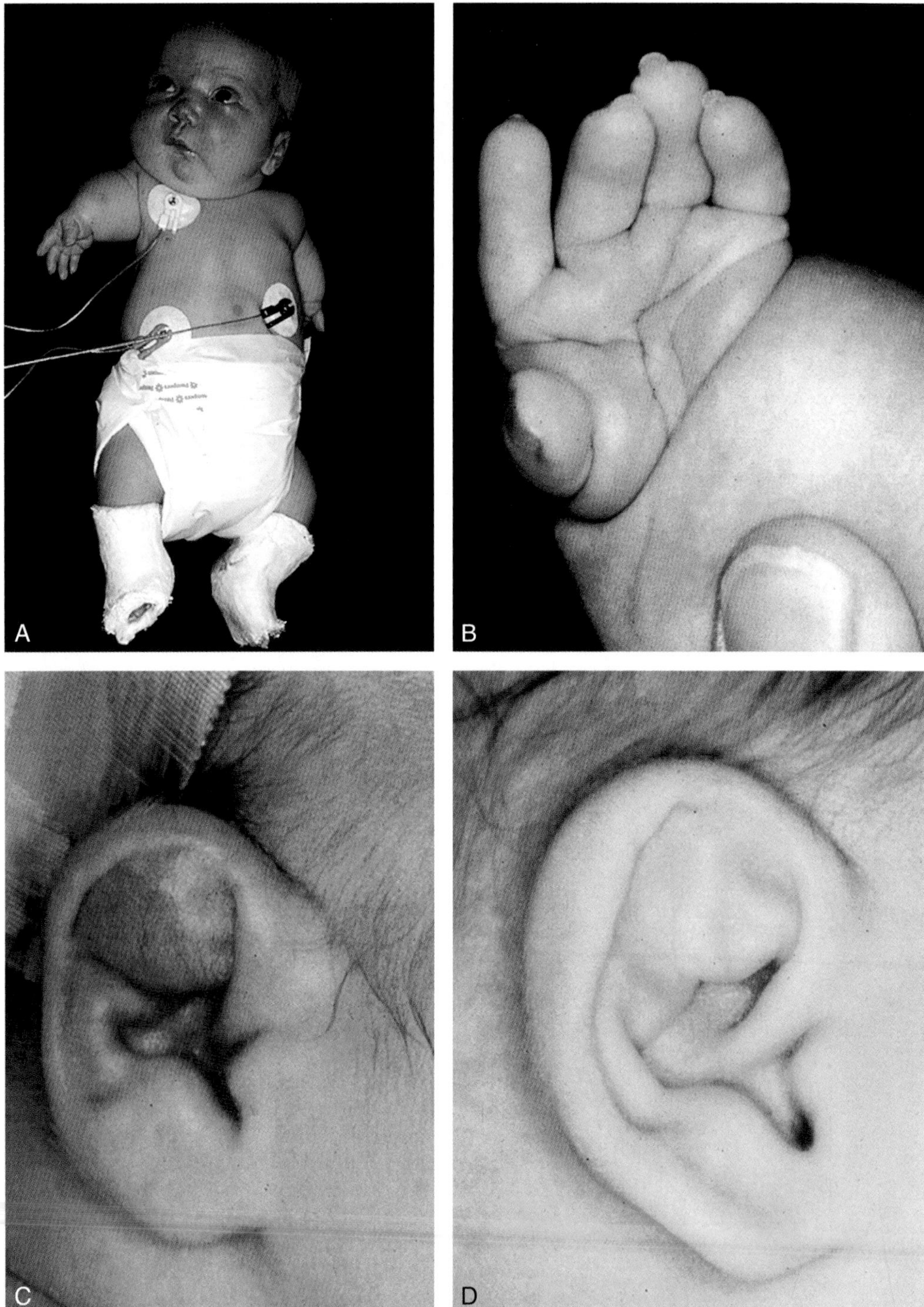

FIGURE 22.11 This child with diastrophic dysplasia (**A** and **B**) developed characteristic ear swellings shortly after birth (**C**), which gradually improved over the first few months without treatment (**D**).

References

1. Aase JM. Structural defects as a consequence of late intrauterine constraint: craniotabes, loose skin, and asymmetric ear size. *Semin Perinatol.* 1983;7:270–273.
2. Chang CS, Bartlett SP. Deformations of the ear and their nonsurgical correction. *Clin Pediatr (Phila).* 2019;58(7):798–805.
3. Matsuo K, Hayashi R, Kiyono M, et al. Nonsurgical correction of congenital auricular deformities. *Clin Plast Surg.* 1990;17:383–395.
4. Lese I, Aldabbas M, Mazeed AS, Bulstrode NW. Lop ear to conchal microtia: an algorithmic surgical approach. *Ann Plast Surg.* 2022;88(2):188–194.
5. Smith DW, Takashima H. Ear muscles and ear form. *Birth Defects Orig Artic Ser.* 1980;16:299–302.
6. Brown FE, Cohen LB, Addante RR, et al. Correction of congenital auricular deformities by splinting in the neonatal period. *Pediatrics.* 1986;78:406–411.
7. Ruder RO, Graham JMJr. Evaluation and treatment of the deformed and malformed auricle. *Clin Pediatr.* 1996;35:461–465.
8. Yotsuyanagi T, Yokoi K, Urushidate S, et al. Nonsurgical correction of congenital auricular deformities in children older than early neonates. *Plast Reconstr Surg.* 1998;101:907–914.
9. Furnas DW. Nonsurgical treatment of auricular deformities in neonates and infants. *Pediatr Ann.* 1999;28:387–390.
10. Chen Y, Wang W, Wang Y, Mao X. Using ear molding to treat congenital auricular deformities. *Front Pediatr.* 2021;9:752981.
11. Yotsuyanagi T. Nonsurgical correction of congenital auricular deformities in children older than early neonates. *Plast Reconstr Surg.* 2004;114:190–191.
12. Wang R, Earl DL, Ruder RO, et al. Syndromic ear anomalies and renal ultrasounds. *Pediatrics.* 2001;108:E32.
13. Wang R, Martinez-Frias ML, Graham JM. Jr: Infants of diabetic mothers are at increased risk for the oculo-auriculo-vertebral sequence: a case-based and case-control approach. *J Pediatr.* 2002;141:611–617.
14. Brent B. The pediatrician's role in caring for patients with congenital microtia and atresia. *Pediatr Ann.* 1999;28:374–383.
15. van Nunen DP, Kolodzynski MN, van den Boogaard MJ, et al. Microtia in the Netherlands: clinical characteristics and associated anomalies. *Int J Pediatr Otorhinolaryngol.* 2014;78(6):954–959.
16. Barisic I, Odak L, Loane M, et al. Prevalence, prenatal diagnosis and clinical features of oculo-auriculo-vertebral spectrum: a registry-based study in Europe. *Eur J Hum Genet.* 2014;22:1026–1033.
17. Slattery WH, Fayad JN. Cochlear implants in children with sensorineural inner ear hearing loss. *Pediatr Ann.* 1999;28:359–363.
18. van Wijk MP, Breugem CC, Kon M. Non-surgical correction of congenital deformities of the auricle: a systematic review of the literature. *J Plast Reconstr Aesthet Surg.* 2012;62:727–736.
19. Feijen MMW, van Cruchten C, Payne PE, van der Hulst RRWJ. Non-surgical correction of congenital ear anomalies: a review of the literature. *Plast Reconstr Surg Glob Open.* 2020;8(11):e3250.

CHAPTER 23

Mandibular Deformation

KEY POINTS

- Congenital compression of the chin can limit jaw growth before birth and result in asymmetric jaw retrusion.
- An asymmetric mandible can be secondary to an altered cranial base or a condylar abnormality secondary to genetic or environmental factors.
- Skin redundancy under the chin suggests pressure-induced growth restriction of the jaw.
- Asymmetric mandibular growth deficiency is often associated with muscular torticollis and can indicate associated congenital muscular torticollis.
- Failure to treat underlying muscular torticollis can result in persistent mandibular asymmetry, facial scoliosis, and rotatory cervical spine subluxation.
- Effective treatment of torticollis can resolve most of the associated jaw asymmetry by the end of the second year.

GENESIS

Intrauterine constraint and positional deformation have been proposed as possible extrinsic causes of mandibular hypoplasia.[1] Congenital compression of the chin against either the chest or intrauterine structures may limit the growth of the jaw before birth; when asymmetric jaw retrusion is more commonly left-sided (Fig. 23.1). If the compression is of prolonged duration, there may be pressure indentation or skin necrosis on the upper thoracic surface. As shown in Fig. 23.1, one deformational cause of asymmetric mandibular growth deficiency is prolonged oligohydramnios. Asymmetric mandibular growth deficiency with a laterally tilted mandible is most commonly the result of head rotation with one side of the mandible compressed against the shoulder or chest, and it is commonly associated with muscular torticollis on the same side as the deficient mandible (Fig. 23.2). Such asymmetric mandibular growth deficiency is often the first indication that an infant might have associated congenital muscular torticollis.[2]

If the ear on the side of the small jaw is dysplastic or microtic, or if there are associated ear tags or epibulbar dermoids, a diagnosis of oculoauriculovertebral sequence (OAVS), Goldenhar syndrome, or craniofacial microsomia should be considered (Fig. 23.3). OAVS is etiologically heterogeneous, and a careful family and gestational history, renal ultrasound, and cervical vertebral radiographs may help evaluate the possibility of an associated syndrome (Figs. 23.4–23.6).[3-5] Muscular torticollis with mandibular asymmetry results from late gestational fetal constraint, whereas OAVS with mandibular asymmetry occurs in early gestation as part of a malformation syndrome. Symmetric undergrowth of the jaw occurs with Pierre Robin malformation sequence with associated posterior cleft palate and glossoptosis (Fig. 23.7).[6] This condition is etiologically heterogeneous, with an estimated incidence of 1 in 8500–14,000 live births.[7] The concept that this may result from intrauterine constraint in some cases is based in part on an increased incidence of Pierre Robin in twins.[8] Skin redundancy under the chin suggests pressure-induced growth restriction of the jaw, especially when there is no associated cleft posterior palate (Fig. 23.8), whereas unilateral mandibular growth deficiency with an associated sulcus that corresponds with compression by the shoulder suggests congenital muscular torticollis (see Fig. 22.3A). In an eloquent study by Parada et al. in 2015, they were able to generate a murine model phenocopy of the human Pierre Robin sequence, culturing maxilla and palate tissue separate from the tongue and mandible.[9] They were able to rescue the tongue and palate phenotype, highlighting the interconnection of early palate, tongue, and mandible development.

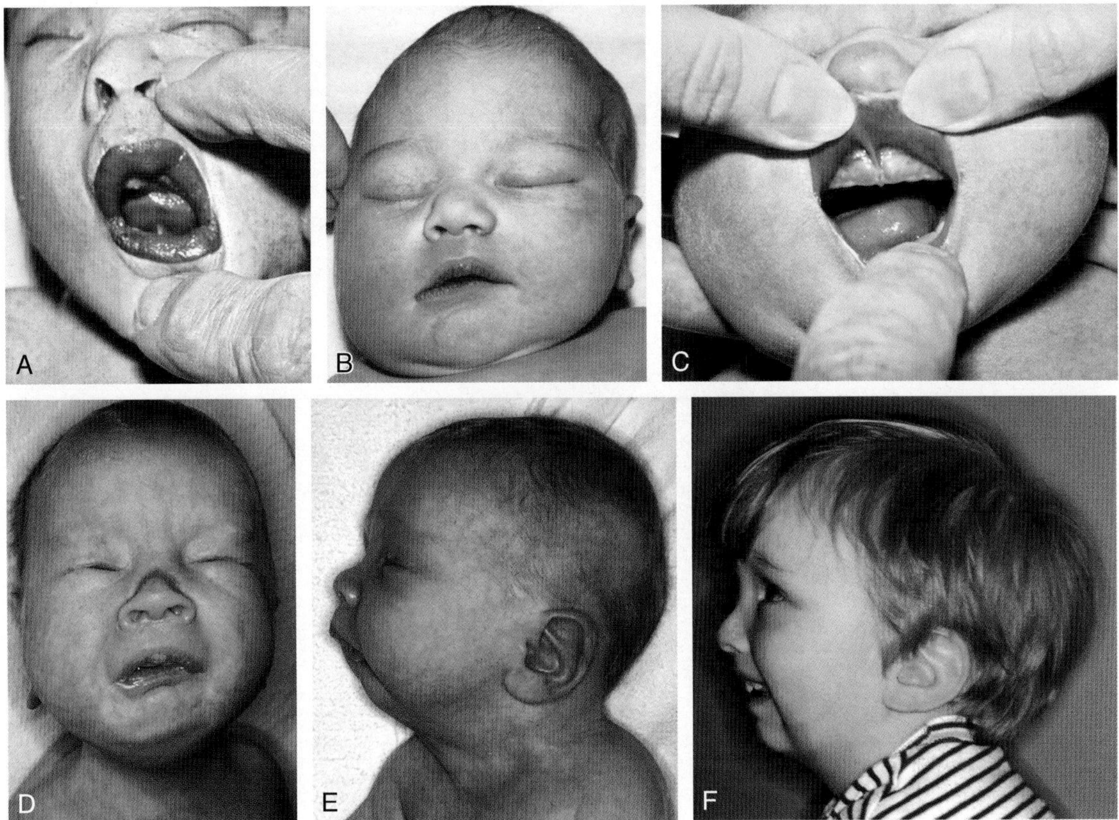

FIGURE 23.1 **A,** This infant was delivered abdominally from an extrauterine location behind the uterus with marked distortion of the face and jaw. Respiratory insufficiency associated with oligohydramnios led to death shortly after birth. **B** and **C,** This infant was also an abdominal pregnancy; her head was under the mother's stomach, and her feet were under the gallbladder. **D–F,** This infant experienced prolonged oligohydramnios with transverse lie owing to premature rupture of the amnion at 26 weeks, with delivery at 36 weeks. **D** and **E,** There is striking mandibular growth restriction with necrotic neck folds. **F,** At age 30 months, mandibular growth deficiency persisted. (**A–C** Courtesy Will Cochran, Beth Israel Hospital and Harvard Medical School, Boston.)

FEATURES

In constraint-related mandibular growth restriction associated with torticollis, the head is often tilted toward the growth-restricted mandible, whereas the chin points toward the other side. The ear on the growth-restricted side is often smaller than the other ear, and there may be a prominent mandibular sulcus, with an upward cant to the mandible on that same side (see Figs. 23.1 and 23.2). Neck rotation is often restricted.[2,10] These features warrant early neck physical therapy once concerns about any possible structural cervical spine anomalies have been resolved through careful physical examination and radiographs, if necessary. With symmetric jaw deficiency resulting from a face presentation or transverse lie, retroflexion of the head with a prominent occipital shelf may be noted. With prolonged compression of the jaw, there may be regional redundancy of the skin owing to constraint-induced overgrowth of the skin in that region (Figs. 23.8 and 23.9). This skin redundancy is usually not present if the mandibular growth deficiency is caused by an underlying syndrome. If there are associated ear malformations or if the neck is wide and short with limited mobility, the possibility of cervical spine anomalies should be considered.

MANAGEMENT AND PROGNOSIS

If there is associated congenital muscular torticollis, early neck physical therapy with frequent variation of the infant's sleeping position should be initiated to prevent the development of secondary deformational

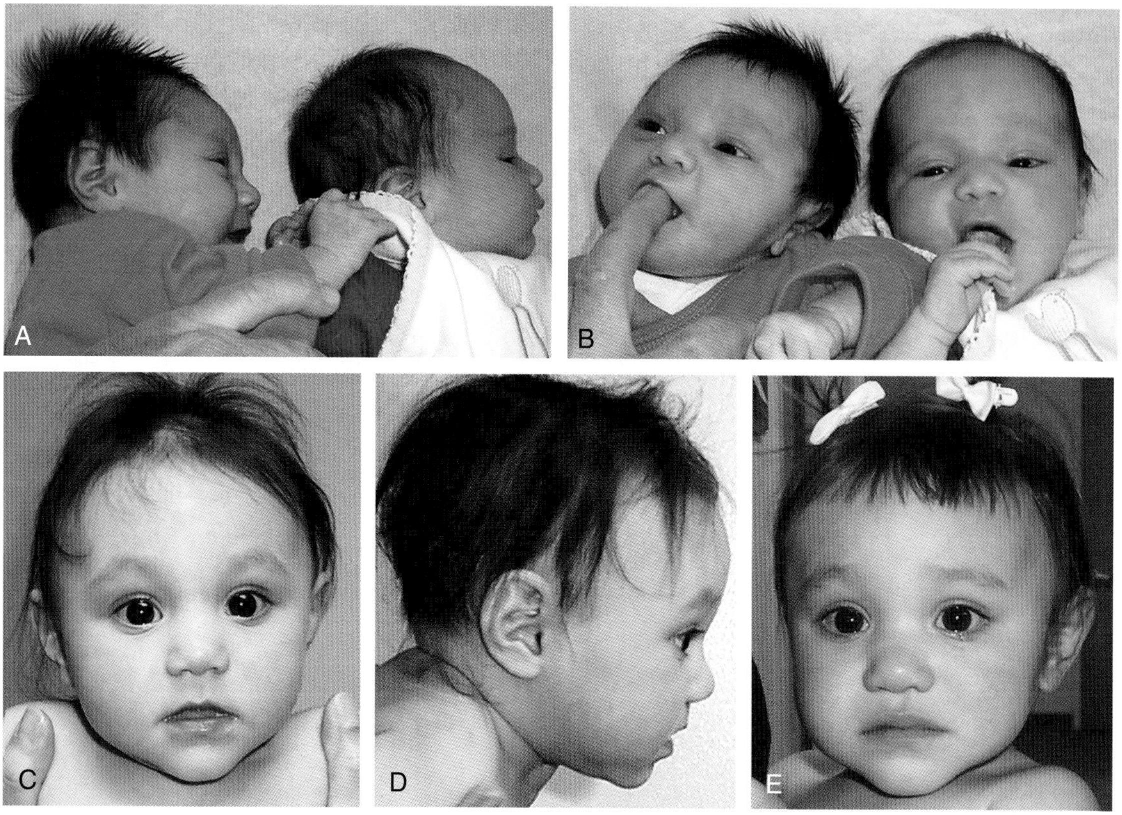

FIGURE 23.2 These twins were born at term to a primigravida woman; the left twin was carried in a prolonged vertex presentation low in the uterus. This twin had severe congenital left muscular torticollis at birth (**A** and **B**), which responded well to neck physical therapy, although mild jaw asymmetry was still evident at age 7 months (**C–E**).

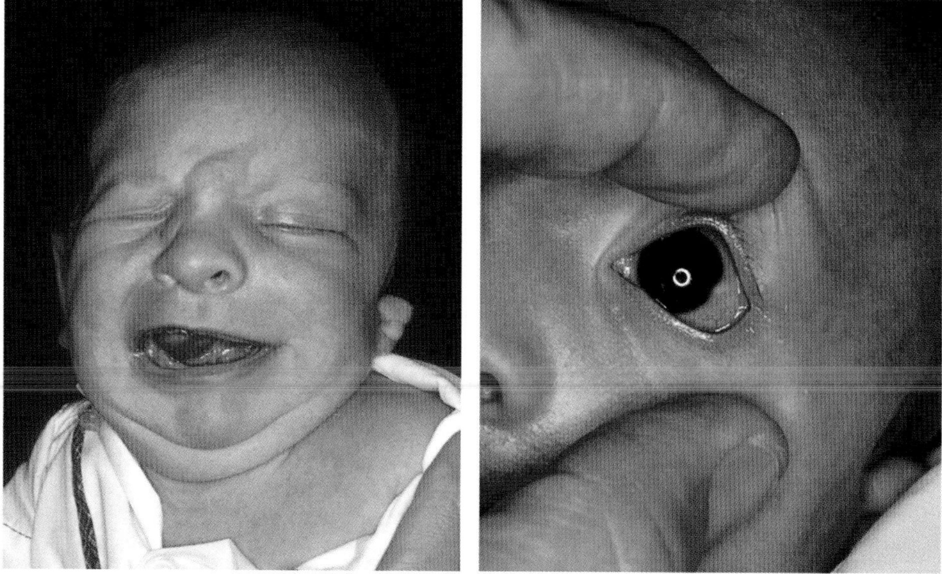

FIGURE 23.3 This infant has left hemifacial microsomia with mandibular growth deficiency, epibulbar dermoid, and microtia on the left.

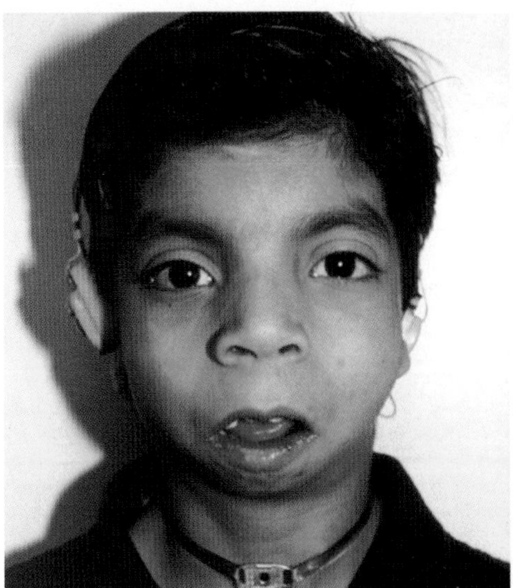
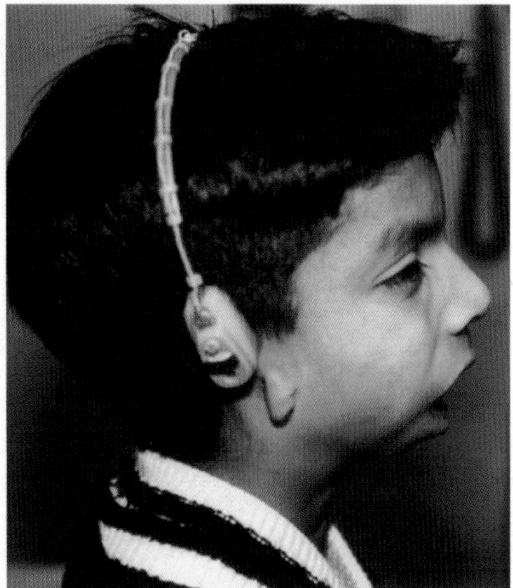

FIGURE 23.4 This child has branchiootorenal syndrome with deafness, bilateral mandibular deficiency, microtia, conjunctival dermoids, and branchial cleft cysts; they were initially diagnosed with familial Goldenhar syndrome.

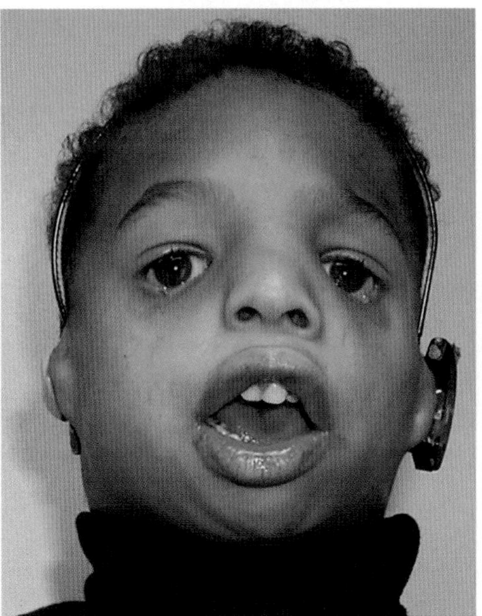
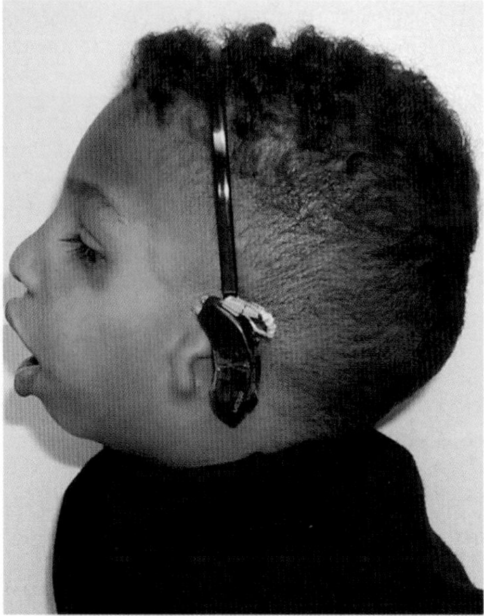

FIGURE 23.5 This child has Treacher Collins syndrome with microtia, deafness, malar clefts, down-slanting palpebral fissures, mandibular growth deficiency, and cleft palate.

posterior plagiocephaly.[2,10,11] Because the infant's neck does not begin to extend vertically until the second half of the first year, asymmetric mandibular growth restriction may be difficult to detect in young infants, but parents may note that the eye on the side of the growth-restricted mandible appears to open less widely because of vertical displacement of the soft tissues of the cheek when the mandible is compressed against the chest on that side.[2,10] Failure to treat muscular torticollis appropriately can result in marked, persistent mandibular asymmetry, facial scoliosis, and rotatory cervical spine subluxation.[11-15] Cranial and cranial base

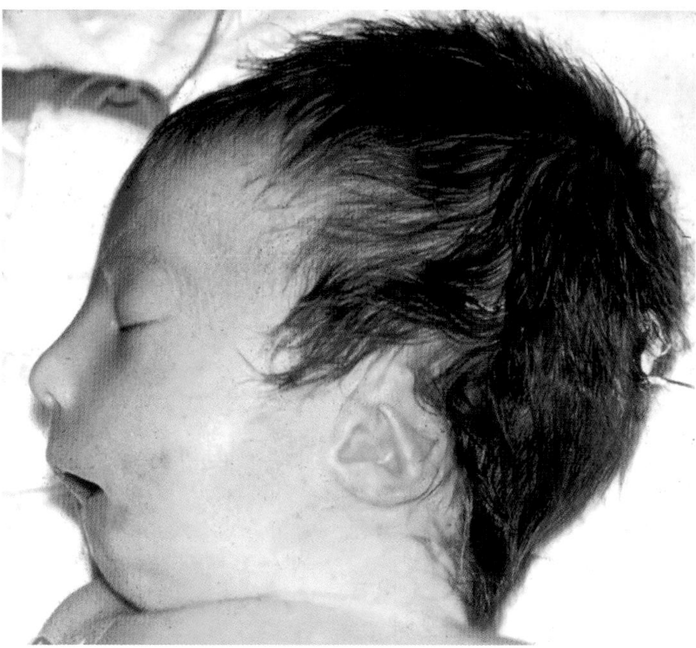

FIGURE 23.6 This child has CHARGE syndrome with characteristic dysplastic ears lacking lobes, sensorineural deafness, bilateral choanal atresia, micrognathia, cleft palate, DiGeorge sequence, genital hypoplasia, and tetralogy of Fallot.

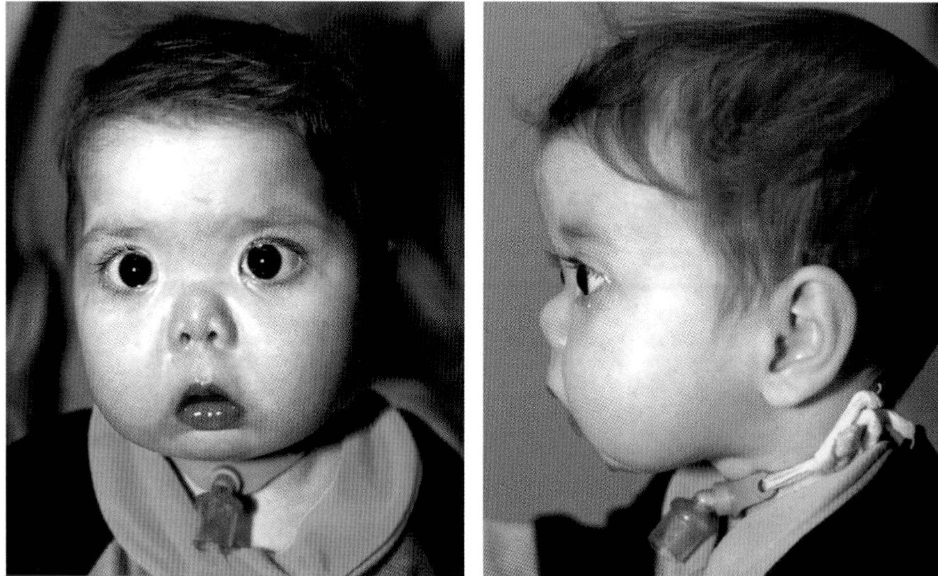

FIGURE 23.7 This child has Stickler syndrome with deafness, Pierre Robin malformation sequence, flat nasal bridge, and severe myopia.

deformity occur early in patients with uncorrected torticollis, followed by facial bone deformity during childhood (Fig. 24.7). The cranial and facial deformity becomes more severe with age, so early release of the muscle restriction is advised in patients with torticollis that has been refractory to physical therapy to prevent progressive craniofacial deformation.[15,16] With effective treatment of the torticollis, most of the associated jaw

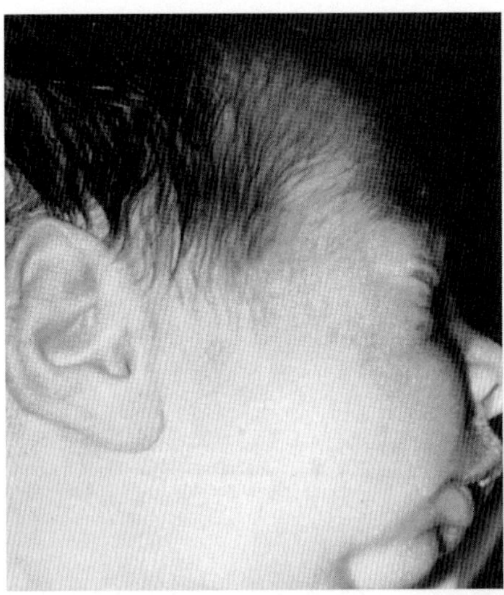
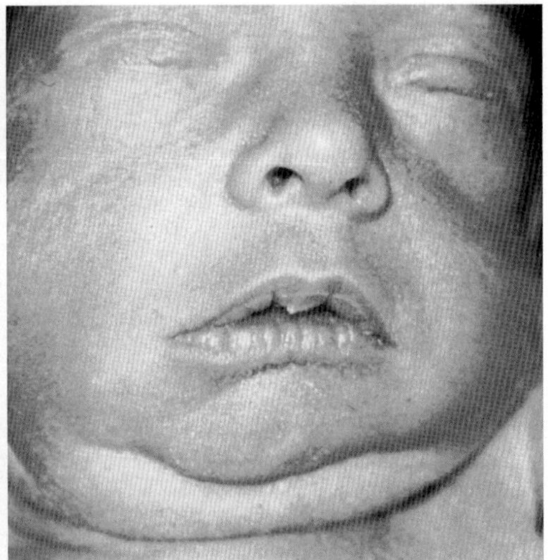

FIGURE 23.8 This infant has mandibular growth deficiency resulting from jaw compression. Note the redundancy of skin secondary to constraint-induced overgrowth of skin.

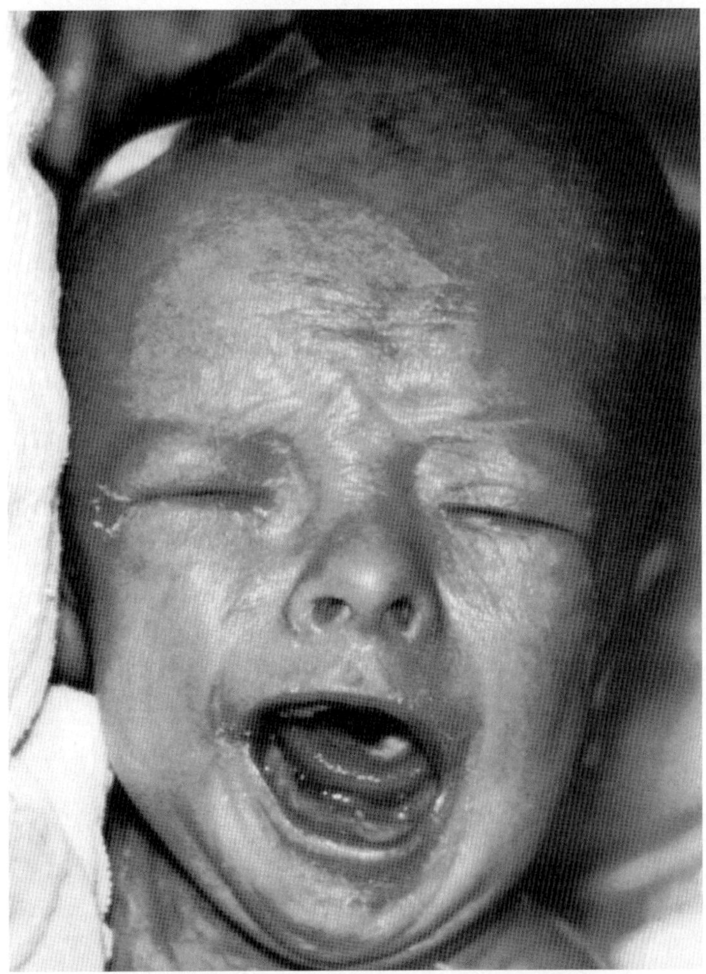

FIGURE 23.9 This neonate has marked jaw asymmetry caused by unilateral shoulder compression in utero.

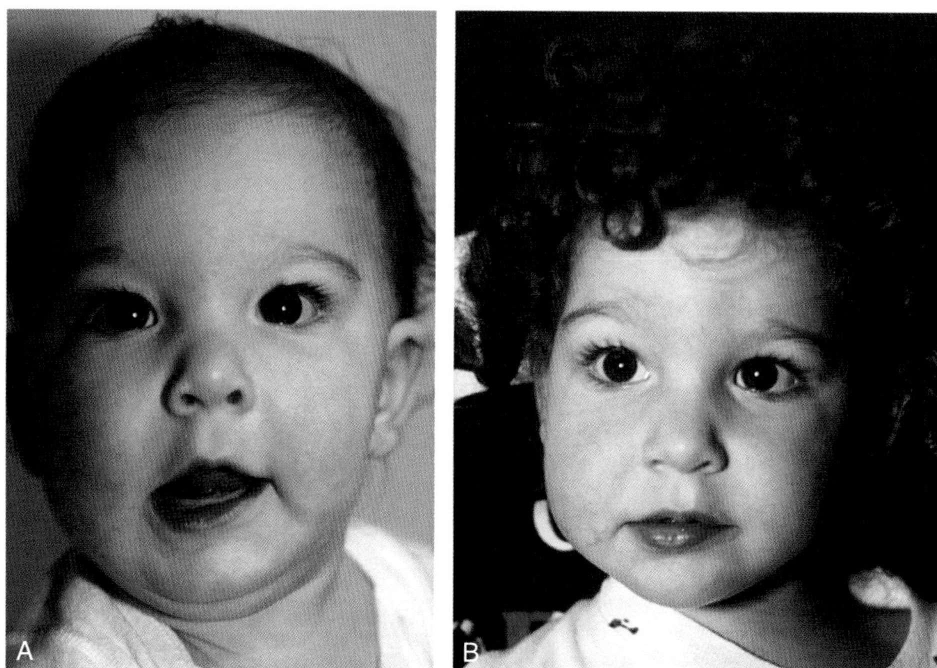

FIGURE 23.10 This child was born with left congenital muscular torticollis and had asymmetric mandibular deficiency on the side of the torticollis (**A**), which resolved by age 2 years (**B**).

asymmetry usually resolves by the end of the second year (Fig. 23.10).

In a study of 80 patients who required surgical release, cephalometry showed improvement in the craniofacial deformity after surgical release, and results were better when surgery was performed before the patient reached 5 years of age. More postsurgical change occurs during the first postoperative year than during the second year.[17] Long-term follow up for 14 years confirmed resolution of the facial asymmetry.[18]

Sternocleidomastoid release has also been beneficial in adults with neglected congenital muscular torticollis, leading to cosmetic and functional improvements and pain relief originating from the muscle imbalance brought about by the long-standing deformity.[18,19]

Among idiopathic cases of laterally deviated mandible, there are two major categories of mandibular asymmetry: (1) altered cranial base from congenital muscular torticollis or unilateral craniosynostosis and (2) condylar abnormality from condylar fractures, condylar hyperplasia, juvenile condylar arthritis, or hemifacial microsomia. Proper diagnosis and subsequent treatment of the underlying abnormality of the deviated mandible ensure appropriate orthognathic reconstruction and decrease the likelihood of skeletal relapse after surgery.[20] There is also an association between hemifacial microsomia and craniofaciocervical scoliosis when associated underlying cervical vertebral anomalies are present.[21] Infants with cervical vertebral anomalies resulting in torticollis benefit from early cranial orthotic therapy in an effort to prevent or at least minimize craniofacial deformation. Such orthotic molding should begin during the first few months and continue through the second year. When mandibular growth deficiency is symmetric and a consequence of abnormal fetal presentation, it may resolve with little more than gentle mandibular massage, but if compression has been prolonged and severe, mandibular growth deficiency may persist (see Fig. 23.1).

Treatment of unilateral or bilateral mandibular insufficiency, such as OAVS or Pierre Robin sequence, is usually accomplished by mandibular distraction osteogenesis.[22-24] For patients with severe mandibular growth deficiency and obstructive sleep apnea, mandibular distraction shortly after birth is recommended.[25,26]

DIFFERENTIAL DIAGNOSIS

Micrognathia is an associated feature in a number of malformation syndromes, with approximately 26–83% of Pierre Robin sequence diagnoses being

BOX 23.1 SYNDROMES MOST FREQUENTLY ASSOCIATED WITH PIERRE ROBIN SEQUENCE

22q11.2 Deletion syndrome
Braddock-Carey syndrome
Campomelic dysplasia
Catel-Manske syndrome
Cornelia De Lange syndrome
Congenital myotonic dystrophy
Carey-Fineman-Ziter syndrome
Fetal alcohol syndrome
Goldenhar syndrome
Hemifacial microsomia
Kabuki syndrome
Kniest dysplasia
Larsen syndrome
Miller syndrome
Moebius syndrome
Nager syndrome
Mandibulofacial dysostosis
Oculoauriculovertebral spectrum
Otopalatodigital syndrome
Russel Silver syndrome
SATB2/Glass syndrome
Spondyloepiphyseal dysplasia
Stickler syndrome
Treacher Collins syndrome

part of an underlying syndrome (see Box 23.1 and Figs. 23.3–23.7).[5,6] Mandibular asymmetry resulting in a laterally deviated mandible can occur with OAVS, congenital muscular torticollis, and several other less frequent conditions.[4,20] Among 56 patients born with developmental dysplasia of the hip (DDH), three-dimensional facial surface images showed significantly more facial asymmetry when compared with healthy controls, suggesting that subtle facial changes might have occurred because of associated congenital muscular torticollis.[27,28] Approximately 10% of children with deformation plagiocephaly and congenital muscular torticollis have mandibular asymmetry.[29] In one study ramal height asymmetry was confirmed via CT scan. Ramal and occlusal cant asymmetry improved in all patients significantly after physical therapy by 7.5 months in their treated cohort. An association between congenital muscular torticollis and DDH has been established in the literature, and among 97 consecutive infants with congenital muscular torticollis who had hip imaging performed, 12% had DDH, all requiring treatment, and 75% (9/12) of the patients with DDH had an abnormal hip exam.[28] Thus in patients with congenital muscular torticollis, an ultrasound or radiograph of the hips should be strongly considered, particularly with breech presentation and an abnormal hip exam.

Striking mandibular growth deficiency can be associated with a posterior cleft palate and glossoptosis in the Pierre Robin malformation sequence, which is etiologically heterogeneous.[5-7] Among 117 patients with Pierre Robin malformation sequence, 31% had an underlying syndrome, and Stickler syndrome, Treacher Collins syndrome, chromosomal disorders, and teratogenic disorders accounted for about half of these syndromes. Another 20% had associated malformations affecting the skeleton, heart, eye, and central nervous system, which resulted in intellectual disability in 67% of these cases, whereas 49% were isolated.[7] These latter cases with an unknown etiology could probably be diagnosed today with the use of more advanced genetic diagnostic tests such as chromosomal microarrays and exome sequencing, as evidenced by the longer list of associated syndromes described by Barisic et al. and Motch Perrine et al.[5,30] Thus a careful search for associated anomalies often reveals the presence of other anomalies that might lead to the diagnosis of an associated syndrome.

References

1. Tan TY, Kilpatrick N, Farlie PG. Developmental and genetic perspectives on Pierre Robin sequence. *Am J Med Genet Part C Semin Med Genet*. 2013;163C:295–305.
2. Kuo AA, Tritasavit S, Graham JM, : Jr Congenital muscular torticollis and positional plagiocephaly. *Pediatr Rev*. 2014;35:79–87.
3. Wang R, Earl DL, Ruder RO, et al. Syndromic ear anomalies and renal ultrasounds. *Pediatrics*. 2001;108:E32.
4. Wang R, Martinez-Frias ML, Graham JM. Jr: Infants of diabetic mothers are at increased risk for the oculo-auriculo-vertebral sequence: a case-based and case-control approach. *J Pediatr*. 2002;141:611–617.
5. Barisic I, Odak L, Loane M, et al. Prevalence, prenatal diagnosis and clinical features of oculo-auriculo-vertebral spectrum: a registry-based study in Europe. *Eur J Hum Genet*. 2014;22:1026–1033.
6. Hsieh ST, Woo AS. Pierre Robin sequence. *Clin Plast Surg*. 2019 Apr;46(2):249–259.
7. Tan TY, Kilpatrick N, Farlie FG. Developmental and genetic perspectives on Pierre Robin sequence. *Am J Med Genet C Semin Med Genet*. 2013;163C:295–305.
8. Holder-Espinasse M, Abadie V, Cormier-Daire V, et al. Pierre Robin sequence: analysis of 117 consecutive cases. *J Pediatr*. 2001;139:588–590.
9. Parada C, Han D, Grimaldi A, et al. Disruption of the ERK/MAPK pathway in neural crest cells as a potential cause of Pierre Robin sequence. *Development*. 2015 Nov 1;142(21):3734–3745. https://doi.org/10.1242/dev.125328. Epub 2015 Sep 22.

10. Graham JM Jr, Gomez M, Halberg A, et al. Management of deformational plagiocephaly: repositioning versus orthotic therapy. *J Pediatr.* 2005;146:258–262.
11. Kane AA, Lo L-J, Vannier MW, et al. Mandibular dysmorphology in unicoronal synostosis and plagiocephaly without synostosis. *Cleft Palate Craniofac J.* 1996;33:418–423.
12. Putnam GG, Postlethwaite KR, Chate RA, et al. Facial scoliosis—a diagnostic dilemma. *Int J Oral Maxillofac Surg.* 1993;22:324–327.
13. Slate RK, Posnick JC, Armstrong DC, et al. Cervical spine subluxation associated with congenital muscular scoliosis and craniofacial asymmetry. *Plast Reconstr Surg.* 1993;91:1187–1195.
14. Poole MD, Briggs M. The cranio-facio-cervical scoliosis complex. *Br J Plast Surg.* 1990;43:670–675.
15. Yu CC, Wong FH, Lo LJ, et al. Craniofacial deformity in patients with uncorrected congenital muscular torticollis: an assessment from three-dimensional computed tomography imaging. *Plast Reconstr Surg.* 2004;113:24–33.
16. Seo SJ, Yim SY, Lee IJ, et al. Is craniofacial asymmetry progressive in untreated congenital muscular torticollis? *Plast Reconstr Surg.* 2013;132:407–413.
17. Lee JK, Moon HJ, Park MS, et al. Change of craniofacial deformity after sternocleidomastoid muscle release in pediatric patients with congenital muscular torticollis. *J Bone Joint Surg Am.* 2012;94:e93.
18. Chate RA. Facial scoliosis from sternocleidomastoid torticollis: long-term postoperative evaluation. *Br J Oral Maxillofac Surg.* 2005;43:428–434.
19. Patwardhan S, Shyam AK, Sancheti P, et al. Adult presentation of congenital muscular torticollis: a series of 12 patients treated with a bipolar release of sternocleidomastoid and Z-lengthening. *J Bone Joint Surg Br.* 2011;93:828–832.
20. Lim KS, Shim JS, Lee YS. Is sternocleidomastoid muscle release effective in adults with neglected congenital muscular torticollis? *Clin Orthop Relat Res.* 2014;472:1271–1278.
21. Kawamoto HK, Kim SS, Jarrahy R, et al. Differential diagnosis of the idiopathic laterally deviated mandible. *Plast Reconstr Surg.* 2009;124:1599–1609.
22. Padwa BL, Bruneteau RJ, Mulliken JB. Association between plagiocephaly and hemifacial microsomia. *Am J Med Genet.* 1993;47:1202–1207.
23. Altug-Atac AT, Grayson BH, McCarthy JG. Comparison of skeletal and soft-tissue changes following unilateral mandibular distraction osteogenesis. *Plast Reconstr Surg.* 2008;121:1751–1759.
24. Dibbs RP, Ferry AM, Sarrami SM, Abu-Ghname A, Dempsey RF, Buchanan EP. Distraction osteogenesis: mandible and maxilla. *Facial Plast Surg.* 2021 Dec;37(6):751–758.
25. Ow AT, Cheung LK. Meta-analysis of mandibular distraction osteogenesis: clinical applications and functional outcomes. *Plast Reconstr Surg.* 2008;121:54e–69e.
26. Hammoudeh J, Bindingnavele VK, Davis B, et al. Neonatal and infant mandibular distraction as an alternative to tracheostomy in severe obstructive sleep apnea. *Cleft Palate Craniofac J.* 2012;49:32–38.
27. Hanis SB, Kau CH, Souccar NM, et al. Facial morphology of Finnish children with and without developmental hip dysplasia using 3D facial templates. *Orthod Craniofac Res.* 2010;13:229–237.
28. Joiner ER, Andras LM, Skaggs DL. Screening for hip dysplasia in congenital muscular torticollis: is physical exam enough? *J Child Orthop.* 2014;8:115–519.
29. Fenton, Gaetani S, MacIsaac Z, Ludwick E, Grunwaldt L. Description of mandibular improvements in a series of infants with congenital muscular torticollis and deformational plagiocephaly treated with physical therapy. *The Cleft Palate-Craniofacial Journal.* 2018;55(9):1282–1288.
30. Motch Perrine SM, Wu M, Holmes G, Bjork BC, Jabs EW, Richtsmeier JT. Phenotypes, developmental basis, and genetics of Pierre Robin complex. *J Dev Biol.* 2020 Dec 5;8(4):30.

CHAPTER 24

Congenital Muscular Torticollis

KEY POINTS

- Congenital muscular torticollis (CMT) must be distinguished from acquired torticollis and underlying structural torticollis (from cervical vertebral anomalies).
- It is most often caused by a congenital asymmetry in the length and/or strength of the sternocleidomastoid (SCM) muscles.
- CMT may be caused by early fetal head descent, an abnormal fetal position, venous occlusion, and/or trauma to the muscle during difficult deliveries.
- Other postnatal causes of torticollis include muscle spasms, trauma, infection, inflammation, neoplasm, dystonic syndromes, drug reactions, and ocular malalignment.
- Most cases of CMT are treated conservatively using active and passive neck-stretching exercises with repositioning.
- Untreated CMT can result in progressive facial asymmetry and positional plagiocephaly.

GENESIS

The term *torticollis* is derived from the Latin terms *torus*, meaning "twisted," and *collum*, meaning "neck," and it refers to the posture that results from the head being twisted and turned to one side.

Torticollis is most often caused by a congenital asymmetry in the length and/or strength of the SCM muscles on each side of the neck, often characterized by the shortening or stiffness of the SCM muscle resulting in ipsilateral lateral flexion of the head with contralateral rotation. CMT must be distinguished from acquired torticollis from structural torticollis resulting from cervical vertebral anomalies (Fig. 24.1).[1] Other postnatal causes of torticollis include muscle spasms, trauma (fracture, dislocation, spinal hematoma, atlantoaxial rotary subluxation), infection, inflammation, neoplasm, dystonic syndromes, drug reactions, and ocular malalignment.[2] Prenatally acquired congenital muscular torticollis (CMT) is the most common type of torticollis, and when it remains partly or completely untreated, it results in progressive facial asymmetry and positional plagiocephaly (see Chapter 25), which may be a presenting feature for the recognition of CMT. The incidence of CMT ranges from 3.9% to 16% of newborns.[3] CMT is thought to be the third congenital orthopedic anomaly requiring intervention/referral, more frequently following congenital hip dysplasia and calcaneovalgus feet. Cheng and colleagues reported a 1.3% incidence of torticollis among Chinese children and studied the outcomes in 1086 children with CMT who were classified into three groups according to severity (from most severe to least severe): 42.7% with a sternomastoid tumor, 30.6% with SCM tightness but no tumor, and 22.1% with postural torticollis who presented with CMT but no demonstrable tightness or tumor.[4]

CMT may occur as a consequence of early fetal head descent or an abnormal fetal position with the head tilted and turned, thereby resulting in muscle imbalance, with occasional associated deformations involving the back, hips, and feet (the intrauterine theory). More severe shortening and fibrosis of the muscle may be caused by venous occlusion from persistent lateral flexion and rotation of the neck (the vascular theory) and/or trauma to the muscle during difficult deliveries (the birth trauma theory).[5] Because there is no difference in the severity of CMT when infants delivered vaginally are compared with those delivered by cesarean section, CMT appears to arise before birth. Among 178 subjects with CMT, there was no significant difference in the rate of surgical release according to the method of childbirth, and for 132 patients less than 6 months of age there was also no significant difference in the rate of stretching exercises.[6] Many clinical studies have demonstrated that infants with CMT are more

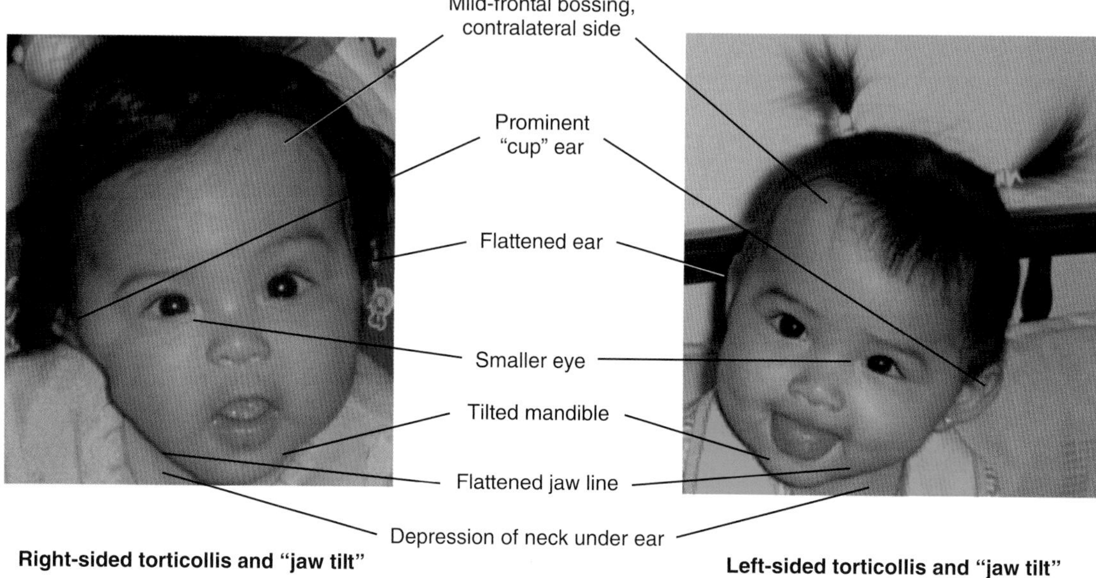

FIGURE 24.1 Examples of the subtle characteristic facial features secondary to right- and left-sided torticollis.

commonly first born and have an increased incidence of other deformations, such as metatarsus adductus, developmental dysplasia of the hip (DDH), and talipes equinovarus.[7]

Histology of affected muscles has demonstrated replacement of muscle by dense fibrous tissue, and when magnetic resonance imaging (MRI) was used to study the affected muscle, altered signal characteristics suggested that severe CMT might be caused by sequelae of an intrauterine or perinatal sternomastoid compartment syndrome.[7] In cadaver studies, flexion with lateral bending and rotation of the head and neck caused the ipsilateral sternomastoid muscle to kink on itself, resulting in ischemia and edema within the sternomastoid muscle compartment. When birth histories were compared with MRI findings, the side of birth presentation correlated with the side of the torticollis.[7] The intrauterine theory concerning the etiology of CMT (which does not exclude the compartment theory) is based on epidemiologic data and emphasizes the concept that CMT is one of a group of associated deformations arising from malposition of the fetus during the third trimester.[5] This theory relies on the association between unilateral hip dislocation, CMT, infantile idiopathic scoliosis, and plagiocephaly. (See Chapter 20 for a discussion of scoliosis and the molded baby syndrome.) It is suggested that the ipsilateral coexistence of a *t*urned head, *a*dduction contracture of the hip, and truncal *c*urvature (TAC syndrome) indicates a specific intrauterine asymmetric posture of the fetus (see Figs. 20.1 and 24.2).[8] Based on a study of 108 infants born with the clinical triad of TAC syndrome, this condition occurs in 5.8 per 1000 live births with a preponderance of females, first born children, winter births, low birth weights, children born to mothers with a small abdominal circumference, and first born children of mothers of advanced maternal age. The frequency of change of position in utero was significantly reduced from that in normal fetuses, and the side of fetal position correlated with the side of the TAC syndrome. When the left side of the fetus in vertex presentation was against the mother's spine, with the back on the left, the hip adduction contracture and torticollis were also on the left; the reverse was true when the back of the fetus was on the mother's right side.[8]

Interstitial fibrosis of the muscle is sometimes palpable as a fusiform fibrous mass or "tumor" that becomes evident within the first 3 weeks after birth and reaches maximum size by 1 month of age.[9] This mass is composed of myoblasts, fibroblasts, myofibroblasts, and mesenchyme-like cells that usually mature and differentiate, resulting in disappearance of the mass over the first 4–8 months of life with variable sequelae.[10] Such masses usually involve the lower two-thirds of the muscle, and their evolution can be followed by ultrasound,[11] which also allows for simultaneous ultrasound screening for hip dysplasia.[12] In a study, DDH occurred in 17% of 47 infants confirmed to have CMT by ultrasound, although only 8.5% of the infants required treatment with a Pavlik harness or surgery.[12] Subsequent studies have confirmed a 12% (12 of 97 consecutive patients with CMT, all requiring orthopedic intervention)[13] to 15% (20 of 133 patients reviewed retrospectively, of whom half required orthopedic intervention)[14] association between CMT and DDH. The difference and ratio of SCM thickness between the normal and abnormal side was significantly greater in DDH patients, and when the SCM ratio was greater than 2.08 and the SCM difference was greater than 6.1 mm, the efficiency of ultrasound for diagnosis of DDH was found to be the best. Because physical examination showed poor sensitivity, hip ultrasound was recommended in 4–6-month-old infants for the diagnosis of DDH associated with CMT when physical examination was positive, or in patients with a large SCM difference.[14]

If myoblasts in the mass differentiate in a normal way, the mass will disappear and conservative treatment with neck physical therapy will have a high likelihood of success; however if the myoblasts degenerate and the remaining fibroblasts produce excess collagen, the result may be a scar-like band that is visible by ultrasound and causes muscular contracture. Myoblasts can be mechanically stimulated to undergo hypertrophy and hyperplasia in vitro by intermittent stretching and relaxation, and the proper orientation of skeletal fibers during myogenesis is maintained by rhythmic contractions.[15–17] Among 28 SCM muscles from 23 subjects with CMT and 5 normal SCMs, gene expression studies showed that 269 genes were differentially expressed within five protein networks relating to fibrosis and collagen and elastin fibrillogenesis, and expression of 8 CMT signature genes showed good correlation with the preoperative severity of the CMT, as determined by MRI.[18] Thus, there is good physiologic justification for the early initiation of neck physical therapy to prevent muscle fibrosis.

A number of associated features suggest that CMT is related to late gestational constraint. The laterality of the birth head position usually matches the laterality of the torticollis. Among 202 infants assessed between 2002 and 2003 for deformational plagiocephaly at around 6 months of age in a craniofacial clinic, 68% were male, 74% were flat on the right occiput, 14% were from a multiple gestation, and 27% were premature.[19] Most parents (93%) did not notice any flattening at birth, but many (92%) noticed a preferential head turn after birth, which tended to improve in 95% of cases. Only 24% of cases had been diagnosed or treated for torticollis, and the mean difference between the cranial diagonal measurements was 12.5 mm (range 8–25 mm), with 97% of infants showing rotational asymmetry of 15 degrees or greater, and younger infants showing more asymmetry, which was correlated with the degree of cranial asymmetry.[19] Because this condition improves rapidly during early infancy, the findings are often subtle and only detected through an unusual head shape with a history of preferential head rotation. Without treatment, the shortened muscle tends to maintain the aberrant posture of the head and neck, with the head tilted toward the affected side and the chin rotated toward the opposite side. There can be associated mild frontal bossing and flattening of the ear on the contralateral side and a prominent ear, flattened jawline, and smaller appearing eye on the side of the torticollis (see Fig. 24.1). This results in deformational posterior plagiocephaly with a rhomboid head shape that can progress in severity if the infant's head remains turned toward one side. Early physical therapy, frequent "tummy time" when the infant is awake and under adult observation, and head repositioning onto the more prominent occiput can prevent many of these secondary positional craniofacial effects.[20–22]

Among the 52 infants with CMT who were 3 months old or less, 46 (88.5%) were successfully managed with only stretching exercises for 1–6 weeks, and 6 infants (11.5%) were managed with botulinum toxin injection, surgical release, or both in addition to stretching exercises. The difference in the SCM thickness between the affected and normal sides was significantly greater in the six children requiring more extensive management, and there was a strong correlation between the total duration of stretching exercise and the thickness of the SCM, with a thicker SCM requiring a longer duration of stretching exercises and other therapeutic interventions.[22] More limited cervical range of motion also corresponds to longer treatment duration, and infants with CMT who were diagnosed earlier and had an earlier intervention had a shorter duration of treatment.[23] Eventually uncorrected torticollis has the potential to result in permanent craniofacial asymmetry, but surgical correction of torticollis need not be attempted until after at least 6 months of neck physical therapy has failed to correct the torticollis, or the muscle has clearly become fibrotic. Among 50 infants less than 3 months of age with a palpable neck mass who were classified by ultrasound according to the severity of fibrosis in the SCM and underwent physical therapy, this treatment was successful in 49 patients (98%). Thus in young infants with CMT, ultrasound can document severity of fibrosis, and an early physiotherapy is effective, even in those with severe fibrosis.[24]

FEATURES

Characteristically the infant manifests lateral head and neck flexion toward one shoulder, with the ear lobule on that side uplifted and the jaw canted upward owing to compression against the shoulder or chest (see Figs. 22.3 and 23.2). The head is tilted toward the tighter, shorter SCM muscle, with the chin turned away. CMT can be difficult to diagnose at birth because of the normal shortness of the neck in a neonate, but it becomes more evident as the neck lengthens during the second 6 months of life. Jaw asymmetry may be the first indication that CMT is present, and there is usually a noticeable upward cant to the alveolar ridge on the side of the torticollis from pressure on the mandible from resting against the chest. Some mothers note that the infant has difficulty turning the head to nurse equally from both breasts or that one eye appears to be more closed than the other because of upward displacement of cheek soft tissues as the jaw rests against the chest on the side of the torticollis (see Figs. 23.2 and 24.3).[21] The ear is usually noticeably smaller on the side of the torticollis, having been relatively protected by the shoulder from the uterine compression experienced by the other ear. When the infant is held in suspension with the head down (see Fig. 24.2), the neck and trunk often flex toward the tight side, as mentioned previously in the discussion of idiopathic infantile scoliosis (see Chapter 20). SCM muscle imbalance is part of a spectrum of CMT that includes muscle length/strength asymmetry at one end and muscle shortening and fibrosis at the other end. With consistent supine positioning, the occiput on the side toward which the head is turned becomes progressively flattened, displacing the ear and forehead forward on the side opposite the torticollis (see Fig. 24.3). When infants previously slept in the prone position, the natural tendency to turn the head toward each side helped correct many cases of postural torticollis. Such a prone sleeping position can only be used if the baby has had sufficient tummy time and physical therapy to gain adequate head control in a prone position. Prone sleepers with an uncorrected, consistent head turn will develop deformational plagiocephaly with frontal flattening on the same side as the torticollis; thus prone positioning without physical therapy is unsafe and ineffective (Fig. 24.4). In the newborn infant with CMT, the position of comfort is usually with the head tilted toward the tight side and the chin turned away. A careful examination for hip dysplasia and truncal curvature is merited so that physical therapy can be directed toward correcting this asymmetric resting position.

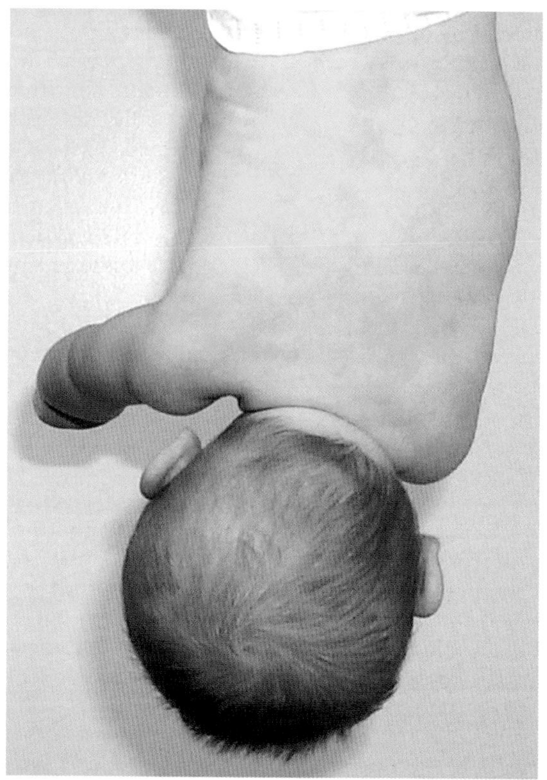

FIGURE 24.2 When a young infant is suspended upside down by holding the feet and ankles securely above an examination table, any generalized tightness of the neck or trunk musculature will cause the infant's neck and body to curve toward the tight side. This infant suspension test can be used to monitor the course of physical therapy, and it will often show differences between multiple gestation infants according to the degree of late gestational constraint each fetus experienced. Normally, an infant with no muscular asymmetry should hang straight down like a plumb bob. This infant has left congenital muscular torticollis with associated curvature of the trunk (idiopathic infantile scoliosis) and mild deformational posterior plagiocephaly. The coexistence of turned head, adduction contracture of the hip, and truncal curvature, TAC, syndrome suggests the specific intrauterine asymmetric posture of this infant as a fetus. He responded well to physical therapy with repositioning.

Dunn has shown that torticollis is commonly associated with plagiocephaly, facial curvature, ipsilateral

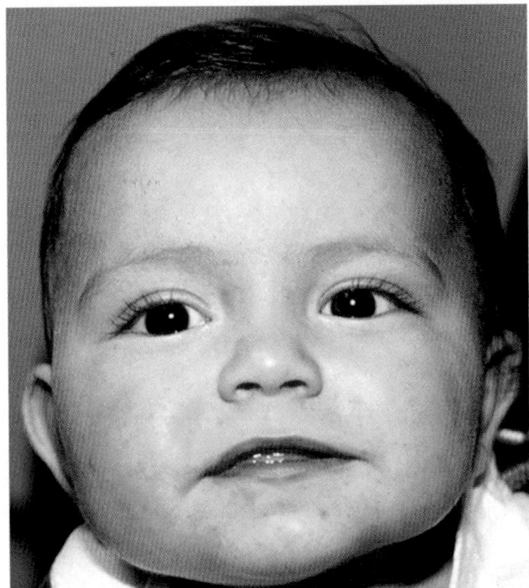

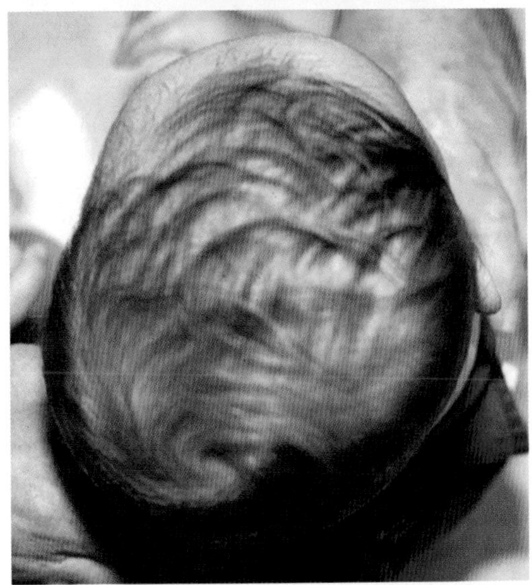

FIGURE 24.3 This infant has untreated left muscular torticollis at 9 months of age, with associated deformational posterior plagiocephaly owing to a persistent head turn to the right and associated left mandibular hypoplasia owing to a persistent head tilt to the left. He responded well to physical therapy and cranial orthotic therapy.

mandibular asymmetry, and positional foot deformities, and among infants with CMT, 56% were first born (vs. an expected 35% frequency) and 20% were in breech presentation (vs. an expected 5% frequency); additionally there was an association with oligohydramnios.[5] As mentioned, DDH that requires orthopedic management occurs in 8–10% of children with CMT.[12-14] These

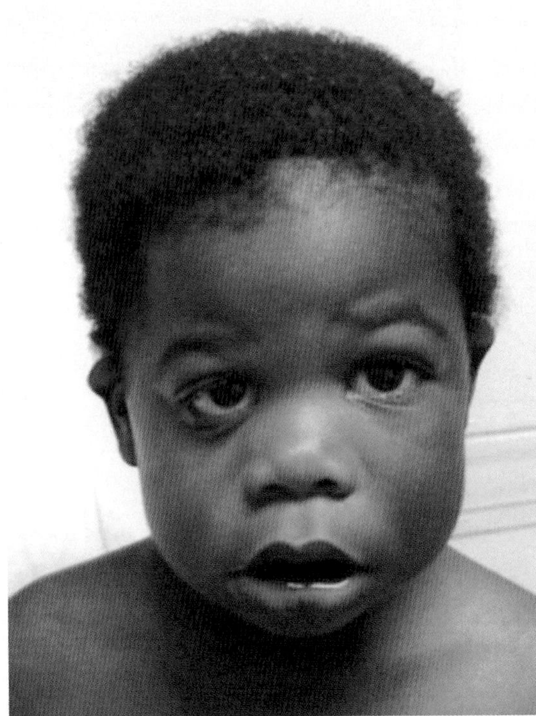

FIGURE 24.4 This 12-month-old boy has untreated right muscular torticollis with right facial flattening because he slept prone with his face turned to the left. He was considered too old to benefit from cranial orthotic therapy, but he responded well to physical therapy, with improved neck range of motion. His parents were instructed to position him for sleep in the prone position with his head turned to the right.

findings implicate late gestational fetal constraint as a primary cause of torticollis, which also occurs frequently with multiple gestation (usually affecting the fetus who is bottom-most in the uterus) and with uterine structural abnormalities.[20,21]

MANAGEMENT AND PROGNOSIS

In 2018, the American Academy of Pediatric Physical Therapy Association published their evidence-based clinical practice guidelines which were re-reviewed in 2023.[3,25] Most cases of CMT are treated conservatively using active and passive neck-stretching exercises with repositioning so as to encourage head turning toward the less preferred side (Fig. 24.5 and Video 24.1).[4,20,21] Because the SCM muscle has a vertical component as well as a horizontal (or rotational) component, the

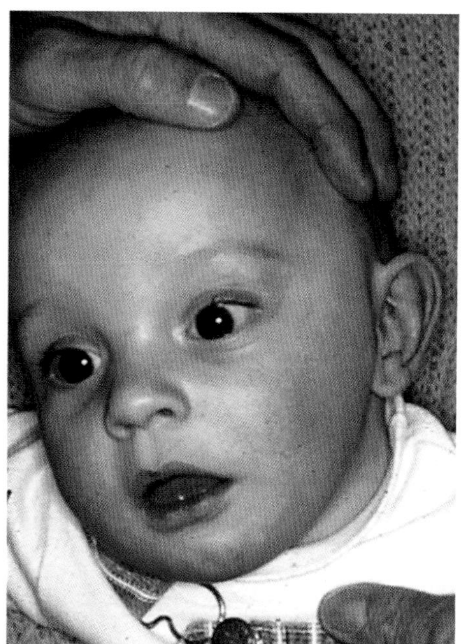
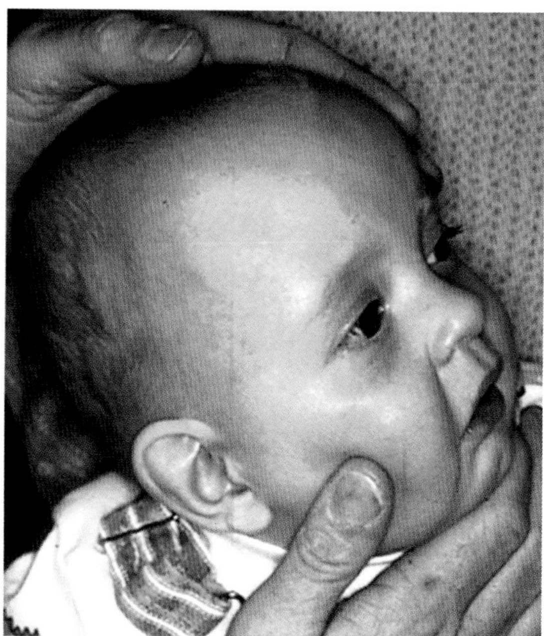

FIGURE 24.5 To restore sternocleidomastoid muscle symmetry and prevent progressive plagiocephaly, neck-stretching exercises should be done at least six times daily, preferably with each diaper change. For left torticollis, gently turn the infant's head toward the left side and try to get the chin slightly past the left shoulder. For the neck stretch, place your right hand on the infant's left shoulder, with your other hand on the left side of the infant's head. Gently stretch the neck, bringing the right ear to the right shoulder. Hold each stretch for at least 20–30 seconds. (Diagrams demonstrating stretching exercises for congenital muscular torticollis can be found on the Orthoseek web site at http://www.orthoseek.com/articles/congenmt.html.)

muscle must be actively stretched in both directions. In most instances it is best to stretch the muscle in both directions on both sides so as to achieve full and symmetric range of motion. For vertical stretching of a tight right CMT, position the infant in a supine position on a firm surface and push down on the right shoulder with one hand while slowly and evenly bringing the left ear toward the left shoulder; reverse the procedure for a tight left CMT. In right torticollis the head is turned to the left, so neck rotation needs to be encouraged by placing a forearm across the upper chest and rotating the chin toward the right shoulder; the procedure is reversed for left torticollis. Each stretch for each of the four directions should be held for 30–60 seconds, and it is best to make it a habit to do these exercises with each diaper change so that the exercises are performed six to eight times per day.[21] Sudden giving way or snapping of the sternomastoid muscle was observed with manual stretching in 8% of 452 patients with a sternomastoid tumor, particularly in infants younger than 1 month with left-sided involvement and associated hip dysplasia. This snapping was associated with clinical signs of bruising and an increased range of motion, suggesting possible release or rupture of the muscle, but it was not associated with any increased need for operative treatment; also 95% of patients with snapping had good or excellent results, which was not significantly different from those patients without snapping.[4]

Video 24.1 Home Exercises for Right Torticollis

Passive neck stretching can be facilitated by placing the infant on his or her stomach and directing the infant's gaze and head up and out on each side so that his or her chin and eyes follow an attractive object in a playful manner. A randomized controlled trial compared the outcomes of 61 infants with CMT younger than 3 months randomized into 1 of 3 groups: passive stretching, handling for active and active-assisted movements, or thermotherapy provided for 30 minutes three times a week, by physical therapists, until the head tilt was 5 degrees or less. After intervention, passive cervical rotation range of motion was significantly improved in the passive stretching group compared with the other two groups, but found no difference in SCM thickness on the affected side or the ratio of SCM thickness on the affected side compared with the nonaffected side.[3] Other forms of neck-stretching exercises consist of cradling the infant in one arm while gently rocking the infant and stretching the neck in each of the four directions. Some infants enjoy being held up by the ankles while gently bending the infant's head away from the shoulder while the head is against a firm surface or mattress. This exercise is especially helpful for vertical stretching, which is sometimes the most difficult direction to stretch. Encouraging the infant to feed toward his or her nonpreferred side is another technique of passive neck stretching. Early encouragement of tummy time facilitates head turning and neck stretching, thereby helping prevent excessive brachycephaly or plagiocephaly as well as facilitating prone motor skills.[21]

If initiated before 3 months of age, conservative treatment is very effective in restoring full range of motion, with minimal infant facial asymmetry in fully compliant families.[5,20,21] Severity of restricted lateral neck rotation and presence of a large palpable tumor are associated with a prolonged need for physical therapy and sometimes with the need for surgical correction. Among infants with CMT, infants with a palpable mass are usually diagnosed earlier at 1–2 months versus 4–5 months for those without a mass. The mean duration of treatment to obtain full range of motion is 4–5 months in infants with no palpable mass, with a longer mean duration of treatment for those presenting with a mass (6–7 months). Among infants with a significant head tilt at 4–5 months, the mean duration of treatment is longer than those without such head tilts. Thus the more severe the neck restriction, the longer the required duration of conservative treatment to achieve full range of motion. In most large series, conservative treatment was successful in 95% of cases, with surgical correction undertaken only in resistant cases.[26,27] One study of kinesiology taping in 28 infants with CMT demonstrated that taping had an immediate effect on muscular imbalance in infants with CMT.[28] Botulinum toxin A injection into the tight SCM muscle has also been used for children with CMT that is resistant to physical therapy as an alternative therapeutic intervention to avoid surgery.[22]

When the severity of CMT was measured by the degree of limitation in passive neck rotation, the need for surgery was associated with patients who completed at least 6 months of manual stretching and still manifested deficits in passive rotation or lateral bending greater than 15 degrees.[4] Infants with a sternomastoid tumor were found to present earlier (within the first 3 months), and this group was associated with the highest incidences of breech presentation (19.5%), difficult labor (56%), and congenital hip dysplasia (6.8%).[29] Severity of limitation in neck rotation was significantly correlated with the presence of a sternomastoid tumor, larger tumor size, hip dysplasia, degree of head tilt, and craniofacial asymmetry. Infants with less than 10 degrees of limitation in passive neck rotation were treated at home with an active stimulation and positioning program, whereas infants with more than 10 degrees of limitation in passive neck rotation were treated with manual stretching three times per week by experienced physiotherapists.[27] Those infants who failed to respond or improve after 6 months of physical therapy with manual stretching were treated surgically with a unipolar open release and partial excision of the clavicular and sternal heads of the sternomastoid muscle. Malpresentation was noted in 14.6% of 1086 cases (13% breech, 1.6% other than breech or vertex presentation), hip dysplasia was found in 4.1%, foot deformations were noted in 6.5%, and craniofacial asymmetry was noted in 90.1%. There was a slight increase in left-sided torticollis (53%) and a 3:2 incidence of males to females.[27] For the sternomastoid tumor group, the tumor occurred in the lower third in 35%, in the middle third in 40.4%, in the upper third in 11.9%, and over the entire muscle in 12.6%. The tumors ranged in size from 1 to 4 cm, and more than 70% of tumors were larger than 2 cm. Tumors were usually detected at 2 weeks, increased in size for the next 2 weeks, and then disappeared by 5–8 months. Cases requiring surgery were associated with late age at presentation, sternomastoid tumor, and more severe limitation in rotation. None of the patients with positional torticollis required surgery, and successful early treatment of CMT prevented secondary plagiocephaly.[26-30] Evidence-based physical therapy guidelines have been created for screening, examination, intervention, and follow-up.[31,32]

Indications for surgery include incorrect head posture persisting after 12 months (Figs. 24.6–24.8) and/or muscle fibrosis persisting after 6 months of age (with reduced activity of the involved muscle demonstrated by electromyography). Ultrasound has been useful in following sternomastoid pseudotumors, and both ultrasound and MRI have been used to confirm fibrous replacement and predict the need for surgical correction (see Fig. 24.8).[22,23,33,34] In most cases ultrasonography is the most cost-effective method for imaging and following sternomastoid changes. Surgical management consists of tenotomy, unipolar or bipolar releases, or complete resection of the fibrotic muscle through incisions near the muscular insertions on the sternum and clavicle or near the origin on the mastoid bone, where the incision can be hidden in the hairline behind the ear.[35-37] Recent techniques emphasize

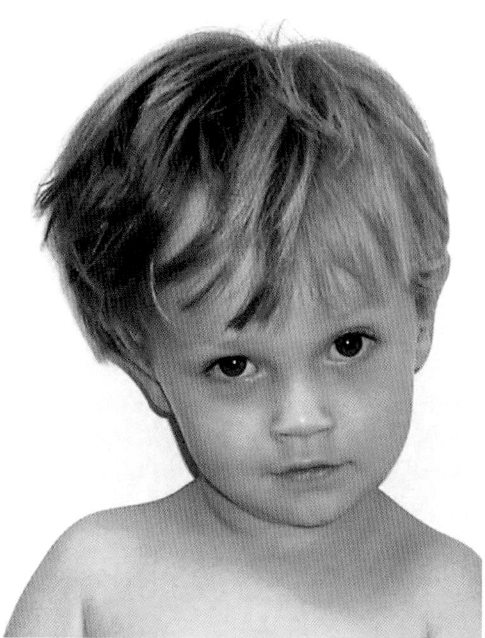
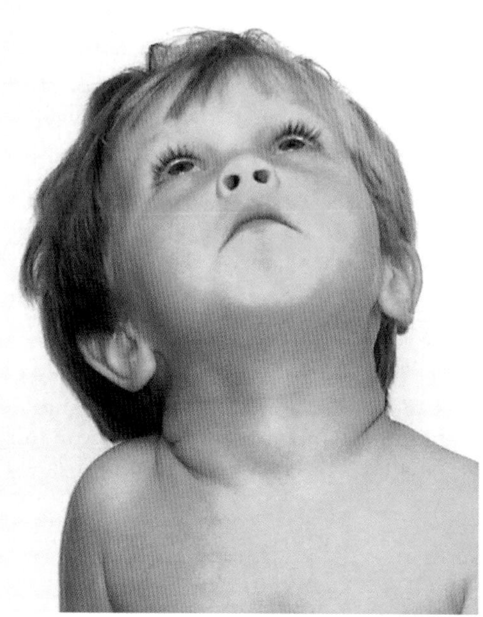

FIGURE 24.6 This boy has partially treated right muscular torticollis at age 18 months. Because the deficits in lateral bending and neck rotation were less than 15 degrees, continued physical therapy was recommended with use of a tubular orthotic.

smaller incisions and minimally invasive techniques via endoscopy, with early institution of postoperative physical therapy and splinting of the neck with a soft cervical collar. Because early physical therapy is effective in the vast majority of CMT cases, there is seldom any indication for surgery before the end of the first year.

Other treatment modalities have been suggested, such as the use of botulinum toxin injection. In one study, 27 children with CMT aged 6–18 months received 30 botulinum toxin type A injections into their SCM or upper trapezius muscle, or both. Twenty of 27 children (74%) had improved cervical rotation or head tilt after the injections, and 2 of 27 (7%) experienced transient adverse events, specifically mild dysphagia and neck weakness.[38] It is clear that physical therapy and persistent repositioning before 5 months can prevent deformational posterior plagiocephaly and that cranial orthotic therapy is effective for most refractory cases after 6 months of age.[20,21]

Failure to treat muscular torticollis can result in persistent mandibular asymmetry, facial scoliosis, deformational plagiocephaly, and rotatory cervical spine subluxation on the side contralateral to the muscular torticollis (see Figs. 24.7 and 24.8).[39–41] Among 80 patients who required surgical release, cephalometry showed improvement in the craniofacial deformity after surgical release, and results were better when surgery was performed before the patient reached 5 years of age. More postsurgical change occurs during the first postoperative year than during the second year.[42] Long-term follow-up for 14 years confirmed resolution of the facial asymmetry.[43] SCM release also has been beneficial in adults with neglected CMT, leading to cosmetic and functional improvements and pain relief originating from the muscle imbalance brought about by the long-standing deformity.[44,45] Use of frontal cephalometric analysis or three-dimensional computed tomography to assess craniofacial deformity in patients with late surgical correction of torticollis suggests that surgical treatment before 5–6 years of age is most effective in preventing severe facial asymmetry, but neck range of motion can be improved by surgical correction at any age.[40,41] With untreated torticollis after 3 years of age, there can be torsional rotation of the lower face toward the affected side, which starts with the mandible, progresses to involve the maxilla, and, ultimately, involves the orbits (see Figs. 24.7 and 24.8).

Among 7609 Dutch infants screened in 1995 for positional plagiocephaly before 6 months of age, the incidence of positional preference was 8.2% (n = 623), with flattening of the occiput noted in 10%, versus a 0.3% incidence of deformational plagiocephaly in Dunn's 1974 study of British infants.[5,46] These findings

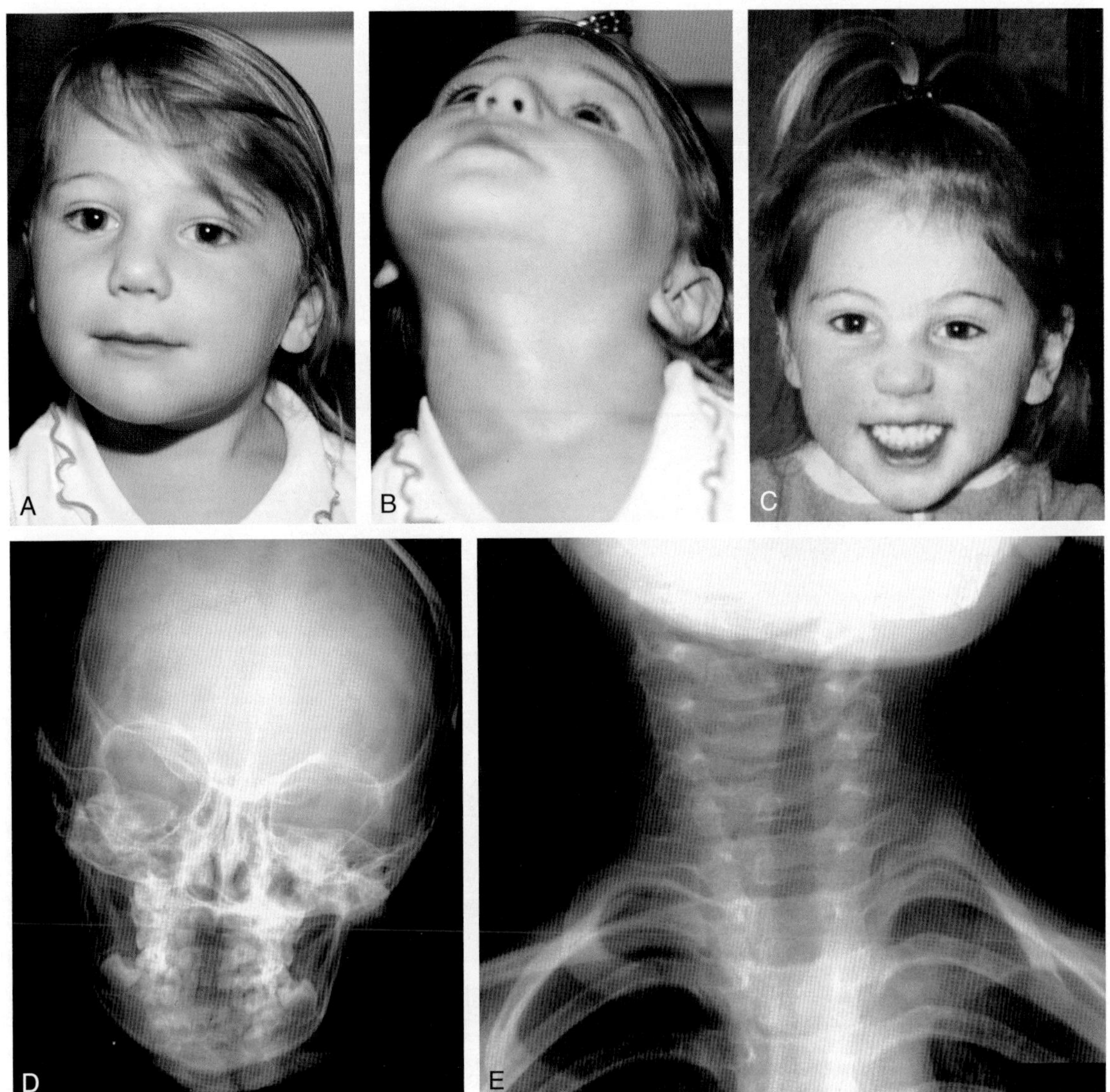

FIGURE 24.7 **A** and **B,** This 3-year-old girl (*top left* and *center*) has untreated severe torticollis-plagiocephaly deformation sequence with a fibrotic left sternocleidomastoid (SCM) muscle and secondary deformation of her left lower face and clavicle. Her cranial diagonal difference was 2 cm with obvious right frontal prominence and a right epicanthal fold. She underwent surgical resection of her fibrotic SCM muscle through a hairline incision near her left mastoid bone. **C,** After surgery she received physical therapy and wore a cervical collar, resulting in much improved neck range of motion. **D** and **E,** Radiographs before surgery (*bottom left* and *right*) demonstrate obvious facial asymmetry with distortion of the left clavicular insertion point for the SCM muscle.

support the opinion that the prevalence of both positional preference and deformational plagiocephaly has risen dramatically in the past decade, with males more frequently affected than females and a head turn to the right more common than to the left.[19,20] This is a direct result of the effort to position children in the supine position to prevent sudden infant death syndrome because prone and side sleeping positions have a protective effect for positional preference, which was noted in only 2.4% of prone-sleeping Swedish infants versus 19% of supine-sleeping infants.[47] Among the 623 infants with positional preference and deformational

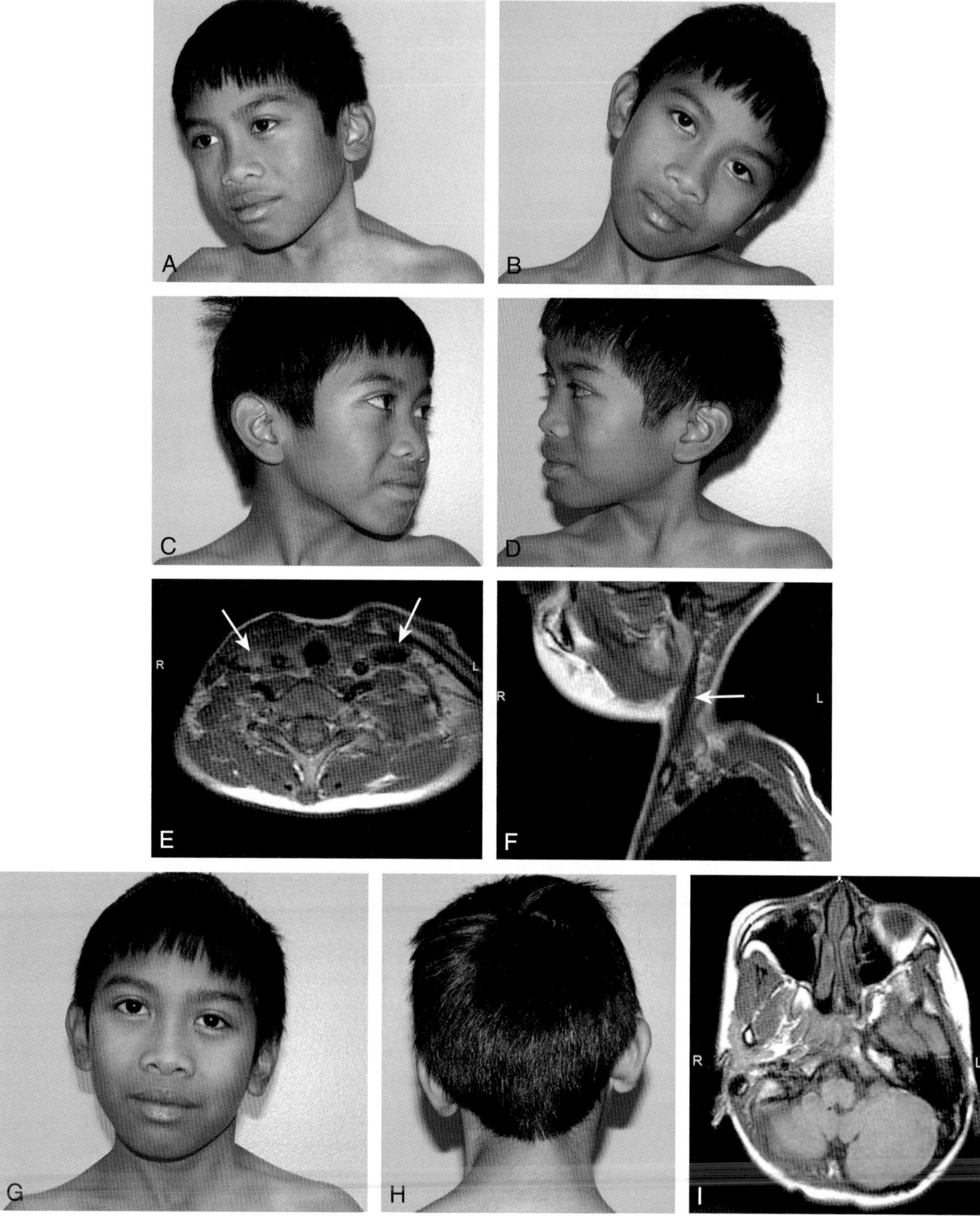

FIGURE 24.8 A–D, This 11-year-old boy has untreated left congenital muscular torticollis with restricted lateral flexion to the right and limited neck rotation to the right. His left clavicle is higher and more prominent than the right clavicle, and the left sternocleidomastoid muscle is cordlike with a palpable mass (*arrows* in **E** and **F**) that is less intense than the contralateral muscle on T1-weighted magnetic resonance imaging, suggesting fibrosis. **G** and **H,** A bipolar release of his left sternocleidomastoid muscle was required to correct his abnormal head posture. **I,** There is obvious persistent deformational plagiocephaly on cranial imaging. (Courtesy Robert M. Bernstein, Cedar Sinai Medical Center, Los Angeles.)

plagiocephaly, these features persisted in nearly one-third when re-examined at 2–3 years of age, resulting in a large number of referrals for additional diagnostic evaluations and/or treatment at much increased medical expense.[46] These findings call for a primary pediatric preventive approach that includes early physical therapy for CMT and encouragement of tummy time when the infant is awake and under direct observation.[20,21] These findings and suggestions should in no way negate the recommendations of the "Back to Sleep" campaign.

DIFFERENTIAL DIAGNOSIS

CMT is the most common type of congenital torticollis, but another cause of torticollis has been attributed to congenital fusion of cervical vertebrae (e.g., as in oculoauriculovertebral sequence or Klippel-Feil sequence), which is estimated to occur in 0.7% of newborns. Klippel-Feil sequence (Fig. 24.9) is found in 5–6% of patients with torticollis and may be associated with scoliosis, elevated scapula (Sprengel deformity), renal anomalies, heart defects, and deafness, whereas CMT usually occurs in otherwise normal children. Acquired torticollis occurs infrequently in children when head and neck infection results in inflammation of cervical joints, with subsequent edema that causes C1–C2 subluxation with atlantoaxial rotatory displacement (Griscelli syndrome), resulting in contralateral stretching and spasm of the sternomastoid muscle (Fig. 24.10).[48] This is usually treated with muscle relaxants and cervical traction in a soft collar for patients who have been symptomatic for less than 1 month, but occasionally posterior spinal fusion is necessary for refractory cases.[46]

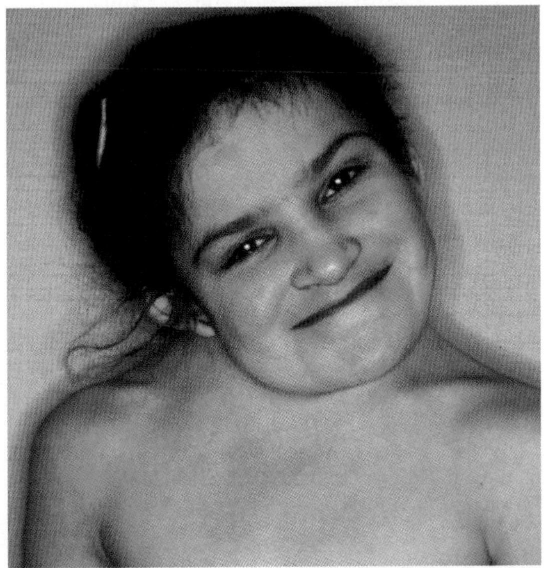

FIGURE 24.9 This girl has Klippel-Feil sequence with an osseous torticollis caused by unbalanced cervical vertebral anomalies. Note her obviously short, wide neck.

Benign paroxysmal torticollis is a self-limited disorder characterized by sudden, stereotypic head-tilting episodes that are often associated with pallor, agitation, nystagmus, and emesis; these episodes are sometimes mistaken for seizures. Episodes can be provoked by changes in position from upright to supine, which suggests a vestibular pathogenesis. Some patients have abnormal audiograms and go on to develop benign paroxysmal vertigo, cerebellar dysfunction, or migraine.[49] Familial spasmodic torticollis may not be distinct from dystonia musculorum because the latter sometimes presents first as torticollis, especially in the dominantly inherited variety. Ocular torticollis develops in some children with vertical ocular dystopia resulting from unilateral coronal synostosis, causing the child to tilt his or her head in a compensatory fashion; however, this does not occur in young infants. Posterior fossa tumors are a rare cause of acquired torticollis and are usually associated with neurologic signs and symptoms in older patients. Among six children with torticollis and central nervous system lesions, all had abnormal neurologic examinations on initial presentation, and the youngest patient was 17 months old.[49] Given the diversity of causes for torticollis,[50] careful etiologic consideration is necessary before initiating treatment, and if uncertainty regarding the diagnosis persists, imaging can be quite useful.[51]

Among 82 infants with CMT who were compared with 40 healthy infants, the CMT group achieved early motor milestones significantly later than the control group until the age of 10 months, but the risk of delay was more strongly associated with little or no time prone when awake than with CMT.[52] When this same group of infants with CMT was followed up at 3.5–5 years, neither CMT nor spending little time as an infant in the prone position when awake had any long-term effects on motor development, and children who had CMT as infants were not at higher risk for a delayed motor development at preschool age.[53] A retrospective study compared the difference in neurodevelopmental outcomes between 1719 children with CMT who did and did not receive physical therapy.[54] Although the authors state infants who did not receive physical therapy intervention had a higher risk of neurodevelopmental delay,

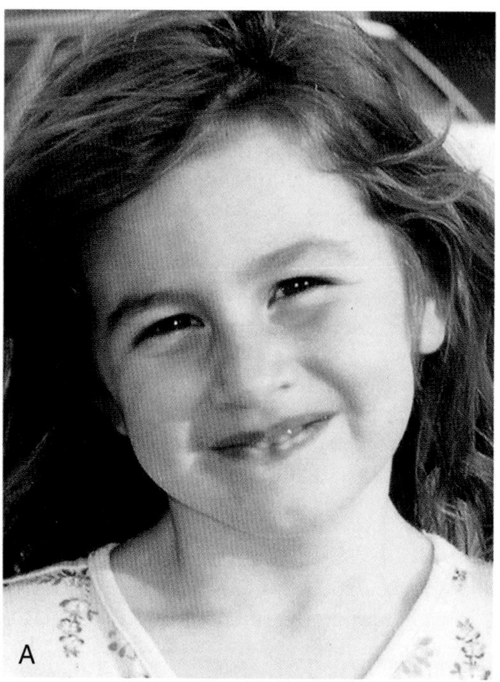

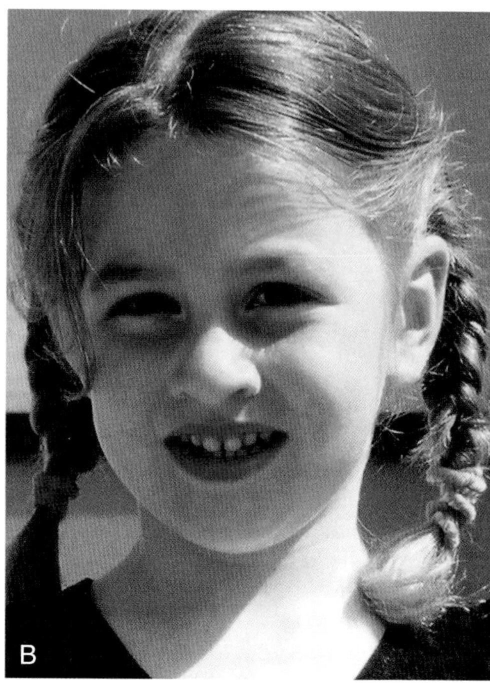

FIGURE 24.10 A, This 6-year-old girl developed right torticollis in association with a cervical abscess (Griscelli syndrome). **B,** The torticollis resolved after treatment of the abscess.

the meta-analysis was not statistically significant and had an adjusted Risk Ratio of 0.97 (95% CI, 0.93–0.99; $P = .10$). CMT should not be considered to be inherited but may recur if constraint-related circumstances remain a factor, and a family history of CMT is found in less than 5% of cases.[29]

References

1. Sargent B, Kaplan SL, Coulter C, Baker C. Congenital muscular torticollis: bridging the gap between research and clinical practice. *Pediatrics*. 2019;144(2):e20190582.
2. Gross PW, Chipman DE, Doyle SM. The tilts, twists, and turns of torticollis. *Curr Opin Pediatr*. 2023;35(1):118–123.
3. Castilla A, Gonzalez M, Kysh L, Sargent B. Informing the physical therapy management of congenital muscular torticollis clinical practice guideline: a systematic review. *Pediatr Phys Ther*. 2023;35(2):190–200.
4. Cheng JCY, Wong MWN, Tang SP, et al. Clinical determinants of outcome of manual stretching in the treatment of congenital muscular torticollis: a prospective study of 821 cases. *J Bone Joint Surg Am*. 2001;83:679–687.
5. Dunn PM. Congenital sternomastoid torticollis: an intrauterine postural deformity. *Arch Dis Child*. 1974;49:824–825.
6. Lee SJ, Han JD, Lee HB, et al. Comparison of clinical severity of congenital muscular torticollis based on the method of childbirth. *Ann Rehabil Med*. 2011;35:641–647.
7. Davids JR, Wenger DR, Mubarak SJ. Congenital muscular torticollis: sequellae of intrauterine or perinatal compartment syndrome. *J Pediatr Orthop*. 1993;13:141–147.
8. Hamanishi C, Tanaka S. Turned head-adducted hip-truncal curvature syndrome. *Arch Dis Child*. 1994;70:515–519.
9. Bredenkamp JK, Hoover LA, Berke GS, et al. Congenital muscular torticollis: a spectrum of disease. *Arch Otolaryngol Head Neck Surg*. 1990;116:212–216.
10. Tang S, Liu Z, Quan X, et al. Sternocleidomastoid pseudotumor of infants and congenital muscular torticollis: fine-structure research. *J Pediatr Orthop*. 1998;18:214–218.
11. Cheng JCY, Metrewell C, Chen TMK, et al. Correlation of ultrasonographic imaging of congenital muscular torticollis with clinical assessment in infants. *Ultrasound Med Biol*. 2000;26:1237–1241.
12. Tien YC, Su JY, Lin GT, et al. Ultrasonographic study of the coexistence of muscular torticollis and dysplasia of the hip. *J Pediatr Orthop*. 2001;21:343–347.
13. Joiner ER, Andras LM, Skaggs DL. Screening for hip dysplasia in congenital muscular torticollis: is physical exam enough? *J Child Orthop*. 2014;8:115–119.
14. Park HK, Kang EY, Lee SH, et al. The utility of ultrasonography for the diagnosis of developmental dysplasia of hip joint in congenital muscular torticollis. *Ann Rehabil Med*. 2013;37:26–32.

15. Carlson BM. The regeneration of skeletal muscle: a review. *Am J Anat.* 1973;173:119–150.
16. Vandenburgh HH, Hatfaludy S, Karlisch P, et al. Skeletal muscle growth is stimulated by intermittent stretch-relaxation in tissue culture. *Am J Physiol.* 1989;256:C674–C682.
17. Levine S, Salzman A. Neogenesis of skeletal muscle in the postinflammatory rat peritoneum. *Exp Mol Pathol.* 1994;60:60–69.
18. Yim SY, Yoon D, Park MC. Integrative analysis of congenital muscular torticollis: from gene expression to clinical significance. *BMC Med Genom.* 2013; 6(Suppl 2):S10.
19. Rogers GF, Oh AK, Mulliken JB. The role of congenital muscular torticollis in the development of deformational plagiocephaly. *Plast Reconstr Surg.* 2009;123:643–652.
20. Graham JM Jr, Gomez M, Halberg A, et al. Management of deformational plagiocephaly: repositioning versus orthotic therapy. *J Pediatr.* 2005;146:258–262.
21. Kuo AA, Tritasavit S, Graham JM Jr. Congenital muscular torticollis and positional plagiocephaly. *Pediatr Rev.* 2014;35:79–87.
22. Han JD, Kim SH, Lee SJ, et al. The thickness of the sternocleidomastoid muscle as a prognostic factor for congenital muscular torticollis. *Ann Rehabil Med.* 2011;35:361–368.
23. Lee JY, Koh SE, Lee IS, et al. The cervical range of motion as a factor affecting outcome in patients with congenital muscular torticollis. *Ann Rehabil Med.* 2013;37:183–190.
24. Lee YT, Yoon K, Kim YB, et al. Clinical features and outcome of physiotherapy in early presenting congenital muscular torticollis with severe fibrosis on ultrasonography: a prospective study. *J Pediatr Surg.* 2011;46:1526–1531.
25. Kaplan SL, Coulter C, Sargent B. Physical therapy management of congenital muscular torticollis: a 2018 evidence-based clinical practice guideline from the APTA Academy of Pediatric Physical Therapy. *Pediatr Phys Ther.* 2018;30(4):240–290.
26. Cheng JC, Au AWY. Infantile torticollis: a review of 624 cases. *J Pediatr Orthop.* 1994;14:802–808.
27. Cheng JCY, Tang SP, Chen TMN, et al. The clinical presentation and outcome of congenital muscular torticollis in infants: a study of 1086 cases. *J Pediatr Surg.* 2000;35:1091–1096.
28. Öhman AM. The immediate effect of kinesiology taping on muscular imbalance for infants with congenital muscular torticollis. *PM R.* 2012;4:504–508.
29. Cheng JCY, Tang SP, Chen TMK. Sternocleidomastoid pseudotumor and congenital muscular torticollis in infants: a prospective study of 510 cases. *J Pediatr.* 1999;134:712–716.
30. Celayir AC. Congenital muscular torticollis: early and intensive treatment is critical: a prospective study. *Pediatr Int.* 2000;42:504–507.
31. Kaplan SL, Coulter C, Fetters L. Physical therapy management of congenital muscular torticollis: an evidence-based clinical practice guideline: from the Section on Pediatrics of the American Physical Therapy Association. *Pediatr Phys Ther.* 2013;25:348–394.
32. Christensen C, Landsettle A, Antoszewski S, et al. Conservative management of congenital muscular torticollis: an evidence-based algorithm and preliminary treatment parameter recommendations. *Phys Occup Ther Pediatr.* 2013;33:453–466.
33. Park HJ, Kim SS, Lee SY, et al. Assessment of follow-up sonography and clinical improvement among infants with congenital muscular torticollis. *AJNR Am J Neuroradiol.* 2013;34:890–894.
34. Hwang JH, Lee HB, Kim JH, et al. Magnetic resonance imaging as a determinant for surgical release of congenital muscular torticollis: correlation with the histopathologic findings. *Ann Rehabil Med.* 2012;36:320–327.
35. Lee IJ, Lim SY, Song HS, et al. Complete tight fibrous band release and resection in congenital muscular torticollis. *J Plast Reconstr Aesthet Surg.* 2010;63:947–953.
36. Lee TG, Rah DK, Kim YO. Endoscopic-assisted surgical correction for congenital muscular torticollis. *J Craniofac Surg.* 2012;23:1832–1834.
37. Ekici NY, Kizilay A, Akarcay M, et al. Congenital muscular torticollis in older children: treatment with Z-plasty technique. *J Craniofac Surg.* 2014;25(5):1867–1869.
38. Oleszek JL, Chang N, Apkon SD, et al. Botulinum toxin type a in the treatment of children with congenital muscular torticollis. *Am J Phys Med Rehabil.* 2005;84(10):813–816.
39. Putnam GG, Postlethwaite KR, Chate RA, et al. Facial scoliosis: a diagnostic dilemma. *Int J Oral Maxillofac Surg.* 1993;22:324–327.
40. Slate RK, Posnick JC, Armstrong DC, et al. Cervical spine subluxation associated with congenital muscular scoliosis and craniofacial asymmetry. *Plast Reconstr Surg.* 1993;91:1187–1195.
41. Seo SJ, Yim SY, Lee IJ, et al. Is craniofacial asymmetry progressive in untreated congenital muscular torticollis? *Plast Reconstr Surg.* 2013;132:407–413.
42. Lee JK, Moon HJ, Park MS, et al. Change of craniofacial deformity after sternocleidomastoid muscle release in pediatric patients with congenital muscular torticollis. *J Bone Joint Surg Am.* 2012;94:e93.
43. Chate RA. Facial scoliosis from sternocleidomastoid torticollis: long-term postoperative evaluation. *Br J Oral Maxillofac Surg.* 2005;43:428–434.
44. Patwardhan S, Shyam AK, Sancheti P, et al. Adult presentation of congenital muscular torticollis: a series of 12 patients treated with a bipolar release of sternocleidomastoid and Z-lengthening. *J Bone Joint Surg Br.* 2011;93:828–832.
45. Lim KS, Shim JS, Lee YS. Is sternocleidomastoid muscle release effective in adults with neglected congenital muscular torticollis? *Clin Orthop Relat Res.* 2014;472:1271–1278.
46. Boere-Boonekamp MMM, van der Linden-Kuiper LT. Positional preference: prevalence in infants and follow-up after two years. *Pediatrics.* 2001;107:339–343.

47. Palmen K. Prevention of congenital dislocation of the hip: the Swedish experience of neonatal treatment of hip joint instability. *Acta Orthop Scand.* 1984;55(Suppl 208):58-67.
48. Kautz SM, Skaggs DL. Getting an angle on spinal deformities, Contemp. *Peds.* 1998;15:111-128.
49. Cataltepe SU, Barron TF. Benign paroxysmal torticollis presenting as "seizures" in infancy. *Clin Pediatr.* 1993;32:564-565.
50. Ballock RT, Song KM. The prevalence of non-muscular causes of torticollis in children. *J Pediatr Orthop.* 1996;16:500-504.
51. Haque S, Bilal Shafi BB, Kaleem M. Imaging of torticollis in children. *Radiographics.* 2012;32:557-571.
52. Ohman A, Nilsso S, Lagerkvist AL, et al. Are infants with torticollis at risk of a delay in early motor milestones compared with a control group of healthy infants? *Dev Med Child Neurol.* 2009;51:545-550.
53. Ohman A, Beckung E. Children who had congenital torticollis as infants are not at higher risk for a delay in motor development at preschool age. *PMR.* 2013;5:850-855.
54. Kim OH, Lee SW, Ha EK, et al. Neurodevelopmental outcomes and comorbidities of children with congenital muscular torticollis: evaluation using the national health screening program for infants and children database. *Clin Exp Pediatr.* 2022;65(6):312-319.

CHAPTER 25

Plagiocephaly

KEY POINTS

- Deformational plagiocephaly is most common in first born, large babies, breech presentation, and multiple-gestation infants.
- Factors associated with asymmetric head deformation include a constraining intrauterine environment, clavicular fracture, cervical/vertebral abnormalities, and incomplete bone mineralization.
- *Nonsynostotic*, *deformational*, and *positional* have been used to distinguish plagiocephaly without synostosis.
- Deformational plagiocephaly is not associated with premature closure of cranial sutures.
- The diagnosis can be challenging when both deformational plagiocephaly and craniosynostosis occur together.
- Placing infants on their backs for sleep, as recommended to reduce the incidence of sudden infant death syndrome (SIDS), has led to an increase in deformational posterior plagiocephaly.
- Much debate still exists over the costs, timing, and benefits of cranial orthotic therapy.
- Outcomes are typically good if the diagnosis is determined early.

GENESIS

Plagiocephaly, which literally translates from the Greek term *plagio kephale* as "oblique head," is a term used to describe asymmetry of the head shape when viewed from the top (Fig. 25.1). It is a nonspecific term that has been used to describe head asymmetry caused by either premature sutural fusion or postnatal head deformation resulting from a positional preference; hence, modifying terms such as *nonsynostotic*, *deformational*, and *positional* have been used to distinguish plagiocephaly without synostosis. The term *deformational plagiocephaly* should suffice to distinguish this type of defect and its proper management. The side of the plagiocephaly is usually indicated by the bone that has been most flattened by the deforming forces (see Figs. 24.3 and 25.2). During late fetal life, the head may become compressed unevenly in utero, but most deformational plagiocephaly occurs after delivery because of an asymmetric resting position. Such inequality of positional gravitational forces may result in asymmetric molding of the head and face.

Torticollis (see Chapter 24) is a condition in which the sternocleidomastoid muscle is shorter and/or tighter on one side of the neck, causing the head to tilt toward the affected muscle and the head to turn away. This is the most frequent cause of deformational plagiocephaly, which results from progressive occipital flattening when an infant with torticollis is placed in the supine position and consistently turns his or her head to one side (see Fig. 25.1). Because the torticollis is usually on the side opposite the head turn, the forehead on the side of the torticollis may appear normal or recessed (see Fig. 24.1), whereas the forehead and ear on the same side as the flattened occiput may become displaced anteriorly. If the infant sleeps on the stomach with a preferential head turn, then the frontal region on the side of the torticollis becomes flattened as the infant turns its head away from the short or tight sternomastoid muscle (see Fig. 24.4). According to Dunn,[1] torticollis occurred with plagiocephaly once in every 300 live births before 1974, when many infants were positioned for sleep on their stomachs. Since the "Back to Sleep" campaign was initiated in 1992 for the prevention of sudden infant death syndrome, the frequency of deformational posterior plagiocephaly has increased dramatically, rising from approximately 5% to upward of 46% at age 7 months. This increase in deformational posterior plagiocephaly was first noted in 1996.[2–5]

Deformational plagiocephaly is not associated with premature closure of cranial sutures, but because craniosynostosis is sometimes associated with fetal head constraint, this diagnosis can be challenging when both deformational plagiocephaly and craniosynostosis occur together.[5,6] Torticollis-plagiocephaly

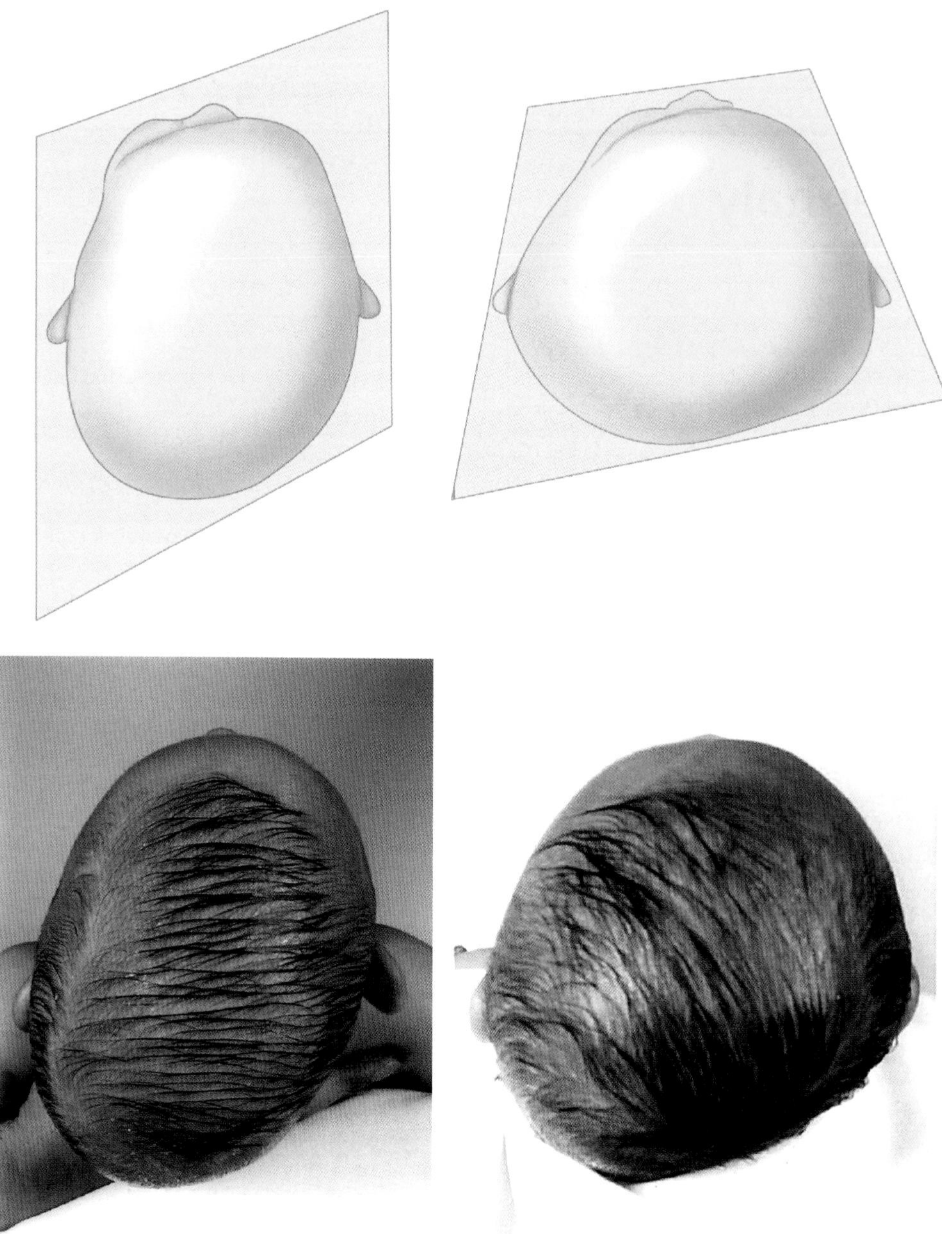

FIGURE 25.1 These infants demonstrate typical head shapes for deformational posterior plagiocephaly when viewed from the top (parallelogram on the *left* and trapezoidal on the *right*). The more brachycephalic head shape on the right suggests very little tummy time. (Adapted from Pomatto JK, Calcaterra J, Kelly KM, et al. A study of family head shape: environment alters cranial shape. *Clin Pediatr.* 2006;45:55–64.)

deformation sequence results from deformation of the infant's skull, as normal postnatal brain growth combines with an asymmetric resting position to result in progressive cranial asymmetry (see Fig. 25.2).[7] Artificial deformation of infant heads has been practiced for years in many cultures throughout the world (Fig. 25.3); hence it is critical to remain cognizant of the lasting impact of postnatal mechanical forces

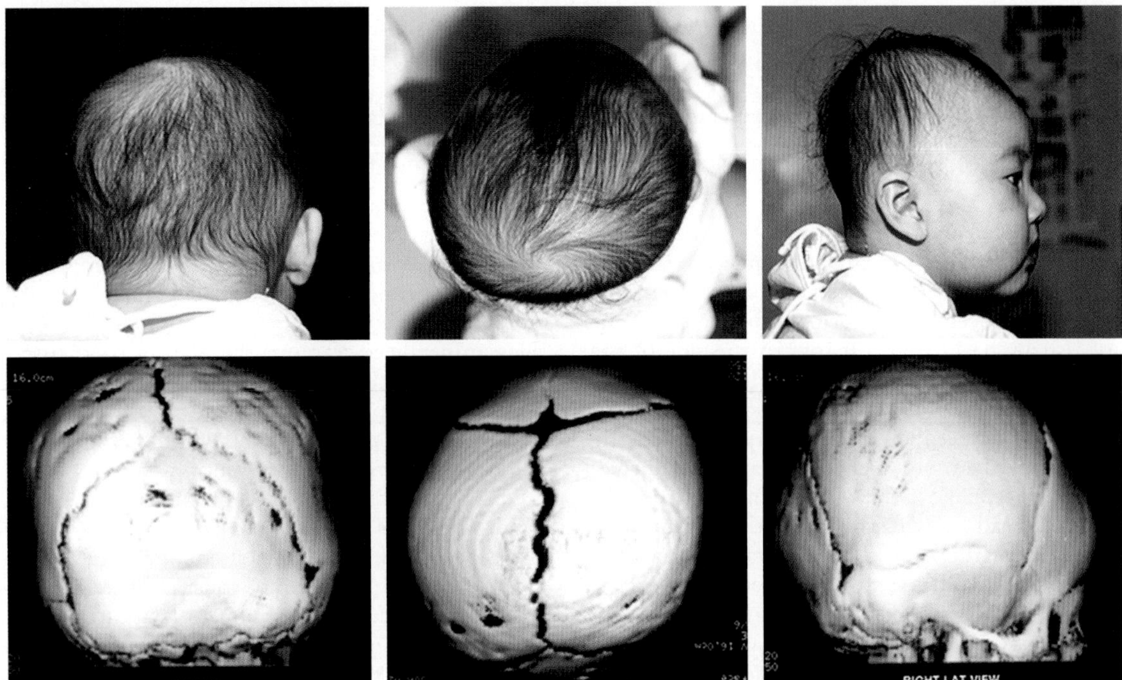

FIGURE 25.2 This 6-month-old infant was referred for an altered head shape resulting from deformational plagiocephaly with left torticollis and associated brachycephaly with right occipital flattening. A cranial 3D computed tomography scan had been done previously and clearly showed patent sutures. She responded well to neck physical therapy and cranial orthotic therapy.

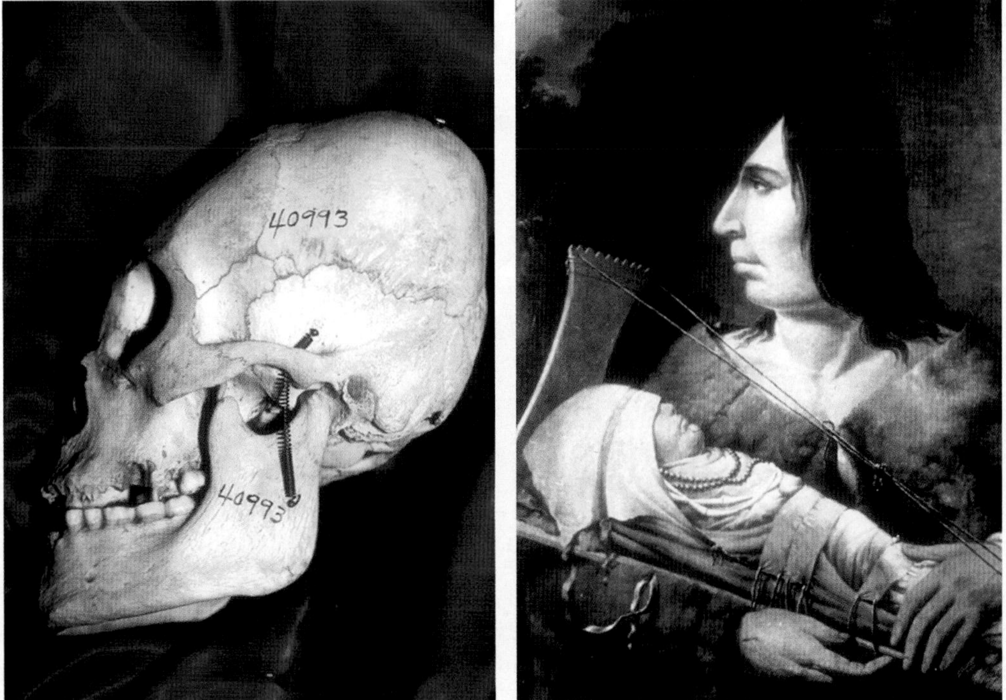

FIGURE 25.3 Northwest Pacific Coast Indians from the Kwakiutl tribe applied boards to the occiput and frontal regions from birth until 8–10 months. Once the boards were removed, the altered calvarial shape would persist for life.

on the shape of an infant's head. Examination of CT scans from 39 deformed pre-Columbian skulls and 19 control skulls revealed that volumes of the cranial cavities were not affected by intentional cranial deformation but that the shapes of the orbits and of the maxillary sinuses were modified in circumferential deformations.[8]

Deformational plagiocephaly is most likely to occur in first born babies, large babies, breech presentation, and among multiple-gestation infants. In the torticollis-plagiocephaly deformation sequence, the infant usually has a head tilt toward the side of the shortened sternomastoid muscle.[7] The growth and development of the brain are usually normal; however, infants with macrocephaly, prematurity, or underlying hypotonia may be more likely to experience deformational plagiocephaly. Other factors associated with asymmetric head deformation include a constraining intrauterine environment, clavicular fracture, cervical/vertebral abnormalities, and incomplete bone mineralization. The importance of intrauterine positioning in determining both the occurrence and the severity of deformational plagiocephaly was demonstrated in a study of 140 twins treated with orthotic devices for positional plagiocephaly.[9,10] Among both discordant and concordant twin pairs, the bottom-most twin was more likely to be affected. The more severely affected twin was more likely to manifest neck involvement and to be in a vertex position, with no observed differences in sleep position (nearly all were supine sleepers) or gender (Fig. 25.4).[10] There was a high incidence of fraternal twins born to older mothers who were pregnant for the first time and using assisted reproductive technologies. Because twins may be born prematurely with a less mineralized cranium, they may be more susceptible to deformational plagiocephaly. Thus intrauterine constraint is a predominant factor in the causation of deformational plagiocephaly, emphasizing the need for early diagnosis and intervention.

To reduce the incidence of sudden infant death syndrome, it is necessary to place infants on their backs for sleep, but infants should be placed on their stomachs for "tummy time" when they are awake and under direct adult supervision to facilitate the development of prone motor skills and to encourage the infant to turn his or her head from side to side. The

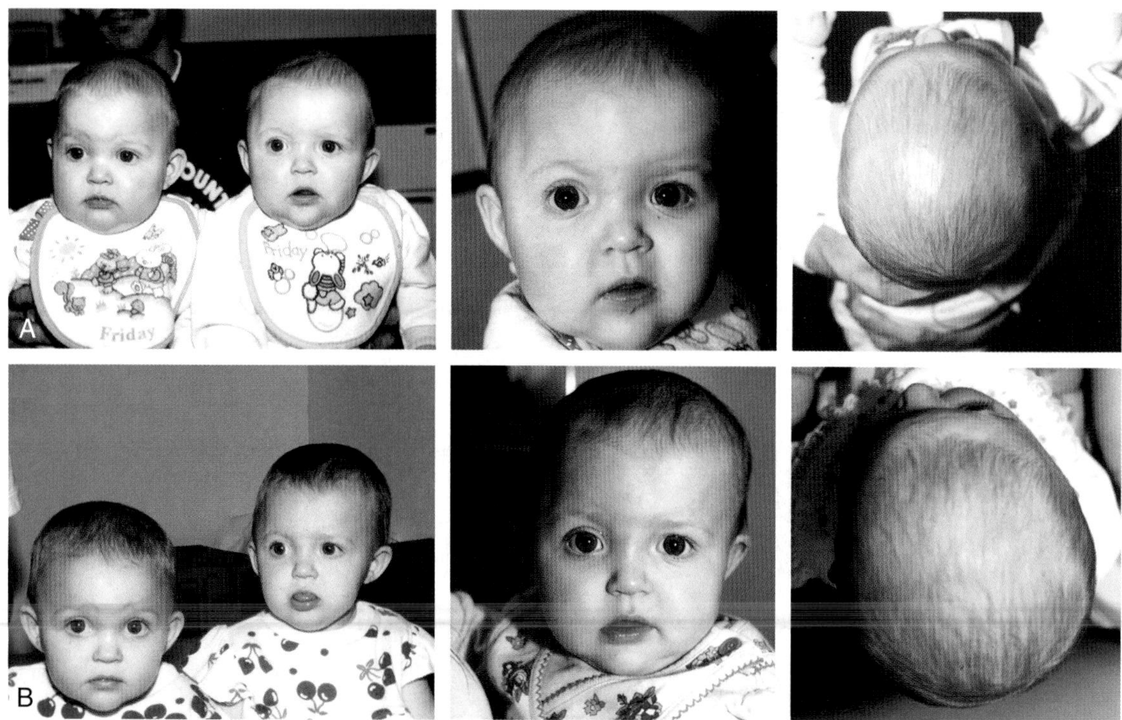

FIGURE 25.4 These monozygotic twins show how residual torticollis-plagiocephaly deformation sequence caused the twin on the right to manifest persistent craniofacial asymmetry between ages 6 (**A**) and 10 months (**B**). The affected twin was beneath her co-twin in vertex presentation with her back to the mother's left side and her head turned to the right.

development of excessive occipital flattening, with or without plagiocephaly, may indicate that parents are not providing their infants with adequate "tummy time." It is important to distinguish between deformational plagiocephaly and plagiocephaly resulting from craniosynostosis, because therapy and management are very different for these conditions.[6] If any uncertainty is present, referral to a craniofacial specialist for evaluation is the next step in determining diagnosis. In both positional deformity and craniosynostosis, outcomes are typically good if the diagnosis is determined early.

FEATURES

Deformational plagiocephaly is caused by oblique molding of the head, and it is often accentuated by the tendency to remain exclusively supine and rest persistently on one side of the occiput. The classical parallelogram-shaped head is a combination of asymmetric flattening of the occiput with ipsilateral prominence of the forehead plus contralateral prominence of the contralateral occiput and recession of the forehead on that same side (see Figs. 24.3, 25.1, and 25.2). This distorts the cranium in such a way that when the cranium is observed from above, it appears to be shaped like a parallelogram instead of having a normal, symmetric oval shape. In cases in which the infant has received little or no tummy time, the head can become excessively flattened and almost trapezoidal in shape (see Fig. 25.1). The eye on the same side as the torticollis may appear to be less open because the soft tissues of the cheek are displaced superiorly on that side due to compression of the chin against the chest and persistent head tilting (see Fig. 25.4). The external ear may protrude and appear displaced anteriorly on the same side as the prominent forehead and flattened occiput, whereas the other ear appears pushed back with an uplifted lobule because of pressure from the shoulder on the side with the recessed forehead, prominent occiput, and tight sternocleidomastoid muscle (Fig. 25.5).[7] This asymmetry of the ears is frequently noted by parents, and the ear on the side with the flattened occiput may also be significantly larger (as a manifestation of prolonged intrauterine compression) when compared with the ear on the side of the torticollis.[11] The position of the ears in deformational plagiocephaly differs from that seen in synostotic plagiocephaly caused by unilateral lambdoid craniosynostosis, in which the ear may be vertically displaced downward on the synostotic side as a result of restricted sutural expansion (Fig. 25.6). Asymmetry of the cranium is most obvious when the head is viewed from above, and such asymmetry may be missed when the infant is examined face to face. The jaw is often pushed up on the side of the torticollis and may appear asymmetric and/or tilted.[7]

Other subtle characteristics may not be particularly noticeable on first glance but have been used to distinguish deformational plagiocephaly from synostotic plagiocephaly. These include asymmetry of the orbits with upward displacement on the side of the synostotic coronal suture, where the forehead and brow appear flattened. The presence of a unilateral epicanthal fold, usually ipsilateral to the side of occipital flattening, should prompt further investigation for torticollis-plagiocephaly deformation sequence.[12] The degree of craniofacial distortion may be sufficient to cause abnormal placement of the eyes,[13] but usually one eye only appears to be less open because of vertical displacement of the soft tissues of the cheek on the side of the torticollis. Infants with torticollis often manifest other deformations such as dislocation of the hips, infantile scoliosis, and positional foot deformations caused by late gestational constraint, especially if the baby was in breech presentation. The position of comfort is with the head tilted toward one side and the chin turned toward the opposite side. Persistence of neck rotation because of lack of physical therapy and/or fibrosis of the muscle on that side will perpetuate the secondary effects of congenital muscular torticollis, but usually this can be prevented with early and persistent physical therapy.[5,14–17] A flattened cranium will foster a tendency for the infant to lie on this flattened area in his or her position of comfort, thus maintaining the deformity.

Among 181 normal infants whose head shapes were observed at regular intervals from birth through 2 years of age in 2002, the prevalence of plagiocephaly or brachycephaly peaked at 4 months at 20% (associated with male gender, firstborn, limited neck rotation, and inability to vary the infant's head position when putting the infant down to sleep), and then fell to 9% by 8 months of age and to 3.3% by 2 years of age.[18] A follow-up study of 129 of these children at 3 and 4 years of age revealed that 61% of abnormal head shapes had reverted to normal, whereas 4% remained severely abnormal at follow-up, with 13% categorized as having poor improvement with continuing parental concern over their child's head shape.[18] Among a cohort of 440 infants examined in 2010, the incidence of plagiocephaly at 7–12 weeks of age was 47%, with 63% affected on the right side and 78% manifesting mild deformation.[19] The prevalence of cranial deformation was assessed in adolescents born after the "Back to Sleep"

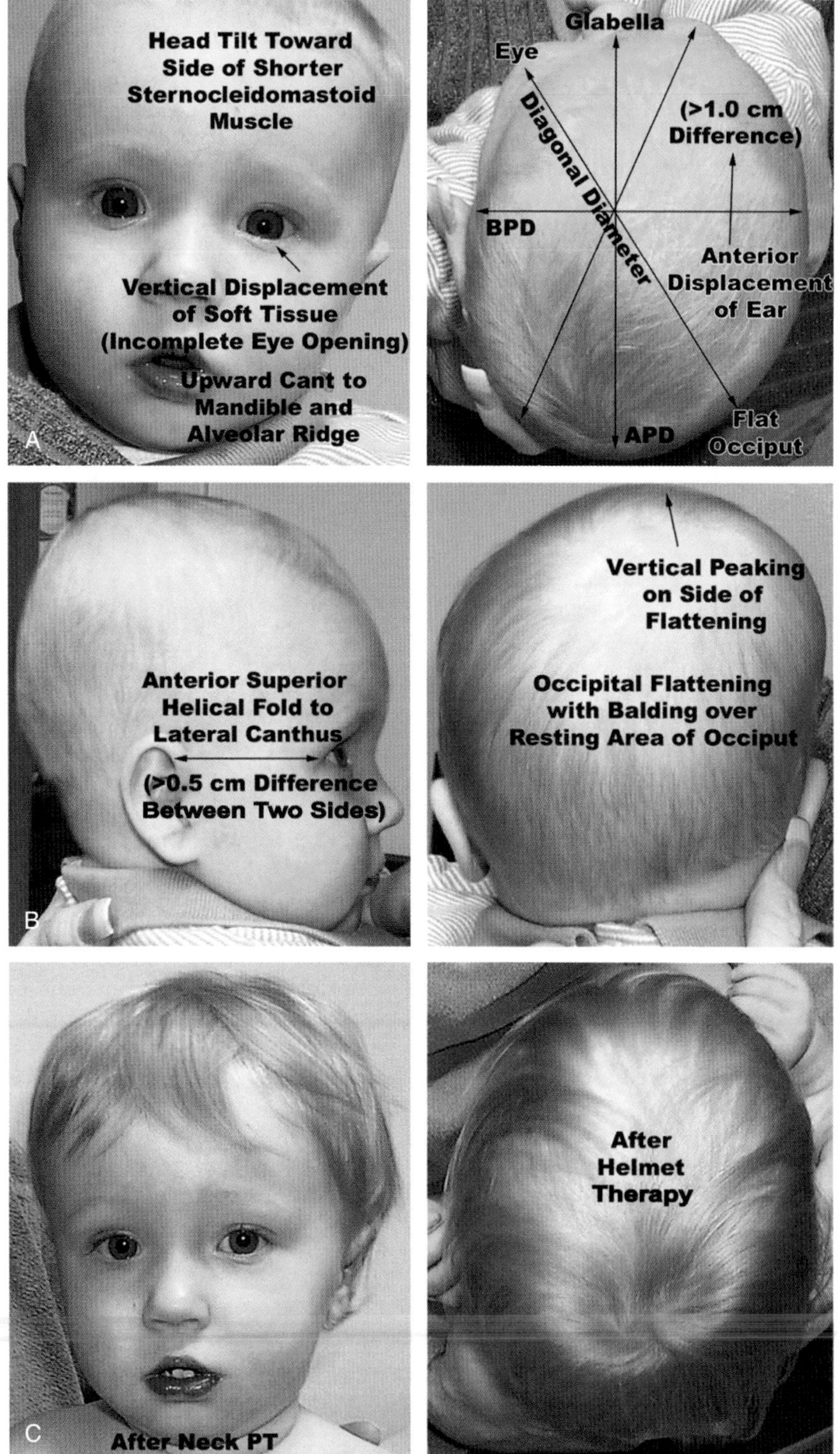

FIGURE 25.5 This infant shows all the key features of torticollis-plagiocephaly deformation sequence, with cranial measurements depicted on the top of his skull, before initiation of helmet therapy at age 5 months (**A** and **B**) and after completion of therapy at 14 months (**C**). *APD*, Anteroposterior diameter; *BPD*, biparietal diameter.

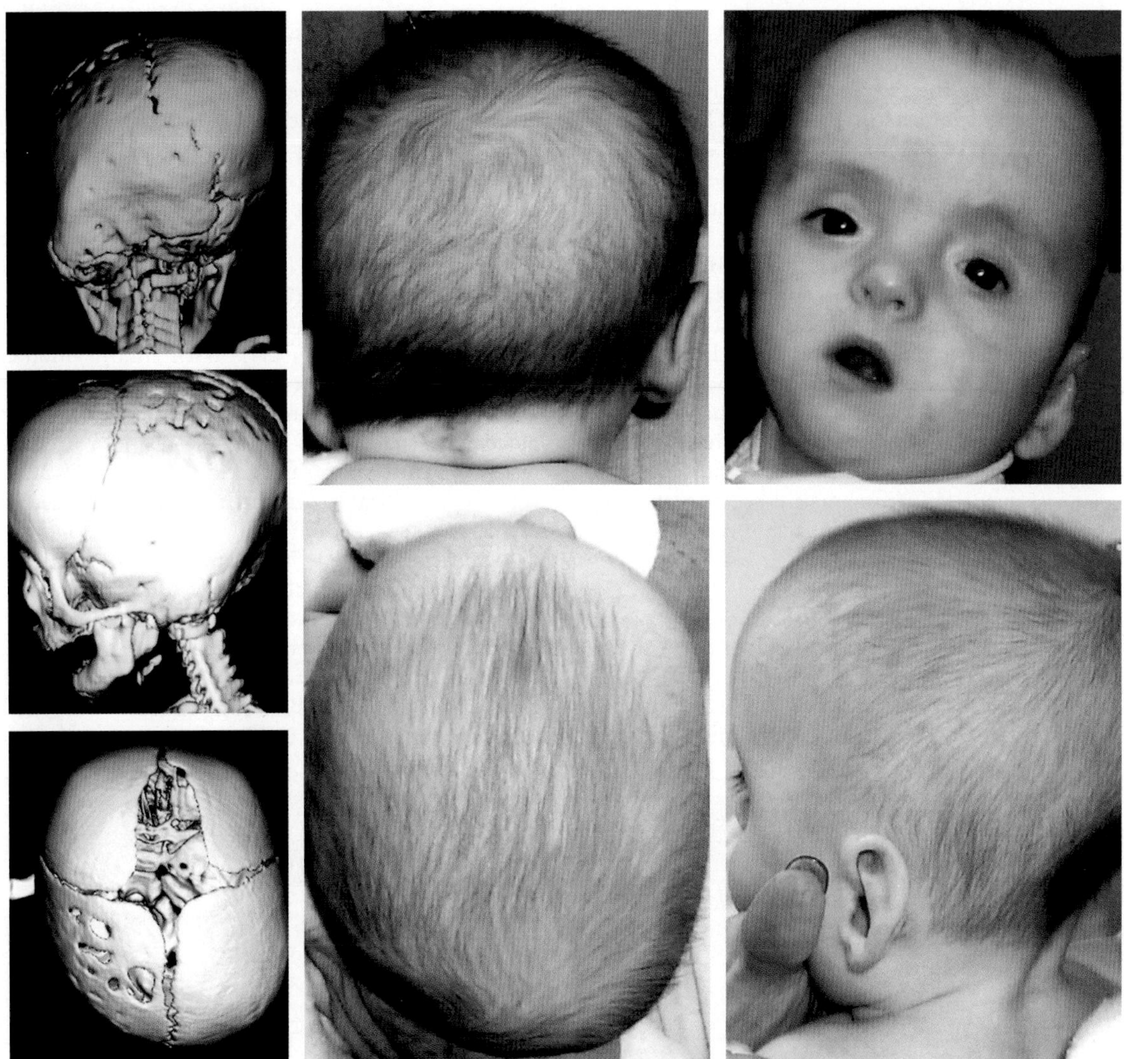

FIGURE 25.6 This infant was born with left lambdoid craniosynostosis and severe right congenital muscular torticollis, resulting in a very distorted cranium that required surgical correction with postoperative cranial orthotic therapy as well as prolonged physical therapy.

program was initiated. Among 1045 high school students (37% male, 63% female) ranging from 12 to 17 years old (average age of 15.7 years), the prevalence of plagiocephaly was 1.1% and the prevalence of brachycephaly was 1.0%, with an overall prevalence of a deformational cranial abnormality of 2.0%.[19] This study was limited by having fewer males, who are affected more often and more severely, and by assuming helmets were not available before 1998, when they were clearly in use after 1980 (but not regulated by the US Food and Drug Administration). Note that Hutchinson found a 4% prevalence of severe brachycephaly or plagiocephaly at 3 and 4 years of age in their longitudinal study that included an excess of males (71% male and 29% female).[20] Among the adolescents with plagiocephaly or brachycephaly, 38.1% were noted to have abnormal facial characteristics.[21]

The impression that most positional head deformations without associated torticollis tend to resolve was confirmed in a small randomized controlled trial of 5–6-month-old Dutch infants with positional plagiocephaly, who were confirmed by physical therapists to have no torticollis and no severe deformation. Of 30 infants who underwent helmet therapy, the mean age of discontinuance of helmet therapy was 10 months. Discontinued use of the helmet before 12 months was either because they were satisfied with the results or because of side effects in 10 cases.[22] There was an unusually high rate of complications (96% skin irritation, 73% poor fit, 33% pain). At 24 months, 79 infants were reevaluated by six physical therapists who were blinded as to their treatment, and among infants who had no treatment, 75% had residual deformity at 24 months; this outcome was not significantly different from that of the infants treated with helmets.[22] Among 410 German infants who were treated with helmets in an experienced craniofacial clinic for moderate-to-severe cranial deformation, 10.5% developed pressure sores, 6.3% had localized erythema, 5.9% had a poorly fitting helmet, 1.2% had skin infections, and 1.2% experienced treatment failure, primarily because of treatment complications resulting in lack of compliance.[23]

MANAGEMENT, PROGNOSIS, AND COUNSEL

In most instances of deformational plagiocephaly with torticollis, observation of the infant's resting position and head shape during the first few weeks after birth will determine whether there is a preferential resting position. During this period of observation, a few procedures are worth considering. The surface upon which the infant's head rests should be firm but soft, and some cultures even use soft rings or pillows for all neonates to prevent infant head deformation (Fig. 25.7). The infant's crib should be placed so that visually attractive objects are on the side opposite to the preferential head turn. The head and neck should be moderately overstretched away from the side of the torticollis (see Chapter 24). With mild-to-moderate torticollis, early neck-stretching exercises usually correct the problem and prevent the postnatal plagiocephaly that would otherwise result from always resting on the same area of the cranium (see Fig. 23.2).[7] A prospective trial to evaluate the impact of stretching exercises versus bedding pillows on positional head deformities included 50 infants aged 5 months or younger with positional head deformity (20 with plagiocephaly, 10 with brachycephaly, and 20 with both). Randomization was performed for treatment with the bedding pillow alone (25) or with stretching exercises (25) for 6 weeks. Bedding pillows and stretching exercises both resulted in improvements in positional

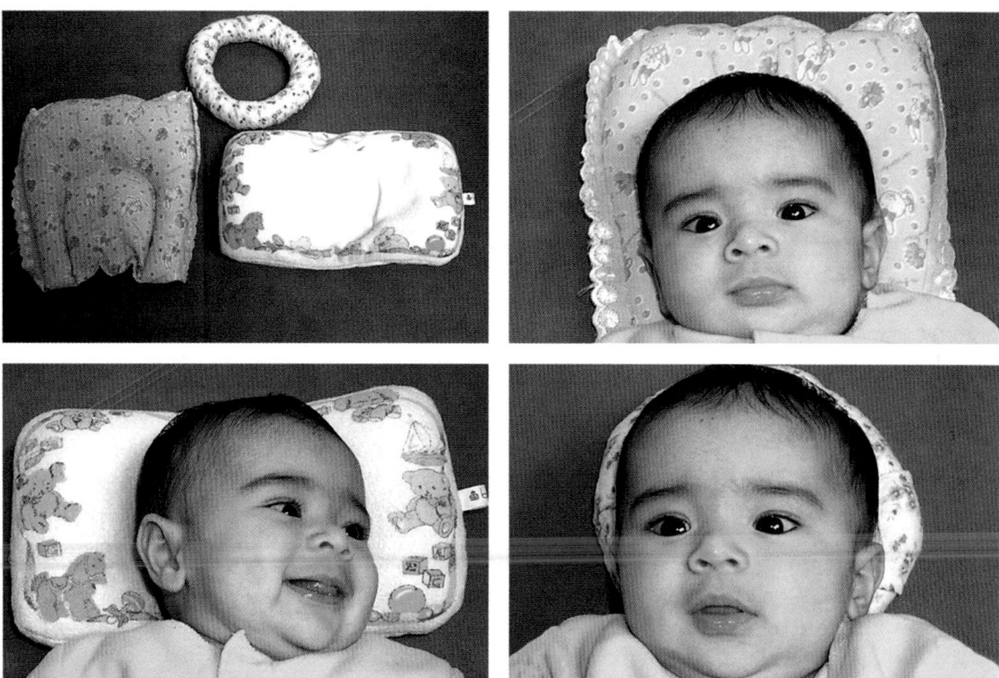

FIGURE 25.7 This infant required only neck physical therapy and head repositioning to maintain her normal head shape. She is shown here with a variety of infant-positioning pillows from various parts of Asia.

cranial deformation, and for infants with combined plagiocephaly and brachycephaly, improvement in cranial asymmetry was slightly greater when using bedding pillows versus stretching.[24]

Inability to nurse equally from both breasts may be the first clue to the presence of torticollis, and early referral to a physical therapist for treatment of torticollis is often the most effective treatment strategy. With torticollis, the head usually tilts to one side and the chin rotates toward the opposite side. For example, with a left torticollis, the head tilts to the left and the face turns to the right. To correct this posture, the neck should be stretched to the right so that the right ear is gradually brought toward the right shoulder and held there for 30–60 seconds. Then the chin should be rotated toward the left so that the chin is brought past the left shoulder and held there for 30–60 seconds (see Fig. 24.5). For the neck stretch to be effective, as the parent faces the baby, the parent's left hand should be on the left side of the baby's face and the right hand should be on the baby's shoulder, where it bears down firmly on the shoulder during the neck stretching. To correct torticollis appropriately, both exercises must be done together and regularly (at least six to eight times each day). After a meal or diaper change is usually a good time to perform these exercises as a regular part of the daily routine. In cases of severe torticollis, it is particularly important to initiate early referral to a physical therapist for neck-stretching exercises to prevent muscle fibrosis and deformational plagiocephaly. Initial management always involves attempts to actively reposition the infant so as to correct any cranial asymmetry in addition to neck physical therapy to correct any associated torticollis (Fig. 25.8).[7]

Parents should be encouraged to correct deformational posterior plagiocephaly by placing the baby in the crib in a three-quarter turn, so that the infant rests on the occiput opposite to the flattened occiput; however, this variation in resting position must be accompanied by neck physical therapy to be effective.[7] Positioning of the infant's head can be maintained through the use of an infant-positioning device (see Fig. 25.8) and facilitated by hanging toys or other stimulating objects in the infant's field of view. By training the child not to lie on the already flattened parts of his or her head, those areas will be allowed to fill out and progression of occipital flattening will be prevented. Once significant occipital flattening occurs, it becomes difficult to reposition the infant, and failure to treat the underlying torticollis with physical therapy will also result in treatment failure.[7] If repositioning is effective, migration of the bald spot from the center of the previously flattened occiput toward the previously prominent occiput can be observed (see Fig. 25.8). It is important to warn the parents to not simply position the infant on the side of the head to prevent further occipital flattening, because this is not an effective way to use positioning and gravity to help correct cranial asymmetry. If the infant has had regular prone experience and is able to sleep safely on his or her front, the parents must be cautioned to be sure the infant sleeps with the head turned toward the side of the torticollis in the nonpreferred position, so that the recessed forehead on that side does not become more recessed. Whenever possible, it is important to use the weight of the infant's head to correct cranial asymmetry by applying gravitational pressure to the prominent areas. The parents should be encouraged to follow through with physical therapy and tummy time at home, particularly if the infant's condition is not being followed by a physical therapist.[7]

Management for infants who do not make progress with exercises and repositioning of the head, as well as for infants with severe plagiocephaly that is still present at 5–6 months of age, involves the use of a corrective helmet or cranial orthotic device, which is most effective if started before 7 months of age but still useful in older infants.[7,25–27] To make serial cranial measurements in 401 infants with a normal head shape and more than 2500 infants with positional cranial deformation (with and without helmet therapy), a nomogram was created for craniofacial norms and objective categorization of positional head deformity. Normative percentiles for all dimensions in cranial vault anthropometric measurements during the first year of life have been published and are illustrated in Fig. 25.9. Children with definite nonsynostotic head deformity were allocated into three different groups: positional plagiocephaly (abnormal Cranial Vault Asymmetry Index [CVAI]), positional brachycephaly (abnormal Cranial Index [CI]), and combined positional plagiocephaly and brachycephaly (abnormal CVAI and CI). These indices are calculated from cranial measurements as follows: CI = width/length × 100 and CVAI = (diagonal A − diagonal B)/diagonal A × 100, where diagonal A < diagonal B. A reliable three-level severity categorization (mild, moderate, and severe) for each group of cranial deformation according to age and gender allowed classification of nonsynostotic early-childhood cranial deformity for decision making regarding the need for cranial orthotic therapy.[28] In general if the difference between cranial diagonal measurements is greater than 1 cm at 6–7 months of age and/or the cephalic index is greater than 95% at 5–6

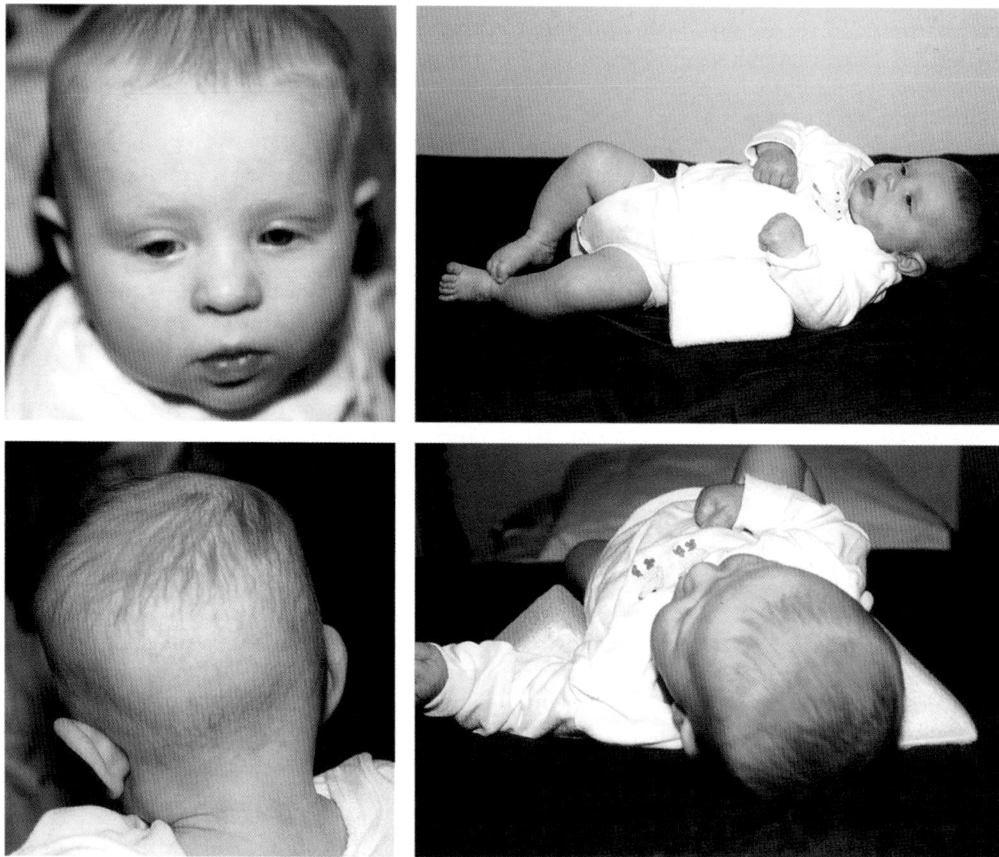

FIGURE 25.8 This female infant with torticollis-plagiocephaly deformation sequence was treated entirely with neck physical therapy and repositioning using an infant-positioning device between 3 and 9 months of age. She is shown here partway through her therapy in a three-fourth turn, resting on her left occiput, with her bald spot shifted from the right, previously flattened occiput to the left occiput.

months of age, then cranial orthotic therapy is a very effective way to correct the abnormal head shape.[7,29]

In a 2015 review of approximately 5000 infants treated with conservative therapy, Steinberg found that these methods sufficiently treated nearly 80% of infants younger than 6 months with a cranial vault asymmetry of less than 1 cm.[30] Current clinical techniques for detecting deformational plagiocephaly are often limited and can rely on subjective measures, such as visual assessments by healthcare providers. New techniques such as three-dimensional imaging, computerized assessments, and other technology have the potential to provide more accurate and objective measurements to classify and monitor plagiocephaly.[31]

Cranial orthotic therapy is intended to remold the infant's head into a more normal, symmetric oval shape as the head grows, and it has been successfully used to correct infant head shapes for more than 30 years. The prominent parts are restrained while normal brain growth provides a corrective mechanical force from within the calvarium to round out the shallow or flattened regions. This method begins by acquiring a three-dimensional (3D) image of the infant's head and creating a computer-generated model of the infant's deformed head (Fig. 25.10). This deformed model is then changed through software to create the shape the cranial orthotic device is to be fabricated around. This includes adding growth room where the infant's head is already flat and applying pressure to the already prominent regions (see Fig. 25.10). This idealized model is then milled to produce a physical model around which the plastic helmet is fabricated. The orthotic with its soft lining is then vacuum formed around the model, computer-generated contour lines showing the shape of the orthotic are created, and the device is carved with a high-precision five-axis

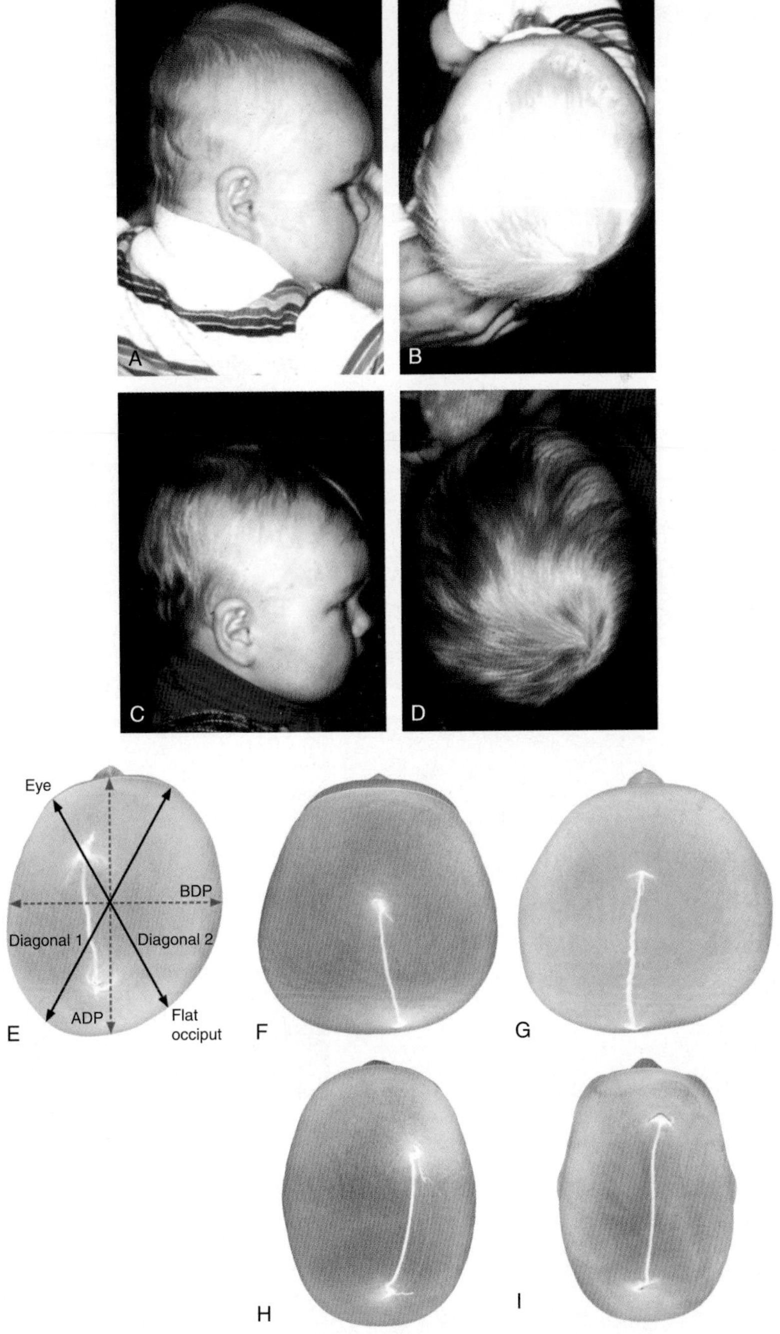

FIGURE 25.9 Before helmet therapy was begun at 6 months, this child had brachycephalic torticollis-plagiocephaly deformation sequence, which was corrected by 4 months of helmet therapy. His head is shown before (**A** and **B**) and after (**C** and **D**) helmet therapy. Measurements can be taken as shown €. Using the normative data published by Wilbrand et al., decisions can be made regarding an infant's head shape: positional plagiocephaly (abnormal Cranial Vault Asymmetry Index [CVAI]), positional brachycephaly (abnormal Cranial Index [CI]), and combined positional plagiocephaly and brachycephaly (abnormal CVAI and CI). These indices are calculated from cranial measurements as follows: CI = width/length × 100, and CVAI = (diagonal A − diagonal B)/diagonal A × 100, where diagonal A < diagonal B. Examples are shown for brachycephaly with CI at 2 standard deviations (SD) above mean for age (**F**), more than 2 SD above mean for age (**G**), and for dolichocephaly with CI at 2 SD below mean for age (**H**) and CI more than 2 SD below mean for age (**I**). *APD*, Anteroposterior diameter; *BPD*, biparietal diameter. (Wilbrand JF, Schmidtberg K, Bierther U, et al. Clinical classification of infant nonsynostotic cranial deformity. *J Pediatr.* 2012;161:1120-1125; images provided courtesy of Tim Littlefield at Cranial Technologies, Inc.)

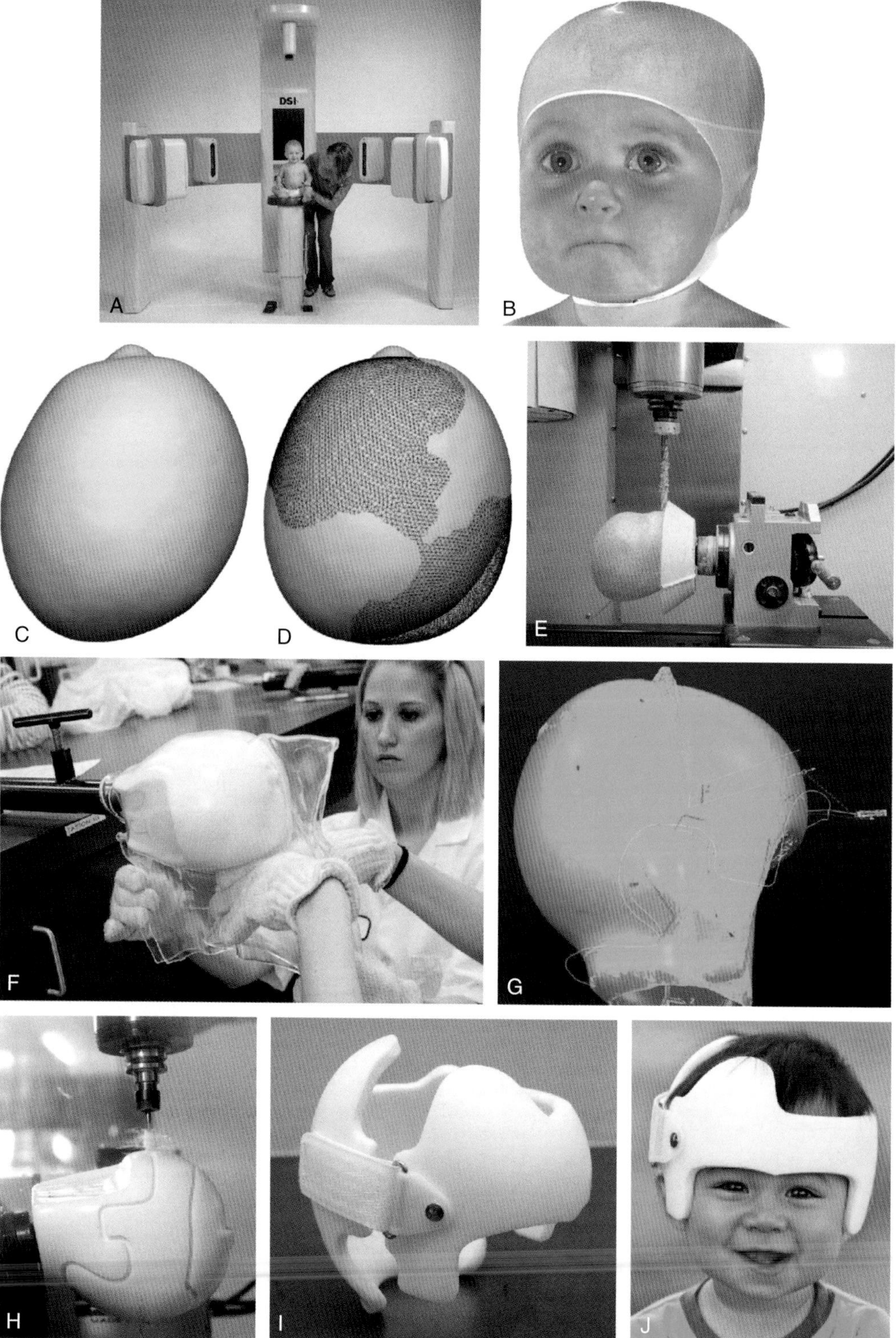

FIGURE 25.10 These figures illustrate procedures for current methods of making a custom cranial orthosis. **A,** Acquire a three-dimensional digital image of infant (Digital Surface Imaging). **B,** Three-dimensional computer image of infant with photographic overlay. **C,** Original vertex view of plagiocephalic deformity. **D,** Computer-modified cranial shape (Black wireframe overlay) for creation of orthosis (Sentient3d). **E,** Milling of idealized physical model in high-speed mill. **F,** Application of foam inner liner and vacuum forming outer plastic shell. **G,** Computer-generated contour lines (Contour3d). **H,** Mill cutting of trim lines. **I,** Finished orthotic device. **J,** Infant wearing DOC Band. (Images provided courtesy of Tim Littlefield at Cranial Technologies, Inc.)

machining center to produce the finished orthotic device. Once brain growth has filled out the helmet, no further management is usually needed and a corrected head shape will persist without further orthotic therapy. If there is residual torticollis, physical therapy is required during and after the orthotic treatment, particularly with early orthotic therapy (Fig. 25.11).[7]

If helmet therapy is initiated by 5–6 months of age, usually only 3–4 months are needed to reform the head to a more normal shape. However, if helmet management is not used until 7–8 months of age, it may take 5–6 months to achieve the desired result. The pace of reformation relates to the rate of brain growth, which is much more rapid during the first 6 months than later in infancy, explaining why a preferential head turn combined with purposeful supine positioning can deform the head so quickly. This type of therapy is typically started at around 5–6 months of age, and the helmet is worn almost constantly for an average of 4 months (only removed for bathing and cleaning the helmet with soapy water and rubbing alcohol). Follow-up must be maintained throughout this period to adjust the inner padding of the helmet to allow for regular growth and to monitor progress.[7] All cranial orthotic techniques use the same principle of using mechanical forces to remold the cranium into a more symmetric shape as the head grows into the symmetric shape of the molding device, and these devices have been cleared by the Food and Drug Administration.[32]

For those children with moderately severe cranial deformation, if intervention is not attempted or is attempted too late, permanent distortion of the head may occur (see Figs. 24.6–24.8).[7] There is concern that residual facial asymmetry may ultimately lead to ocular disturbances. These ocular problems differ from those seen in craniosynostotic plagiocephaly, in which vertical displacement of the orbit occurs.[33] Unlike synostotic plagiocephaly, which is sometimes associated

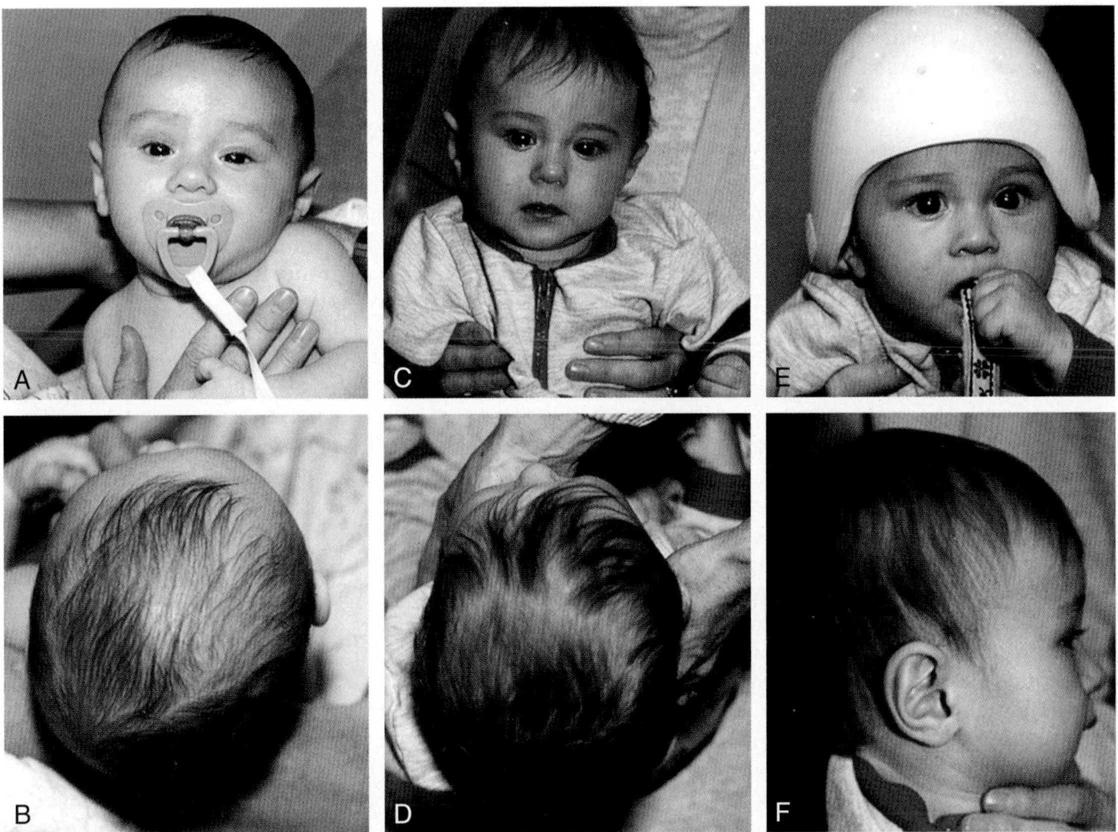

FIGURE 25.11 This infant with left torticollis is shown before (**A–C**) and after (**D–F**) helmet therapy for deformational plagiocephaly. Even though his head shape is fully corrected at 10 months of age, he still needs continued neck physical therapy to correct his torticollis.

with genetic syndromes, deformational plagiocephaly is not a heritable disorder, and recurrence rates are usually low unless an underlying uterine factor, such as a bicornuate uterus, has caused the fetal head constraint. The average length of treatment with helmet orthosis is 4.5 months for infants who average 6.5 months of age at the start of treatment, but younger infants can be successfully treated with repositioning and physical therapy alone.[7] Orthotic treatment does not restrict cranial growth but rather redirects growth into a symmetric shape. Efficacy of treatment is related to both the initial degree of asymmetry and the age at which orthosis is initiated, with earlier treatment more successful and late treatment of little or no benefit (Fig. 25.12). The practice of artificial postnatal head deformation is an ancient one that has been practiced by many older cultures (see Fig. 25.3).[34] These cultural practices confirm that head shape differences secondary to early infantile head deformation can persist throughout life if not managed appropriately.[7]

Failure to treat muscular torticollis can result in persistent facial asymmetry, cervical scoliosis, and deformational plagiocephaly (see Chapter 24).[35,36] A strict definition for congenital muscular torticollis (CMT) requires the presence of muscle fibrosis or a palpable knot, but this knot is not usually palpable after the first month or so; however muscle imbalance is common, and this is the most common reason for an asymmetric resting position.[7,14] Among 232 patients with CMT, 82% had the diagnosis first established before 3 months of age,[36] thus it is extremely important to treat any underlying CMT as soon as cranial asymmetry is noted. For infants without a sternomastoid tumor, the parents' presenting complaint is often head shape rather than neck range of motion. Breech presentation has been reported in 28% of patients with CMT, and this finding should alert the birth pediatrician to check for CMT before the head becomes asymmetric.[37] Among 7609 Dutch infants screened in 1995 for positional plagiocephaly before age of 6 months, 8.6% manifested positional preference with resultant deformational plagiocephaly, whereas an additional 10% manifested occipital flattening, and 45% of these affected infants showed persistent asymmetric occipital flattening at 2–3 years of age.[38] These findings support the opinion that the prevalence of both positional preference and deformational plagiocephaly has risen dramatically in the past decade, with males slightly more frequently affected than females, and a head turn to the right more common than to the left.[38] In addition, these Dutch children in the 1995 cohort had incurred a large number of referrals for additional diagnostic evaluations and/or treatment at much additional medical expense.[38]

Much debate still exists among pediatricians over the monetary and psychosocial costs of cranial orthotic therapy. Thus early diagnosis and appropriate conservative and preventive management of positional plagiocephaly can both benefit the child's well-being and minimize the potential financial burden on families. Healthcare providers should be aware of costs associated with the diagnosis and management of this condition and work with families to identify the most effective and cost-efficient treatment options.[39] Orthotic devices clearly correct abnormal head shapes that could be prevented by more prompt recognition and treatment of torticollis with early physical therapy. To assess changes in head shape in infancy and at 18 months of age in children with and without plagiocephaly or brachycephaly, three-dimensional surface imaging was used to assess and compare head shapes in 233 cases of deformational plagiocephaly or brachycephaly and 167 unaffected controls. Cases had greater skull flattening and asymmetry than unaffected controls at both time points, and symmetry was more improved for those who received orthotic treatment.[40] In a randomized controlled trial of 126 New Zealand infants presenting to a plagiocephaly clinic, infants were randomized to either positioning or to positioning plus the use of a swaddling positioning wrap and followed. There was no difference in head-shape outcomes for the two treatment groups after 12 months of age, with 42% of infants having normal head shapes by that time and 80% showing good improvement. Those that had poor improvement were more likely to have both plagiocephaly and brachycephaly, and to have presented later to the clinic.[41] In a longitudinal cohort study of 126 infants with deformational plagiocephaly from this same outpatient clinic, development was assessed 3, 6, and 12 months later, and initially 30% manifested delays.[42] These delays were primarily gross motor in type but had reduced to approach the expected level by the time of the 12-month follow-up, at a mean age of 17 months.[20] Among 129 children from this same clinic who had long-term follow-up at a mean age of 4 years, 61% of head-shape measurements reverted to the normal range but 4% remained severe at follow-up. Initially, 85% of parents reported being "somewhat" or "very" concerned, and this decreased to 13% at follow-up. The percentage of children with motor delay decreased from 41% initially to 11% at follow-up. Overall, head shape measurements, parental concern, and developmental delays in infancy showed a dramatic improvement when remeasured at 3 and 4 years of age.[20]

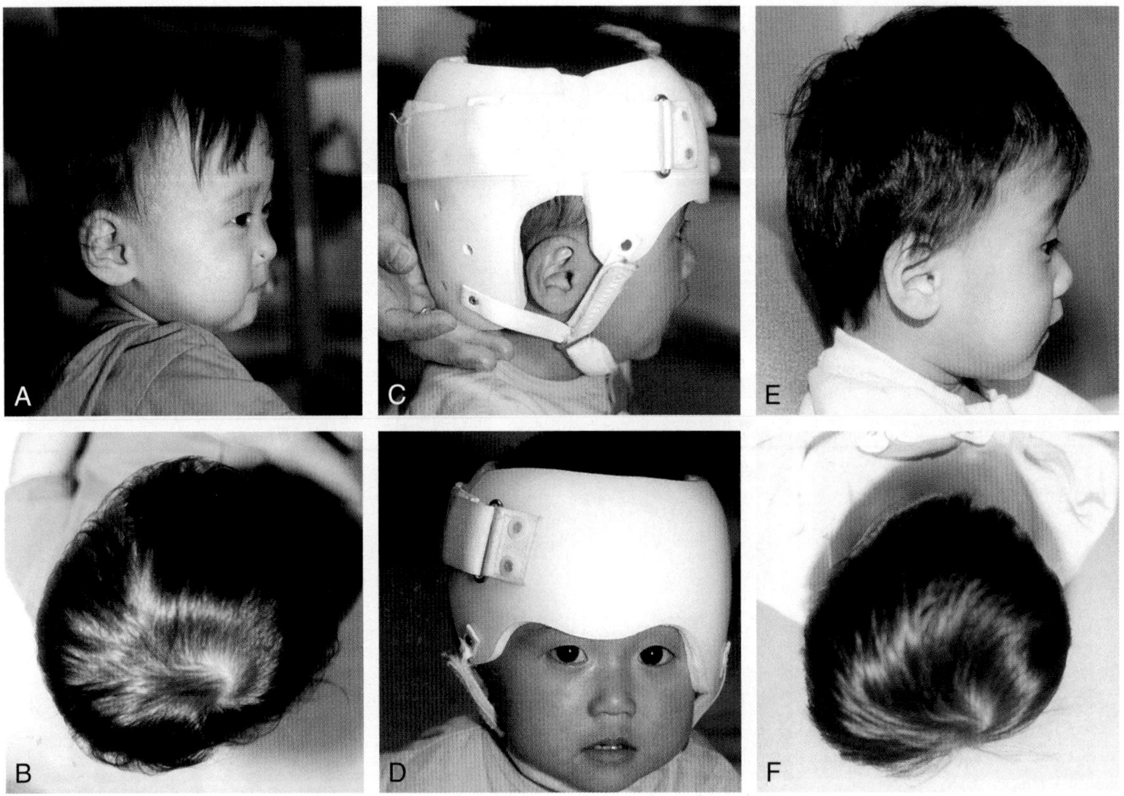

FIGURE 25.12 Helmet treatment was initiated at 15 months (**A** and **B**) and continued for the next 9 months (**C** and **D**), but this only reduced the cranial diameters from 2.0 to 1.5 cm, and the resultant cranial asymmetry persisted thereafter (**E** and **F**).

DIFFERENTIAL DIAGNOSIS

Deformational plagiocephaly, unilateral coronal craniosynostosis, and lambdoid craniosynostosis all cause oblique deformities of the skull, with clear differences in physical findings and radiologic findings, and markedly different treatments.[43] High-frequency ultrasound has been used to confirm the diagnosis of positional plagiocephaly and exclude true synostosis.[44,45] Overlapping bone plates may be seen on the affected side of the skull in infants with deformational plagiocephaly, but this has no prognostic value regarding early fusion of sutures and should not affect treatment decisions. Lambdoidal craniosynostosis accounts for about 2% of all cases of craniosynostosis and deformational posterior plagiocephaly has previously been confused with lambdoid synostosis, leading to unnecessary surgery and falsely elevated statistics concerning the frequency of lambdoid synostosis; however the distinction between these conditions can now be made with certainty. Clinical features of lambdoid craniosynostosis include a thick bony ridge over the fused lambdoid suture, with contralateral parietal and frontal bulging and an ipsilateral occipitomastoid bulge leading to tilting of the ipsilateral skull base and a downward displacement of the ear on the synostotic side. These changes result in a trapezoidal head shape when viewed from above (see Chapter 33).[46] In contrast, children with deformational, nonsynostotic posterior plagiocephaly had a parallelogram-shaped head, with forward displacement of the ear and frontal bossing on the side ipsilateral to the occipitoparietal flattening, accompanied by contralateral occipital bossing. Craniometric measurements in nine patients with unilateral lambdoid synostosis were compared with 12 patients with deformational plagiocephaly. All lambdoid synostosis patients had deviation of the posterior cranial fossa toward the affected side, whereas deformational plagiocephaly patients had variable deflection. All lambdoid synostosis patients demonstrated marked posterior displacement of the contralateral temporomandibular joint, whereas deformational

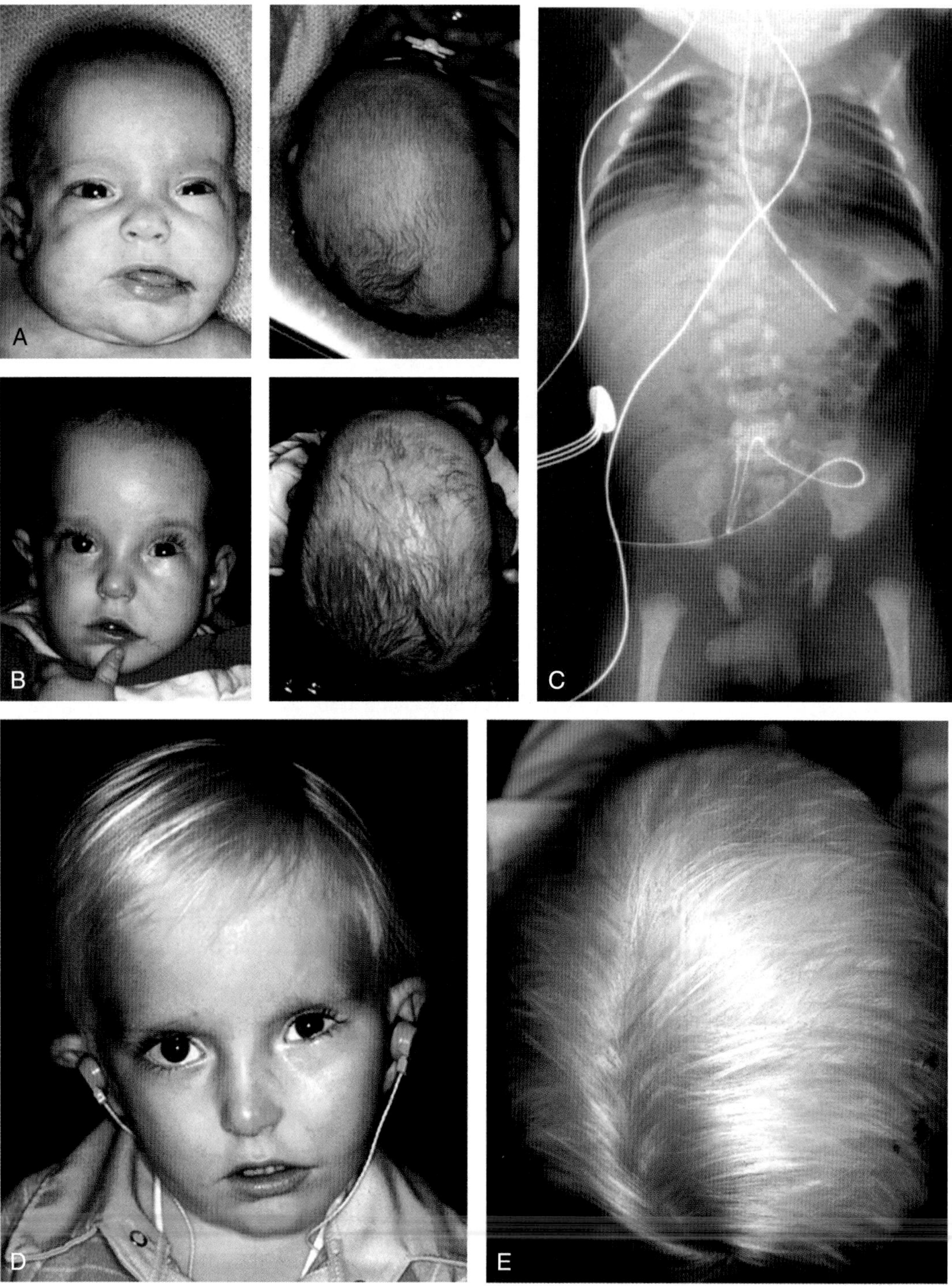

FIGURE 25.13 This infant with oculoauriculovertebral dysplasia (**A**) had severe cervical vertebral anomalies (**B**) that resulted in a persistent head turn to the right. **C,** By 3 months of age, he had developed marked plagiocephaly as a consequence of his asymmetric resting position. Because his cervical vertebral anomalies could not be corrected, he was fitted with two consecutive helmets to maintain normal cranial symmetry during the period of most rapid head growth (through 2 years of age). **D** and **E,** At 3 years of age, he had a persistent head turn and head tilt but relatively normal cranial symmetry.

plagiocephaly patients had either symmetric temporomandibular joint position (75%) or slight contralateral posterior displacement (25%).[47] As shown in Fig. 25.6, some patients present with both unilateral lambdoid synostosis and torticollis-plagiocephaly deformation sequence, which suggests that both types of problems can result from fetal head constraint in utero and mandates a treatment program that includes surgery, physical therapy, and cranial orthotic therapy. Among patients with positional plagiocephaly, 39% were noted to have some form of metopic suture abnormality,[48] suggesting some patients with deformational plagiocephaly have mild metopic ridging that may be related to fetal head constraint.

A malformation of the cervical vertebrae can be the primary cause of the head being turned to one side, in which case the deformational plagiocephaly and torticollis would be secondary to an intrinsic malformation problem (Fig. 25.13). In such infants, it is usually necessary to use more than one helmet to achieve the desired cranial symmetry because the torticollis does not respond to physical therapy. In severe bone dysplasias resulting in osteopenia, such as osteogenesis imperfecta type III or severe hypophosphatasia, the calvarium may be extremely soft and too undermineralized to maintain its normal protective shape, with the result that the brain is actually compressed in an anteroposterior dimension, sometimes leading to communicating hydrocephalus. In such instances, prolonged helmet therapy may be helpful.

A primary neuromuscular disorder may also be the primary cause of the torticollis, as in spastic torticollis, but these disorders are quite rare. After birth, neuromuscular disorders predisposing toward hypotonia and (occasionally) severe neglect may cause an infant to lie in one position long enough to give rise to asymmetric molding of the head. This can usually be distinguished from CMT by physical examination and history. Prematurely born infants may have poor muscle tone with a relatively malleable cranium. If such an infant lies persistently on a firm surface with the head turned to one side, he or she may develop deformational plagiocephaly. Such cases can usually be distinguished from postnatal constraint deformation by the history.

References

1. Dunn PM. Congenital sternomastoid torticollis: an intrauterine postural deformity. *Arch Dis Child.* 1974;49:824–825.
2. Argenta LC, David LR, Wilson JA, et al. An increase in infant cranial deformity with supine sleeping position. *J Craniofac Surg.* 1996;7:5–11.
3. Turk AE, McCarthy JG, Thorne CHM, et al. The "Back to Sleep Campaign" and deformational plagiocephaly: is there cause for concern? *J Craniofac Surg.* 1996;7:12–18.
4. Kane AA, Mitchell LE, Craven KP, et al. Observations on a recent increase in plagiocephaly without synostosis. *Pediatrics.* 1996;97:877–885.
5. Santiago GS, Santiago CN, Chwa ES, Purnell CA. Positional plagiocephaly and craniosynostosis. *Pediatr Ann.* 2023 Jan;52(1):e10–e17.
6. Di Chiara A, La Rosa E, Ramieri V, Vellone V, Cascone P. Treatment of deformational plagiocephaly with physiotherapy. *J Craniofac Surg.* 2019;30(7):2008–2013.
7. Graham JM Jr, Gomez M, Halberg A, et al. Management of deformational plagiocephaly: repositioning versus orthotic therapy. *J Pediatr.* 2005;146:258–262.
8. Khonsari RH, Friess M, Nysjö J, et al. Shape and volume of craniofacial cavities in intentional skull deformations. *Am J Phys Anthropol.* 2013;151:110–119.
9. Littlefield TR, Kelly KM, Pomatto JK, et al. Multiple-birth infants at higher risk for development of deformational plagiocephaly. *Pediatrics.* 1999;103:565–569.
10. Littlefield TR, Kelly KM, Pomatto JK, et al. Multiple-birth infants at higher risk for development of deformational plagiocephaly. II. Is one twin at greater risk? *Pediatrics.* 2002;109:19–25.
11. Aase JM. Structural defects as a consequence of late intrauterine constraint: craniotabes, loose skin, and asymmetric ear size. *Semin Perinatol.* 1983;7:270–273.
12. Jones MC. Unilateral epicanthal fold: diagnostic significance. *J Pediatr.* 1986;108:702–704.
13. Frederick DR, Mulliken JB, Robb RM. Ocular manifestations of deformational frontal plagiocephaly. *J Pediatr Ophthalmol Strab.* 1993;30:92–95.
14. Kuo AA, Tritasavit S, Graham JM, Jr. Congenital muscular torticollis and positional plagiocephaly. *Pediatr Rev.* 2014;35:79–87.
15. Wilbrand JF, Seidl M, Wilbrand M, et al. A prospective randomized trial on preventative methods for positional head deformity: physiotherapy versus a positioning pillow. *J Pediatr.* 2013;162:1216–1221.
16. Hutchison BL, Stewart AW, De Chalain TB, et al. A randomized controlled trial of positioning treatments in infants with positional head shape deformities. *Acta Paediatr.* 2010;99:1556–1560.
17. van Vlimmeren LA, van der Graaf Y, Boere-Boonekamp MM, et al. Effect of pediatric physical therapy on deformational plagiocephaly in children with positional preference: a randomized controlled trial. *Arch Pediatr Adolesc Med.* 2008;162:712–718.
18. Hutchinson BL, Hutchinson LAD, Thompson JMD, et al. Plagiocephaly and brachycephaly in the first two years of life: a prospective cohort study. *Pediatrics.* 2004;114:970–980.
19. Mawji A, Vollman AR, Hatfield J, et al. The incidence of positional plagiocephaly: a cohort study. *Pediatrics.* 2013;132:298–304.
20. Hutchison BL, Stewart AW, Mitchell EA. Deformational plagiocephaly: a follow-up of head shape, parental

concern and neurodevelopment at ages 3 and 4 years. *Arch Dis Child.* 2011;96:85–90.

21. Roby BB, Finkelstein M, Tibesar RJ, et al. Prevalence of positional plagiocephaly in teens born after the "Back to Sleep" campaign. *Otolaryngol Head Neck Surg.* 2014;146:823–828.
22. van Wijk RM, van Vlimmeren LA, Groothuis-Oudshoorn CG, et al. Helmet therapy in infants with positional skull deformation: randomised controlled trial. *BMJ.* 2014;348:g2741. https://doi.org/10.1136/bmj.g2741.
23. Wilbrand JF, Wilbrand M, Malik CY, et al. Complications in helmet therapy. *J Cranio-Maxillo-Fac Surg.* 2012;40:341–346.
24. Wilbrand JF, Seidl M, Wilbrand M, et al. A prospective randomized trial on preventative methods for positional head deformity: physiotherapy versus a positioning pillow. *J Pediatr.* 2013;162:1216–1221.
25. Moghaddam MB, Brown TM, Clausen A, et al. Outcome analysis after helmet therapy using 3D photogrammetry in patients with deformational plagiocephaly: the role of root mean square. *J Plast Reconstr Aesthet Surg.* 2014;67:159–165.
26. Couture DE, Crantford JC, Somasundaram A, et al. Efficacy of passive helmet therapy for deformational plagiocephaly: report of 1050 cases. *Neurosurg Focus.* 2013;35:E4.
27. Goh JL, Bauer DF, Durham SR, et al. Orthotic (helmet) therapy in the treatment of plagiocephaly. *Neurosurg Focus.* 2013;35:E2.
28. Wilbrand JF, Schmidtberg K, Bierther U, et al. Clinical classification of infant nonsynostotic cranial deformity. *J Pediatr.* 2012;161:1120–1125.
29. Graham JM Jr, Kreutzman J, Earl D, et al. Deformational brachycephaly in supine-sleeping infants. *J Pediatr.* 2005;146:253–257.
30. Steinberg JP, Rawlani R, Humphries LS, Rawlani V, Vicari FA. Effectiveness of conservative therapy and helmet therapy for positional cranial deformation. *Plast Reconstr Surg.* 2015;135(3):833–842.
31. Watt A, Zammit D, Lee J, Gilardino M. Novel screening and monitoring techniques for deformational plagiocephaly: a systematic review. *Pediatrics.* 2022;149(2):e2021051736.
32. Littlefield TR. Food and Drug Administration regulation of orthotic cranioplasty. *Cleft Palate Craniofac J.* 2001;38:337–340.
33. Greenberg MF, Pollard ZF. Ocular plagiocephaly: ocular torticollis with skull and facial asymmetry. *Ophthalmology.* 2000;107:173–179.
34. Fitzsimmons E, Prost JH, Peniston S. Infant head molding: a cultural practice. *Arch Fam Med.* 1998;7:88–90.
35. Putnam GD, Postlethwaite KR, Chate RA, et al. Facial scoliosis: a diagnostic dilemma. *Int J Oral Maxillofac Surg.* 1993;22:324–327.
36. Slate RK, Posnick JC, Armstrong DC, et al. Cervical spine subluxation associated with congenital muscular scoliosis and craniofacial asymmetry. *Plast Reconstr Surg.* 1993;91:1187–1195.
37. Morrison DL, MacEwen GD. Congenital muscular torticollis: observations regarding clinical findings, associated conditions, and results of treatment. *J Pediatr Orthop.* 1982;2:500–505.
38. Boere-Boonekamp MMM, van der Linden-Kuiper LT. Positional preference: prevalence in infants and follow-up after two years. *Pediatrics.* 2001;107:339–343.
39. Watt A, Alabdulkarim A, Lee J, Gilardino M. Practical review of the cost of diagnosis and management of positional plagiocephaly. *Plast Reconstr Surg Glob Open.* 2022;10(5).
40. Collett BR, Heike CL, Atmosukarto I, et al. Longitudinal, three-dimensional analysis of head shape in children with and without deformational plagiocephaly or brachycephaly. *J Pediatr.* 2012;160:673–678.
41. Hutchison BL, Stewart AW, De Chalain TB, et al. A randomized controlled trial of positioning treatments in infants with positional head shape deformities. *Acta Paediatr.* 2010;99:1556–1560.
42. Hutchison BL, Stewart AW, de Chalain T, et al. Serial developmental assessments in infants with deformational plagiocephaly. *J Paediatr Child Health.* 2012;48:274–278.
43. Liu Y, Kadlub N, da Silva Freitas R, et al. The misdiagnosis of craniosynostosis as deformational plagiocephaly. *J Craniofac Surg.* 2008;19:132–136.
44. Regelsberger J, Delling G, Tsokos M, et al. High-frequency ultrasound confirmation of positional plagiocephaly. *J Neurosurg.* 2006;105(5 Suppl):413–417.
45. Krimmel M, Will B, Wolff M, et al. Value of high-resolution ultrasound in the differential diagnosis of scaphocephaly and occipital plagiocephaly. *Int J Oral Maxillofac Surg.* 2012;41:797–800.
46. Matushita H, Alonso N, Cardeal DD, et al. Major clinical features of synostotic occipital plagiocephaly: mechanisms of cranial deformations. *Childs Nerv Syst.* 2014;30:1217–1224.
47. Smartt JM Jr, Elliott RM, Reid RR, et al. Analysis of differences in the cranial base and facial skeleton of patients with lambdoid synostosis and deformational plagiocephaly. *Plast Reconstr Surg.* 2011;127:303–312.
48. Fisher DC, Kornrumpf BP, Couture D, et al. Increased incidence of metopic suture abnormalities in children with positional plagiocephaly. *J Craniofac Surg.* 2011;22:89–95.

CHAPTER 26

Infant Sleeping Position and Sudden Infant Death Syndrome

KEY POINTS

- Sudden infant death syndrome (SIDS) has a multifactorial and heterogeneous etiology with a triple-risk hypothesis proposed: (1) exogenous/environmental stressor, (2) early infancy, and (3) an underlying vulnerability or genetic susceptibility.
- Metabolic conditions have historically been thought to be a substantial proportion of SIDS cases, but many are now detected early through newborn screening programs.
- Infant sleeping position has emerged as a major risk factor for SIDS, with prone sleeping associated with a significantly higher risk.
- Despite education and intervention efforts, thousands of infants still die of SIDS annually.
- The leading model of SIDS is the "triple-risk model," which postulates that SIDS occurs in a biologically vulnerable infant during a critical developmental period, when triggered by a stressor or external risk factor.

GENESIS

The postmortem diagnosis of sudden infant death syndrome (SIDS), once known as "cot death," was introduced midway through the 20th century, but its association with infant sleeping position was not established until the 1990s. SIDS is considered to have a multifactorial and heterogeneous basis whereby some infants are born with risk factors that make them more vulnerable to dying during infancy with additive subtle risk factors. There is a growing body of evidence suggesting that a proportion of SIDS has a genetic underpinning, including a four- to five fold relative risk of SIDS in subsequent siblings and an increased SIDS risk in monozygotic twins compared to dizygotic.[1,2] Historically, metabolic conditions have been thought to be a substantial proportion of SIDS cases, many of which are now being detected early and treated after the introduction of tandem mass spectrometry-based newborn screening programs. Although morbidity and mortality of conditions such as medium-chain acyl-CoA dehydrogenase (MCAD) deficiency has significantly reduced, neonatal death in individuals with early disease manifestation and severe hypoglycemia may still occur. Decompensation due to MCAD deficiency has been reported in the first hours and days of life before any metabolic screening results become available, with episodes that lead to death in up to 5% of affected patients.[3] Rigorous cardiac genetic evaluations have not been historically recommended unless the circumstances at the time of death or family history are suggestive of an arrhythmic death.[4]

Although rates of SIDS have decreased by 50% since the 1990s, African-American and Native-American infants are more than twice as likely to die of SIDS than are White babies.[5] A metaanalysis of 217 articles found 7 qualitative studies that surveyed African-American mothers and found several themes: many tended to believe that SIDS is a random occurrence and is not preventable, so they may feel that there was little reason to make their infant sleep in a cold, hard crib when they could sleep in a warm, comfortable bed with them.[6] In a 2022 retrospective study of infant mortality in the District of Columbia, 89% were African American and 63% involved bed sharing, despite more than half of those cases having a known safe sleep surface available.[7] Nurses should work with Black mothers to understand their cultural beliefs while educating them about safe sleep practices. Some genetic variants have been proposed as risk factors for SIDS; for example, the carnitine palmitoyltransferase 1 (*CPT1A*) p.P479L variant common in Aboriginal populations on the west and north coasts of Alaska and Canada and in northeast Siberia and Greenland, although the association may be more prevalent on the basis of drift, positive selection, or a founder effect, and more likely has a noncausal association with infant death owing to a range of social and environmental risk factors that also occur at higher rates in the population.[8] Currently, whole-exome or whole-genome sequencing techniques are largely used postmortem in an otherwise healthy infant. These broad tests do not have adequate predictive value and are still cost-prohibitive for universal use after the death of an infant.

The leading model of SIDS is the "triple-risk model," which postulates that SIDS occurs in a biologically vulnerable infant during a critical developmental period when triggered by a stressor or external risk factor. Infant sleeping position has emerged as a major risk factor for SIDS. It has been hypothesized that abnormalities in the arcuate nucleus, which controls breathing and waking, might be involved in some cases of SIDS. Normal infants sense inadequate air intake, which triggers them to awaken, cry, and change cardiorespiratory function to compensate for insufficient oxygen and excess carbon dioxide. This situation might result from infants sleeping on their stomachs and rebreathing exhaled air that is trapped in underlying bedding, and a baby with defective functioning of the arcuate nucleus might lack this protective mechanism and succumb to SIDS. There are also other predisposing factors for SIDS, such as chronic hypoxia induced by maternal cigarette smoking during pregnancy or concurrent respiratory infection in the infant. Also, more SIDS cases occur in the colder months, when such infections are more common. Increases in cellular and protein immune responses also have been suggested to play a role, along with the microbiome in the gut. Arousal thresholds are significantly higher in both active and quiet sleep when infants sleep prone at 2–3 weeks or 2–3 months (the age of peak susceptibility to SIDS) but not at 5–6 months (the age when susceptibility to SIDS is decreased). Thus the prone position significantly impairs arousal from sleep during the time when infants are most likely to die from SIDS, which is the major cause of death for infants between 1 and 12 months of age.[9]

FEATURES

Between 1989 and 1991, epidemiologic studies showed a strong association between infants sleeping on their stomachs and death from SIDS.[10–14] In 1992, the American Academy of Pediatrics formed a Task Force on Infant Positioning and SIDS, which determined that infants who slept prone on their stomachs had as much as an 11.7-times higher risk for SIDS than infants who slept supine on their backs. Hence in 1992, the recommendation was made to position infants on their backs or sides for sleep, except in cases of prematurity, gastroesophageal reflux, or obstructive sleep apnea.[15] By 1993, similar risk-reduction efforts in Australia, the UK, and New Zealand had resulted in a 50% reduction in SIDS deaths over a 1–2-year period.[16–18] In addition, there was no apparent increase in doctor visits or adverse respiratory events for infants placed on their sides or backs.[19,20] When side positioning was compared with placing infants on their backs, it became evident that the risk for SIDS was greater when infants were placed on their sides, possibly because of a higher likelihood of spontaneously turning onto their stomachs. Thus in 1996, the recommendation was revised to avoid side positioning.[21] In 2022, further recommendations were made to position babies on a firm surface free of soft bedding, pillows, or comforters because sleeping with these items also increases the risk of SIDS (and possibly explains the increased frequency of SIDS during the colder months).[5,22,23]

As a consequence of the "Back to Sleep" campaign, the predominant sleeping pattern in the United States changed from 70% prone in 1992 to 24% prone in 1996, with a concomitant 38% decrease in SIDS during the same time interval.[24,25] Between 1994 and 1998, prone placement declined from 44% to 17% among White infants and from 53% to 32% among Black infants, with supine positioning increasing from 27% to 58% among White infants and from 17% to 31% among Black infants.[26] In 2001, the prevalence of prone positioning among White infants was 11% (compared with 21% among Black infants), and the rate of SIDS among Black infants was 2.5 times that of White infants.[27] This decrease in supine positioning among Black versus White infants may account for the increased frequency of SIDS among Black infants. Despite recommendations for supine sleep positioning, some caregivers persist with prone positioning because they believe the infant is more comfortable and sleeps better. Side and prone sleeping positions both increase the risk of SIDS, particularly in infants who are unused to prone sleeping, with an adjusted odds ratio (OR) of 6.9 and 8.2, respectively.[28] The end result of this public education effort was a decline in the prevalence of prone sleeping position from 70% in 1992 to 13% in 2004, with a concomitant reduction in the rate of SIDS from 1.2 per 1000 in 1992 to 0.56 per 1000 in 2001 (a decrease of 53% over this 10-year period).[27] During this same time period, for specific subgroups the risk of SIDS for low-birth-weight infants rose from an OR of 2.1 to 3.6; for infants born to smoking mothers, from 2.7 to 3.7; for infants born to unmarried mothers, from 1.4 to 2.5; for infants born to Black mothers, from 1.4 to 2.5; and for infants born to mothers with limited prenatal care, from 1.5 to 2.5. Thus the reduction in SIDS deaths associated with changes in sleeping practices has strengthened the association of SIDS with these other risk factors. These findings emphasize the interplay between SIDS, lung disease, socioeconomic factors, and exposure to tobacco smoke, and suggest that some population subgroups remain unaware of medical advice regarding optimal sleep positioning for infants.[29]

MANAGEMENT

Given the strong association between prone sleeping positioning and SIDS, it is advisable to position infants on their backs for sleep except in cases of prematurity, gastroesophageal reflux, or obstructive sleep apnea. The key to effective management is to position infants in the supine position, with regular variation in the position of the infant's head so as to avoid undue flattening.[27,30,31] Aberrant head shapes can be avoided by early initiation of neck physical therapy at the first sign of positional asymmetry or brachycephaly, with effective positioning to both sides of the occiput. Supine sleepers attain several motor milestones later than prone sleepers (e.g., rolling prone to supine, tripod sitting, creeping, crawling, and pulling to stand); however all milestones are eventually attained within the expected normal range.[32]

Encouraging "tummy time" when infants are awake and under observation may help to minimize these differences in normal motor development by strengthening the infant's neck muscles and facilitating prone motor activities.[33] In a 2020 review of over 4237 participants, tummy time was positively associated with better gross motor and overall development, a reduction in body mass index z-score, prevention of brachycephaly, and the ability to move while prone, supine, crawling, and rolling.[34] Because supine-sleeping infants are unused to viewing their world from the stomach, they need prone visual experience to facilitate their motor development. Studies have shown that 53% of SIDS victims who had always slept in a nonprone position died shortly after they were placed prone by a parent or other caretaker, and in 56% of these cases a secondary caretaker other than the parents was responsible for the change.[34] This emphasizes the importance of stressing proper infant sleep positioning to everyone involved in the care of infants, as well as the importance of giving infants adequate "tummy time" experience while they are awake so as to facilitate development of head turning while prone as a key protective mechanism in case the infant turns from supine to prone during sleep.[30-37] Taking all these data together, it is clear that the "Back to Sleep" campaign has been one of the modern triumphs of preventive medicine in reducing the incidence of SIDS by more than 50%, but primary care providers should deliver a broader message and consider other causes of infant mortality for further risk reduction. It is essential to place infants on their backs for sleep, except in cases of prematurity, gastroesophageal reflux, or obstructive sleep apnea, but infants should be on their stomachs whenever they are awake and under direct adult supervision to develop their prone motor skills and full range of neck motion.

DIFFERENTIAL DIAGNOSIS

Rarely, an underlying genetic disease causes SIDS, such as certain metabolic or genetic diseases. MCAD deficiency may be mistaken as SIDS. This deficiency prevents proper processing of fatty acids, leading to build-up of fatty acid metabolites that disrupt cardiorespiratory function. Up to 50% of infants who died of SIDS had prolonged QT on electrocardiograms performed during the first week of life.[37] Evidence from clinical correlations between long QT syndrome and SIDS, as well as genetic analyses in cohorts of SIDS victims, have revealed a large number of mutations in ion channel–related genes that are linked to inheritable arrhythmogenic syndromes, particularly long QT syndrome, short QT syndrome, Brugada syndrome, and catecholaminergic polymorphic ventricular tachycardia. Data from population-based cohort studies suggest that at least one in five SIDS victims carries a mutation in a cardiac ion channel–related gene and that the majority of these mutations are of a known malignant phenotype.[38] An investigation of genetic risk factors involved in the autonomous nervous system among 195 Dutch unclassified sudden infant death or SIDS cases (onset of the fatal episode apparently occurring during sleep) and 846 Dutch, age-matched healthy controls revealed DNA variants from 11 genes involved in serotonin metabolism or in congenital central hypoventilation syndrome, some of which were previously associated with SIDS. Of all DNA variants considered, only the length variation of the polyalanine repeat in exon 3 of the *PHOX2B* gene was found to be statistically significant, with contraction of the *PHOX2B* exon 3 polyalanine repeat in six of 160 cases versus six of 814 controls, suggesting this might be a genetic risk factor in the Dutch population.[39]

Despite a major decrease in the incidence of SIDS after 1992, this decline has plateaued in recent years and other causes of sleep-related deaths have become more prominent, including suffocation, asphyxia, entrapment, and ill-defined or unspecified causes of death. Current recommendations to reduce the risk of sleep-related infant deaths include supine positioning, use of a firm sleep surface, breastfeeding, room sharing without bed sharing, routine immunization, consideration of a pacifier, and avoidance of soft bedding, overheating, and exposure to tobacco smoke, alcohol, and illicit drugs.[40] An Irish population-based case control study examined alcohol consumption and maternal smoking during pregnancy and the risk of SIDS. Mothers who smoked were three times more likely to have a SIDS case, and a dose response effect was apparent. Similarly, mothers who drank were three times more likely to have a SIDS case, and a dose response with frequency of drinking was apparent.[41]

The proportion of sudden unexpected infant deaths in neonates less than 7 days old has increased among all sudden unexpected infant death cases during the first year of life. Among neonates who died within 24 hours after birth, 52% of the incidents occurred while the mother and her newborn were still hospitalized, and 48% had been sleeping in the parents' bed, with another 11% in a sofa-sharing situation.[42] Between 1993 and 2010, bed sharing increased from 6.5% to 13.5%, especially among Black and Hispanic infants.[43] A metaanalysis of 11 studies confirmed that bed sharing is a risk factor for SIDS, with especially enhanced risks in smoking parents and in very young infants.[44] Bed sharing increases the risk for SIDS, as well as the risk for accidental suffocation/asphyxia of the baby, and mothers should be instructed not to bed share.

Among 215 sleep-related sudden infant deaths in Florida in 2008, 47.9% resulted from accidental suffocation and strangulation in bed, 35.4% were of unknown or undetermined cause, and 16.7% resulted from SIDS. Sleep-related sudden infant deaths occurred most frequently in an adult bed (50.2%) with 54.4% infants sharing a sleep surface, 38.1% placed nonsupine, 24.2% placed on a pillow, and 10.2% having a head covering. Thus approximately 80% of sleep-related sudden infant deaths were related to unsafe sleeping environments.[45] Among 3136 sleep-related sudden unexpected infant deaths from 2005 to 2008, only 25% of infants were sleeping in a crib or on their back when found, and 70% were on a surface not intended for infant sleep (e.g., an adult bed), with 64% of infants sharing a sleep surface and almost half of these infants sleeping with an adult. Infants whose deaths were classified as suffocation or of undetermined cause were significantly more likely to be found on a surface not intended for infant sleep and to be sharing that sleep surface than were infants whose deaths were classified as SIDS.[46] Analysis of events reported to the Consumer Product Safety Commission between 2004 and 2012 revealed 36 incidents involving wearable blankets and swaddle wraps, including 10 deaths (median age at death 3.5 months), and 80% of these deaths were attributed to positional asphyxia related to prone sleeping, with 70% involving additional risk factors, usually soft bedding. Among 12 incidents involving swaddling in blankets that resulted in death (median age at death, 2 months), 58% of deaths were attributed to positional asphyxia related to prone sleeping, and 92% involved additional risk factors, most commonly soft bedding. Reports of sudden unexpected death in swaddled infants are rare, and risks can be reduced by placing infants supine and discontinuing swaddling as soon as infants attempt to roll over, with further risk reduction achieved by removing soft bedding and bumper pads from the infant's sleeping environment.[47]

Epidemiologic studies have shown that pacifier use decreases the risk of SIDS, even when infants sleep prone, but pacifier use did not alter infant spontaneous arousability in 30 term infants studied at three time periods during the first 6 months, in both the prone and supine sleeping position.[48] Over a 3-year period from 2005 to 2007, there were 5203 postneonatal out-of-hospital deaths attributable to SIDS in the United States; 2010 attributable to other sudden deaths; 1270 attributable to suffocation in bed; and

3681 attributable to other causes. The rate of SIDS among the most preterm infants (24–28 weeks' gestation) was significantly increased compared with term infants, and despite a marked decrease in the incidence of SIDS over the past two decades, the risk for SIDS among very preterm infants has remained elevated. Other causes of sudden infant death for which SIDS is often mistaken manifest similar levels of increased risk among preterm infants.[49] Cerebral oxygenation is reduced in the prone position in preterm infants (and lower compared with age-matched term infants), especially when mean arterial pressure is already reduced in the prone position, and this may contribute to their increased SIDS risk.[50] The major SIDS risk factor for infants younger than 3 months is bed sharing, whereas rolling into objects in the sleep area is the major risk factor for infants greater than 3 months of age, so parents should be warned about the dangers of these specific risk factors appropriate to their infant's age.[51] Prone sleeping impairs arousal from sleep and cardiovascular control in infants at 2–3 months, coinciding with the highest risk period for SIDS. Absence of the vasodilatory response during quiet sleep at 2–3 months may underlie the decreased arousability from sleep and increase the risk for SIDS at this age.[52]

Clearly the risk for SIDS has dropped with a reduction in prone infant sleeping positions, but there are many other opportunities to reduce infant mortality. A 1983–2006 Swedish retrospective nationwide cohort study of singleton nonmalformed infants born at 37 gestational weeks or later revealed a 0.12% infant mortality rate.[53] Compared with infants born at 40 weeks, the risk of infant mortality was increased among early-term infants (37 weeks), and compared with infants with normal birth weight, very small for gestational age (less than the third percentile) infants had twice the risk for infant mortality. SIDS was the most common cause of death, accounting for 39% of all infant mortality. In 1987, the SIDS rate in the United States was 1.2 per 1000 live births, and by 2005 the SIDS rate had dropped more than half to approximately 0.5 per 1000 live births. In 1987, the risk of SIDS was 2.32 times greater for extremely premature infants (24–28 weeks' gestation) compared with term infants. Over a 3-year period (2005–2007), the risk for SIDS among the most preterm infants remained 2.57-times greater compared with term infants, so despite this marked drop in the incidence of SIDS since 1987, the risk for SIDS among very preterm infants remains elevated.[49] With improved neonatal care and management of gestational age in the United States between 1995–1996 and 2004–2005, the SIDS rate declined from 8.3 to 5.6 per 10,000 live births among singletons and from 14.2 to 10.6 per 10,000 live births among twins, but there are opportunities for further improvement.[53] Further reductions in infant mortality can be achieved by encouraging a supine infant sleep position on a firm sleep surface, breastfeeding, room sharing without bed sharing, routine immunization, and avoidance of soft bedding, overheating, and exposure to tobacco smoke, alcohol, and illicit drugs.[40]

References

1. Keywan C, Poduri AH, Goldstein RD, Holm IA. Genetic factors underlying sudden infant death syndrome. *Appl Clin Genet.* 2021;14:61–76.
2. Scheers NJ, Daytron M, Kemp JS. Sudden infant death with external airways covered: case-comparison study of 206 deaths in the United States. *Arch Pediatr Adolesc Med.* 1998;152:540–547.
3. Mütze U, Nennstiel U, Odenwald B, et al. Sudden neonatal death in individuals with medium-chain acyl-coenzyme A dehydrogenase deficiency: limit of newborn screening. *Eur J Pediatr.* 2022;181:2415–2422.
4. Erickson CC, Salerno JC, Berger S, et al. Section on Cardiology and Cardiac Surgery, Pediatric and Congenital Electrophysiology Society (PACES) Task Force on Prevention of Sudden Death in the Young. Sudden death in the young: information for the primary care provider. *Pediatrics.* 2021;148(1):e2021052044.
5. Zundo K, Richards EA, Ahmed AH, Codington JA. Factors associated with parental compliance with supine infant sleep: an integrative review. *Pediatr Nurs.* 2017;43(2):83–91.
6. Stiffler D, Ayres B, Fauvergue C, Cullen D. Sudden infant death and sleep practices in the Black community. *J Spec Pediatr Nurs.* 2018;23(2):e12213.
7. Isbey SC, Howard MB, Abdulrahman E, Giese K, Cuchara B, Gourishankar A. Characteristics and geographic variation in sudden unexpected infant deaths in the District of Columbia. *Am J Forensic Med Pathol.* 2022 Dec 1;43(4):328–333.
8. Fohner AE, Garrison NA, Austin MA, Burke W. Carnitine palmitoyltransferase 1A P479L and infant death: policy implications of emerging data. *Genet Med.* 2017;19(8):851–857.
9. Horne RC, Ferens D, Watts AM, et al. The prone sleeping position impairs arousability in term infants. *J Pediatr.* 2001;138:811–816.
10. Lee NN, Chan YF, Davies DP, et al. Sudden infant death in Hong Kong: confirmation of low incidence. *Br Med J.* 1989;298:721.
11. Fleming PJ, Gilbert R, Azaz Y, et al. Interaction between bedding and sleeping position in the sudden infant death syndrome: a population-based case-control study. *Br Med J.* 1990;301:85–89.

12. Mitchell EA, Scragg R, Stewart AW, et al. Results from the first year of the New Zealand cot death study. *NZ Med J*. 1991;104:71–76.
13. Dwyer T, Ponsonby A-L, Newman NM, et al. Prospective cohort study of prone sleeping position and sudden infant death syndrome. *Lancet*. 1991;337:1244–1247.
14. Dwyer T, Ponsonby A-L, Newman NM, et al. Prone sleeping position and SIDS: evidence from recent case-control and cohort studies in Tasmania. *J Paediatr Child Health*. 1993;27:340–343.
15. Task AAP. Force on Infant Positioning and SIDS: Positioning and SIDS. *Pediatrics*. 1992;89:1120–1126.
16. Dwyer T, Ponsonby A-L, Blizzard L, et al. The contribution of changes in prevalence of prone sleeping position to the decline in sudden infant death syndrome in Tasmania. *JAMA*. 1995;273:783–789.
17. Gilbert R. The changing epidemiology of SIDS. *Arch Dis Child*. 1994;70:445–449.
18. Mitchell EA, Brunt JM, Everard CM. Reduction in mortality from sudden infant death syndrome in New Zealand: 1986–1992. *Arch Dis Child*. 1994;70:291–294.
19. Ponsonby A-L, Dwyer T, Cooper D. Sleeping position, infant apnea, and cyanosis: a population-based study. *Pediatrics*. 1997;99:e3.
20. Willinger M, Hoffman HJ, Hartford RB. Infant sleep position and risk for sudden infant death syndrome: report of meeting held January 13–14, 1994, *National Institutes of Health*. 93. Bethesda, MD: Pediatrics; 1994:814–820.
21. Task AAP. Force on Infant Positioning and SIDS: Positioning and sudden infant death syndrome (SIDS). *Pediatrics*. 1996;92:1216–1218.
22. Glinge C, Rossetti S, Oestergaard LB, et al. Risk of sudden infant death syndrome among siblings of children who died of sudden infant death syndrome in Denmark. *JAMA Netw Open*. 2023;6:1.
23. Moon RY, Carlin RF, Hand I. Task Force on Sudden Infant Death Syndrome and the Committee on Fetus and Newborn. Evidence base for 2022 updated recommendations for a safe infant sleeping environment to reduce the risk of sleep-related infant deaths. *Pediatrics*. 2022;150(1):e2022057991.
24. Willinger M, Hoffman HJ, Wu K-T, et al. Factors associated with the transition to nonprone sleep positions of infants in the United States. *JAMA*. 1999;280:329–335.
25. Willinger M, Ko C-W, Hoffman HJ, et al. Factors associated with caregiver's choice of infant sleep position: 1994–1998. *JAMA*. 2000;283:2135–2142.
26. Task AAP. Force on Sudden Infant Death Syndrome: The changing concept of sudden infant death syndrome: diagnostic coding shifts, controversies regarding the sleep environment, and new variables to consider in reducing risk. *Pediatrics*. 2005;116:1245–1255.
27. Li DK, Petitti DB, Willinger M, et al. Infant sleeping position and the risk of sudden infant death syndrome in California, 1997–2000. *Am J Epidemiol*. 2003;157:446–455.
28. Paris C, Remler R, Daling JR. Risk factors for sudden infant death syndrome: changes associated with sleep position recommendations. *J Pediatr*. 2001;139:771–777.
29. Persing J, James H, Swanson J, et al. Prevention and management of positional skull deformities in infants. *Pediatrics*. 2003;112:199–202. [Letters to the editor, *Pediatrics* 113:422–424.
30. Graham M, Gomez JM Jr, Halberg A, et al. Management of deformational plagiocephaly: repositioning versus orthotic therapy. *J Pediatr*. 2005;146:258–262.
31. Graham J, Kreutzman JM Jr, Earl D, et al. Deformational brachycephaly in supine-sleeping infants. *J Pediatr*. 2005;146:253–257.
32. Graham JM, Jr. Tummy time is important. *Clin Pediatr*. 2006;45:119–221.
33. Cote A, Gerez T, Brouillette RT, et al. Circumstances leading to a change to prone sleeping in sudden infant death syndrome victims. *Pediatrics*. 2000;106:e86.
34. Hewitt L, Kerr E, Stanley RM, Okely AD. Tummy time and infant health outcomes: a systematic review. *Pediatrics.*. 2020;145:6.
35. Davis BE, Moon RY, Sachs HC, et al. Effects of sleep position on infant motor development. *Pediatrics*. 1998;102:135–140.
36. Schwartz PJ, Stramba-Badiale M, Segantini A, et al. Prolongation of QT interval and the sudden infant death syndrome. *N Engl J Med*. 1998;338:1709–1714.
37. Wilders R. Cardiac ion channelopathies and the sudden infant death syndrome. *ISRN Cardiol*. 2012;846171 https://doi.org/10.5402/2012/846171.
38. Liebrechts-Akkerman G, Liu F, Lao O, et al. *PHOX2B* polyalanine repeat length is associated with sudden infant death syndrome and unclassified sudden infant death in the Dutch population. *Int J Legal Med*. 2014;128:621–629.
39. Task Force on Sudden Infant Death Syndrome Moon RY. SIDS and other sleep-related infant deaths: expansion of recommendations for a safe infant sleeping environment. *Pediatrics*. 2011;128:e1341–e1367.
40. McDonnell-Naughton M, McGarvey C, O'Regan M, et al. Maternal smoking and alcohol consumption during pregnancy as risk factors for sudden infant death. *Ir Med J*. 2012;105:105–108.
41. Hoffend C, Sperhake JP. Sudden unexpected death in infancy in the early neonatal period: the role of bed-sharing. *Forensic Sci Med Pathol*. 2014;10:157–162.
42. Colson ER, Willinger M, Rybin D, et al. Trends and factors associated with infant bed sharing, 1993-2010: the National Infant Sleep Position Study. *JAMA Pediatr*. 2013;167:1032–1037.
43. Vennemann MM, Hense HW, Bajanowski T, et al. Bed sharing and the risk of sudden infant death syndrome: can we resolve the debate? *J Pediatr*. 2012;160:44–48. e2.
44. Sauber-Schatz E.K., Sappenfield W.M., Shapiro-Mendoza C.K. Comprehensive review of sleep-related sudden unexpected infant deaths and their investigations:

Florida 2008, Matern Child Health J June 5, 2014. [Epub ahead of print]

45. Schnitzer PG, Covington TM, Dykstra HK. Sudden unexpected infant deaths: sleep environment and circumstances. *Am J Public Health*. 2012;102:1204–1212.
46. McDonnell E, Moon RY. Infant deaths and injuries associated with wearable blankets, swaddle wraps, and swaddling. *J Pediatr*. 2014;164:1152–1156.
47. Odoi A, Andrew S, Wong FY, et al. Pacifier use does not alter sleep and spontaneous arousal patterns in healthy term-born infants. *Acta Paediatr*. 2014. https://doi.org/10.1111/apa.12790. [Epub ahead of print].
48. Malloy MH. Prematurity and sudden infant death syndrome: United States 2005–2007. *J Perinatol*. 2013;33:470–475.
49. Fyfe KL, Yiallourou SR, Wong FY, et al. Cerebral oxygenation in preterm infants. *Pediatrics*. 2014. pii: peds.2014–0773. [Epub ahead of print].
50. Colvin JD, Collie-Akers V, Schunn C, et al. Sleep environment risks for younger and older infants. *Pediatrics*. 2014;134:e406–e412.
51. Wong F, Yiallourou SR, Odoi A, et al. Cerebrovascular control is altered in healthy term infants when they sleep prone. *Sleep*. 2013;36:1911–1918.
52. Altman M, Edstedt Bonamy AM, Wikström AK, et al. Cause-specific infant mortality in a population-based Swedish study of term and post-term births: the contribution of gestational age and birth weight. *BMJ Open*. 2012;2e001152.
53. Lisonkova S, Hutcheon HA, Joseph KS. Sudden infant death syndrome: a re-examination of temporal trends. *BMC Pregnancy Childbirth*. 2012;12:59.

CHAPTER 27

Positional Brachycephaly

KEY POINTS

- Brachycephaly is defined as a shortened, wide head, often caused by constant supine positioning during infancy.
- Infants should be placed on their backs for sleep but on their stomachs during awake time under adult supervision to encourage neck rotation and motor skills.
- Routine use of repositioning and tummy time during the first 6 weeks and thereafter should prevent brachycephaly.
- The "Back to Sleep" campaign to prevent sudden infant death syndrome (SIDS) has led to a decrease in prone sleeping and a rise in positional head deformities.
- Measuring the cephalic index can help classify the severity and assist with medical decision making regarding the need for cranial orthotic therapy versus monitoring.
- For severe persistent brachycephaly, use of an orthotic helmet will improve the brachycephaly and any associated plagiocephaly.

GENESIS

Brachycephaly translates literally to "short head" and refers to a head that is shortened in the anteroposterior dimension and wide between the biparietal eminences when viewed from above. The most frequent cause of brachycephaly is constant supine positioning during infancy (Fig. 27.1). The increasing prevalence of brachycephaly in recent years is a consequence of the success of efforts to prevent sudden infant death syndrome (SIDS). The "Back to Sleep" campaign was initiated by the American Academy of Pediatrics in June 1992, with the initial recommendation to place infants to sleep on their sides or backs to prevent SIDS. After 1996, the more stringent recommendation for only supine sleep positioning was made because it was recognized that some side-sleeping infants were still dying from SIDS after assuming a prone sleeping position during the night.[1] The end result of this public education effort was a decline in the prevalence of prone sleeping position from 70% in 1992 to 13% in 2004, with a concomitant reduction in the rate of SIDS from 1.2 per 1000 in 1992 to 0.56 per 1000 in 2001 (a decrease of 53% over this 10-year period).[2] Unfortunately, strict supine sleep-positioning campaigns have also increased the rate of positional head deformities by 400–600%.[3] When infants remain in a persistently supine position without any preferential head turn because of torticollis and without the developmental benefits of turning their heads from side to side during regular periods of "tummy time" while awake and under direct adult observation, their heads become progressively flattened through the impact of gravity and persistent occipital mechanical pressure.

A 1995 study of 7609 Dutch infants, who were screened for positional preference before 6 months of age, revealed that 8.6% manifested positional preference with resultant deformational plagiocephaly; an additional 10% manifested occipital flattening, 45% of whom showed persistent asymmetric occipital flattening at 2–3 years of age.[4] Among 181 otherwise normal New Zealand infants whose head shapes were followed at regular intervals from birth through 2 years of age in 2002, the prevalence of plagiocephaly or brachycephaly peaked at 4 months at 20% (associated with male gender, first born, limited neck rotation, and inability of caregivers to vary the infant's head position when putting the infant down to sleep) and then fell to 9% by 8 months of age and 3.3% by 2 years of age. Despite continued advice by family doctors and community child health nurses to encourage neck rotation, tummy time, and repositioning, 33% of the 8-month-old infants with abnormal head shapes were still abnormal at 2 years of age.[5] The supine-sleeping infants in this 2002 cohort were significantly more brachycephalic at

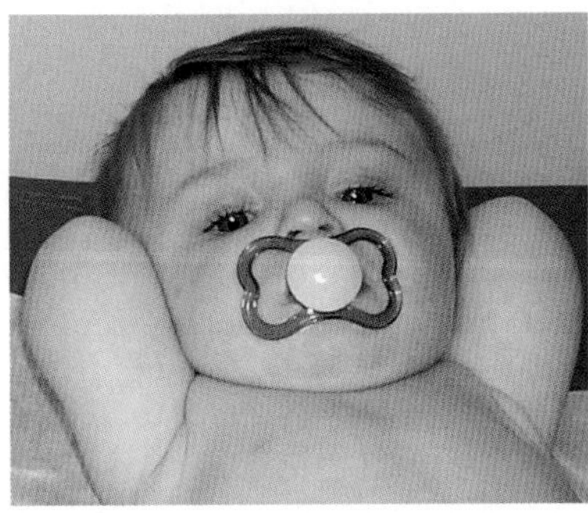
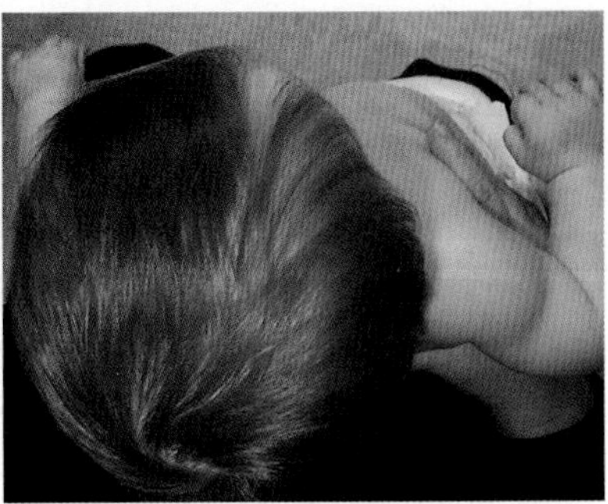

FIGURE 27.1 This 9-month-old boy was one of a set of quadruplets who were delivered close to term, and his position of comfort after birth was with both arms positioned behind his head. Persistent prone positioning resulted in brachycephaly with a cranial index of 98%.

each assessment interval (cephalic index 4–5%), greater than a 1977 cohort of prone-sleeping infants, and these investigators used a cephalic index cutoff of 93% as the point at which the abnormal head shape was obvious. A follow-up study of 129 of these children at 3 and 4 years of age revealed that 61% of abnormal head shapes had reverted to normal, whereas 4% remained severely abnormal at follow-up, with 13% categorized as having poor improvement with continuing parental concern over their child's head shape.[6]

Among 1045 high school students (37% male, 63% female) ranging from 12 to 17 years old (average age, 15.7 years), the prevalence of plagiocephaly was 1.1% and the prevalence of brachycephaly was 1.0%, with an overall prevalence of a deformational cranial abnormality of 2.0%.[7] This study was limited by having fewer males, who are affected more often and more severely, and by assuming helmets were not available before 1998, when they were clearly in use after 1980 (but not regulated by the US Food and Drug Administration). Among the adolescents with plagiocephaly or brachycephaly, 38.1% were noted to have abnormal facial characteristics.[8] Note that Hutchinson found a 4% prevalence of severe brachycephaly or plagiocephaly at 3 and 4 years of age in her longitudinal study that included an excess of males (71% male, 29% female).[6]

Taking all of these data together, it is clear that the "Back to Sleep" campaign has been a major success in reducing the incidence of SIDS by more than 50%, but primary care providers also need to emphasize the importance of tummy time to parents. It is essential to place infants on their backs for sleep, except in cases of prematurity, gastroesophageal reflux, or obstructive sleep apnea. Infants should be placed on their stomachs whenever they are awake and under direct adult supervision so as to develop their prone motor skills and to encourage the full range of neck rotation. The development of positional brachycephaly, with or without plagiocephaly, is an indication that parents may not be providing their infants with adequate tummy time.

FEATURES

Using serial cranial measurements from 401 infants with a normal head shape and more than 2500 infants with positional cranial deformation (with and without helmet therapy), a nomogram was created for craniofacial norms and objective categorization of positional head deformity. Normative percentiles for all dimensions in cranial vault anthropometric measurements during the first year of life have been published.[8] Children with definite nonsynostotic head deformity were allocated into three different groups: positional plagiocephaly (abnormal Cranial Vault Asymmetry Index [CVAI]), positional brachycephaly (abnormal Cranial Index [CI]), and combined positional plagiocephaly and brachycephaly (abnormal CVAI and CI). These indices are calculated from cranial measurements as follows: CI = width/length × 100 and CVAI = (diagonal A − diagonal B)/diagonal A × 100, where diagonal A < diagonal B. A reliable three-level severity categorization (mild, moderate, and severe) for each group of cranial deformation according to age and gender allowed evidence-based classification of nonsynostotic cranial deformity for decision making regarding the need for cranial orthotic therapy.[8]

Normal brain growth combined with a constant supine postnatal resting position can result in progressive cranial widening with occipital flattening (see Fig. 27.1). The malleable neonatal cranium, which arises from within the dura mater surrounding the growing brain, reflects the mechanical interaction between internal brain growth and external deforming forces. Although excessive brachycephaly is considered abnormal today, it may not have been so in the past. The purposeful use of external mechanical forces to deform the shape of an infant's head was practiced by various cultures for thousands of years, and a variety of head shapes were intentionally created using various external shaping devices (Fig. 27.2).[9,10] Six main techniques were used for intentional cranial deformation: manual cranial massage, wooden boards, banding, pads, stones, and cradle boards. Positioning infants in hard wooden cradles may also have unintentionally created brachycephalic heads in some Middle Eastern cultures,[10] and binding an infant's head to a stiff surface has similarly altered head shapes in many primitive cultures throughout the world.[11]

Certain wooden cribs and cradle boards with flat bottoms were particularly likely to deform an infant's head. Other cultures used pads and bindings to create deforming devices made from various materials. In some regions of the world, manual massaging of the infant's head was done to achieve a perfectly round effect. In addition, brachycephaly has a worldwide distribution because of supine positioning on a hard surface. Immobility or cradling also resulted in brachycephaly because many cultures bound their infants in

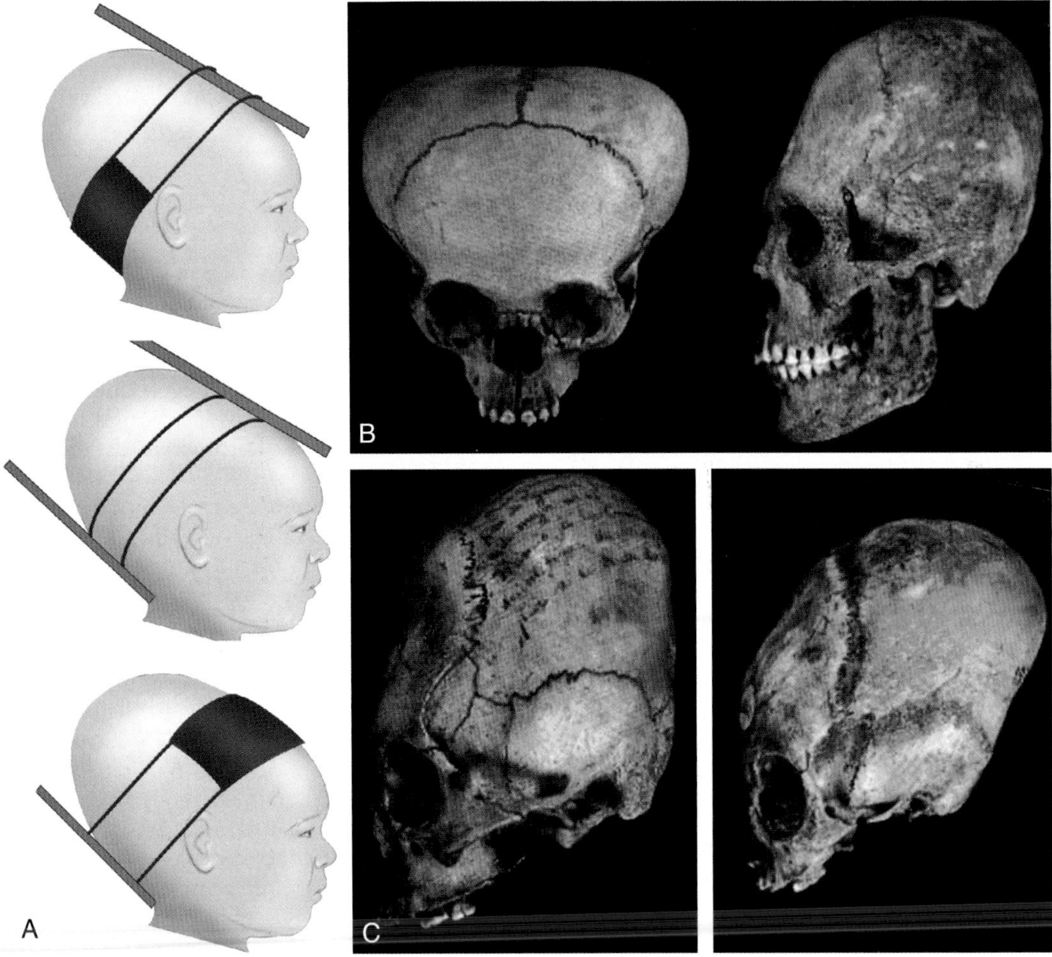

FIGURE 27.2 **A,** A variety of devices used by Peruvian Indians to achieve brachycephalic skull shapes, as demonstrated by adult skulls from these cultures. Highland Peruvians apparently applied circumferential bandages to the calvarium to achieve a conical head shape (**B**), whereas Coastal Peruvians applied boards to the occiput and pads to the frontal region, along with circumferential banding (**C**). (Adapted from Dingwall EJ. *Artificial Cranial Deformation. A Contribution to the Study of Ethnic Mutilation.* London: John Bale, Sons, & Danielson; 1931.)

a supine position. The inability of a swaddled infant to reposition itself, combined with constant supine positioning on a firm surface, often resulted in brachycephaly.[10] Because both unintentional and deliberate cranial deformations persist throughout life, it is essential for pediatricians to recognize the impact of postnatal mechanical forces in shaping infant heads. Primitive practices of head molding from older cultures also provide the basis of current therapy for infants who have developed misshapen heads. The typical brachycephalic head shape is flat in the back and quite wide, with peaking of the vertex. Sometimes the head is so flattened that it is wider than it is long, with a confidence interval greater than 100% in the most severe cases.

Cultures in which infants are placed for sleeping in the supine position have a higher incidence of brachycephaly than do cultures in which infants are placed in the prone position.[11] The confidence interval is 80% for term neonates delivered by cesarean section, which is similar to that of prone-sleeping cultures. The confidence interval during infancy in India (where infants sleep supine) is higher than during later childhood. Of note, child-rearing practices in India promote frequent tummy time when the infant is awake and under observation. Prone-sleeping cultures have a normocephalic confidence interval (mean confidence interval = 80%, with a range from 76% to 81%), whereas school children in Japan and Korea (supine-sleeping cultures) are brachycephalic (85–91%).[11] With the continued success of the "Back to Sleep" campaign, infants will have a more rounded head shape than was seen among cultures that put their infants to sleep on their stomachs. The current normative confidence interval is 86–88%, and it is relatively rare to encounter a case of dolichocephaly among infants who sleep supine unless the infant has sagittal craniosynostosis, a breech head, or congenital hypotonia. In a study of 39 infants with plagiocephaly, 30% of the infants had head widths more than 2 standard deviations above the mean for age, and 4.6% exceeded three standard deviations.[12] The mean confidence interval for these infants was 88.5% (whereas the mean confidence interval for their fathers was 75% and the mean confidence interval for their mothers was 74%), and 14% of the infants had a confidence interval greater than 100%.[12] Thus infants who sleep supine have significantly more brachycephaly than their prone-sleeping parents.

Some parents who become concerned about their infant's positional brachycephaly from prolonged supine positioning consider positioning their infant in a side-sleeping position, which is a dangerous sleep position for SIDS in an infant who has had little or no tummy time. Infants who experience little or no consistent tummy time become very distressed when placed in the prone position, and their parents readily agree that their infant has never tolerated being on their stomach. The best management is to institute regular periods of tummy time beginning in early infancy while the infant is awake and under direct observation.[13]

MANAGEMENT, PROGNOSIS, AND COUNSEL

Because the primary cause of brachycephaly is constant supine positioning, the most important method of treatment is to vary the infant's head position during sleep. Repositioning may be accomplished with the use of an infant-positioning device, and toys and other stimulating objects can be placed in the infant's field of view to encourage them to turn from side to side during sleep. Another essential form of treatment is providing the infant with adequate tummy time each day throughout infancy. Although it is recommended that infants sleep on their backs, placing an infant on their stomach (under adult supervision) is an excellent method to not only prevent cranial flattening but also facilitate good neck muscle rotation and tone while stimulating the development of prone motor skills. Many brachycephalic infants in our clinic were deprived of tummy time by well-meaning parents who followed advice to keep infants on their backs to prevent SIDS. Such infants experienced no periods of regular tummy time and became very distressed when placed in the prone position. The cure is to institute regular periods of tummy time throughout each day, beginning shortly after birth, while the infant is awake and under direct observation.

Among 292 infants at a mean age of 6 months who were treated with cranial orthotic therapy (64 for positional brachycephaly and 248 for posterior positional plagiocephaly), cranial measurements were made before initiation of therapy and at 2-month intervals until the completion of therapy, and statistically significant improvements were seen in all patients. Among 33 infants with brachycephaly (average age 4.6 ± 1.5 months, treated for 4.5 ± 1.5 months) who were treated with orthotics, younger infants improved slightly more than older infants (less than 6 months, the average confidence interval decreased from 94% to 91%; greater than 6 months, the average confidence interval decreased from 92% to 90%). Overall, the children with posterior plagiocephaly normalized their head shapes; however, the head shapes of the children with positional brachycephaly remained slightly brachycephalic despite statistically significant improvements in their confidence interval.[14] Among 92 infants with positional brachycephaly (confidence interval greater than or equal to 90%), 37 were treated with positioning alone at a mean age of 4.5 months for an average of 3.1 months, with improvement in the confidence interval from 94% to 91%. Among the other 55 infants treated with cranial orthotics at a mean age of 5.7 months for an average of 3.9 months, their confidence interval improved from 97.5% to 92%.[11] Among 1206 cases of positional brachycephaly treated with cranial orthotics at a mean age of 5.9 months for an average of 3.3 months, the CI improved from 95% to 89%.[15] Cephalic index improved by 5.9%, 5.5%, and 4.8% in the greater than 3 to less than 6, greater than 6 to less than 9, and greater than 9 to less than 12-month groups, respectively. There was a statistically significant relationship between entrance age and treatment time ($p < .001$), with shorter treatment times at young ages (2.8 months, 3.9 months, and 4.4 months, respectively).[15]

Cranial orthotic therapy has proven to be effective in correcting deformational posterior plagiocephaly, and it has also been used to correct brachycephaly. With extreme occipital flattening, a helmet can often be difficult to fit or require prolonged treatment, thus prevention is of paramount importance. At the first sign of occipital flattening, repositioning and tummy time should be promptly initiated to correct brachycephaly, and routine use of these practices during the first 6 weeks and thereafter should prevent this deformity.[13,16] For those infants who do not make progress with repositioning and tummy time and have severe persistent brachycephaly (confidence interval greater than 90%) at 5 months of age, use of an orthotic helmet will improve the brachycephaly (Fig. 27.3 younger infant; Fig. 27.4 older infant) and any associated plagiocephaly (Fig. 27.5).[11,15] The confidence interval

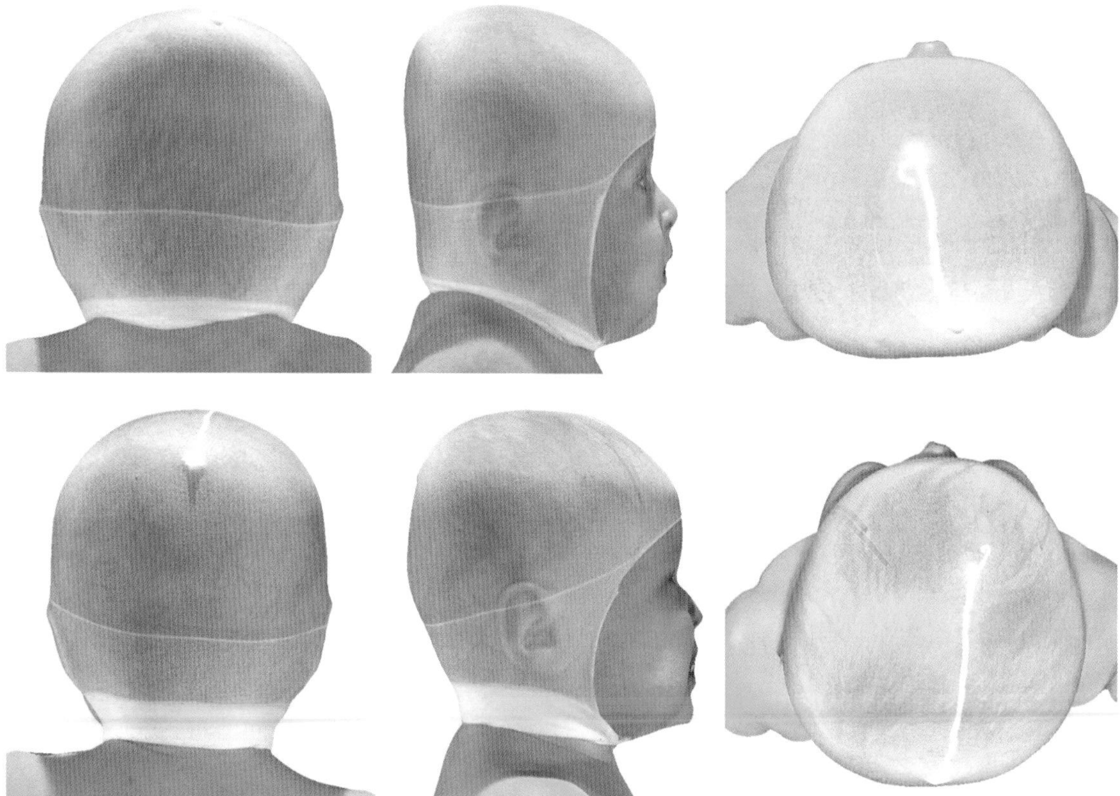

FIGURE 27.3 Positional brachycephaly before treatment and a confidence interval of 109% at age 3 months (*top*), with a confidence interval of 88% at 5 months of age after treatment with a cranial orthotic (*bottom*). (Images provided courtesy of Tim Littlefield MS at Cranial Technologies, Inc.)

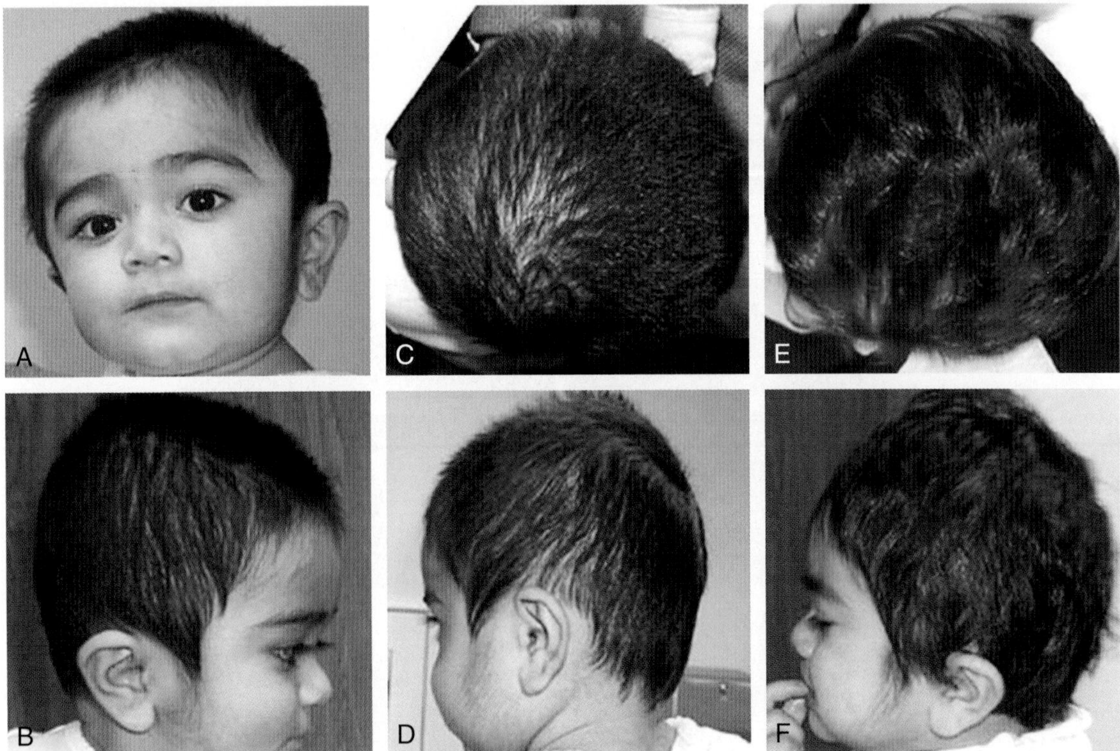

FIGURE 27.4 At 10.5 months, this male infant presented with a confidence interval of 103% (**A–D**). After 5 months of orthotic helmet therapy, his confidence interval was brought into the normal range (**E** and **F**).

cutoff for clinical abnormality in one study was 93%,[5] but attempts to reposition brachycephalic heads after 5 months of age demonstrated only slight improvement in CI;[11] hence significant brachycephaly at 5–6 months of age is likely to persist without cranial orthotic therapy. Reassurance may be appropriate for parents of those infants with a confidence interval less than 90% at 5 months of age because positional brachycephaly is unlikely to develop or worsen after this age.[11] Helmet therapy can remold the infant's head into a more normal, symmetric oval shape, and it has been successfully used to correct infant head shapes for more than 35 years. The prominent lateral parts of the infant's head are restrained from becoming any wider while normal brain growth provides the corrective mechanical anteroposterior forces from within the calvarium to round out the shallow or flattened regions. Positional brachycephaly and plagiocephaly persist without early treatment (see Figs. 25.12 and 27.6), and this can result a head shape that is dramatically different from either parent (Fig. 27.7). As shown in Fig. 27.8, cranial orthotic therapy for deformational brachycephaly at 3–6 months is more effective and takes a shorter treatment time than treatment at 9–12 months, but even at older ages, cranial orthotic therapy can result in significant improvement (see Fig. 27.4).

DIFFERENTIAL DIAGNOSIS

Brachycephaly can be associated with bilateral coronal craniosynostosis, and cranial orthotic therapy after corrective surgery can be helpful in directing head growth into a more optimal shape. Some surgical techniques for bicoronal synostosis actually duplicate the mechanical effects of helmet molding by surgically producing transverse tension across the skull and letting it expand anteriorly through a superiorly hinged fronto-orbital flap and expand posteriorly via an inferiorly based occipital flap. This may be particularly useful for genetic types of bicoronal synostoses with defective fibroblast growth factor receptor responses.[17,18] It is important to distinguish deformational brachycephaly from bilateral coronal

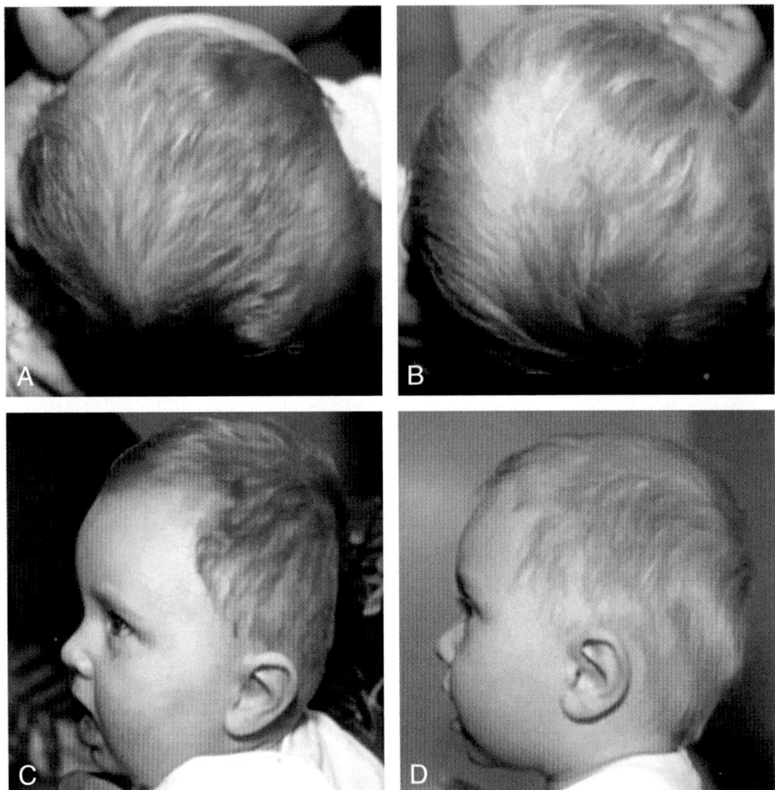

FIGURE 27.5 A, B, This 7-month-old male infant with right torticollis had a cephalic index of 93% with a diagonal difference (DD) of 1.5 cm. **C, D,** After 5 months of helmet orthotic therapy, his confidence interval was improved to 91% and his DD was reduced to 0.5 cm.

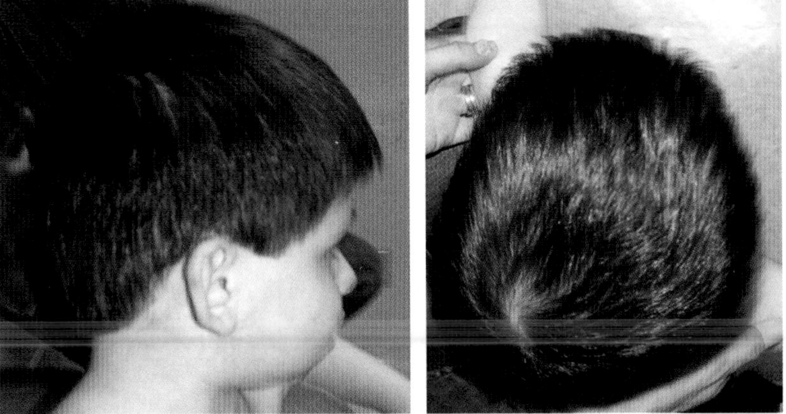

FIGURE 27.6 This child was adopted from a Russian orphanage where brachycephalic plagiocephaly was not managed, resulting in a 95% confidence interval and 1-cm diagonal difference at 18 months of age.

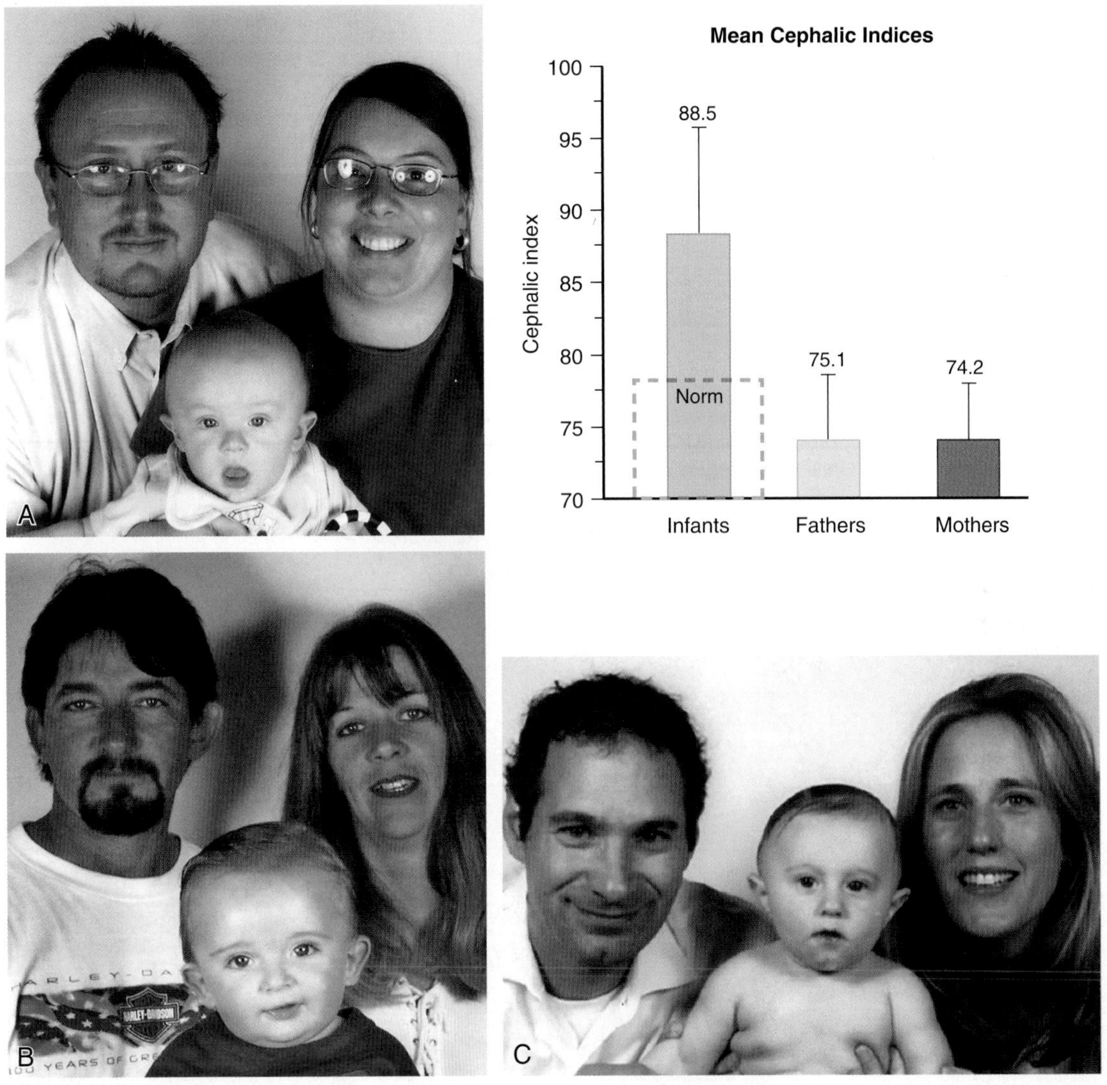

FIGURE 27.7 These infants with brachycephalic plagiocephaly had a confidence interval that was dramatically different from that of their parents. (Adapted from Pomatto JK, Littlefield TR, Calcaterra J, et al. A study of family head shape: environment alters cranial shape. *Clin Pediatr*. 2006;45:55-63.)

craniosynostosis because therapy and management are very different for each condition. It is also important to note that brachycephaly may be associated with various syndromes that increase pliability of the infant skull through calvarial demineralization or increase an infant's tendency to remain recumbent for prolonged periods of time. Thus conditions associated with skull demineralization, such as osteogenesis imperfecta or hypophosphatasia, can lead to deformational brachycephaly because the cranium is much more malleable (Fig. 27.9). Conditions resulting in congenital hypotonia, such as Down syndrome, can also lead to brachycephaly, as do conditions associated with limited neck mobility, such as Klippel-Feil sequence (see Fig. 24.9).

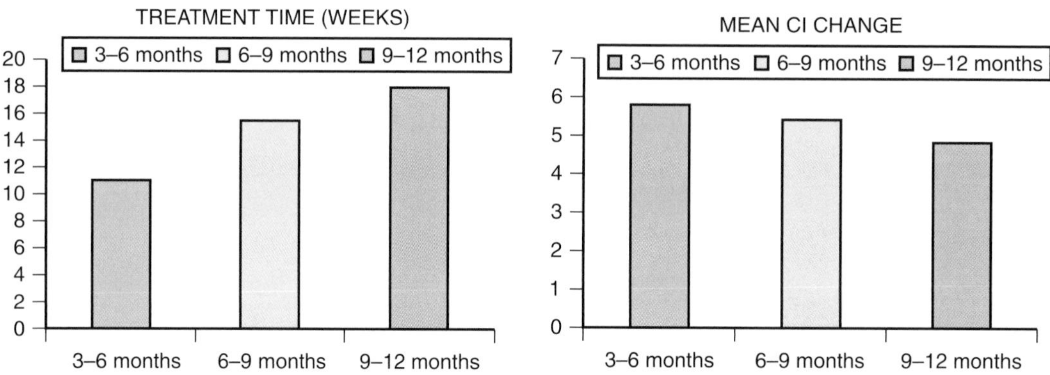

FIGURE 27.8 In a study of 1206 infants with an average confidence interval of 95%, infants treated at a younger age with cranial orthotic therapy had a greater improvement and a shorter treatment time than infants treated at older ages. (Adapted from data provided by Tim Littlefield of Cranial Technologies.)

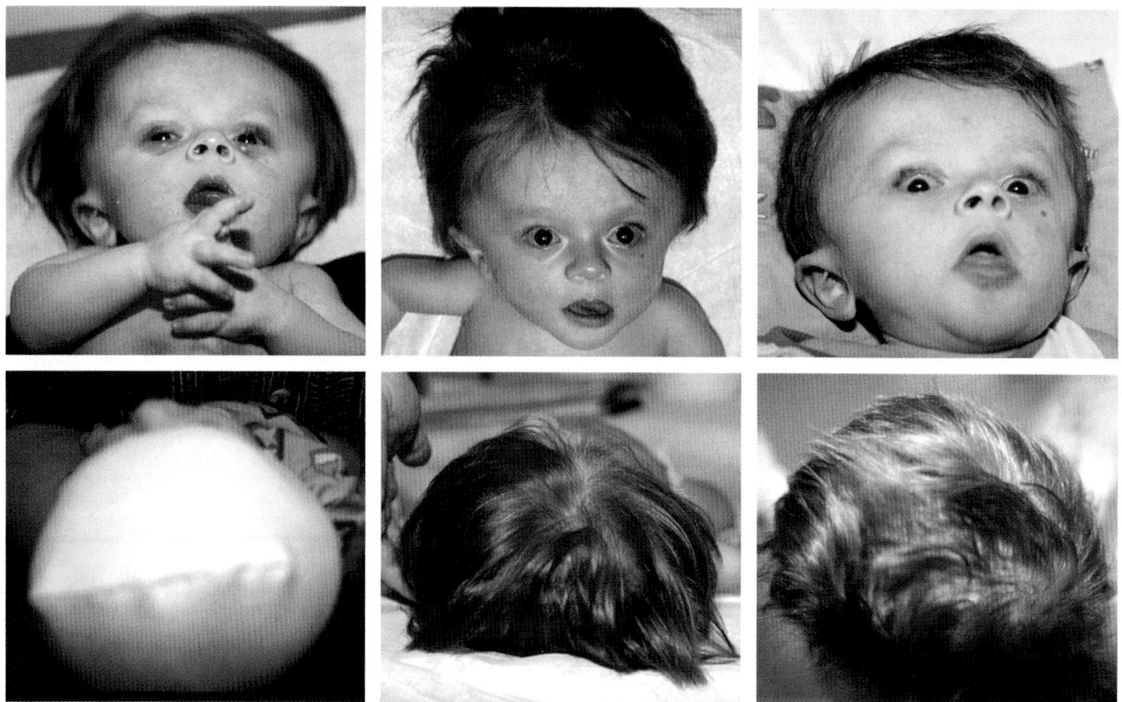

FIGURE 27.9 Severe brachycephaly in an infant with osteogenesis imperfecta type III and associated communicating hydrocephalus. The infant was first treated at age 11 months, and over the course of the next year his neurologic state improved after initiation of helmet therapy.

References

1. Task AAP. Force on Infant Positioning and SIDS. Positioning and sudden infant death syndrome (SIDS). *Pediatrics*. 1996;92:1216–1218.
2. Task AAP. Force on Sudden Infant Death Syndrome. The changing concept of sudden infant death syndrome: diagnostic coding shifts, controversies regarding the sleep environment, and new variables to consider in reducing risk. *Pediatrics*. 2005;116:1245–1255.
3. Marshall JM, Shahzad F. Safe sleep, plagiocephaly, and brachycephaly: assessment, risks, treatment, and when to refer. *Pediatr Ann*. 2020;49(10):e440–e447.

4. Boere-Boonekamp MM, van der Linden-Kuiper LT. Positional preference: prevalence in infants and follow-up after two years. *Pediatrics*. 2001;107:339–343.
5. Hutchinson BL, Hutchinson LA, Thompson JM, et al. Plagiocephaly and brachycephaly in the first two years of life: a prospective cohort study. *Pediatrics*. 2004;114:970–980.
6. Hutchison BL, Stewart AW, Mitchell EA. Deformational plagiocephaly: a follow-up of head shape, parental concern and neurodevelopment at ages 3 and 4 years. *Arch Dis Child*. 2011;96:85–90.
7. Roby BB, Finkelstein M, Tibesar RJ, Sidman JD. Prevalence of positional plagiocephaly in teens born after the "Back to Sleep" campaign. Otolaryngol Head Neck Surg. 2012 May;146(5):823-8.
8. Wilbrand JF, Schmidtberg K, Bierther U, et al. Clinical classification of infant nonsynostotic cranial deformity. *J Pediatr*. 2012;161:1120–1125.
9. Dingwall EJ. *Artificial cranial deformation*. London: John Bale, Sons, & Danielson; 1931.
10. Ewing JF. *Hyperbrachycephaly as influenced by cultural conditioning. Papers of the Peabody Museum of American Archaeology & Ethnology*. vol. XXIII. Cambridge, MA: Harvard University; 1950.
11. Graham JM Jr, Kreutzman J, Earl D, et al. Deformational brachycephaly in supine-sleeping infants. *J Pediatr*. 2005;146:253–257.
12. Pomatto JK, Littlefield TR, Calcaterra J, et al. A study of family head shape: environment alters cranial shape. *Clin Pediatr*. 2006;45:55–63.
13. Graham JM Jr. Tummy time is important. *Clin Pediatr*. 2006;45:119–122.
14. Teichgraeber JF, Seymour-Dempsey K, Baumgartner JE, et al. Molding helmet therapy in the treatment of brachycephaly and plagiocephaly. *J Craniofac Surg*. 2004;15:118–123.
15. Kelly KM, Joganic E, Beals SP, Riggs JA, McGuire MK, Littlefield TR. A Prospective study of cranial orthotic treatment of infants with isolated deformational brachycephaly. Canadian prosthetics & orthotics journal, Volume 1, issue 2, 2018; Abstract, oral presentation at the Aopa's 101st National Assembly, Sept. 26-29, Vancouver, canada, 2018. https://doi.org/10.33137/cpoj.v1i2.32024.
16. Graham JM Jr, Gomez M, Halberg A, et al. Management of deformational plagiocephaly: repositioning versus orthotic therapy. *J Pediatr*. 2005;146:258–262.
17. Lauritzen C, Friede H, Elander A, et al. Dynamic cranioplasty for brachycephaly. *Plast Reconstr Surg*. 2006;98:7–14.
18. Guimaraes-Ferreira J, Gewall F, Sahlin P, et al. Dynamic cranioplasty for brachycephaly in Apert syndrome: long-term follow-up study. *J Neurosurg*. 2001;94:757–764.

CHAPTER 28

Other Postnatal Head Deformations

KEY POINTS

- Premature infants and infants with a neurologic deficiency who are unable to change position are at high risk of head shape abnormalities.
- Intubation and major surgical procedures can reduce repositioning efforts, monitoring, and routine care. Severe plagiocephaly at discharge is predictive of persistent deformation.
- Flattening on both sides of the head can result in a narrow, dolichocephalic head shape that may persist into adulthood.
- Careful positioning on water-filled cushions or pressure-relief mattresses can minimize the risk of deformation.
- Measuring the cephalic index and cranial vault asymmetry index can help classify the severity and assist with medical decision making and use of cranial orthotics.
- Refer to a specialist with expertise in craniofacial malformations in severe cases or if there is suspicion of premature suture fusion.

PREMATURE INFANT

The liability toward cranial deformation depends on the magnitude and duration of the forces applied and the pliability of the fetus. The prematurely born infant is more malleable than the term baby, and before the "Back to Sleep" campaign, postnatal cranial deformation was primarily a problem of premature infants, resulting in lasting parental concerns.[1,2] The premature infant is less active and more likely to persistently lie in one position, and if the surface on which the infant lies is relatively firm, often the premature infant will develop flattening on both sides of the head, resulting in a dolichocephalic, narrow head shape (Figs. 28.1 and 28.2). This head shape can persist into adulthood and inhibit parental attachment and bonding in some cases,[1-4] and it can be avoided by placing premature infants on pressure-relief mattresses or waterbeds to prevent adverse molding.[2,5,6] Early studies documented that preterm infants in prone position with resultant lateral flattening had more dolichocephaly than term infants.[7] Because infants were positioned on their backs to prevent sudden infant death syndrome in 1994, the incidence of dolichocephaly related to prematurity has markedly decreased, but other unusual head shapes have occurred, such as plagiocephaly in infants with torticollis, oxycephaly in infants with persistent vertex molding, and brachycephaly in infants with constant supine positioning. The risk for such deformations in prematurely born infants can be minimized to some extent by careful positioning of premature infants on water-filled cushions or pressure-relief mattresses rather than the relatively firm surfaces in standard incubators.[2,5,6]

Developmental care of prematurely born infants has become standard in today's modern neonatal intensive care units, in which skilled nurses rotate the infant's head position on a regular basis, especially for those neonates who cannot do so themselves.[7] Without such changes in resting position, the premature baby may lie persistently on one side of the head and develop plagiocephaly as a result. This is particularly likely to occur in premature infants who undergo surgical procedures that limit their opportunities for repositioning or in neurologically damaged infants. Obviously, gentle physical therapy and repositioning can help prevent some postnatal deformations in premature infants, but continued vigilance is necessary. There are a growing number of supporting devices for premature infants in the neonatal intensive care unit (NICU). Prone and side-lying positions, as well as supported sitting positions, have been found to have had some beneficial impact on a premature infant's physiological and developmental outcome.[8]

The cranial vault asymmetry index (CVAI) and cranial index (CI) were both calculated from routine head scans with a laser scanner and categorized in 195 infants for three different groups of gestational age. Most very preterm (73%) and some late preterm (28%) infants had dolichocephaly, compared with term babies (11%), at term equivalent age (TEA). The CI was lowest in very (71.4%) and late (77.2%) preterm infants compared with term infants (80.0%), reflecting more extreme dolichocephaly in very early preterm infants at TEA. The prevalence of deformational plagiocephaly was 38% in very preterm infants, and CVAI

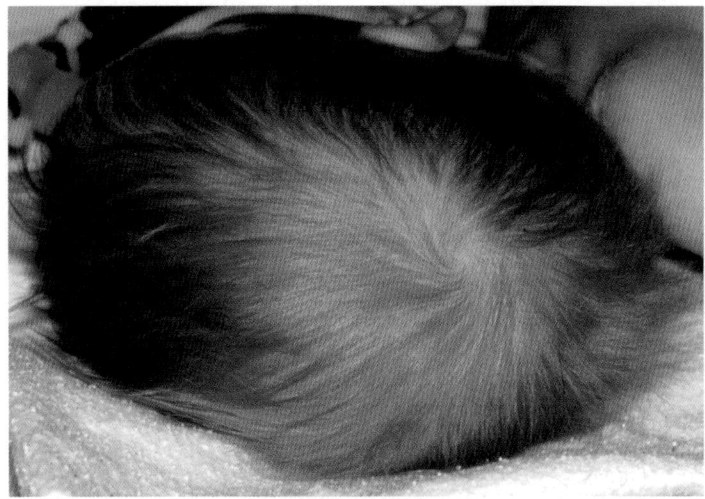

FIGURE 28.1 This is a fairly typical premature infant head shape from 30 years ago, long and narrow, with a cranial index less than 76%.

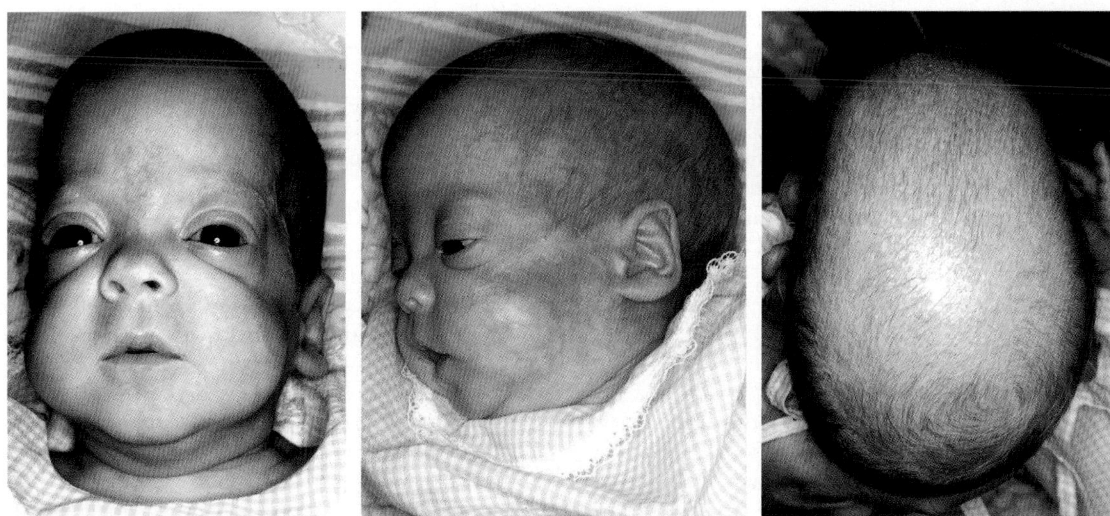

FIGURE 28.2 This infant was born prematurely at 28 weeks and positioned on the sides of her head for most of her first few months because of the need for respiratory therapy and venous access. As she rested on one side or the other, her head became progressively more dolichocephalic, with frontal bossing. As her head became longer and narrower, she lacked sufficient neck strength to rest on her occiput without a positioning ring. This is about as close as infants come today to a true premature infant head shape.

at TEA was higher in very preterm compared with term and late preterm infants, reflecting more head asymmetry in very preterm infants at TEA.[9] To quantify the course of cranial symmetry at corrected age 6 months, 56 infants born at less than 32 gestational weeks were examined at discharge and corrected age 3 and 6 months. Cranial proportion and symmetry were quantified using a three-dimensional laser scanner and classified using age-related reference values. The prevalence of dolichocephaly was highest at discharge (77%) and subsequently decreased, whereas the prevalence of plagiocephaly was 34% at discharge, 46% at 3 months, and 27% at 6 months corrected age. CI was 71.4% at discharge and improved over the examination period. Severe plagiocephaly at discharge was predictive of persistent deformation, whereas 46% of infants without plagiocephaly at discharge developed it by 6 months corrected age.[10] Among 192 infants born at a gestational age 32 weeks or less, the prevalence of a positional preference of the head at TEA was 44.8%, and 10.4% had a plagiocephaly at TEA, whereas 13% had plagiocephaly at 6 months corrected age. Gross motor maturity at 6 months was less developed in infants with a positional preference at TEA compared with preterm norms. This high prevalence of a positional preference in infants born preterm at TEA requires extra alertness to prevent the development of plagiocephaly, especially in boys and twins.[11]

It has been noted that premature infants with deformational plagiocephaly required longer durations of head orthosis therapy to achieve a similar degree of cranial symmetry compared to full-term infants with the same condition. Additionally, premature infants demonstrated a slower rate of cranial growth during the treatment period, and therefore prematurity should be taken into account when planning treatment for infants with deformational plagiocephaly, as it can impact the duration and effectiveness of head orthosis therapy.[12]

FULL-TERM INFANT

Pediatricians must be able to properly differentiate infants with benign skull deformities from those with craniosynostosis, educate parents on methods to proactively decrease the likelihood of the development of occipital flattening, initiate appropriate management, and make appropriate referrals when necessary. A 2011 report from the American Academy of Pediatrics Committee on Practice and Ambulatory Medicine and the section on neurological surgery provides guidance for the prevention, diagnosis, and management of positional skull deformity in an otherwise normal infant without evidence of associated anomalies, syndromes, or spinal disease.[11] Cranial orthotics should be reserved for severe cases of deformity or for the infant with significant torticollis whose deformity does not improve after 6 months of age. Referral to a specialist with expertise in craniofacial malformations should be considered if there is progression or lack of improvement after a trial of repositioning or any suspicion of craniosynostosis. There is one case report of a preterm infant at 29 weeks of gestation who gradually developed a Chiari I malformation (acquired tonsillar herniation through the foramen magnum) with hydrocephalus and premature unilateral fusion of the posterior intraoccipital synchondrosis. Brain ultrasonography was initially normal, but follow-up ultrasonography showed the progressive development of hydrocephalus, and brain magnetic resonance imaging demonstrated the presence of a tonsillar ectopia and a deformation of the occipital bone. A computed tomography scan confirmed closure of the right posterior intraoccipital synchondrosis, resulting in a deformation of the posterior cranial fossa and demonstrating the close relationship between a malformation of the skull base and Chiari I malformation.[13]

A term infant with a neurologic deficiency or who is unable to change positions or is neglected may tend to lie in one position and may develop asymmetric flattening on one side of the head (Fig. 28.3). Thumb sucking seldom causes deformation in early infancy; however once the teeth have developed, thumb sucking can deform the upper jaw. This is especially true when the child "pulls out" on the teeth. Growth of the mandible tends to catch up to that of the maxilla during the first few years, and the mandibular teeth normally conform to the maxillary teeth. Supernumerary teeth or the absence of teeth can lead to mild deformation, including malocclusions between the maxilla and mandible. Nowhere have the principles of mechanical treatment been more effectively used than in the mouth. Once the teeth have fully erupted, they may be used as anchors for a variety of devices to alter the growth and/or alignment of the maxilla, mandible, or both. Intraoral devices that provide rather small pressures on developing teeth can have a considerable effect on form. In India, mothers often massage infants' alveolae in an effort to help align the unerupted teeth buds into an even row. Current anthropologic data also indicate

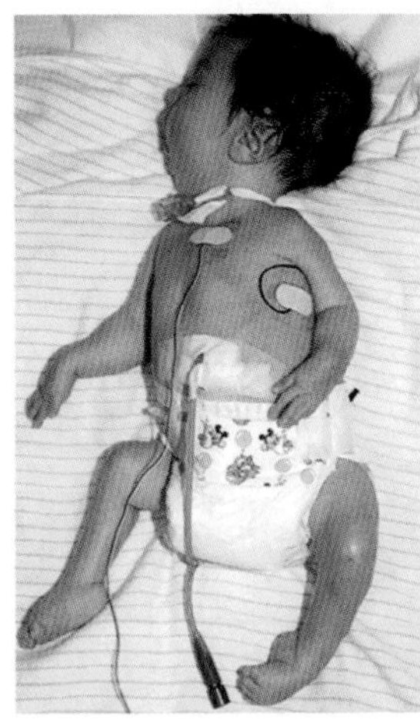
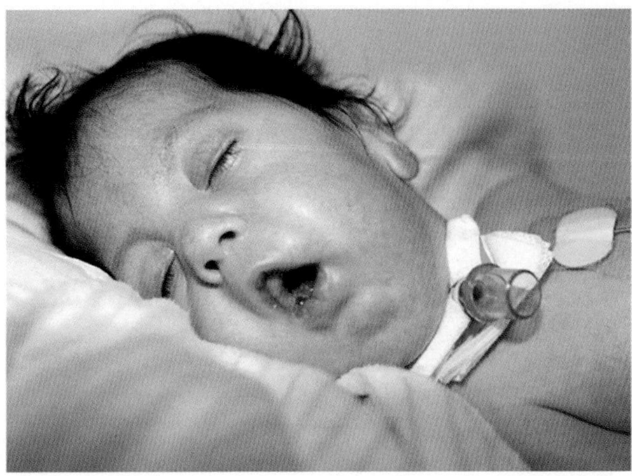

FIGURE 28.3 This infant was born with profound congenital hypotonia of undetermined etiology. The head is turned on one side or the other and has become progressively flattened because of the infant's inability to move. This infant is at risk for idiopathic infantile scoliosis with inability to suck or swallow; prominent lateral palatine ridges because of lack of tongue movement; inability to control secretions, necessitating tracheostomy; and a poor long-term prognosis.

that infant head molding, through the application of pressure or bindings to the cranial bones to alter their shapes, is still prevalent among certain Caribbean, Latino, European, African-American, Asian, and Native American groups.[14] The use of cranial orthotics to correct aberrant head shapes is discussed in Chapters 25 and 27.

References

1. Budreau G. Postnatal cranial molding and infant attractiveness: implications for nursing. *Neonat Netw*. 1987;4:13–19.
2. Chan J, Kelley M, Khan J. The effects of pressure relief mattress on postnatal head molding in very low birth weight infants. *Neonat Netw*. 1993;12:19–22.
3. Chan J, Kelley M, Khan J. Predictors of postnatal head molding in very low birth weight infants. *Neonat Netw*. 1995;14:47–52.
4. Baum J, Searls D. Head shape and size of preterm low-birth-weight infants. *Dev Med Child Neurol*. 1971;13:576–581.
5. Hemingway MM, Oliver SK. Waterbed therapy and cranial molding of the sick preterm infant. *Neonat Netw*. 1991;10:53–56.
6. Schwirian PM, Eesley T, Cuellar L. Use of water pillows in reducing head shape distortion in preterm infants. *Res Nurs Health*. 1986;9:203–207.
7. Largo RN, Duc G. Head growth changes in head configuration in healthy preterm and term infants during the first six months of life. *Helv Paediatr Acta*. 1977;32:431–442.
8. Yang L, Fu H, Zhang L. A systematic review of improved positions and supporting devices for premature infants in the NICU. *Heliyon*. 2023;9(3):e14388.
9. Ifflaender S, Rüdiger M, Konstantelos D, et al. Prevalence of head deformities in preterm infants at term equivalent age. *Early Hum Dev*. 2013;89:1041–1047.
10. Ifflaender S, Rüdiger M, Konstantelos D, et al. Individual course of cranial symmetry and proportion in preterm infants up to 6 months of corrected age. *Early Hum Dev*. 2014;90:511–515.
11. Nuysink J, van Haastert IC, Eijsermans MJ, et al. Prevalence and predictors of idiopathic asymmetry in infants born preterm. *Early Hum Dev*. 2013;88:387–392.
12. Yang L, Fu H, Zhang L. A systematic review of improved positions and supporting devices for premature infants in the NICU. *Heliyon*. 2023;9(3):e14388.
13. Laughlin J, Luerssen TG, Dias MS. the Committee on Practice and Ambulatory Medicine, Section on Neurological Surgery: Prevention and management of positional skull deformities in infants. *Pediatrics*. 2011;128:1236.
14. Kanavaki A, Jenny B, Hanquinet S. Chiari I malformation associated with premature unilateral closure of the posterior intraoccipital synchondrosis in a preterm infant. *J Neurosurg Pediatr*. 2013;11:658–660.

Section VIII
Craniosynostosis

CHAPTER 29

Craniosynostosis

General

KEY POINTS

- Differentiating between craniosynostosis and primary cranial deformation is critical to determining the proper mode of treatment.
- It is important for pediatric and primary care providers to know the normal range and timing of fontanel and cranial suture closure.
- Craniosynostosis can occur due to prenatal limitation of normal growth stretch across a suture during late fetal life or a deficit in brain growth, among other causes.
- Mild craniostenosis may not require surgery, but early surgery may be necessary to restore normal craniofacial shape and growth and reduce complications associated with increased intracranial pressure.
- Various neurosurgical techniques exist for treating craniosynostosis, including partial calvarectomy and endoscopic repair.
- Many syndromic disorders associated with craniosynostosis are genetically determined and can be diagnosed through mutational analysis and/or chromosome microarray.
- Early rickets, hyperthyroidism, hypercalcemia, storage disorders, and hematologic disorders can also cause craniosynostosis.

GENESIS

The term *craniostenosis* (literally translating as "cranial narrowing") is used to describe the abnormal head shape that results from premature fusion of one or more sutures, whereas *craniosynostosis* is the process of premature sutural fusion that results in craniostenosis. The term *craniosynostosis* is used more widely, perhaps in an effort to distinguish deformational nonsynostotic head shapes from those caused by underlying sutural synostosis, but the two terms can be used interchangeably. Plagiocephaly is a nonspecific term used to describe an asymmetric head shape that can result from either craniosynostosis or cranial deformation, and differentiation between these two processes is critical to determining the proper mode of treatment (i.e., surgery versus physical techniques). Synostotic plagiocephaly is usually corrected by a neurosurgical procedure, whereas deformational plagiocephaly responds to early physical therapy, repositioning, and cranial orthotic therapy if these early measures are unsuccessful.

General pediatricians often refer patients for a concern of craniosynostosis when they cannot detect the anterior fontanel or when there is concern for an abnormal head shape with subtle sutural ridging. On average, the anterior fontanel closes at 1 year ± 4 months, the posterior fontanel closes at birth ± 2 months, and the metopic suture by 6 months ± 3 months (10% of adults have an open metopic suture).[1,2] Clinical closure of sutures is perceived at 6–12 months of age and anatomic closure of sutures by 30th year. In a study of normal infants followed from birth to 24 months, the anterior fontanel was closed in 11% at 3 months of age, 32% at 6 months, 56% at 9 months, 81% at 12 months, 96% at 18 months, and 100% by 24 months (Fig. 29.1).[2]

In an otherwise normal fetus, prenatal limitation of normal growth stretch across a suture during late fetal life can result in craniosynostosis (Fig. 29.2). Craniosynostosis can also occur when the lack of growth stretch is caused by a deficit in brain growth, as in severe primary microcephaly. Experimental prolongation of gestation, which resulted in fetal crowding after installation of a cervical clip in pregnant mice, has been shown to lead to craniosynostosis.[3] The frequency of craniosynostosis was greatest among mouse

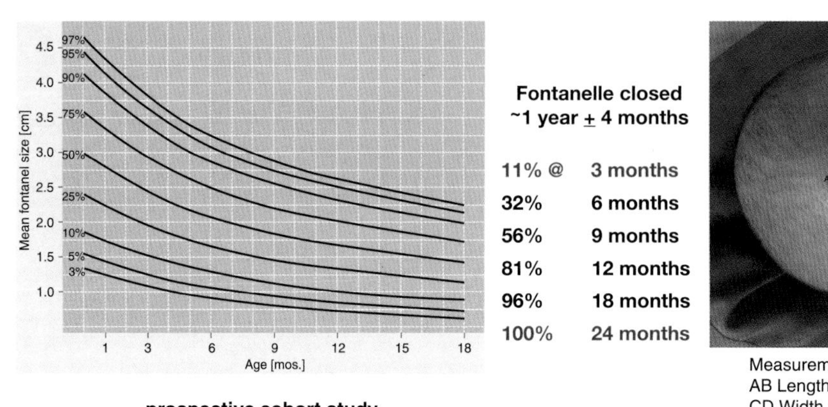

FIGURE 29.1 Growth chart of the mean fontanel size of healthy term babies (by age) (Left). Table of the percent of infants and children with a closed anterior fontanel (by age) (Center). Method to calculate mean fontanel size (Right). (Adapted from Boran P, Oğuz F, Furman A, Sakarya S. Evaluation of fontanel size variation and closure time in children followed up from birth to 24 months. *J Neurosurg Pediatr.* 2018;22:323–329.)

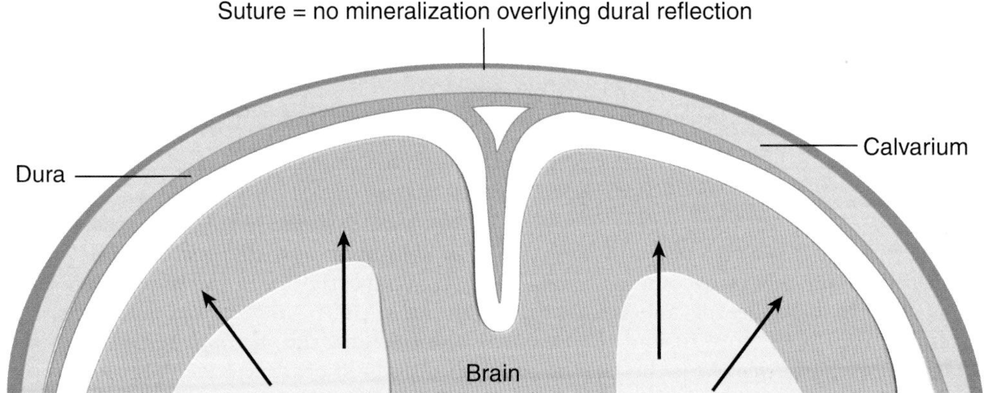

FIGURE 29.2 As long as there is continued growth stretch from the expanding brain, the sites over the dural reflections remain unossified, thereby forming the sutures.

fetuses located proximally in the uterine horns, where the crowding was most severe. The most common cause of craniosynostosis in an otherwise normal infant is constraint of the fetal head in utero.[4-9] Factors influencing fetal head constraint can include multiple gestation, macrosomia, oligohydramnios, primigravida, and maternal uterine malformations.[10,11] When external fetal head constraint limits growth stretch across a cranial sutural area between the constraining points, it may lead to craniosynostosis of an intervening suture (see Fig. 29.2). With sagittal craniosynostosis (the most common type), this event usually occurs in an otherwise normal child. The constrained suture tends to develop a bony ridge, especially at the point of maximum constraint between the biparietal eminences. Such ridging can easily be palpated or visualized on skull radiographs, and three-dimensional cranial computed tomography (3D-CT) allows the ridge to be seen even more clearly.

In general, craniosynostosis begins at one point and then spreads along a suture.[8,12] At the center of the fused suture, there is complete sutural obliteration with nonlamellar bone extending completely across the sutural space, while further away from the initial site of fusion, the sutural margins are closely approximated with ossifying connective tissue. The longer the time before the craniosynostosis is surgically corrected, the greater the tendency for more of the suture

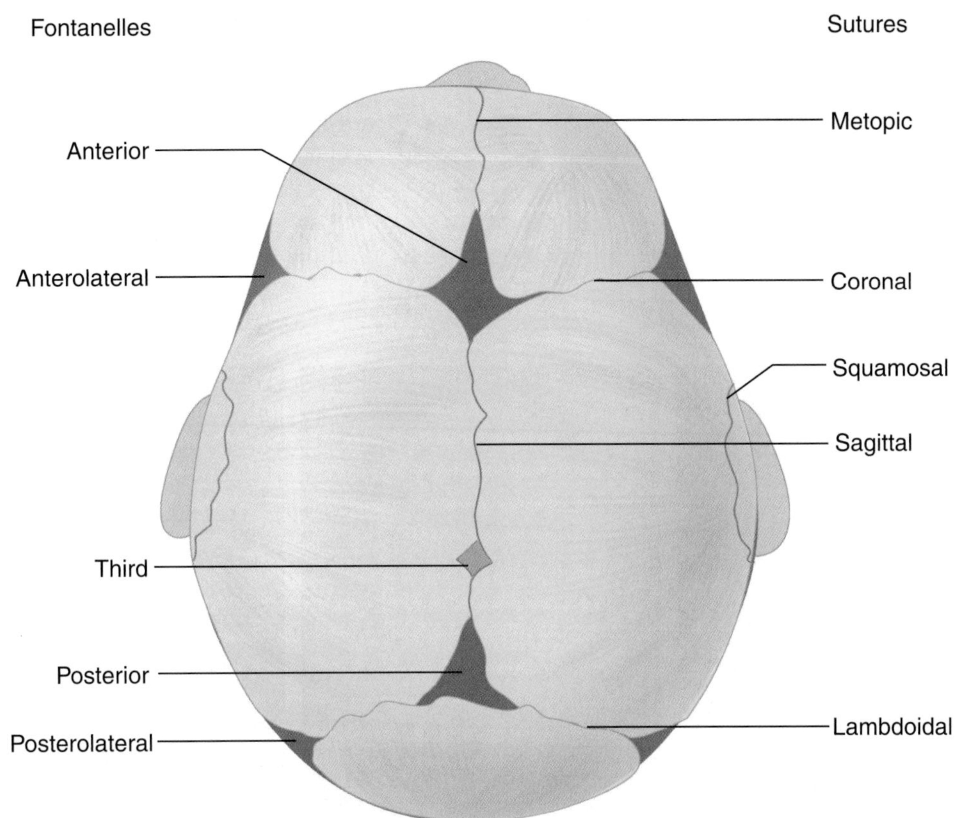

FIGURE 29.3 Diagram showing the named cranial sutures and fontanelles.

to become synostotic, with synostosis beginning at only one location in most cases.[6] Pronounced sutural ridging tends to occur primarily over midline end-to-end sutures (i.e., in sagittal and metopic synostosis). Ridging also occurs with coronal and lambdoidal synostosis, but it may be less prominent than that seen with synostotic midline end-to-end sutures. Synostosis prevents future expansion at that site, and the rapidly growing brain then distorts the calvarium into an aberrant shape, depending on which sutures have become synostotic. The various sutures and fontanels are shown in Fig. 29.3, and the specific head shapes that result from each type of sutural fusion are shown in Figs. 29.4 and 29.5. The earlier the synostosis takes place, the greater the effect on skull shape, but the precise mechanisms that lead to sutural synostosis are heterogeneous and incompletely understood. For example, craniosynostosis may result from mutant gene function, storage disorders, hyperthyroidism, or failure of normal brain growth. The topic of craniosynostosis has been comprehensively reviewed by Cohen and MacLean.[12] Molecular characterization of a large cohort of patients evaluated at a single center is summarized by Wilkie et al.[13] Although many patients with a genetically determined cause harbor a variant in one of just seven genes (EFNB1, ERF, FGFR2, FGFR3, SMAD6, TCF12, and TWIST1), over 60 genes are known to be recurrently mutated and often impact the FGF/MAPK, BMP, Wnt, hedgehog, retinoic acid, STAT, and ephrin signaling pathways.[14,15] Chromosomal aberrations (mostly microdeletions) account for about 6.7–40% of cases of syndromic craniosynostoses and often present with premature fusion of metopic or sagittal sutures plus additional clinical findings.[16]

The frequency of craniosynostosis is 1 per 2000–2500 live births, and it is usually an isolated, sporadic anomaly in an otherwise normal child. Most cases, approximately 73–85%, are isolated and nonsyndromic, while the other 15–27% are recognized as part of an underlying syndrome or are suspected to be syndromic.[14,17,18] About 8–15% of all craniosynostosis

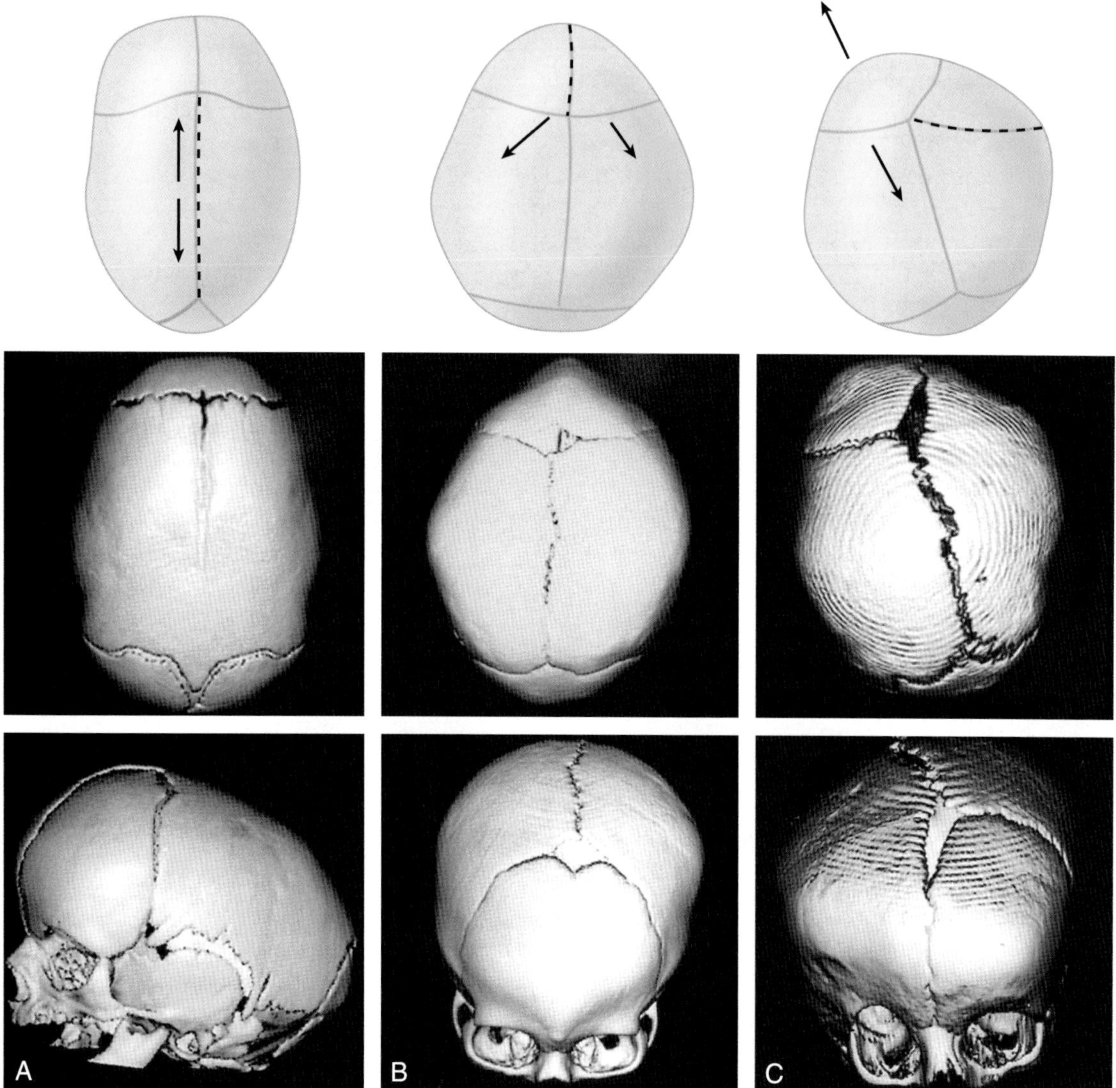

FIGURE 29.4 Diagrams and three-dimensional cranial computed tomography scans depicting sagittal (A), metopic (B), and right coronal (C) synostosis.

cases are familial.[19,20] Familial types of craniosynostosis occur most frequently in coronal synostosis and account for 14.4–22.2% of coronal synostosis, 4–8% of sagittal synostosis, and 5–12.7% of metopic synostosis.[20-23] Lambdoidal synostosis is almost never familial but has been reported.[24] The frequency of associated twinning is increased and most twin pairs are discordant, especially in sagittal and metopic synostosis; this would tend to support fetal crowding as a cause of these types of synostosis, whereas concordance for coronal synostosis is much higher for monozygotic twins than for dizygotic twins.[12] In 2014, Greenwood et al. reported on 660 mutation-negative nonsyndromic craniosynostosis cases and found that the incidence rate for first-degree relatives of probands was 6.4% for metopic, 4.9% for complex craniosynostosis, 3.8% for sagittal, 3.9% for lambdoid, and 0.7% for coronal cases.[19] Familial craniosynostosis is usually transmitted as an autosomal dominant trait with incomplete penetrance and variable expressivity.

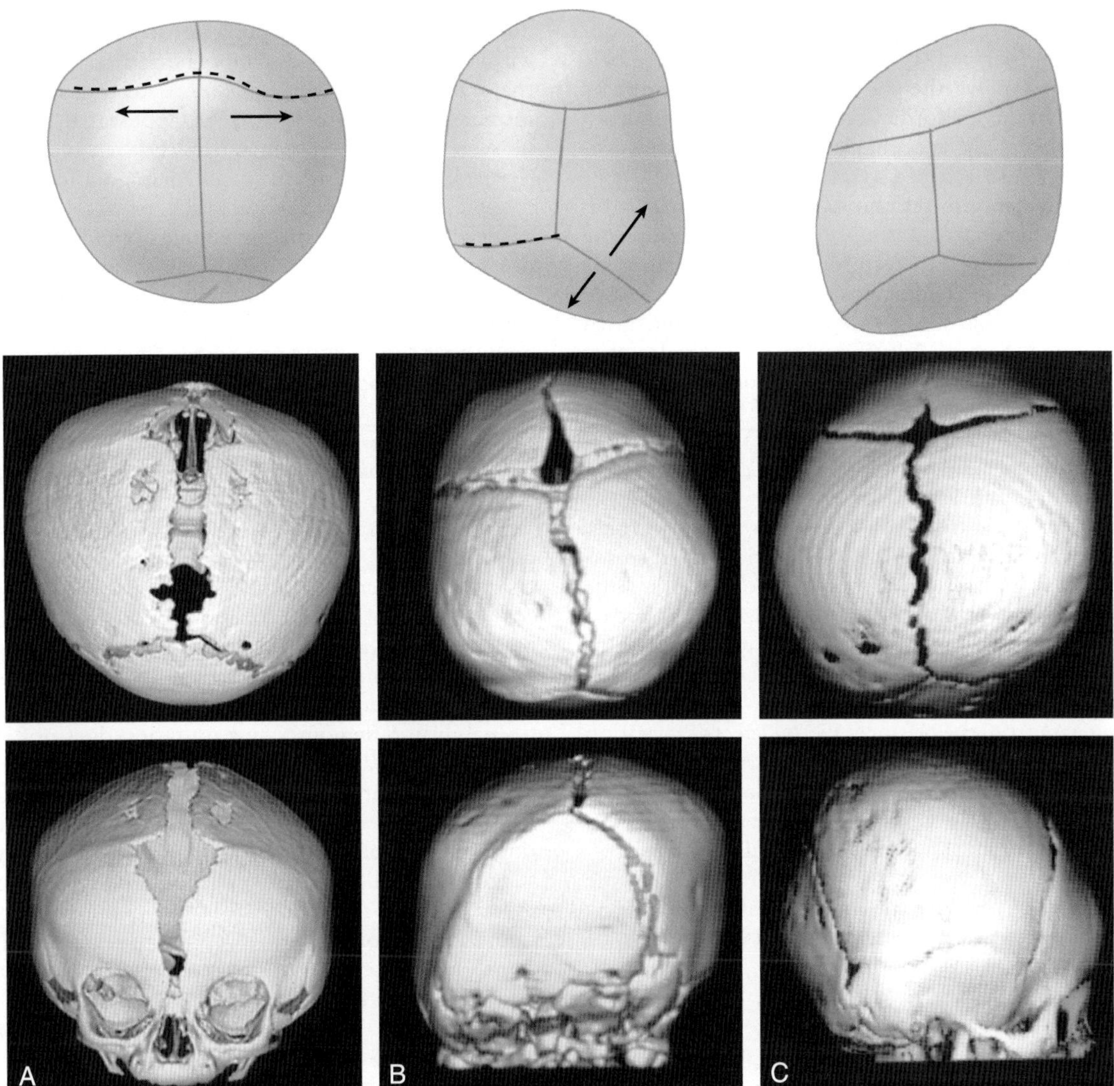

FIGURE 29.5 Diagrams and three-dimensional cranial computed tomography scans depicting bilateral coronal synostosis (A), left lambdoid synostosis (B), and right occipital deformational plagiocephaly (C).

A wide variety of chromosomal anomalies have also been associated with craniosynostosis, a fact that emphasizes the importance of karyotype and chromosome microarray analysis for those patients with syndromic craniosynostosis in whom a recognizable monogenic syndrome is not apparent, particularly when there is associated developmental delay and growth deficiency. In addition, craniosynostosis can also occur as a component of numerous syndromes, many of which manifest phenotypic overlap and genetic heterogeneity.

Named syndromes with a demonstrated mutational basis include Apert syndrome, Crouzon syndrome, Pfeiffer syndrome, Saethre-Chotzen syndrome, Jackson-Weiss syndrome, Boston craniosynostosis, Beare-Stevenson cutis gyrata syndrome, and Muenke syndrome. New craniosynostosis-related genes continue to be uncovered as exome sequencing becomes a routine part of evaluation in unrecognized syndromes.[25-28]

Secondary craniosynostosis can occur with certain primary metabolic disorders (e.g., hyperthyroidism, rickets), storage disorders (e.g., mucopolysaccharidosis), hematologic disorders (e.g., thalassemia, sickle cell anemia, polycythemia vera, congenital hemolytic icterus), brain malformations (e.g., holoprosencephaly, microcephaly, encephalocele, overshunted hydrocephalus), and selected teratogenic exposures (e.g., diphenylhydantoin, retinoic acid, valproic acid, aminopterin, fluconazole, cyclophosphamide, clomiphene citrate).[12,29] There are recurrent gain-of-function de novo variants in retinoic acid receptor alpha (RARA; c.865 G>A [p.Gly289Arg]) identified in probands with similar phenotypes.[15] Future studies may help decipher potential gene-environment interactions. Recent epidemiologic studies have expanded the knowledge and impact of environmental risk factors in craniosynostosis.[30] Maternal smoking appears to be the greatest risk (odds ratio [OR], 1.6) to the developing fetus after the first trimester, and the risk increases with the number of cigarettes smoked per day.[31] Gestational diabetes is seen at a significantly higher rate in mothers of infants with craniosynostosis than mothers of nonaffected infants.[32] The rates of maternal or gestational diabetes-diagnosed mothers of children with craniosynostosis ranges from 3% to over than 10%.[33,34] A 2023 study using data from the National Birth Defects Prevention Study demonstrated that mothers who consume high amounts of caffeine (≥300 mg per day) have an elevated adjusted OR (1.3 [95% confidence interval (CI) 1.1–1.6]) of having an infant with craniosynostosis.[35,36] Rasmussen et al. found that maternal thyroid disease was associated with craniosynostosis after controlling for maternal age with an adjusted OR of 2.47 (95% CI 1.46–4.18).[37,38]

FEATURES

The impact of craniosynostosis on skull shape is dependent on which sutures are synostotic, the extent of the craniosynostosis, and the timing of the problem. The earlier the fusion, the more profound its impact on subsequent craniofacial development. Craniosynostosis of multiple sutures may limit overall brain growth and result in increased intracranial pressure.[9] Elevated intracranial pressure occurs more commonly with syndromic craniosynostosis and multiple sutural synostosis. On skull radiographs, increased intracranial pressure due to craniosynostosis may be associated with a "beaten copper" appearance. The precise reason for this phenomenon is not known, but it may be the result of the altered magnitude and direction of forces on the bony trabecular organization within the calvarium. A copper-beaten appearance of the skull has poor sensitivity in detecting increased intracranial pressure, as such an appearance can also be seen in normal patients.[39] In children older than 8 years, the finding of papilledema indicates the presence of increased intracranial pressure, but the absence of papilledema in younger children is not predictive of normal pressure. Pronounced sutural ridging occurs primarily in sagittal and metopic synostosis, and these midline, end-to-end sutures may be predisposed toward ridging when they become synostotic.[12] It is important to distinguish craniosynostosis in normal-appearing infants from that which occurs in association with genetic syndromes.[12,21–23] Ridging of one lambdoid suture occurs commonly with lambdoid synostosis, and such ridging helps distinguish lambdoidal synostosis from deformational posterior plagiocephaly.[40–43] Ridging occurs infrequently in unilateral coronal craniosynostosis, suggesting that some of these cases may have a constraint-related phenotype, but unless a mutation is detected, it is virtually impossible to distinguish between coronal synostosis due to fetal head constraint and genetic craniosynostosis.

Inability to demonstrate a mutation does not rule out a genetic basis for the craniosynostosis, and not every person with a mutation manifests craniosynostosis. Bilateral coronal synostosis often lacks sutural ridging and usually has a genetic pathogenesis, which suggests that all such patients should be screened for mutations. Approximately 25–30% of craniosynostosis cases are syndromic, defined by the presence of additional anomalies, developmental delay, intellectual disability, or other major findings. As the costs of genetic testing has decreased, many large academic centers have begun advocating for comprehensive whole-exome/whole-genome testing as a first-tier test to screen for rare or novel genetic causes of syndromic craniosynostosis yet the majority of craniofacial centers continue to rely on a tiered systematic clinical approach starting with a comprehensive examination, gene panel, and microarray before considering broader testing.[14,44,45] At a minimum, mutation analysis should be performed in all patients with coronal synostosis.

MANAGEMENT AND PROGNOSIS

Mild degrees of craniostenosis may not always require surgery; however early surgical therapy is usually warranted in most cases.[46,47] With the exception of instances in which both the coronal and sagittal sutures are synostotic (thereby impairing brain growth early in infancy), the predominant indication for surgery is the restoration of normal craniofacial shape and growth, thus reducing neurologic and ophthalmologic complications associated with increased intracranial pressure and inadequate orbital volume as well as improving childhood psychosocial development.[48] A variety of neurosurgical techniques have been developed for the treatment of craniosynostosis.[12] Most of these techniques involve removing the aberrant portion of the bony calvarium from its underlying dura, including the area that surrounds the synostotic suture(s). If this is done within the first few months after birth, a new bony calvarium usually develops within the remaining dura mater, following the same principles that normally guide prenatal calvarial morphogenesis.[8] As long as there is continued growth stretch from the expanding brain, the sites over the dural reflections remain unossified, thereby forming the sutures (see Fig. 29.2). Thus the calvarium and its sutures usually develop normally after a partial calvarectomy for constraint-induced craniosynostosis. The new bony calvarium begins to develop within 2–3 weeks after surgery and is usually firm by 5–8 weeks. If the procedure is performed after 3–4 months of age the approach is similar, with the exception that pieces of the calvarium are usually replaced in a mosaic over the dura mater to act as niduses for the mineralization of new calvarium.

In 1994, Vicari et al. described the first minimally invasive "endoscopic" craniosynostosis repair.[49] Since then, newer endoscopic repair techniques have been developed (Fig. 29.6) as well as postoperative orthotic molding techniques (Fig. 29.7); such procedures are most effective if done relatively early in infancy.[49] These techniques are most useful in otherwise normal infants who do not manifest a syndromic type of craniosynostosis with impaired responses to normal growth factors. With or without endoscopic surgical techniques, the use of postsurgical cranial remodeling devices has improved cosmetic results and in some circumstances has avoided the need for a second surgical procedure.[50,51]

After early surgery for isolated craniosynostosis (primary fronto-orbital advancement and/or calvarial vault remodeling at a mean age of 8 months), only 13% of 104 patients (10 bilateral coronal, 57 unilateral coronal, 29 metopic, and 8 sagittal) required a second cranial vault operation for residual defects at a mean age of 23 months. Perioperative complications were minimal (5%), with 87.5% of patients considered to have at least satisfactory craniofacial form and with low rates of hydrocephalus (3.8%), shunt placement (1%), and seizures (2.9%). Among cases of isolated craniosynostosis, unilateral coronal synostosis was the most problematic type due to vertical orbital dystopia,

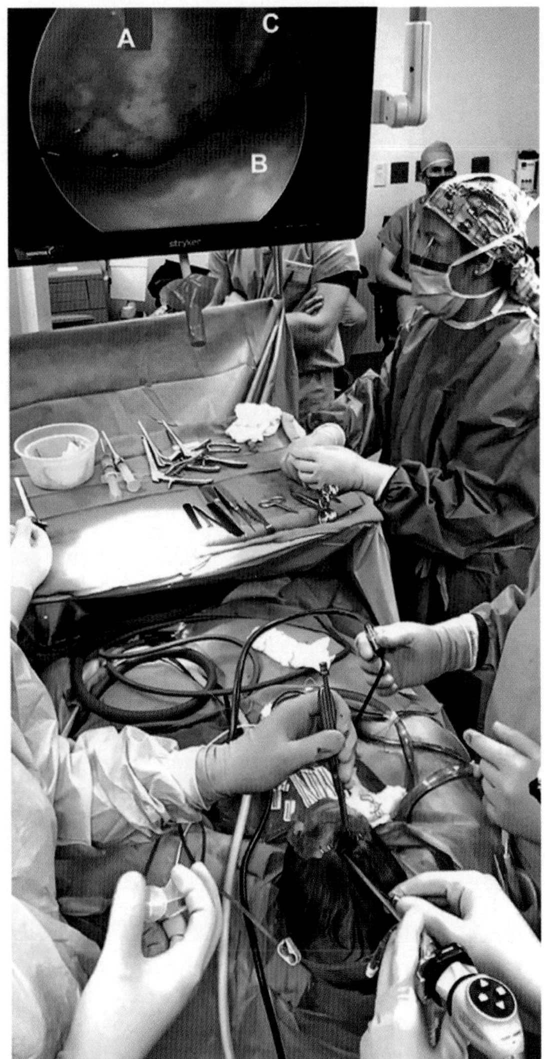

FIGURE 29.6 Epidural dissection in the patient with sagittal craniosynostosis. The bone *(A)* and the dura *(B)* are easily visualized on the monitor, and an insulated suction in 'the surgeon's right hand *(C)* is advanced in front of the endoscope, which is placed under the bone and advanced posteriorly. (From Jimenez DF, Moon HS. Endoscopic approaches to craniosynostosis. *Atlas Oral Maxillofacial Surg Clin N Am.* 2022;30:63–73.)

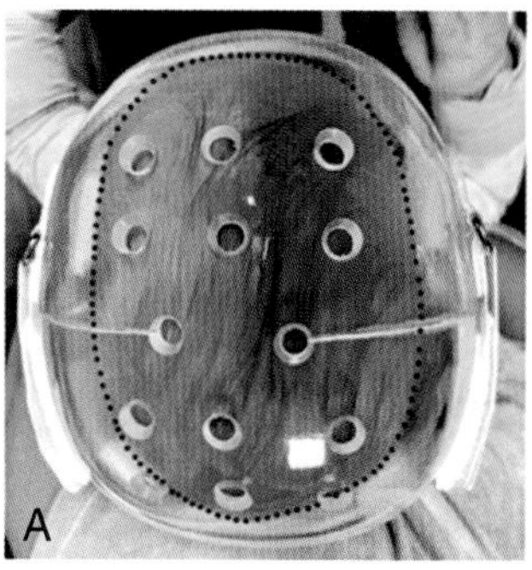

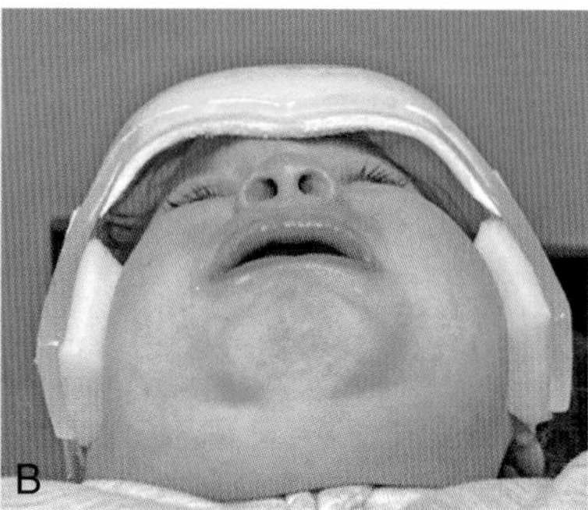

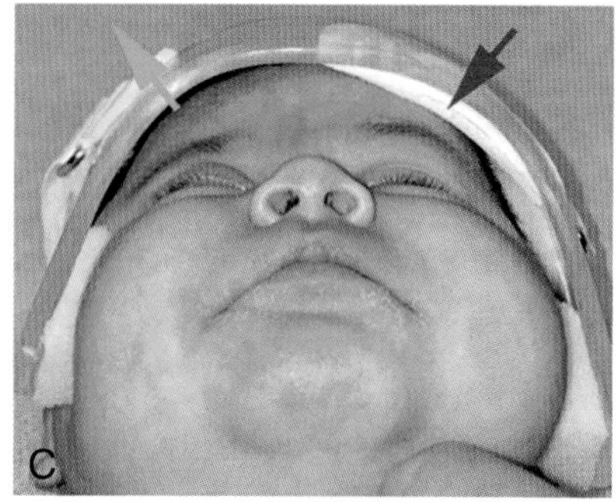

FIGURE 29.7 A, Postoperative cranial remolding helmet in a patient with sagittal craniosynostosis and scaphocephaly. The contour of the head is marked with black dots. There is contact anteriorly and posteriorly, whereas there is ample space bilaterally for cranial expansion and correction of deformity. B, Helmet in a patient with trigonocephaly. There is a contact on a midforehead area and space on the sides for expansion of the forehead and correction of deformity. C, Helmet in a patient with right coronal craniosynostosis. The padded helmet makes direct contact on the left forehead *(red arrow)* as there is space over the right forehead for expansion and correction of deformity. (From Jimenez DF, Moon HS. Endoscopic approaches to craniosynostosis. *Atlas Oral Maxillofacial Surg Clin N Am.* 2022;30:63–73.)

nasal tip deviation, and altered craniofacial growth problems with residual craniofacial asymmetry.[52,53] In a second study of 167 children with both nonsyndromal (isolated) and syndromal craniosynostosis (12 bilateral coronal, 18 unilateral coronal, 39 metopic, and 46 sagittal), reoperation was necessary in only 7%, with reoperation occurring more often in syndromic cases (27.3%) than in cases of nonsyndromic craniosynostosis (5.6%).[17] One series of 256 patients underwent endoscopic-assisted craniectomies for craniosynostosis (134 sagittal, 57 coronal, 50 metopic, and 9 lambdoid) followed by postoperative helmet therapy.[17] Of the patients with sagittal synostosis, 87% had excellent results with a Cephalic Index (CI) >75, and only 4.3% had poor results with a CI <70 (mostly attributed to poor parental compliance with helmet therapy). Helmet therapy consisted of three phases: the first helmet was worn for 1–2 months after surgery to achieve a normal CI, the second helmet was worn for 3–6 months to overcorrect the CI, and the third helmet was worn for 7–12 months to maintain a normal CI.[54]

Although intracranial pressure can be elevated in patients with nonsyndromic craniosynostosis, they usually do not have decreased cranial volumes either before or after surgical repair, and as a group they show slightly larger intracranial volumes when compared with normal controls.[19] This could reflect the impact of fetal constraint on fetuses with larger heads, or it might relate to the known association of macrocephaly with nonsyndromic coronal craniosynostosis due to the common Pro250Arg mutation in FGFR3 (which was not analyzed in these studies). Hydrocephalus occurs in 4–10% of patients with craniosynostosis and is more common with syndromic and multiple sutural craniosynostosis. In nonsyndromic patients, the rate of cerebral ventricular dilatation is the same as that observed in the general population and appears to be related to venous hypertension induced by jugular foramen stenosis, which usually stabilizes spontaneously and rarely requires shunting. Some cases of progressive hydrocephalus among syndromic craniosynostosis cases were related to multiple sutural involvement that constricted cranial volume as well as to alterations in the skull base, crowding in the posterior fossa, and jugular foraminal stenosis.[55] These findings were most frequent among patients with Crouzon, Pfeiffer, or Apert syndromes, especially in association with cloverleaf skull abnormalities. A diffuse, beaten copper pattern on skull radiographs, in addition to obliteration of anterior sulci or narrowing of basal cisterns in children younger than 18 months of age, is predictive of increased intracranial pressure in more than 95% of cases.[56]

In large cohort survey of 660 mutation-negative nonsyndromic craniosynostosis, Greenwood et al. reported that ear infections, palate abnormalities, and hearing problems were more common in complex craniosynostosis patients. Visual problems were more common in coronal craniosynostosis, and metopic craniosynostosis patients noted increased frequency of chronic cough.

In 2014, Knight et al. summarized a systematic review of 33 papers in 27 cohorts on neurodevelopmental outcomes in children with single-suture craniosynostosis.[57] In general, these children are at elevated risk for developmental difficulties during infancy and childhood. Although there is growing evidence supporting an elevated risk for adverse developmental functioning during infancy and early childhood, the extent of neurodevelopmental difficulties and factors contributing to outcome are not yet clear.[58,59]

It is possible to visualize cranial sutures and fontanels at 15–16 weeks of gestation, but the sagittal suture is difficult to visualize using two-dimensional ultrasonography, and three-dimensional ultrasonography appears to be the best method for its demonstration.[60] It is unlikely that most cases of isolated craniosynostosis arise this early in gestation. Very few cases of craniosynostosis have been diagnosed prenatally, and in most of these cases, the diagnosis was made through association with other malformations.[61–64]

DIFFERENTIAL DIAGNOSIS

The numerous causes of craniostenosis can be divided into several general categories, such as problems of the brain or mesenchymal tissues and metabolic disorders.[21,23] In the 1990s there were apparent "epidemics" of craniosynostosis in Colorado, where the birth prevalence was more than twice that found in Atlanta, Georgia, highlight the impact of differing diagnostic techniques and illustrate how misdiagnosis can lead to inappropriate surgery.[12,40,41,65] In Colorado and York-Selby, United Kingdom, almost half of all craniosynostosis cases were diagnosed as having lambdoid synostosis, a type that usually constitutes less than 5% of all cases. Overdiagnosis of nonsynostotic deformational posterior plagiocephaly as unilateral lambdoid synostosis accounted for most instances of this misdiagnosis. Thus it is critically important to validate the diagnosis of posterior craniosynostosis, either through an independent second opinion or via 3D-CT scan. Categorization of the craniosynostosis (i.e., as isolated or syndromic, sporadic or familial, and primary or secondary) can also help clarify the diagnosis in most cases. There are several categorical causes for craniosynostosis.

Brain Problems

Basic problems in early brain morphogenesis may cause a lack of dural reflection and hence the lack of a suture, thereby resulting in the inability of the calvarium to grow laterally in that region.[22] Observed examples[3] include holoprosencephaly (single ventricle) with no anterior interhemispheric fissure and consequently no metopic suture[4]; unilateral deficiency of the early cerebrum with no insular sulcus and hence no sphenoid wing; or unilateral deficiency of the dural reflection and hence no coronal suture. Deficit of brain growth, such as occurs in severe microcephaly, may result in a lack of expansile brain force, with craniostenosis as a secondary consequence. More localized brain growth deficiency may cause a particular suture to become prematurely craniostenotic; for example, frontal brain growth deficiency may result in metopic craniostenosis. Excessive shunting of hydrocephalus may also result in lack of growth stretch at the suture lines, enhancing the tendency toward craniostenosis.[21]

Mesenchymal Tissue Problems

In a number of disorders, various types of craniosynostosis occur because of an aberration in mesenchymal tissues. In many of these syndromes, there are associated anomalies in limbs, such as syndactyly, brachydactyly, or broad deviated thumbs and halluces, suggesting a specific syndrome with a known pathogenesis and natural history (e.g., Apert, Crouzon, Pfeiffer, or Saethre-Chotzen syndromes). Most of these syndromic disorders are genetically determined, and mutational analysis for disorders resulting from mutations in FGFR1, FGFR2, FGFR3, and TWIST is now available through several clinical molecular genetic testing facilities. It is beyond the scope of this text to discuss these syndromes in detail, and the reader is referred to other sources.[12]

Metabolic Problems

Early rickets, regardless of its cause, can result in craniosynostosis in about one third of cases. In a 2021 study of 50 patients with hypophosphatemic rickets, 52% had craniosynostosis, with 73% of these affecting the sagittal suture and the remainder affecting multiple sutures.[66] The prolonged use of aluminum-containing antacids along with the ingestion of soy-based formulas, both of which prevent phosphate absorption and lead to rickets, has been reported to cause secondary craniosynostosis.[67,68] In rare instances, early hyperthyroidism has also caused craniosynostosis, as has hypercalcemia.[21] Secondary craniosynostosis can also occur with storage disorders, such as mucopolysaccharidosis, and with various hematologic disorders, such as thalassemia, sickle cell anemia, polycythemia vera, and congenital hemolytic icterus.[69–71]

References

1. Boran P, Oguz F, Furman A, Sakarya S. Evaluation of fontanel size variation and closure time in children followed up from birth to 24 months. *J Neurosurg Pediatr.* 2018;22(3):323–329.
2. Goodman RM, Gorlin RJ. *Atlas of the Face in Genetic Disorders.* 2d ed. Saint Louis: Mosby; 1977.
3. Koshkinen-Moffett L, Moffet BC. Sutures and intrauterine deformation. In: Pershing JA, Edgerton MT, Jane JA, eds. *Scientific Foundations and Surgical Treatment of Craniosynostosis.* Baltimore: Williams & Wilkins; 1989:96–106.
4. Graham JM Jr, deSaxe M, Smith DW. Sagittal craniostenosis: fetal head constraint as one possible cause. *J Pediatr.* 1979;95(5 Pt 1):747–750.
5. Graham JM Jr, Badura RJ, Smith DW. Coronal craniostenosis: fetal head constraint as one possible cause. *Pediatrics.* 1980;65(5):995–999.
6. Graham JM Jr, Smith DW. Metopic craniostenosis as a consequence of fetal head constraint: two interesting experiments of nature. *Pediatrics.* 1980;65(5):1000–1002.
7. Higginbottom MC, Jones KL, James HE. Intrauterine constraint and craniosynostosis. *Neurosurgery.* 1980;6(1):39–44.
8. Koskinen-Moffett LK, Moffet BC, Graham JM Jr. Cranial synostostosis and intra-uterine compression: a developmental study of human sutures. In: Dixon AD, Sarnat BG, eds. *Factors and Mechanisms Influencing Bone Growth.* New York: Alan R. Liss; 1982:365–378.
9. Graham JM Jr. Craniofacial deformation. *Ballier Clin Pediatr.* 1988;6:293–315.
10. Sanchez-Lara PA, Carmichael SL, Graham JM Jr, et al. Fetal constraint as a potential risk factor for craniosynostosis. *Am J Med Genet A.* 2010;152A(2):394–400.
11. Lakin GE, Sinkin JC, Chen R, Koltz PF, Girotto JA. Genetic and epigenetic influences of twins on the pathogenesis of craniosynostosis: a meta-analysis. *Plast Reconstr Surg.* 2012;129(4):945–954.
12. Cohen MM, MacLean RE. *Craniosynostosis: Diagnosis. Evaluation, and Management.* 2nd ed. New York: Oxford University Press; 2000.
13. Wilkie AO, Byren JC, Hurst JA, et al. Prevalence and complications of single-gene and chromosomal disorders in craniosynostosis. *Pediatrics.* 2010;126(2):e391–e400.
14. Tooze RS, Calpena E, Weber A, Wilson LC, Twigg SRF, Wilkie AOM. Review of recurrently mutated genes in craniosynostosis supports expansion of diagnostic gene panels. *Genes (Basel).* 2023;14(3).
15. Timberlake AT, McGee S, Allington G, et al. De novo variants implicate chromatin modification, transcriptional regulation, and retinoic acid signaling in syndromic craniosynostosis. *Am J Hum Genet.* 2023;110(5):846–862.
16. Kutkowska-Ka-mierczak A, Gos M, Obersztyn E. Craniosynostosis as a clinical and diagnostic problem: molecular pathology and genetic counseling. *J Appl Genet.* 2018;59(2):133–147.
17. Yapijakis C, Pachis N, Sotiriadou T, Vaila C, Michopoulou V, Vassiliou S. Molecular mechanisms involved in craniosynostosis. *In Vivo.* 2023;37(1):36–46.
18. Tønne E, Due-Tønnessen BJ, Wiig U, et al. Epidemiology of craniosynostosis in Norway. *J Neurosurg Pediatr.* 2020;26(1):68–75.
19. Greenwood J, Flodman P, Osann K, Boyadjiev SA, Kimonis V. Familial incidence and associated symptoms in a population of individuals with nonsyndromic craniosynostosis. *Genet Med.* 2014;16(4):302–310.
20. Kalantar-Hormozi H, Abbaszadeh-Kasbi A, Sharifi G, Davai NR, Kalantar-Hormozi A. Incidence of familial craniosynostosis among patients with nonsyndromic craniosynostosis. *J Craniofac Surg.* 2019;30(6):e514–e517.
21. Lajeunie E, Le Merrer M, Bonaiti-Pellie C, Marchac D, Renier D. Genetic study of nonsyndromic coronal craniosynostosis. *Am J Med Genet.* 1995;55(4):500–504.
22. Lajeunie E, Le Merrer M, Bonaiti-Pellie C, Marchac D, Renier D. Genetic study of scaphocephaly. *Am J Med Genet.* 1996;62(3):282–285.
23. Lajeunie E, Le Merrer M, Marchac D, Renier D. Syndromal and nonsyndromal primary trigonocephaly: analysis of a series of 237 patients. *Am J Med Genet.* 1998;75(2):211–215.
24. Kadlub N, Persing JA, da Silva Freitas R, Shin JH. Familial lambdoid craniosynostosis between father and son. *J Craniofac Surg.* 2008;19(3):850–854.
25. Twigg SR, Vorgia E, McGowan SJ, et al. Reduced dosage of ERF causes complex craniosynostosis in humans and mice and links ERK1/2 signaling to regulation of osteogenesis. *Nat Genet.* 2013;45(3):308–313.
26. Sharma VP, Fenwick AL, Brockop MS, et al. Mutations in *TCF12*, encoding a basic helix-loop-helix partner of *TWIST1*, are a frequent cause of coronal craniosynostosis. *Nat Genet.* 2013;45(3):304–307.
27. Zollino M, Lattante S, Orteschi D, et al. Syndromic craniosynostosis can define new candidate genes for suture development or result from the non-specifc effects of pleiotropic genes: rasopathies and chromatinopathies as examples. *Front Neurosci.* 2017;11:587.
28. Sanchez-Lara PA. Clinical and genomic approaches for the diagnosis of craniofacial disorders. *Curr Top Dev Biol.* 2015;115:543–559.
29. Kalantar-Hormozi A, Moradi E, Hashemi SZ, Kalantar-Hormozi H, Abbaszadeh-Kasbi A. The effect of using in vitro fertilization (IVF) on increasing the prevalence of craniosynostosis. *J Craniofac Surg.* 2022;33(1):26–28.
30. Rasmussen SA, Yazdy MM, Frias JL, Honein MA. Priorities for public health research on craniosynostosis: summary and recommendations from a Centers for Disease Control and Prevention-sponsored meeting. *Am J Med Genet A.* 2008;146A(2):149–158.
31. Carmichael SL, Ma C, Rasmussen SA, Honein MA, Lammer EJ, Shaw GM. Craniosynostosis and maternal smoking. *Birth Defects Res A Clin Mol Teratol.* 2008;82(2):78–85.
32. Sergesketter AR, Elsamadicy AA, Lubkin DT, Krucoff KB, Krucoff MO, Muh CR. Characterization of

perinatal risk factors and complications associated with nonsyndromic craniosynostosis. *J Craniofac Surg.* 2019;30(2):334–338.

33. Ardalan M, Rafati A, Nejat F, Farazmand B, Majed M, El Khashab M. Risk factors associated with craniosynostosis: a case control study. *Pediatr Neurosurg.* 2012;48(3):152–156.
34. Stanton E, Urata M, Chen JF, Chai Y. The clinical manifestations, molecular mechanisms and treatment of craniosynostosis. *Dis Model Mech.* 2022;15(4):dmm049390.
35. Browne ML, Hoyt AT, Feldkamp ML, et al. Maternal caffeine intake and risk of selected birth defects in the National Birth Defects Prevention Study. *Birth Defects Res A Clin Mol Teratol.* 2011;91(2):93–101.
36. Williford EM, Howley MM, Fisher SC, et al. Maternal dietary caffeine consumption and risk of birth defects in the National Birth Defects Prevention Study, 1997-2011. *Birth Defects Res.* 2023;115(9):921–932.
37. Rasmussen SA, Yazdy MM, Carmichael SL, Jamieson DJ, Canfield MA, Honein MA. Maternal thyroid disease as a risk factor for craniosynostosis. *Obstet Gynecol.* 2007;110(2 Pt 1):369–377.
38. Carmichael SL, Ma C, Rasmussen SA, et al. Craniosynostosis and risk factors related to thyroid dysfunction. *Am J Med Genet A.* 2015;167a(4):701–707.
39. Desai V, Priyadarshini SR, Sharma R. Copper beaten skull! Can it be a usual appearance? *Int J Clin Pediatr Dent.* 2014;7(1):47–49.
40. Huang MH, Gruss JS, Clarren SK, et al. The differential diagnosis of posterior plagiocephaly: true lambdoid synostosis versus positional molding. *Plast Reconstr Surg.* 1996;98(5):765–774. discussion 775–766.
41. Dias MS, Klein DM, Backstrom JW. Occipital plagiocephaly: deformation or lambdoid synostosis? I. Morphometric analysis and results of unilateral lambdoid craniectomy. *Pediatr Neurosurg.* 1996;24(2):61–68.
42. Dias MS, Klein DM. Occipital plagiocephaly: deformation or lambdoid synostosis? II. A unifying theory regarding pathogenesis. *Pediatr Neurosurg.* 1996;24(2):69–73.
43. Haas-Lude K, Wolff M, Will B, Bender B, Krimmel M. Clinical and imaging findings in children with non-syndromic lambdoid synostosis. *Eur J Pediatr.* 2014;173(4):435–440.
44. Tønne E, Due-Tønnessen BJ, Vigeland MD, et al. Whole-exome sequencing in syndromic craniosynostosis increases diagnostic yield and identifies candidate genes in osteogenic signaling pathways. *Am J Med Genet A.* 2022;188(5):1464–1475.
45. Armand T, Schaefer E, Di Rocco F, Edery P, Collet C, Rossi M. Genetic bases of craniosynostoses: an update. *Neurochirurgie.* 2019;65(5):196–201.
46. Persing JA. MOC-PS(SM) CME article: management considerations in the treatment of craniosynostosis. *Plast Reconstr Surg.* 2008;121(4 Suppl):1–11.
47. McCarthy JG, Warren SM, Bernstein J, et al. Parameters of care for craniosynostosis. *Cleft Palate Craniofac J.* 2012;49(Suppl:):1S–24S.
48. McCarthy JG, Warren SM, Bernstein J, et al. Parameters of care for craniosynostosis. *Cleft Palate Craniofac J.* 2012;49 Suppl(10):1S–24S.
49. MacKinnon S, Proctor MR, Rogers GF, Meara JG, Whitecross S, Dagi LR. Improving ophthalmic outcomes in children with unilateral coronal synostosis by treatment with endoscopic strip craniectomy and helmet therapy rather than fronto-orbital advancement. *J Aapos.* 2013;17(3):259–265.
50. Littlefield TR. Cranial remodeling devices: treatment of deformational plagiocephaly and postsurgical applications. *Semin Pediatr Neurol.* 2004;11(4):268–277.
51. Wolfswinkel EM, Sanchez-Lara PA, Jacob L, Urata MM. Postoperative helmet therapy following fronto-orbital advancement and cranial vault remodeling in patients with unilateral coronal synostosis. *Am J Med Genet A.* 2021;185(9):2670–2675.
52. McCarthy JG, Glasberg SB, Cutting CB, et al. Twenty-year experience with early surgery for craniosynostosis: I. Isolated craniofacial synostosis--results and unsolved problems. *Plast Reconstr Surg.* 1995;96(2):272–283.
53. McCarthy JG, Glasberg SB, Cutting CB, et al. Twenty-year experience with early surgery for craniosynostosis: II. The craniofacial synostosis syndromes and pansynostosis--results and unsolved problems. *Plast Reconstr Surg.* 1995;96(2):284–295. discussion 296–288.
54. Jimenez DF, Barone CM, McGee ME. Design and care of helmets in postoperative craniosynostosis patients: our personal approach. *Clin Plast Surg.* 2004;31(3):481–487. vii.
55. Cinalli G, Sainte-Rose C, Kollar EM, et al. Hydrocephalus and craniosynostosis. *J Neurosurg.* 1998;88(2):209–214.
56. Tuite GF, Evanson J, Chong WK, et al. The beaten copper cranium: a correlation between intracranial pressure, cranial radiographs, and computed tomographic scans in children with craniosynostosis. *Neurosurgery.* 1996;39(4):691–699.
57. Knight SJ, Anderson VA, Spencer-Smith MM, Da Costa AC. Neurodevelopmental outcomes in infants and children with single-suture craniosynostosis: a systematic review. *Dev Neuropsychol.* 2014;39(3):159–186.
58. Kapp-Simon KA, Leroux B, Cunningham M, Speltz ML. Multisite study of infants with single-suture craniosynostosis: preliminary report of presurgery development. *Cleft Palate Craniofac J.* 2005;42(4):377–384.
59. Kapp-Simon KA, Speltz ML, Cunningham ML, Patel PK, Tomita T. Neurodevelopment of children with single suture craniosynostosis: a review. *Childs Nerv Syst.* 2007;23(3):269–281.
60. Ginath S, Debby A, Malinger G. Demonstration of cranial sutures and fontanelles at 15 to 16 weeks of gestation: a comparison between two-dimensional and three-dimensional ultrasonography. *Prenat Diagn.* 2004;24(10):812–815.
61. Miller C, Losken HW, Towbin R, et al. Ultrasound diagnosis of craniosynostosis. *Cleft Palate Craniofac J.* 2002;39(1):73–80.

62. Regelsberger J, Delling G, Helmke K, et al. Ultrasound in the diagnosis of craniosynostosis. *J Craniofac Surg.* 2006;17(4):623–625. discussion 626–628.
63. Delahaye S, Bernard JP, Renier D, Ville Y. Prenatal ultrasound diagnosis of fetal craniosynostosis. *Ultrasound Obstet Gynecol.* 2003;21(4):347–353.
64. Tonni G, Panteghini M, Rossi A, et al. Craniosynostosis: prenatal diagnosis by means of ultrasound and SSSE-MRI. Family series with report of neurodevelopmental outcome and review of the literature. *Arch Gynecol Obstet.* 2011;283(4):909–916.
65. Alderman BW, Fernbach SK, Greene C, Mangione EJ, Ferguson SW. Diagnostic practice and the estimated prevalence of craniosynostosis in Colorado. *Arch Pediatr Adolesc Med.* 1997;151(2):159–164.
66. Arenas MA, Jaimovich S, Perez Garrido N, et al. Hereditary hypophosphatemic rickets and craniosynostosis. *J Pediatr Endocrinol Metab.* 2021;34(9):1105–1113.
67. Inman PC, Mukundan Jr. S, Fuchs HE, Marcus JR. Craniosynostosis and rickets. *Plast Reconstr Surg.* 2008;121(4):217e–218e.
68. Pivnick EK, Kerr NC, Kaufman RA, Jones DP, Chesney RW. Rickets secondary to phosphate depletion. A sequela of antacid use in infancy. *Clin Pediatr (Phila).* 1995;34(2):73–78.
69. Di Rocco F, Rothenbuhler A, Cormier Daire V, et al. Craniosynostosis and metabolic bone disorder. A review. *Neurochirurgie.* 2019;65(5):258–263.
70. Manrique M, Toro-Tobon S, Bade Y, et al. Sickle cell disease association with premature suture fusion in young children. *Plast Reconstr Surg Glob Open.* 2022;10(10):e4620.
71. Cohen MM Jr. Etiopathogenesis of craniosynostosis. *Neurosurg Clin N Am.* 1991;2(3):507–513.

CHAPTER 30

Sagittal Craniosynostosis

KEY POINTS

- Sagittal craniosynostosis limits lateral cranial expansion, with progressive frontal and/or occipital prominence and ridging along the mid-posterior portion of the skull.
- Sagittal synostosis can result from fetal head constraint secondary to factors such as twining, oligohydramnios, or early descent of the fetal head into the maternal pelvis with fetal head entrapment, resulting in biparietal constraint.
- Various surgical techniques have been used to correct sagittal craniosynostosis, and can include minimally invasive endoscopic surgery and extended strip craniectomy.
- Isolated sagittal synostosis does not affect the neurologic function of the infant or toddler, and surgical intervention may be difficult to resolve whether it is necessary or not.

GENESIS

Early descent of the fetal head into the maternal pelvis (as early as 4–6 weeks before delivery) with fetal head entrapment that results in biparietal constraint is considered the most common cause of sagittal craniostenosis.[1-3] This mode of genesis is shown in Fig. 29.2. Synostosis limits lateral cranial expansion, resulting in dolichocephaly with progressive frontal and/or occipital prominence (Fig. 30.1), and ridging is usually palpable along the posterior portion of the sagittal suture (Fig. 30.2). The platypelloid pelvis, which is relatively small in the anteroposterior dimension compared with its lateral dimensions, would hypothetically constitute the greatest risk for this type of entrapment head constraint. Prolongation of gestation in pregnant mice via placement of a cervical clip resulted in fetal crowding and craniosynostosis.[4] Further support for the importance of biomechanical forces in sagittal craniosynostosis derives from a study of sutural histology in completely synostotic and nonsynostotic sagittal sutures that were removed at the time of surgery. There is a definite qualitative difference in the trabecular pattern for both the vector and direction of suture fusion initiation for the partially and completely synostotic suture compared with the open portion of the same suture (Fig. 30.3). Within the synostotic suture, the trabecular pattern is more disorganized and less polarized than it is within the open suture, where trabeculae are oriented parallel to the direction of biomechanical growth-stretch forces.[5,6] Bony ridging is most prominent in the posterior half of the synostotic sagittal suture (in the plane of the widest cranial diameter), consistent with this being the initiation site of synostosis and the site of the most longstanding sutural fusion.[5]

Sagittal craniosynostosis is the most common type of synostosis, accounting for 50–60% of cases and occurring in 1.9 per 10,000 births, with a 3.5:1 male:female gender ratio.[7] Only 6% of cases are familial, with 72% of cases sporadic and no paternal or maternal age effects noted. Twinning occurred in 4.8% of 366 cases, with only one monozygotic twin pair being concordant, and intrauterine constraint was considered a likely cause in many cases.[7] The predilection for occurrence in males has been attributed to the more rapid rate of head growth in the male fetus during the last trimester of gestation.[1,2] The larger head is more likely to become seriously constrained, and the associated twinning also contributes toward fetal head constraint.[8]

FEATURES

The head is long and narrow (dolichocephalic) with a prominent forehead and occiput (see Fig. 30.1). There is usually a ridge along the mid- to posterior sagittal

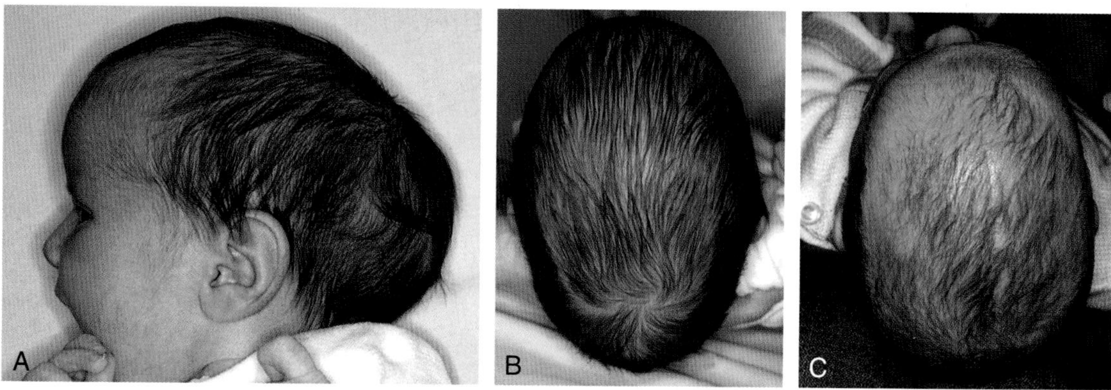

FIGURE 30.1 Side (A) and top (B) views of sagittal craniosynostosis, demonstrating a prominent occipital bulge with prominent forehead resulting in dolichocephaly. C, Postoperative top view of this same infant, demonstrating resolution of the initial dolichocephaly.

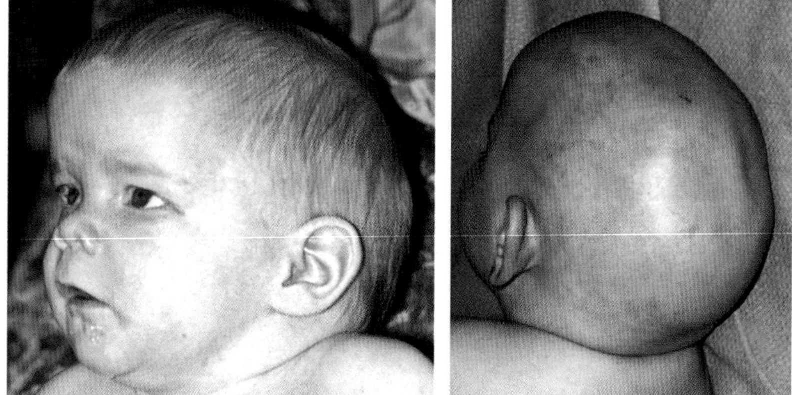

FIGURE 30.2 Prominent forehead with ridging of the sagittal suture along the posterior sagittal suture between the biparietal eminences in the plane of presumed lateral head constraint.

suture that is most prominent between the biparietal eminences (see Fig. 30.2). The term *scaphocephaly* comes from the Greek word *scaphos*, which refers to the keel of a boat. In older children, endocranial ridging is sometimes observed on skull radiographs, suggesting a change in the distribution of intracranial and extracranial biomechanical forces over time; this may be accompanied by calvarial thinning just lateral to the most ridged suture. Relatively excessive anteroposterior growth may partially spread the coronal, temporosquamosal, and/or lambdoidal sutures (Fig. 30.4), and restraint of growth along the posterior sagittal suture may result in flattening between the occiput and the vertex (see Fig. 30.1). The head circumference may appear to be falsely increased, providing a mistaken impression of macrocephaly or possibly even hydrocephalus. Histologic examination of the synostotic suture reveals complete obliteration of the sutural ligament with endocranial bone resorption and ectocranial bone deposition (see Fig. 30.3).[5,6] Skull radiographs show obliteration and hyperostosis of the sagittal suture (Fig. 30.5).

MANAGEMENT, PROGNOSIS, AND COUNSEL

(See also Chapter 29.) Craniosynostosis of the sagittal suture alone imposes a moderate cranial structural problem, and it may sometimes be difficult for the parents and physicians to resolve the question of whether surgical intervention is indicated.[3,9] Sagittal synostosis does not affect the neurologic function of the infant or toddler.[10] However, older children may

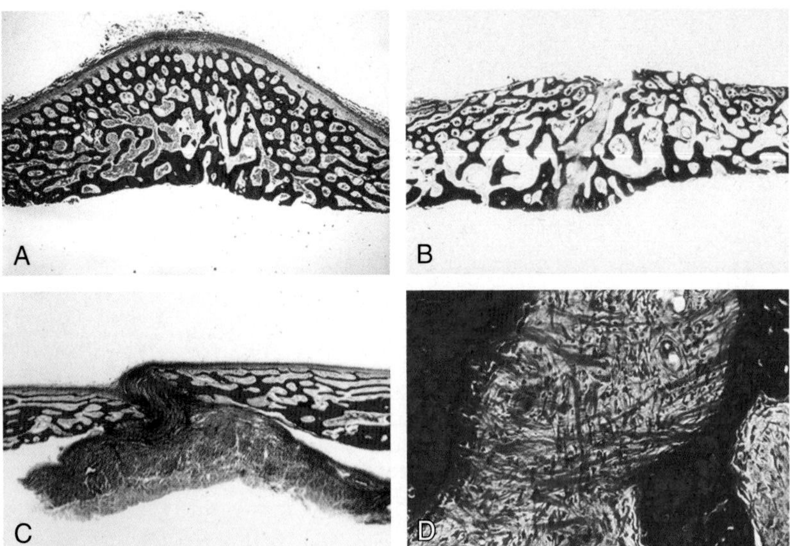

FIGURE 30.3 There is a definite qualitative difference in the trabecular pattern for both the vector and direction of suture fusion initiation for the partially and completely synostotic suture (A) versus the open portion of the same suture (B). Within the closing suture (C), the trabecular pattern was more disorganized and less polarized than it was within a completely open sagittal suture from an infant who died of an unrelated cause. In this normal open sagittal suture (D), the trabeculae were oriented parallel to the direction of biomechanical growth–stretch forces.

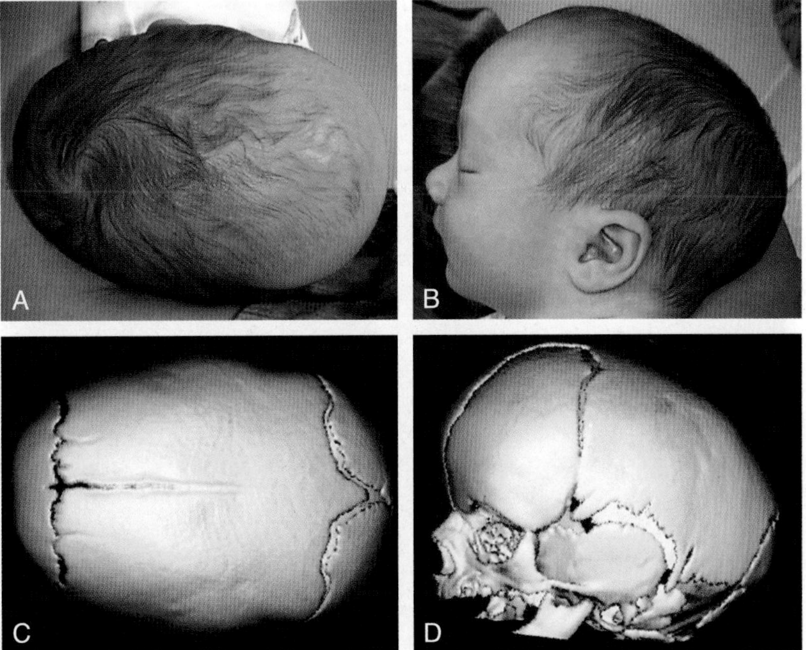

FIGURE 30.4 A, B, This 6-week-old infant has typical features of sagittal synostosis with a palpable ridge along the posterior sagittal suture. C, D, Three-dimensional cranial computed tomography scans demonstrating obliteration of the posterior sagittal suture with compensatory expansion of other cranial sutures.

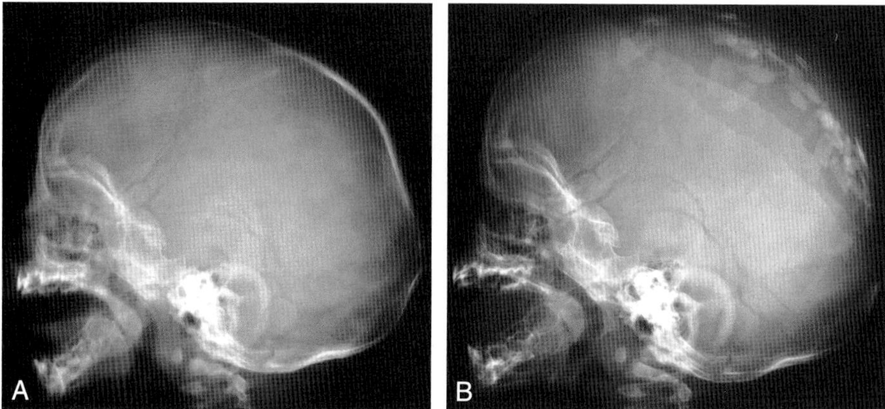

FIGURE 30.5 A, Skull radiographs before surgical correction, demonstrating scaphocephaly with hyperostosis of the sagittal suture. B, Skull radiographs after subtotal calvarectomy. Pieces of cranial bone are placed over the dura to serve as niduses for the reformation of new cranial bones with reformation of a new sagittal suture.

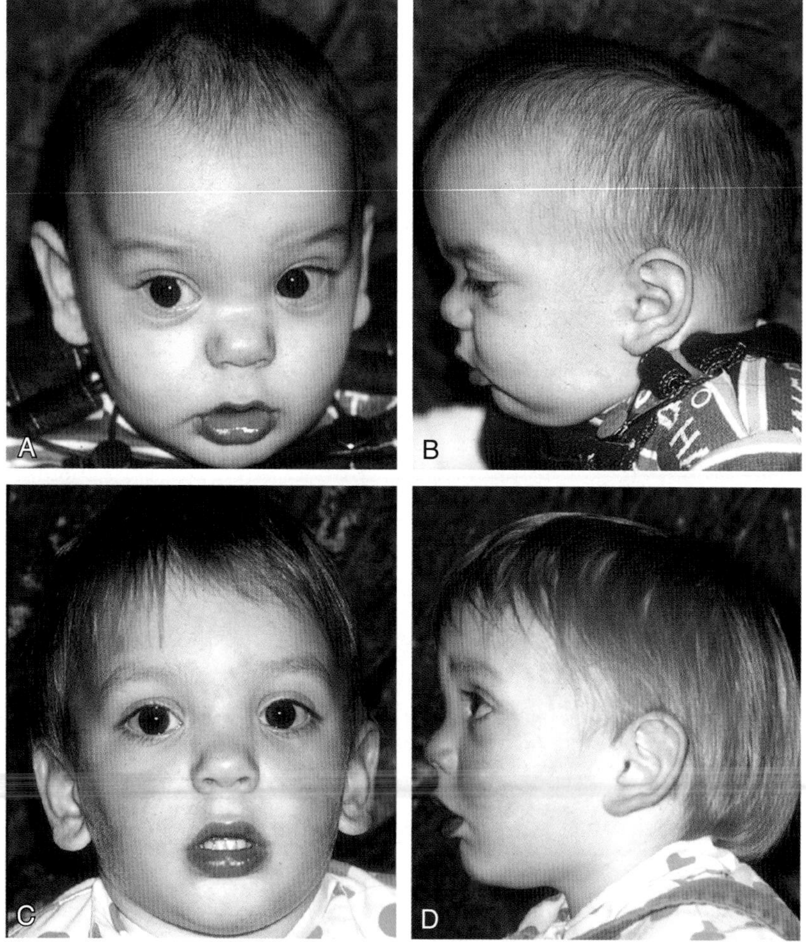

FIGURE 30.6 Infant with sagittal synostosis before (A, B) (age 6 months) and after surgery (C, D) (age 10 months). Note the dramatic change in the bifrontal versus biparietal dimensions in the top view of the head.

demonstrate moderately severe speech and language difficulties, with rates of neurocognitive risk ranging from 35% to 50% of school-aged children with isolated single suture craniosynostosis.[11,12] In as many as 37% of cases the tendency toward such problems is associated with a positive family history for such difficulties and later age of surgical correction.[13-15] In a study of 30 older untreated children (average age, 9.25 years) with sagittal synostosis, almost all patients and parents were pleased with their decision, and the affected children demonstrated normal cognitive and school performance as well as normal behavior and psychological adjustment on standardized testing.[11] In a study by Beiriger et al., of 108 patients with late-presenting sagittal craniosynostosis (after 1 year of age), only 11.1% were found to undergo surgery following their initial consultation. Of the remaining children who initially chose conservative treatment, only 4% of those ultimately required surgery.[9] In a 2020 literature review of over 190 publications on cognitive outcomes and sagittal craniosynostosis, Thiele-Nygaard et al. did not find evidence in support an association between

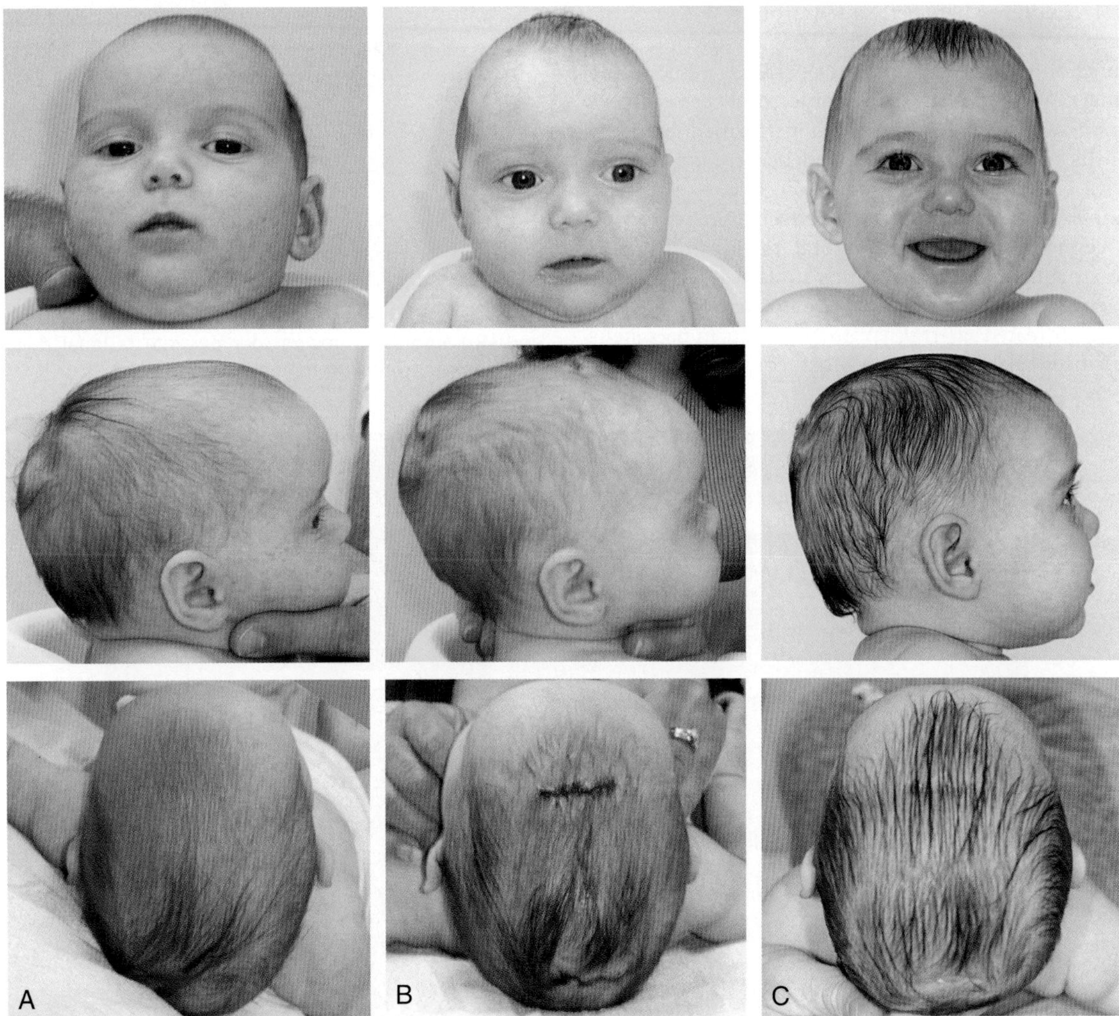

FIGURE 30.7 A, This infant with sagittal synostosis is shown just prior to endoscopic strip craniectomy at 2.5 months with a cephalic index of 73% and frontal bossing. B, Two weeks after surgery, she had persistent frontal bossing with a cephalic index of 75%, at which time she was fitted with a cranial orthotic. C, After 3 months of orthotic therapy, her frontal bossing had resolved and her cephalic index had improved to 76%, and the orthotic was discontinued. She maintained her correction with a cephalic index of 75% at 9 months of age.

increased intracranial pressure and negative global cognitive outcome measures in patients with sagittal craniosynostosis.[16]

Various surgical techniques have been used to correct sagittal craniosynostosis.[17] With extended strip craniectomy, an H-shaped strip of calvarium is excised along the sagittal suture, just above the lambdoid sutures and just behind the coronal sutures. With subtotal calvarectomy and cranial vault remodeling, the excised frontal, parietal, and occipital bones are trimmed, reshaped, and relocated using absorbable sutures (see Figs. 30.1, 30.5, and 30.6). Subtotal calvarectomy will normalize head shape for the majority of children when performed around 4–6 months of age.[14,18,19] Another technique uses endoscopic strip craniectomy with postoperative cranial remodeling helmets.[20,21] Extended strip craniectomy can achieve a comparable head shape when performed before 4 months of age and accompanied by prompt postoperative orthotic molding (Fig. 30.7). It is still unclear whether strip craniectomy is as effective in correcting the cephalic index as is subtotal calvarectomy, and comparison studies are currently underway.[22–24] Timely surgery corrects the craniofacial deformation, whereas late or untreated sagittal synostosis results in persistent dolichocephaly (Fig. 30.8). Most constraint-induced instances of sagittal craniosynostosis are sporadic; however there are some rare instances of familial sagittal craniosynostosis (Fig. 30.9).[25,26] It is not clear whether such familial cases are a consequence of inherited pelvic type, large head size, or a gene that specifically affects the sagittal suture and results in early closure.

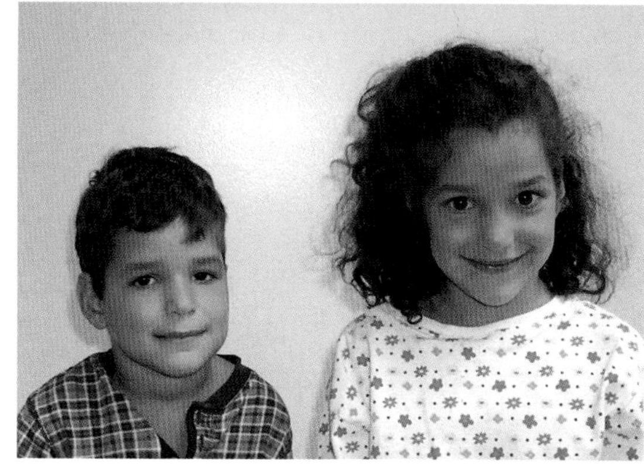

FIGURE 30.9 This brother and sister with sagittal synostosis and late surgical correction demonstrate residual dolichocephaly with frontal prominence.

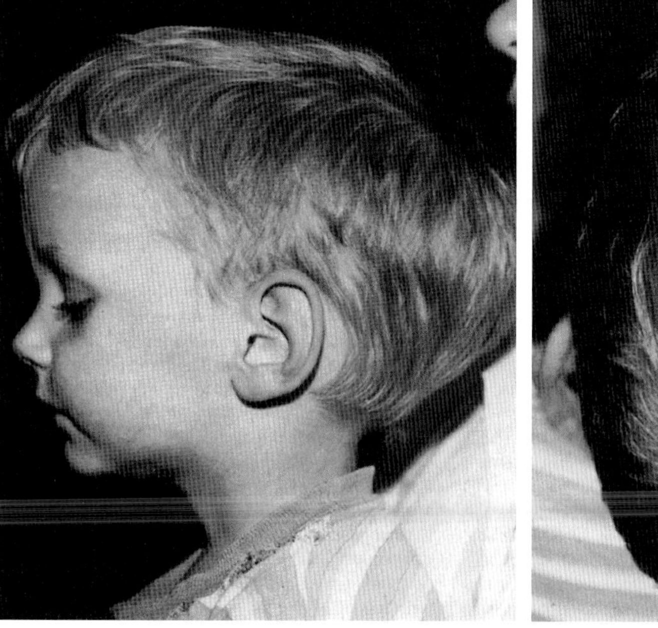

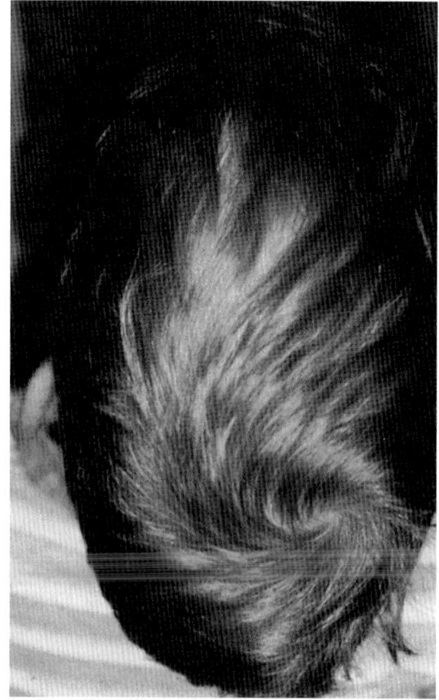

FIGURE 30.8 This 6-year-old boy has unoperated sagittal craniosynostosis (note scaphocephaly with prominent occipital bulge).

References

1. Graham JM Jr. deSaxe M, Smith DW. Sagittal craniostenosis: fetal head constraint as one possible cause. *J Pediatr*. 1979;95(5 Pt 1):747–750.
2. Graham JM Jr. Craniofacial deformation. *Ballier Clin Pediatr*. 1988;6:293–315.
3. Manrique M, Mantilla-Rivas E, Rana MS, et al. Normocephalic sagittal craniosynostosis in young children is common and unrecognized. *Childs Nerv Syst*. 2022;38(8):1549–1556.
4. Koshkinen-Moffett L, Moffet BC. Sutures and intrauterine deformation. In: Pershing JA, Edgerton MT, Jane JA, eds. *Scientific Foundations and Surgical Treatment of Craniosynostosis*. Baltimore: Williams & Wilkins; 1989:96–106.
5. Koskinen-Moffett LK, Moffet BC, Graham JM Jr. Cranial synostostosis and intra-uterine compression: a developmental study of human sutures. In: Dixon AD, Sarnat BG, eds. *Factors and Mechanisms Influencing Bone Growth*. New York: Alan R. Liss; 1982:365–378.
6. Ozaki W, Buchman SR, Muraszko KM, Coleman D. Investigation of the influences of biomechanical force on the ultrastructure of human sagittal craniosynostosis. *Plast Reconstr Surg*. 1998;102(5):1385–1394.
7. Lajeunie E, Le Merrer M, Bonaiti-Pellie C, Marchac D, Renier D. Genetic study of scaphocephaly. *Am J Med Genet*. 1996;62(3):282–285.
8. Sanchez-Lara PA, Carmichael SL, Graham JM, et al. Fetal constraint as a potential risk factor for craniosynostosis. *American Journal of Medical Genetics Part a*. 2010;152A(2):394–400.
9. Beiriger JW, Bruce MK, Mak A, et al. Late presenting sagittal craniosynostosis: an update to a standardized treatment protocol. *Plast Reconstr Surg*. 2023
10. Kapp-Simon KA, Figueroa A, Jocher CA, Schafer M. Longitudinal assessment of mental development in infants with nonsyndromic craniosynostosis with and without cranial release and reconstruction. *Plast Reconstr Surg*. 1993;92(5):831–839. discussion 840-831.
11. Kapp-Simon KA, Speltz ML, Cunningham ML, Patel PK, Tomita T. Neurodevelopment of children with single suture craniosynostosis: a review. *Childs Nerv Syst*. 2007;23(3):269–281.
12. Kapp-Simon KA, Leroux B, Cunningham M, Speltz ML. Multisite study of infants with single-suture craniosynostosis: preliminary report of presurgery development. *Cleft Palate Craniofac J*. 2005;42(4):377–384.
13. Virtanen R, Korhonen T, Fagerholm J, Viljanto J. Neurocognitive sequelae of scaphocephaly. *Pediatrics*. 1999;103(4 Pt 1):791–795.
14. Panchal J, Marsh JL, Park TS, Kaufman B, Pilgram T, Huang SH. Sagittal craniosynostosis outcome assessment for two methods and timings of intervention. *Plast Reconstr Surg*. 1999;103(6):1574–1584.
15. Shipster C, Hearst D, Somerville A, Stackhouse J, Hayward R, Wade A. Speech, language, and cognitive development in children with isolated sagittal synostosis. *Dev Med Child Neurol*. 2003;45(1):34–43.
16. Thiele-Nygaard AE, Foss-Skiftesvik J, Juhler M. Intracranial pressure, brain morphology and cognitive outcome in children with sagittal craniosynostosis. *Childs Nerv Syst*. 2020;36(4):689–695.
17. Persing JA. MOC-PS(SM) CME article: management considerations in the treatment of craniosynostosis. *Plast Reconstr Surg*. 2008;121(4 Suppl):1–11.
18. Panchal J, Marsh JL, Park TS, Kaufman B, Pilgram T. Photographic assessment of head shape following sagittal synostosis surgery. *Plast Reconstr Surg*. 1999;103(6):1585–1591.
19. Jimenez DF, Barone CM, McGee ME. Design and care of helmets in postoperative craniosynostosis patients: our personal approach. *Clin Plast Surg*. 2004;31(3):481–487.
20. Ridgway EB, Berry-Candelario J, Grondin RT, Rogers GF, Proctor MR. The management of sagittal synostosis using endoscopic suturectomy and postoperative helmet therapy. *J Neurosurg Pediatr*. 2011;7(6):620–626.
21. Shakir S, Roy M, Lee A, Birgfeld CB. Management of sagittal and lambdoid craniosynostosis: minimally invasive approaches. *Oral Maxillofac Surg Clin North Am*. 2022;34(3):421–433.
22. Proctor MR. Endoscopic cranial suture release for the treatment of craniosynostosis: is it the future? *J Craniofac Surg*. 2012;23(1):225–228.
23. Chan JW, Stewart CL, Stalder St MW, Hilaire H, McBride L, Moses MH. Endoscope-assisted versus open repair of craniosynostosis: a comparison of perioperative cost and risk. *J Craniofac Surg*. 2013;24(1):170–174.
24. Vogel TW, Woo AS, Kane AA, Patel KB, Naidoo SD, Smyth MD. A comparison of costs associated with endoscope-assisted craniectomy versus open cranial vault repair for infants with sagittal synostosis. *J Neurosurg Pediatr*. 2014;13(3):324–331.
25. McGillivray G, Savarirayan R, Cox TC, et al. Familial scaphocephaly syndrome caused by a novel mutation in the FGFR2 tyrosine kinase domain. *J Med Genet*. 2005;42(8):656–662.
26. Kitabata R, Sakamoto Y, Miwa T, Yoshida K, Kishi K. Delayed-onset familial sagittal suture synostosis. *J Craniofac Surg*. 2020;31(5):e475–e477.

CHAPTER 31

Coronal Craniosynostosis

KEY POINTS

- Coronal craniosynostosis may occur as an isolated finding or as part of several genetic disorders.
- Coronal craniosynostosis can be unilateral or bilateral and can be caused by early descent of the fetal head into a constraining position, or aberrant fetal lie, or constraint within a bicornuate uterus.
- Late gestational constraint may cause an appearance similar to coronal synostosis at birth, but spontaneous restitution occurs within a few postnatal weeks if the coronal sutures are not fused.
- In unilateral coronal craniosynostosis, the forehead on the affected side is tall and flattened, with vertical upward displacement of the orbit and ear on that side, and the nasal root deviates toward the flattened side.
- Limb defects, such as syndactyly, brachydactyly, or broad, deviated thumbs and halluces, suggest the presence of an underlying syndrome.

GENESIS

Coronal craniosynostosis is the second most common type of craniosynostosis, accounting for 20–30% of cases.[1-3] Constraint-induced unilateral coronal craniosynostosis can be secondary to early descent of the fetal head into a constraining pelvis, aberrant fetal lie, or constraint within a bicornuate uterus.[4-7] It is known that the majority (67–71%) of unilateral coronal craniosynostosis is right-sided,[8,9] and this nonrandom predilection may relate to the fact that 67% of vertex presentations are in the left occiput transverse position, with the left coronal suture against the sacral prominence.[4] If the fetal head descends early and is maintained in the most common position (i.e., left occiput transverse), the result may be more constraint across the right coronal suture as it lies against the pubic bone compared with the left coronal suture as it lies against the sacral prominence. This may explain the increased prevalence of right-sided, unilateral coronal craniosynostosis. Nonsyndromic coronal craniosynostosis occurs in 0.94 per 10,000 births, with 61% of cases sporadic and 14.4% of 180 pedigrees familial. Bilateral cases occur much more frequently than unilateral cases, and coronal synostosis is more common in females (male:female ratio, 1:2). The paternal age is significantly older than average (32.7 years), with an average paternal age of 26 to 27 years and the advent of testicular aging at 30 years of age. Most sperm banks discourage donors over 40 years of age. These data have been interpreted as being consistent with autosomal dominant inheritance, with 60% penetrance when the synostosis has a genetic basis.[10]

Defects in postmigratory neural crest cells can result in pre- or postossification defects in the developing craniofacial skeleton and craniosynostosis.[11] When craniosynostosis occurs as part of a syndrome, it is most important to examine the patient carefully for associated anomalies. Evaluation of the limbs, ears, eyes, and cardiovascular system yields the most significant data for diagnosing syndromes associated with craniosynostosis. Limb defects such as syndactyly, brachydactyly, or broad, deviated thumbs and halluces suggest the presence of an associated syndrome. It is also important to examine both parents for digital anomalies, carpal coalition, and/or facial asymmetry because these findings may represent variable expression of an altered gene in a parent.

Bilateral coronal synostosis often lacks sutural ridging and usually has a genetic basis, which suggests that all such patients should be screened for mutations. Among 57 patients with bilateral coronal synostosis, mutations were found in fibroblast growth factor receptor (*FRGR*) genes for all 38 patients who had a syndromic form of craniosynostosis. Among 19 patients with unclassified brachycephaly, mutations in or near exon 9 of *FGFR2* were found in four patients, and a common Pro250Arg mutation in exon 7 of *FGFR3* was detected in 10 patients. Only five patients (9%) manifested brachycephaly without a detectable mutation in *FGFR1*, *2*, or *3*.[12] In a study of 233 individuals, whose previous testing had not identified a causative variant within *FGFR1–3* or *TWIST1*, pathogenic or likely pathogenic variants in non-FGFR genes were identified in 43 individuals, with diagnostic yields of ~15% and variants most frequently identified in *TCF12* and *EFNB1*.[13] These findings suggest that mutation analysis of *FGFR1–3*, *TWIST1*, *TCF12*, and *EFNB1* genes should be considered in all patients with coronal synostosis. Tooze et al. describe the expansion and diagnostic yield of gene panels in craniosynostosis.[14]

It is also important to obtain hand and foot radiographs in older children and their parents, because subtle digital changes and carpal/tarsal coalition can be seen in individuals with the Pro250Arg mutation in *FGFR3*, even if they lack findings of coronal craniosynostosis.[15] An estimated 10% of patients with unilateral coronal synostosis carry this mutation; some parents carry this mutation but demonstrate few clinical manifestations.[16] In a prospective study of 47 patients with synostotic frontal plagiocephaly (unilateral coronal synostosis), mutations were found in eight patients (17%): two with *FGFR2*, three with *FGFR3* Pro250Arg, and three with *TWIST* mutations.[17] Two clinical features were strongly associated with mutation detection: (1) asymmetric brachycephaly with retrusion of both orbital rims; and (2) orbital hypertelorism. More recently, a study by Sharma et al. of 28 bicoronal and 115 unicoronal craniosynostosis cases found a *TCF12* gene mutation in 32% of bilateral and 10% of unicoronal cases.[18] In addition, several patients were carriers of a mutation but did not express signs of craniosynostosis. It is also important to emphasize that inability to demonstrate a mutation does not rule out a genetic cause for the craniosynostosis, and not every person with a mutation manifests craniosynostosis.

FEATURES

In patients with bilateral coronal craniosynostosis, the forehead is high and broad. The impact of bilateral coronal synostosis on the craniofacial region is summarized in Figs. 31.1 and 31.2. When there is unilateral

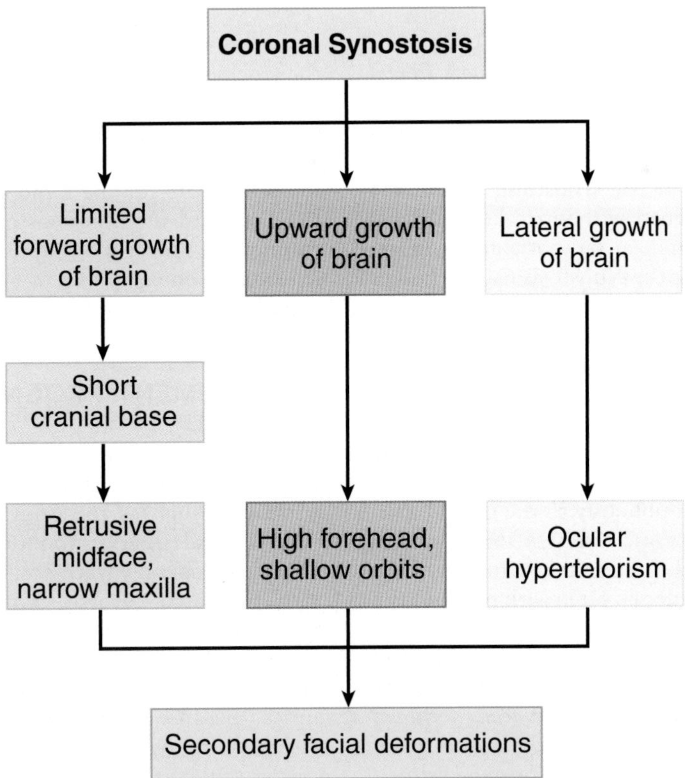

FIGURE 31.1 Diagram depicting the manner in which bilateral coronal craniostenosis results in secondary facial effects.

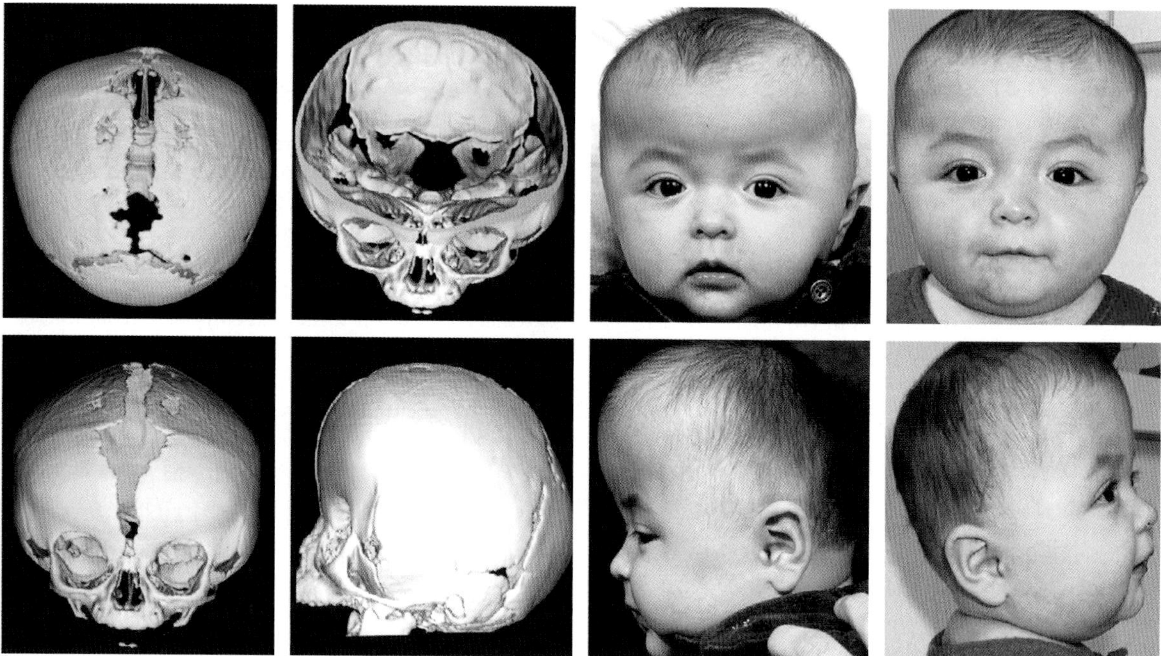

FIGURE 31.2 As shown on this three-dimensional cranial computed tomography scan, there is complete obliteration of both coronal sutures, resulting in a high, broad forehead with brachycephaly and ocular hypertelorism.

coronal craniosynostosis (also termed *synostotic frontal plagiocephaly*), the impact on the facial structures is asymmetric, resulting in significant facial distortion that may complicate surgical correction (Figs. 31.3 and 31.4). On the side of the synostotic suture, the forehead is tall and flattened, with vertical upward displacement of the orbit and ear on that side. The forehead on the side opposite the synostosis usually bulges forward, and the nasal root deviates toward the flattened side. The affected supraorbital rim is retruded, elevated, and slightly displaced laterally on the side of the flattened forehead. These features persist and worsen in patients who are not treated surgically, with orbital distortion affecting the visual system. There may be marked thickening and up-tilting of the sphenoid wings, with an oval obliquity to the orbital margins (called the *harlequin sign*). With syndromes such as Crouzon, Pfeiffer (Fig. 31.5), and Apert syndromes, the orbits are shallow and wide-set, often with pronounced proptosis. The synostosis is often initiated at the lower end of the coronal suture (near the sphenoid wing) and progresses superiorly. There is a head tilt toward the nonsynostotic side (sometimes termed *ocular torticollis* or *pseudopalsy of the superior oblique muscle*) in about half the affected children because the foreshortened superomedial orbital wall on the affected side displaces the trochlea posteriorly, which weakens the action of the superior oblique tendon. This results in relative overactivity of the inferior oblique muscle compared with the superior oblique muscle. Thus in an attempt to compensate for the diplopia, the head may begin to tilt toward the nonsynostotic side. Astigmatism is common in unicoronal craniosynostosis and has been reported in one eye in up to 54%, with the majority of these being in the contralateral eye.[19]

MANAGEMENT, PROGNOSIS, AND COUNSEL

The impact of coronal synostosis on adjacent facial structures, such as the orbit, is of such magnitude that surgical intervention during the first half of infancy is generally warranted. Furthermore the child with untreated coronal craniosynostosis may have a restricted nasopharynx fostering middle ear infections, an abnormal oral cavity contributing to speech problems, dental malocclusion, and obstructive sleep apnea. Because intracranial volume almost triples within the first year and by 2 years of age is four times greater than the cranial capacity at birth, asymmetric cranial expansion due to unilateral coronal synostosis

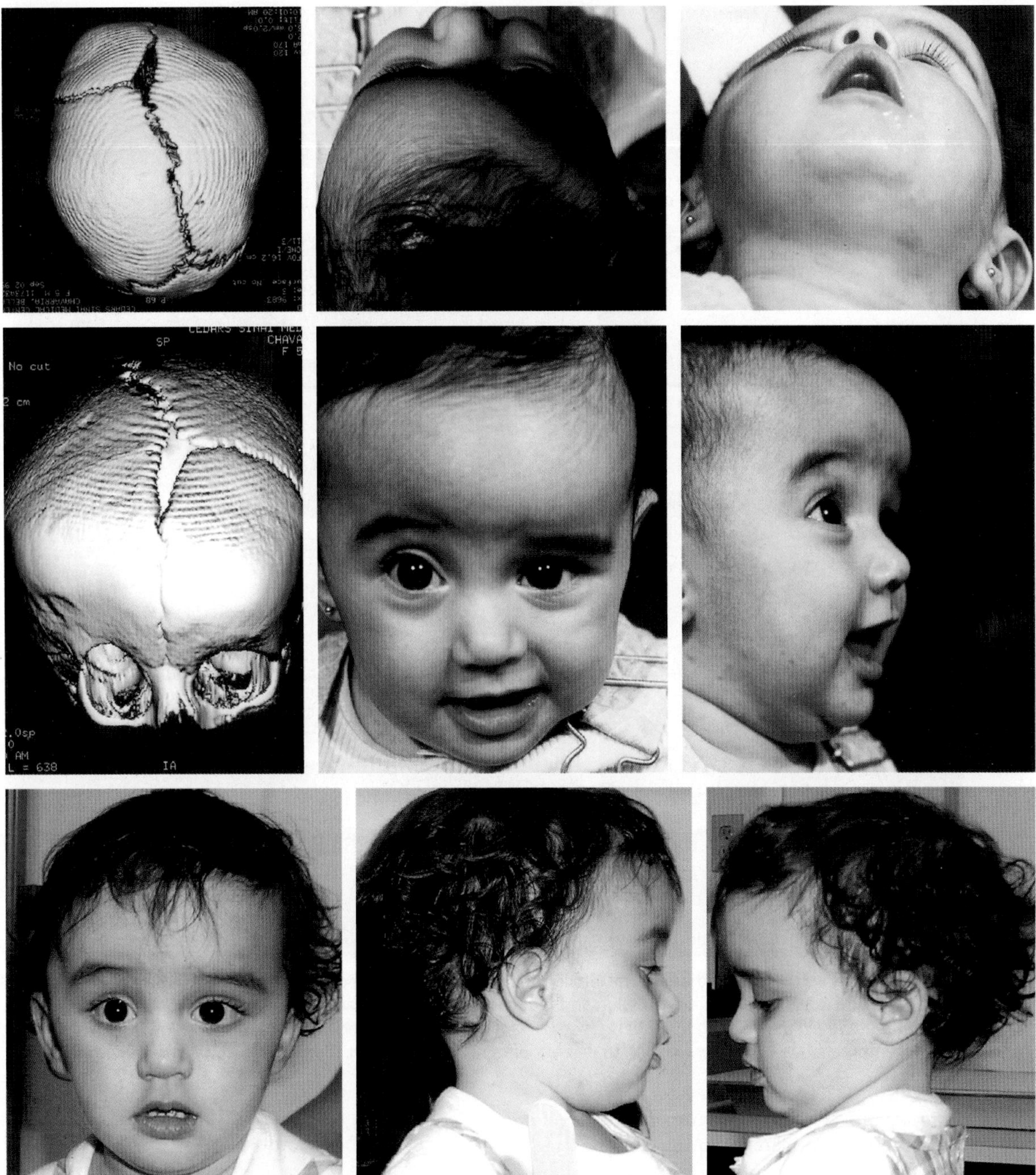

FIGURE 31.3 This girl has right coronal synostosis with a tall, flattened forehead on the side of the synostotic suture, resulting in vertical upward displacement of the orbit and ear on that side. The forehead on the side opposite the synostosis is prominent, and the nasal root deviates toward the flattened side. The supraorbital rim on the side of the flattened forehead is retruded, elevated, and laterally displaced.

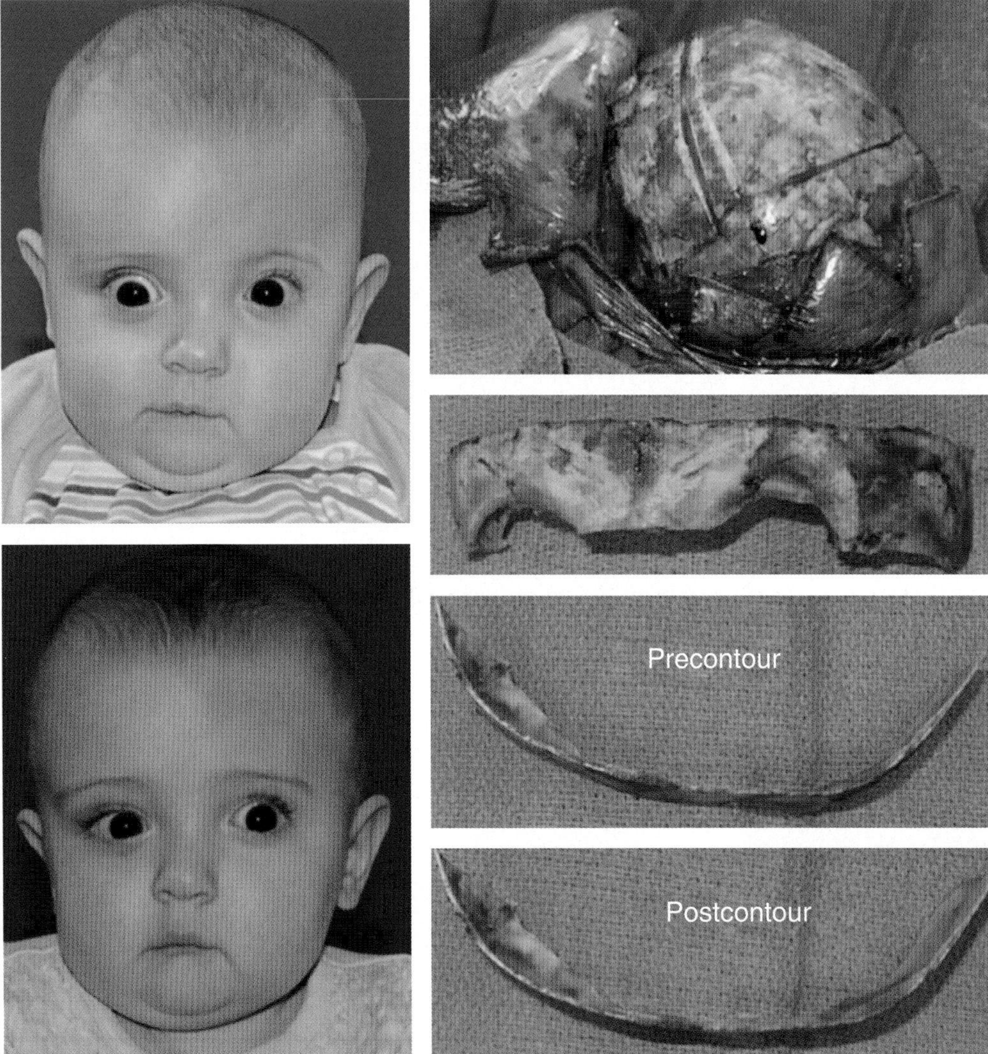

FIGURE 31.4 Eight-month-old female with unilateral left coronal craniosynostosis demonstrating palpable ridging over her synostotic left coronal suture *(top left image)* and recession and reduction of the bossed area after calvarial recontouring with orbital rim advancement *(bottom left image)*. *(Right images)* Open calvarial vault remodeling with bifrontal craniotomy with pre- and post-contour of the frontal bone. (Courtesy Mark M. Urata and Jeffrey A. Hammoudeh, Children's Hospital Los Angeles, CA, USA.)

can have a major impact on the symmetry of facial structures. Surgery for unilateral coronal craniosynostosis (or synostotic frontal plagiocephaly) seeks to correct the progressive distortions affecting the forehead and orbits and to align the nasal root. The basic variations in surgical techniques have evolved over the years (listed in order of their development):

1. Unilateral fronto-orbital advancement
2. Bilateral fronto-orbital advancement without nasal straightening
3. Bilateral fronto-orbital advancement with closing wedge nasal osteotomy[20]
4. Endoscopic strip craniectomy and helmet therapy[21]
5. Forehead remodeling with bone graft.[22]

Measurable postoperative fronto-orbital asymmetry remains most marked in the first group, which leads most surgeons to advance both sides even though only one side may be synostotic. Postoperative symmetry is most ideal with slight overcorrection of the vertical and anteroposterior supraorbital rim deformity on the

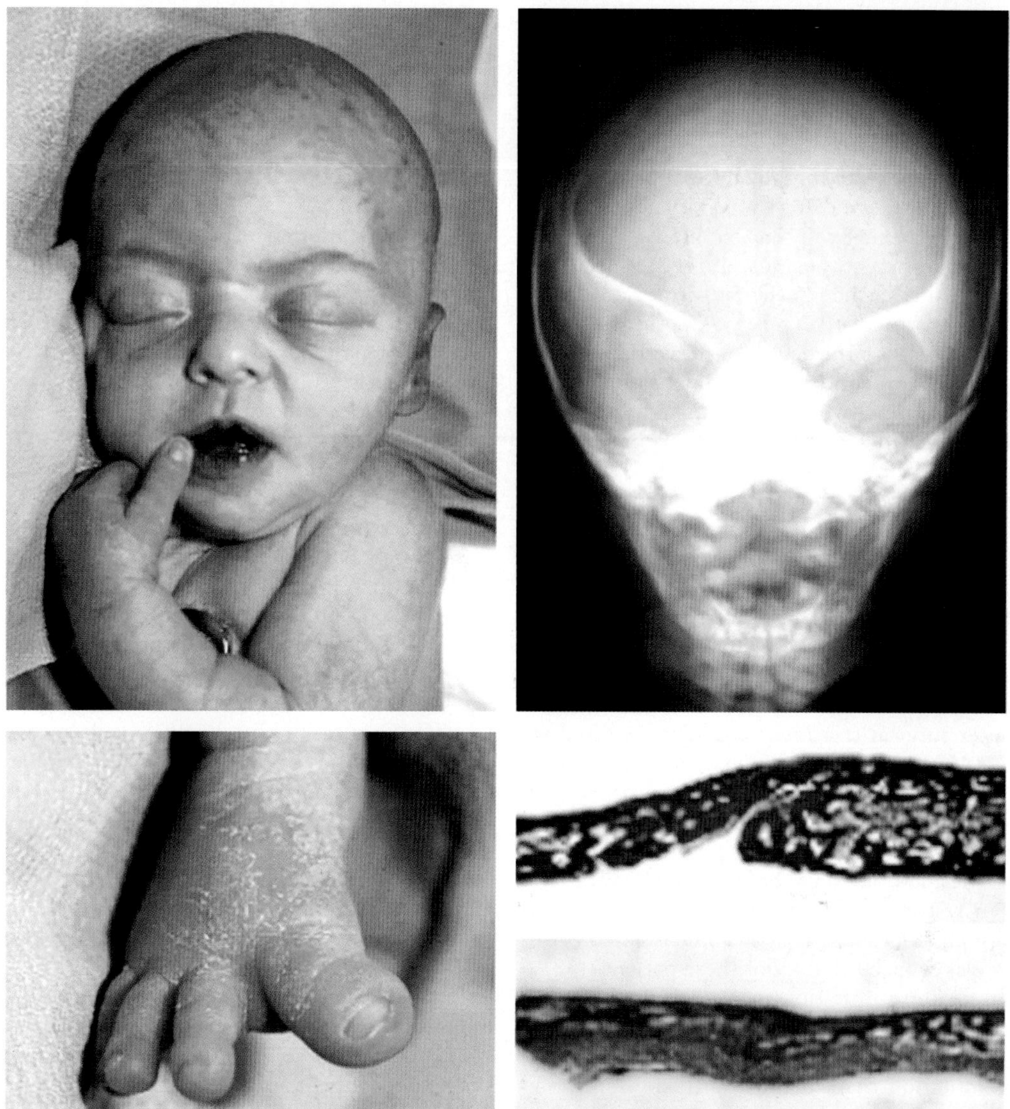

FIGURE 31.5 This infant with Pfeiffer syndrome shows laterally deviated thumbs and halluces with a bilateral harlequin sign on skull radiographs. (Note the facial differences compared with the infants shown in Figs. 31.2–31.4, who have nonsyndromic bilateral coronal synostosis.)

affected side, along with nasal straightening.[20] In children with bilateral coronal craniosynostosis, particularly when it occurs as part of a syndrome (e.g., Pfeiffer, Apert, or Crouzon syndromes), primary fronto-orbital advancement during infancy must be exaggerated to compensate for diminished frontal growth potential.[23]

Because binocular vision develops at 3 months when the retina reaches maturity and because the eye reaches its adult size by 3 years of age, with a doubling of ocular volume during the first 12 months, early surgical correction of plagiocephaly is necessary to prevent strabismus due to synostosis-related traction on the ocular globe. Even when surgery is undertaken between 3 and 6 months of age, the ocular problems are not always prevented or alleviated, and careful ophthalmologic follow-up is indicated.[24] In a study of 39 children with unicoronal synostosis, vertical strabismus was explained by initial traction on the lateral rectus muscles, with secondary stretching of the inferior oblique muscle and associated underaction of the superior oblique muscle on the side of the synostosis. When strabismus was followed over time and correlated with time of surgical repair, it was clear that strabismus was initially horizontal and then became vertical if the synostosis was not released early. Children who were surgically treated after 11 months of age showed vertical strabismus, and those surgically treated before this age had horizontal strabismus. The later that reconstructive surgery was performed, the more pronounced was the degree of measurable astigmatism because of continuing compensatory bone growth.[25] Thus primary fronto-orbital advancement is usually performed between 3 and 9 months of age; some surgeons operate as early as 3 months due to the increased pliability of cranial bone and predictable reossification of cranial defects, and others wait until 6–9 months, when bone is stronger and fixation is more stable.[26,27] Early surgery allows the cranial base (the roof of the face) to grow forward, carrying the midface with it. The forward growth of the cranial base is normally 56% complete by birth and 70% complete by 2 years of age. Delayed synostoses of uninvolved sutures after surgical treatment has been reported in 2.1% (3 of 145) patients undergoing open craniosynostosis surgery and 1.7% (2 of 121) patients undergoing endoscopic surgery.[28]

When mutations in FGFR genes limit the forward growth of the anterior cranial base, surgery may be less effective in restoring facial features to normal.[29,30] A study of 76 patients with nonsyndromic isolated coronal synostosis revealed that 29 of these patients (38%) had the Pro250Arg mutation in *FGFR3*. Reoperation for functional reasons (raised intracranial pressure) was nearly five times more common in the patients with this mutation than in those with no mutation. Within the entire group of 76 patients, the reoperation rate was 11.8% (10.5% for functional reasons). Presence of the Pro250Arg mutation in *FGFR3* was the only factor that reached significance for predicting reoperation. This suggests that the risk of functional sequelae and thus the need for reoperation is higher in syndromic craniosynostosis as well as in nonsyndromic coronal synostosis with the Pro250Arg mutation in *FGFR3*.[30] For these reasons, preoperative mutation evaluation is strongly recommended. Syndromic craniosynostosis has been associated with mutations in *FGFR1*, *FGFR2*, *FGFR3*, *TWIST*, *MSX2*, and *EFNB1*, and nonsyndromic coronal craniosynostosis has been associated with the Pro250Arg mutation in *FGFR3* and *EFNB4*, and with mutations in *TCF12*.[31–33]

DIFFERENTIAL DIAGNOSIS

Coronal synostosis may occur as an isolated finding or as part of a variety of genetic disorders that affect the growth of craniofacial structures and limbs.[17,30,34] It is beyond the scope of this text to review these syndromes in any detail; the reader is referred to Cohen and MacLean's comprehensive book on craniosynostosis for an extensive discussion of this topic.[18] Mutations are found in virtually all patients with Apert, Crouzon, or Pfeiffer syndrome, and a mutation was also found in 75% of patients with unclassified brachycephaly.[12] Mutations in *TWIST* are found in 80% of patients with Saethre-Chotzen syndrome (Fig. 31.6).[17] Patients with macrocephaly; a high, broad forehead; down-slanting palpebral fissure; distal brachydactyly; and/or anomalous toes may demonstrate the *FGFR3* Pro250Arg mutation (Figs. 31.7 and 31.8).[15] Patients with unilateral coronal synostosis have a 6%–11% likelihood of demonstrating this mutation.[16,17] Approximately 54% of patients with craniofrontonasal syndrome (Fig. 31.9) demonstrate synostotic frontal plagiocephaly,[30] and mutations have been found in the X-linked gene *EFNB1*, which is located at Xq13.1.[35] Loss-of-function mutations in *EFNB1* result in a paradoxically greater severity in heterozygous females than in hemizygous males (which may be one of the factors that explains much of the observed female excess in coronal craniosynostosis).[36] For this condition, males who are mosaic for the mutation express more similar severity to females.[31,36] Constraint limitation of craniofacial growth in late gestation may occasionally yield an appearance at birth quite similar to that of coronal synostosis, especially in patients with face presentations or persistent transverse lie, or who were constrained in one horn of a bicornuate uterus. If the coronal sutures are not fused, such patients demonstrate rapid spontaneous restitution toward normal form in the first few postnatal weeks, which would not be expected with coronal craniosynostosis. For this single reason, it is probably best to wait a few weeks before making a decision about calvarial surgery unless the problem is obvious and severe with evidence of increased intracranial pressure. The discovery of a common point mutation in *FGFR3* (Pro250Arg) in patients with "nonsyndromic" coronal craniosynostosis warrants consideration in any patient with this disorder (see Figs. 31.7 and 31.8). In a study of 62 familial and sporadic cases of nonsyndromal coronal craniosynostosis, this mutation was found in 42% of cases. Among 35 sporadic cases, 17% had the *FGFR3* Pro250Arg mutation (with an average paternal age of

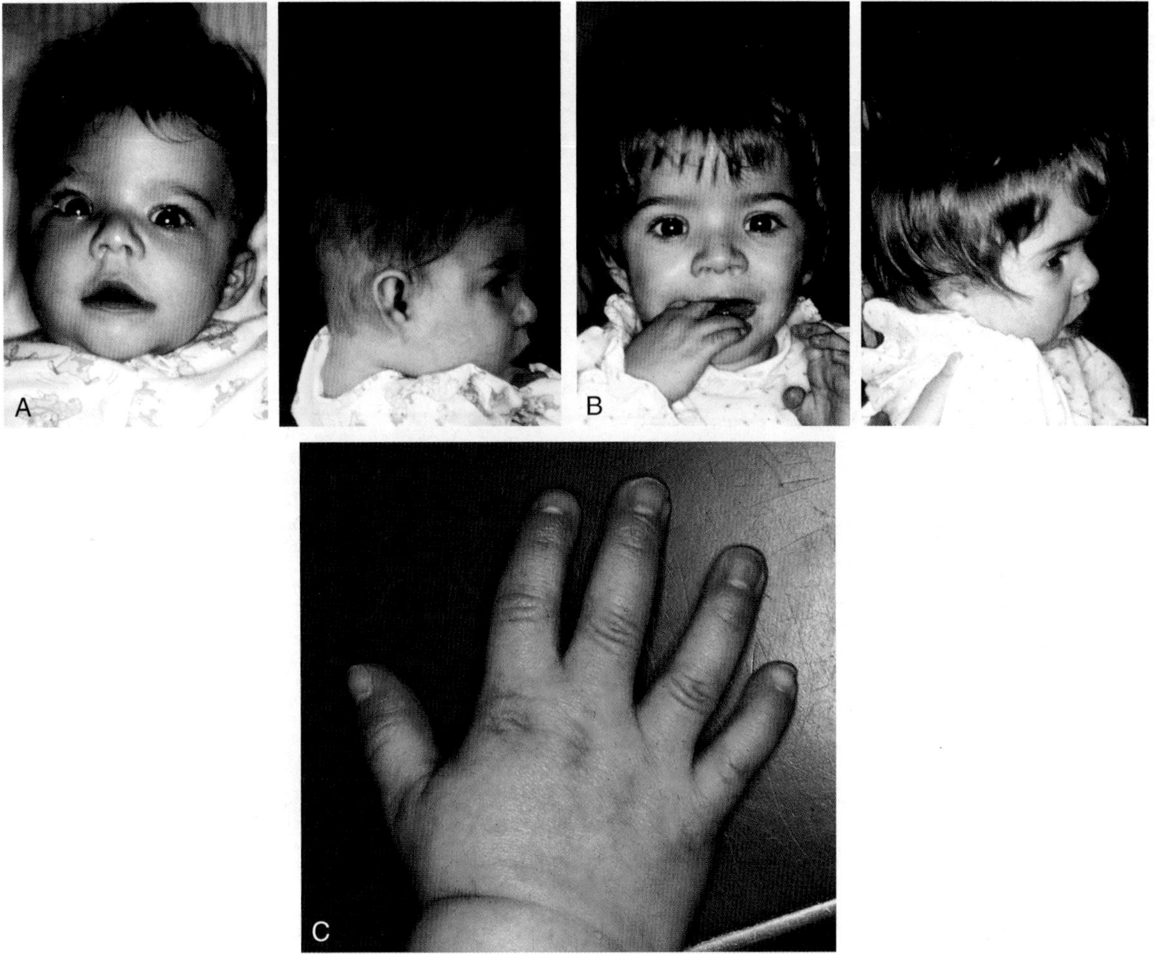

FIGURE 31.6 This girl with Saethre-Chotzen syndrome is shown (A) before and (B) after surgical reconstruction. C, Note partial syndactyly with fifth-finger clinodactyly.

39.7 years at the time of birth, which suggests fresh dominant mutation) whereas 74% of 27 familial cases revealed this mutation. Of the 62 cases, 30% had plagiocephaly and 70% had brachycephaly.

When associated findings were examined, many patients manifested severe forehead retrusion with hypertelorism and bulging of the temporal fossae (possibly reflecting poorer postoperative results in older patients who underwent outdated surgical procedures). The mean intelligence quotient (IQ) among affected persons was 97, but 26 patients had an IQ less than 80, and one patient with associated hydrocephalus had an IQ of 63. No effort was made to correlate efficacy of surgical repair with cognitive outcomes. In a 2022 systematic review and meta-analysis by Fotouhi et al., they found that patients with unicoronal craniosynostosis scored 1 standard deviation below the normative data in neurodevelopment (in verbal, psychomotor, and mathematic outcome assessments), although scores generally remained within the normal range.[37] Brachydactyly was observed in 22 of 32 cases, most commonly affecting the middle phalanges; carpal fusion was noted in only three of 22 radiographs, with tarsal fusion in two cases and calcaneo-cuboid fusion in one case. In one familial case, both parents had normal skull radiographs and craniofacial examinations, but both the proband and her father carried the mutation and demonstrated carpal and tarsal fusions on radiographs. Among 4 of 37 patients with unicoronal synostosis due to this *FGFR3* mutation, 3 fathers were

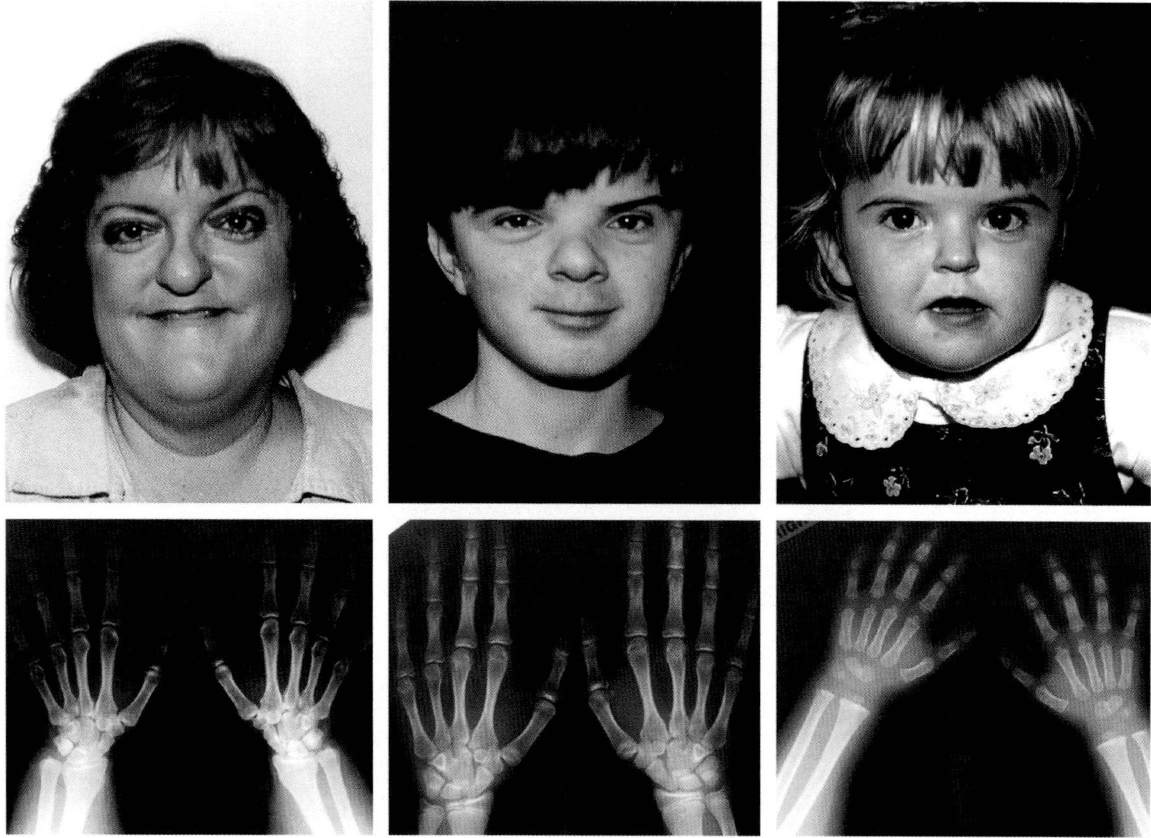

FIGURE 31.7 This mother and her two children have the *FGFR3* Pro250Arg mutation that results in macrocephaly with variable coronal synostosis and capitate-hamate coalition.

identified as carrying the same mutation but had only subtle hand radiographic findings and no craniofacial findings.[16] Thus, not only should this mutation be searched for in patients with nonsyndromic coronal craniosynostosis, but both parents should also be analyzed if the mutation is found, even if they appear clinically normal. If mutation screening is negative for this common mutation in *FGFR3*, screening for *FGFR1*, *FGFR2*, and *TWIST* should be done because mutations in these genes can also cause coronal craniosynostosis with variable, subtle associated facial and distal limb anomalies. Saethre-Chotzen syndrome is caused by mutations that result in haploinsufficiency for *TWIST*, and it can usually be distinguished on clinical grounds from Muenke syndrome, which results from a gain-of-function mutation in *FGFR3* due to the point mutation Pro250Arg.[38,39] Patients with Saethre-Chotzen syndrome have a low frontal hairline, microcephaly (37%), ptosis, small ears, dilated parietal foramina, intradigital webbing, hallux valgus, and/or broad great toes with a wide distal phalanx. They must be observed for progressive multi-suture fusion, which occurs in 53% of patients and can lead to intracranial hypertension (35% of patients at a median age of 30 months).[39] The presence of intracranial hypertension leads to reoperation in 18% of patients with Saethre-Chotzen syndrome, and papilledema was the most frequent sign of this complication. In five patients who were not treated early enough, visual loss occurred due to irreversible optic nerve damage; therefore such patients should be observed with annual eye exams.[39] Patients with Muenke syndrome had mild to moderate intellectual disability in 34% of cases, with sensorineural hearing loss in 32% of cases; thus these patients should receive early intervention and annual hearing exams.[38]

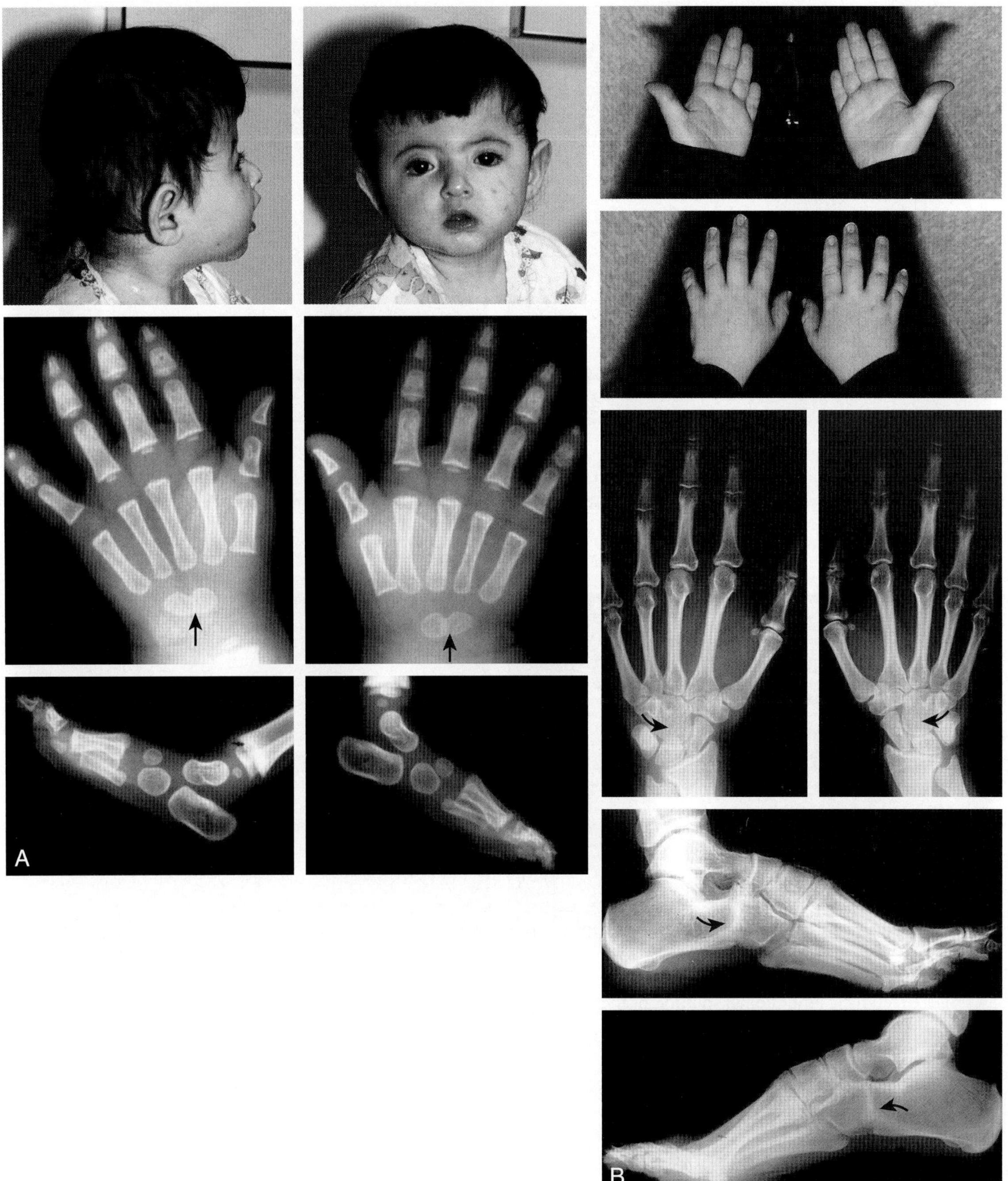

FIGURE 31.8 This infant with the *FGFR3* Pro250Arg mutation has coronal synostosis and capitate-hamate coalitions with hypoplastic distal phalanges (A). Her affected mother also required surgery for bilateral coronal synostosis and demonstrates capitate-hamate coalitions, calcaneo-cuboid coalitions, and hypoplastic distal phalanges (B).

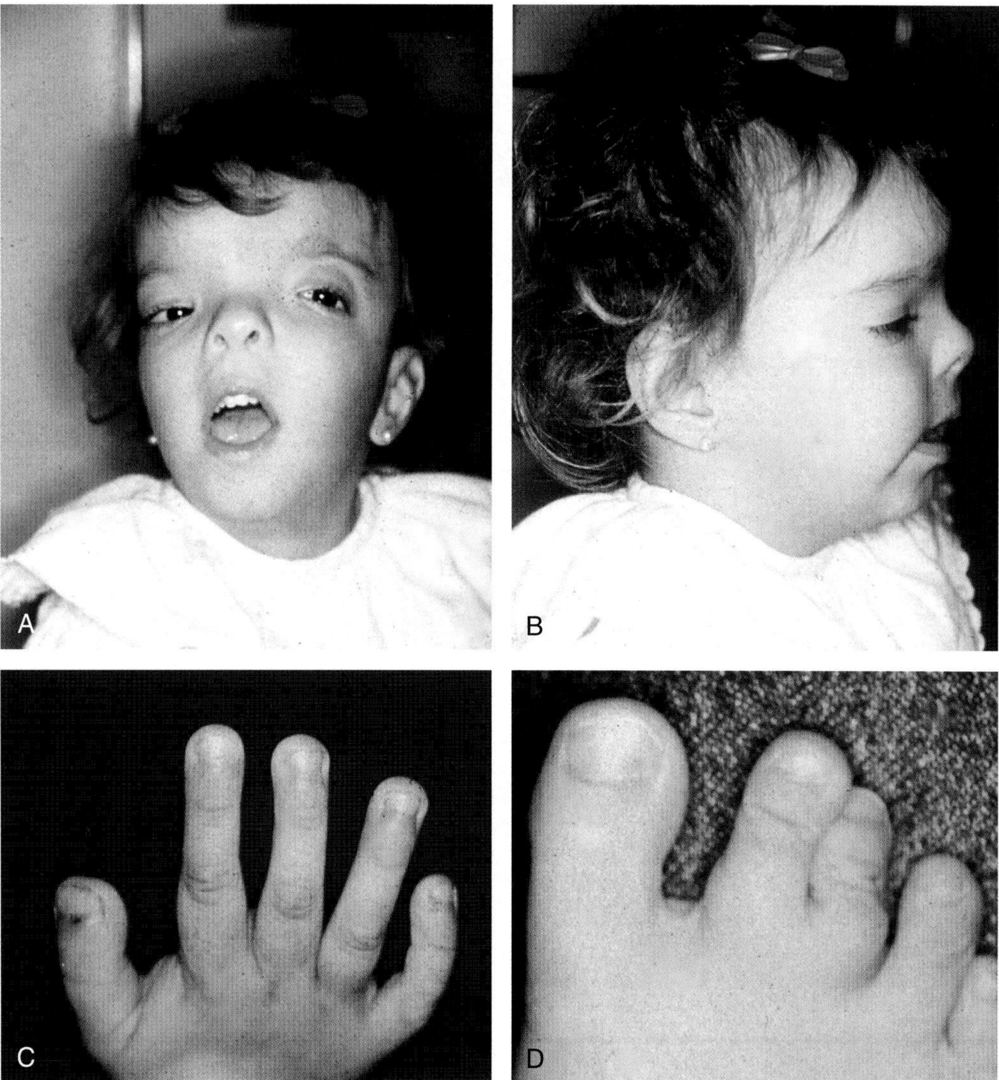

FIGURE 31.9 This girl with craniofrontonasal syndrome demonstrates left coronal synostosis with severe ocular hypertelorism (A and B), characteristic longitudinal splitting of the nails (C), and partial syndactyly of the second and third toes (D).

References

1. Marbate T, Kedia S, Gupta DK. Evaluation and management of nonsyndromic craniosynostosis. *J Pediatr Neurosci*. 2022;17(Suppl 1):S77–S91.
2. Gonzalez SR, Light JG, Golinko MS. Assessment of epidemiological trends in craniosynostosis: limitations of the current classification system. *Plast Reconstr Surg Glob Open*. 2020;8(3):e2597.
3. Stanton E, Urata M, Chen JF, Chai Y. The clinical manifestations, molecular mechanisms and treatment of craniosynostosis. *Dis Model Mech*. 2022 Apr 1;15(4):dmm049390.
4. Graham JM Jr, Badura RJ, Smith DW. Coronal craniostenosis: fetal head constraint as one possible cause. *Pediatrics*. 1980;65(5):995–999.
5. Sanchez-Lara PA, Carmichael SL, Graham JM Jr, et al. Fetal constraint as a potential risk factor for craniosynostosis. *American Journal of Medical Genetics Part a*. 2010;152A(2):394–400.
6. Higginbottom MC, Jones KL, James HE. Intrauterine constraint and craniosynostosis. *Neurosurgery*. 1980;6(1):39–44.
7. Graham JM Jr. Craniofacial deformation. *Ballier Clin Pediatr*. 1988;6:293–315.

8. Hunter AG, Rudd NL. Craniosynostosis. II. Coronal synostosis: its familial characteristics and associated clinical findings in 109 patients lacking bilateral polysyndactyly or syndactyly. *Teratology*. 1977;15(3):301–309.
9. Boulet SL, Rasmussen SA, Honein MA. A population-based study of craniosynostosis in metropolitan Atlanta, 1989-2003. *Am J Med Genet A*. 2008;146A(8):984–991.
10. Lajeunie E, Le Merrer M, Bonaiti-Pellie C, Marchac D, Renier D. Genetic study of nonsyndromic coronal craniosynostosis. *Am J Med Genet*. 1995;55(4):500–504.
11. Siismets EM, Hatch NE. Cranial neural crest cells and their role in the pathogenesis of craniofacial anomalies and coronal craniosynostosis. *J Dev Biol*. 2020;8:3.
12. Mulliken JB, Steinberger D, Kunze S, Muller U. Molecular diagnosis of bilateral coronal synostosis. *Plastic and Reconstructive Surgery*. 1999;104(6):1603–1615.
13. Lee E, Le T, Zhu Y, et al. A craniosynostosis massively parallel sequencing panel study in 309 Australian and New Zealand patients: findings and recommendations. *Genet Med*. 2018;20(9):1061–1068.
14. Tooze RS, Calpena E, Weber A, Wilson LC, Twigg SRF, Wilkie AOM. Review of recurrently mutated genes in craniosynostosis supports expansion of diagnostic gene panels. *Genes (Basel)*. 2023;14(3).
15. Graham JM Jr, Braddock SR, Mortier GR, Lachman R, Van Dop C, Jabs EW. Syndrome of coronal craniosynostosis with brachydactyly and carpal/tarsal coalition due to Pro250Arg mutation in *FGFR3* gene. *Am J Med Genet*. 1998;77(4):322–329.
16. Gripp KW, McDonald-McGinn DM, Gaudenz K, et al. Identification of a genetic cause for isolated unilateral coronal synostosis: a unique mutation in the fibroblast growth factor receptor 3. *J Pediatr*. 1998;132(4):714–716.
17. Mulliken JB, Gripp KW, Stolle CA, Steinberger D, Muller U. Molecular analysis of patients with synostotic frontal plagiocephaly (unilateral coronal synostosis). *Plast Reconstr Surg*. 2004;113(7):1899–1909.
18. Sharma VP, Fenwick AL, Brockop MS, et al. Mutations in *TCF12*, encoding a basic helix-loop-helix partner of *TWIST1*, are a frequent cause of coronal craniosynostosis (vol 45, pg 304, 2013). *Nature Genet*. 2013;45(10):1261-1261.
19. Levy RL, Rogers GF, Mulliken JB, Proctor MR, Dagi LR. Astigmatism in unilateral coronal synostosis: incidence and laterality. *J Aapos*. 2007;11(4):367–372.
20. Hansen M, Padwa BL, Scott RM, Stieg PE, Mulliken JB. Synostotic frontal plagiocephaly: anthropometric comparison of three techniques for surgical correction. *Plastic and Reconstructive Surgery*. 1997;100(6):1387–1395.
21. Tan SPK, Proctor MR, Mulliken JB, Rogers GF. Early frontofacial symmetry after correction of unilateral coronal synostosis: frontoorbital advancement vs endoscopic strip craniectomy and helmet therapy. *J Craniofac Surg*. 2013;24(4):1190–1194.
22. Maltese G, Tarnow P, Lindstrom A, et al. New objective measurement of forehead symmetry in unicoronal craniosynostosis - comparison between fronto-orbital advancement and forehead remodelling with a bone graft. *J Plast Surg Hand Surg*. 2014;48(1):59–62.
23. Pai L, Kohout MP, Mulliken JB. Prospective anthropometric analysis of sagittal orbital-globe relationship following fronto-orbital advancement in childhood. *Plast Reconstr Surg*. 1999;103(5):1341–1346.
24. Rosenberg JB, Tepper OM, Medow NB. Strabismus in craniosynostosis. *J Pediatr Ophthalmol Strabismus*. 2013;50(3):140–148.
25. Denis D, Genitori L, Conrath J, Lena G, Choux M. Ocular findings in children operated on for plagiocephaly and trigonocephaly. *Childs Nerv Syst*. 1996;12(11):683–689.
26. Pai L, Kohout MP, Mulliken JB. Prospective anthropometric analysis of sagittal orbital-globe relationship following fronto-orbital advancement in childhood. *Plastic and Reconstructive Surgery*. 1999;103(5):1341–1346.
27. Posnick JC. Unilateral coronal synostosis (anterior plagiocephaly): current clinical perspectives. *Ann Plast Surg*. 1996;36(4):430–447.
28. Yarbrough CK, Smyth MD, Holekamp TF, et al. Delayed synostoses of uninvolved sutures after surgical treatment of nonsyndromic craniosynostosis. *J Craniofac Surg*. 2014;25(1):119–123.
29. Reinhart E, Muhling J, Michel C, Collmann H, Pistner H, Reuther J. Craniofacial growth characteristics after bilateral fronto-orbital advancement in children with premature craniosynostosis. *Childs Nerv Syst*. 1996;12(11):690–694.
30. Thomas GP, Wilkie AO, Richards PG, Wall SA. *FGFR3* P250R mutation increases the risk of reoperation in apparent 'nonsyndromic' coronal craniosynostosis. *J Craniofac Surg*. 2005;16(3):347–352; discussion 353-344.
31. van den Elzen ME, Twigg SR, Goos JA, et al. Phenotypes of craniofrontonasal syndrome in patients with a pathogenic mutation in *EFNB1*. *Eur J Hum Genet*. 2014;22(8):995–1001.
32. Lajeunie E, Lemerrer M, Bonaitipellie C, Marchac D, Renier D. Genetic study of nonsyndromic coronal craniosynostosis. *Am J Med Genet*. 1995;55(4):500–504.
33. Sharma VP, Fenwick AL, Brockop MS, et al. Mutations in *TCF12*, encoding a basic helix-loop-helix partner of *TWIST1*, are a frequent cause of coronal craniosynostosis. *Nature Genet*. 2013;45(3):304–307.
34. Mulliken JB, Steinberger D, Kunze S, Muller U. Molecular diagnosis of bilateral coronal synostosis. *Plast Reconstr Surg*. 1999;104(6):1603–1615.
35. Cohen MM, MacLean RE. *Craniosynostosis: Diagnosis. Evaluation, and Management*. 2nd ed. New York: Oxford University Press; 2000.
36. Twigg SR, Kan R, Babbs C, et al. Mutations of ephrin-B1 (*EFNB1*), a marker of tissue boundary formation, cause craniofrontonasal syndrome. *Proc Natl Acad Sci U S A*. 2004;101(23):8652–8657.
37. Fotouhi AR, Chiang SN, Peterson AM, et al. Neurodevelopment in unilateral coronal craniosynostosis: a

systematic review and meta-analysis. *J Neurosurg Pediatr.* 2023;31(1):16–23.
38. Lajeunie E, El Ghouzzi V, Le Merrer M, Munnich A, Bonaventure J, Renier D. Sex related expressivity of the phenotype in coronal craniosynostosis caused by the recurrent P250R *FGFR3* mutation. *J Med Genet.* 1999;36(1):9–13.
39. Kress W, Schropp C, Lieb G, et al. Saethre-Chotzen syndrome caused by *TWIST 1* gene mutations: functional differentiation from Muenke coronal synostosis syndrome. *Eur J Hum Genet.* 2006;14(1):39–48.

CHAPTER 32

Metopic Craniosynostosis

KEY POINTS

- The metopic suture is the first cranial suture to close and normally closes by 8 to 9 months.
- Mild degrees of metopic ridging occur frequently at birth, but unless there is progressive distortion of the orbits, it usually resolves.
- Metopic synostosis is characterized by trigonocephaly, lateral supraorbital retrusion, and hypotelorism.
- Trigonocephaly can occur as an isolated anomaly or as part of a syndrome or chromosome abnormality.
- Prenatal lateral constraint of the frontal part of the head is a frequent cause of metopic craniosynostosis.

GENESIS

The range of incidence of metopic synostosis occurs in about 0.67–14 per 10,000 births.[1] It accounts for 10–20% of patients requiring calvarial surgery, making it the third most common type of craniosynostosis in the clinic.[2] It is characterized by trigonocephaly, lateral supraorbital retrusion, and hypotelorism.[3] Like sagittal synostosis, metopic synostosis occurs more frequently in males, with a 2–6.5:1 male:female ratio reported with no maternal or paternal age effect.[4] Only 5.6% of cases have been familial.[5] The frequency of associated twinning was 7.8% of 179 pedigrees studied, with two twin monozygotic pairs concordant.[5,6] The similarity of epidemiologic features in sagittal and metopic craniosynostosis suggests that prenatal lateral constraint of the frontal part of the head is a frequent cause of metopic craniosynostosis (Figs. 32.1–32.4). Examples of constraint-induced metopic synostosis have included a monozygotic triplet whose forehead was wedged between the buttocks of her two co-triplets in utero (see Fig. 32.3) and an infant whose head was compressed within one horn of his mother's bicornuate uterus (see Fig. 32.4).[7] There is also some evidence to suggest that fetal head constraint can induce chondrocyte apoptosis and alter the expression of transforming growth factor beta and fibroblast growth factor receptors, resulting in nonsyndromic craniosynostosis.[8,9]

The metopic suture is the first cranial suture to close, and analysis of computed tomography scans in patients with and without metopic synostosis demonstrated that the metopic suture normally begins to close at 3 to 4 months and is usually completely closed by 8 to 9 months.[10] Fusion can be normal and completed as early as 2 months, and can also stay patent and persist into adulthood.[11] Normal fusion commences at the nasion and proceeds superiorly, concluding at the anterior fontanelle.[12,13]

Trigonocephaly is usually an isolated anomaly in an otherwise normal child, but it can occur as part of a syndrome in about 35% of cases.[14,15] Examples include Baller-Gerold, Saethre-Chotzen, Say-Mayer, and Opitz C trigonocephaly syndrome (Fig. 32.5), or result from a wide range of chromosome abnormalities, such as deletions of 9p22-p24 or 11q23-q24, the latter deletion also called *Jacobsen syndrome* (Fig. 32.6).[16–18] In a study of 25 infants with trigonocephaly and metopic synostosis, 6% were familial, 16 (64%) had isolated metopic synostosis, two (8%) had metopic synostosis combined with sagittal synostosis, and seven (28%) had metopic synostosis as part of a syndrome (two with Jacobsen syndrome due to chromosomal deletion of 11q23-q24, one with Opitz C trigonocephaly syndrome, one with Say-Meyer trigonocephaly syndrome, one with I-cell disease, and two others with unknown syndromes).[17] In a study of 76 unrelated patients with syndromic (36 patients) and nonsyndromic trigonocephaly (40 patients) caused by metopic synostosis, molecular screening for microdeletions at 9p22-p24 and 11q23-q24 revealed deletions in seven syndromic patients (19.4%), but no deletions were found in the nonsyndromic patients.[19] The ratio of affected males to females was 5:1 in the syndromic group and 1.8:1 in the nonsyndromic group, which suggests that genes in

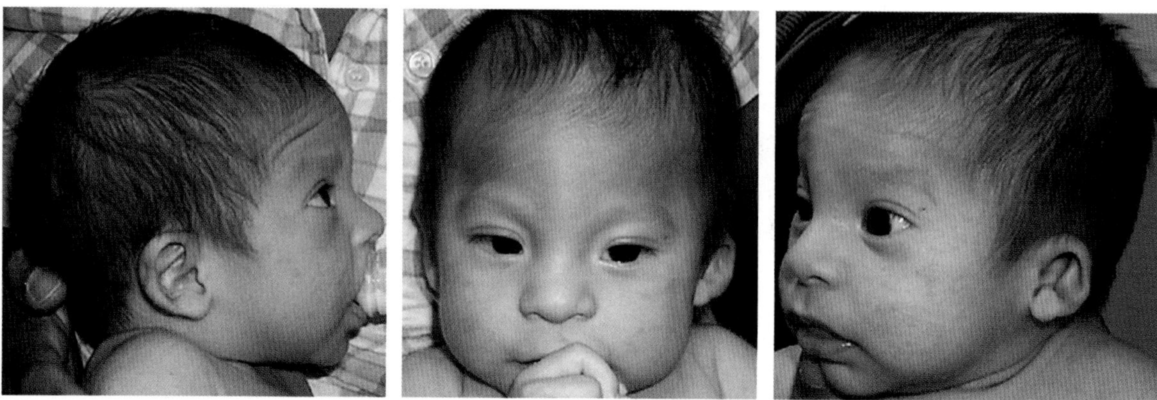

FIGURE 32.1 This child shows characteristic features of metopic craniosynostosis. Findings include bitemporal narrowing and a palpable midline ridge from the nasion to the anterior fontanelle over the site of the fused suture, resulting in a prow-shaped, triangular anterior cranial vault (termed *trigonocephaly*). There is also upslanting of the palpebral fissures with ocular hypotelorism.

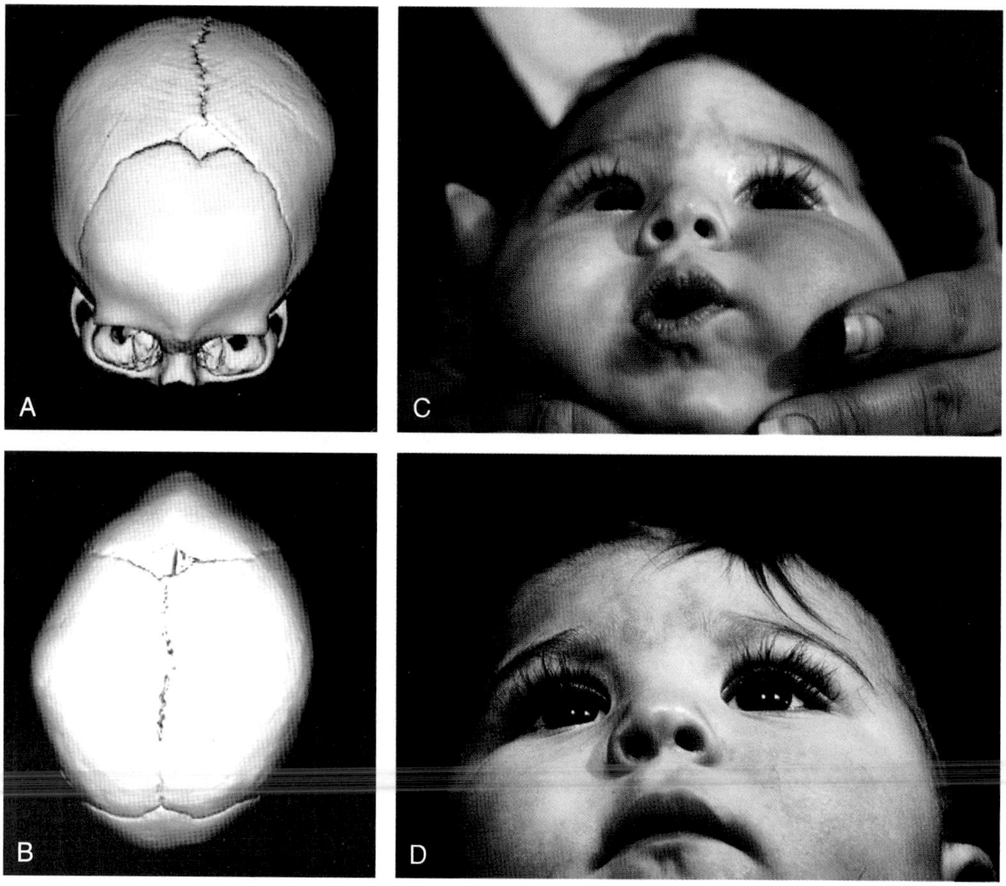

A C B D

FIGURE 32-2 Three-dimensional computed tomography scans (**A** and **B**) demonstrating the ridged metopic suture, which is most evident in the worm's-eye view of this patient before (**C**) and after (**D**) surgery.

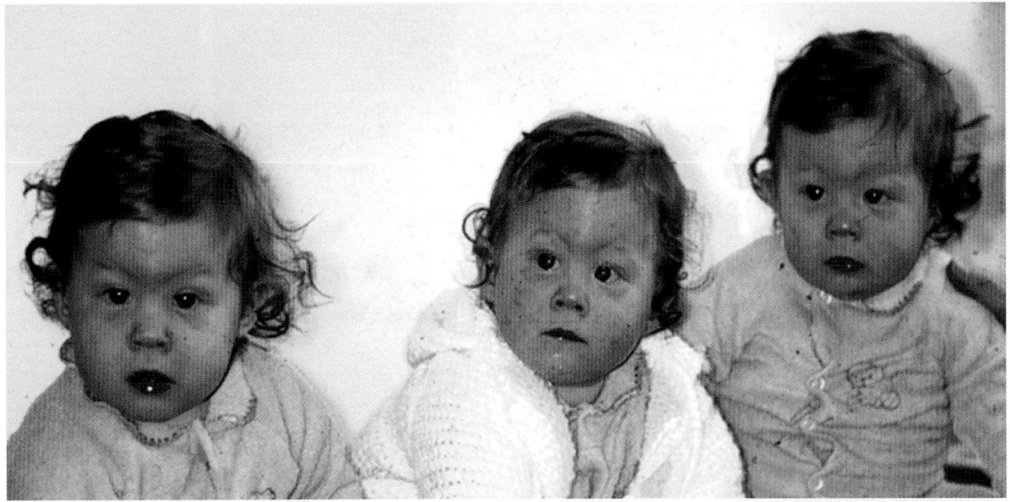

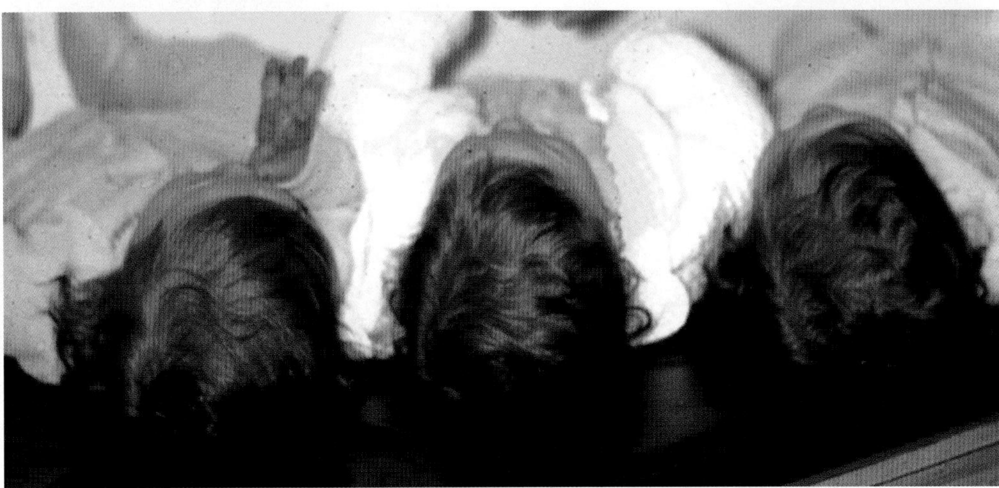

FIGURE 32.3 One of monozygotic triplets born to a 104-lb (prepregnancy weight) woman who gained 64 pounds during the pregnancy. Prenatal radiographs had shown this triplet to have the frontal portion of her head wedged between the buttocks of her co-triplets. This was considered the source of the constraint that yielded the metopic craniostenosis with secondary narrowed forehead and upslanting palpebral fissures, features that were not shared by her monozygotic co-triplets. (From Graham JM Jr, Smith DW. Metopic craniostenosis as a consequence of fetal head constraint. Two interesting experiments of nature. *Pediatrics*. 1980;65:1000.)

these deleted regions and on the X-chromosome play a major role in syndromic trigonocephaly.[19]

In another study of 278 cases of metopic synostosis, 75% were nonsyndromic and 6% were familial.[1] Metopic synostosis has also been associated with fetal exposure to valproic acid but not with exposure to other anticonvulsants.[20] The mean intelligence quotient of 17 patients with metopic synostosis was 75; significantly higher intelligence quotients were noted in infants who were surgically treated before 6 months of age.[20]

FEATURES

The diagnosis of metopic synostosis is made clinically and confirmed by radiographic studies. Findings include bitemporal narrowing, a palpable midline ridge from the nasion to the anterior fontanelle over the site of the fused suture, and a prow-shaped, triangular anterior cranial vault (termed *trigonocephaly*). There may be progressive upslanting of the palpebral fissures with ocular hypotelorism (see Figs. 32.1 to 32.4). Normal metopic sutural closure is usually associated

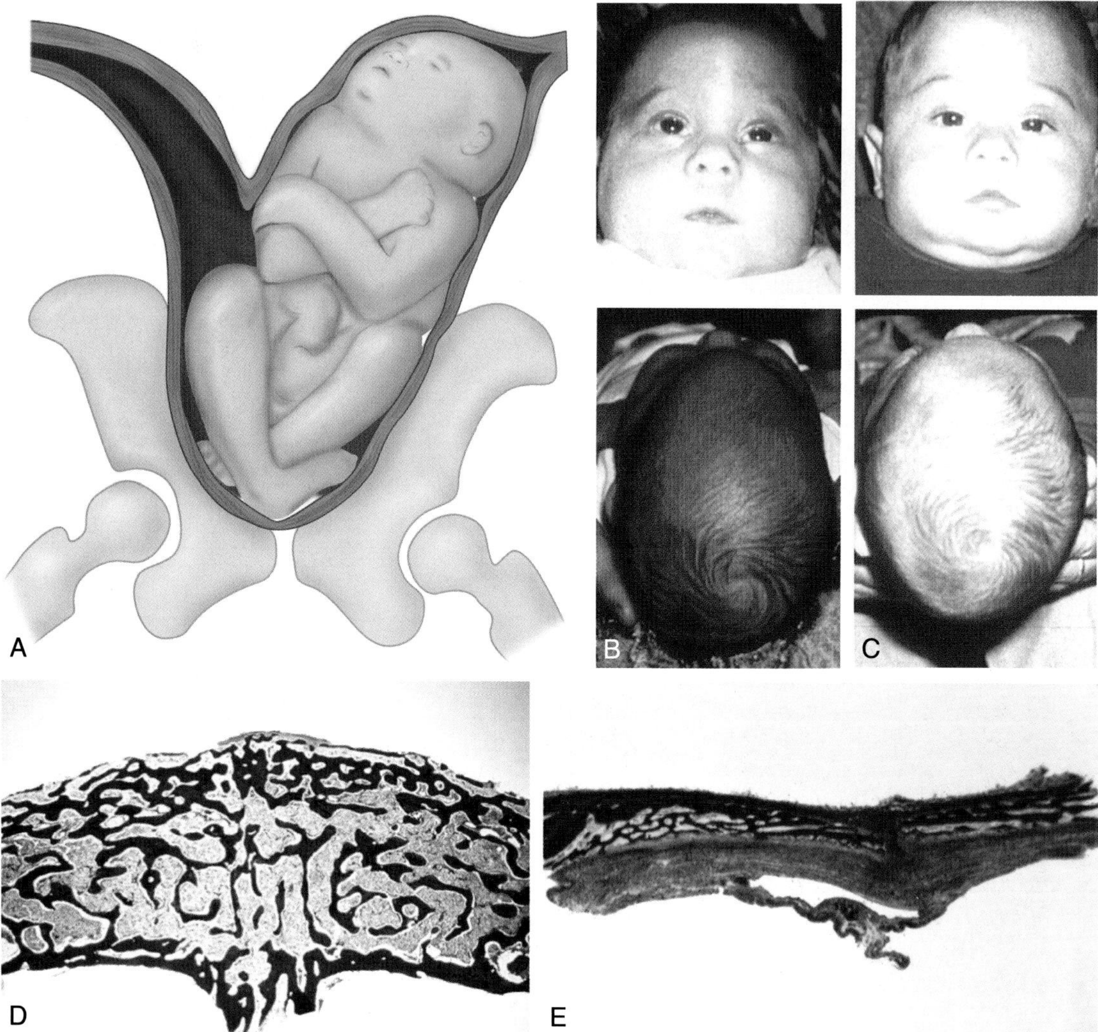

FIGURE 32.4 Metopic craniostenosis in an infant who was reared in a bicornuate uterus (B). During cesarean section, it took several minutes to dislodge the head from its tightly entrapped position in one upper uterine horn (illustrated in A). C, Postoperative status of the infant following calvarectomy of the frontal bone region down to the supraorbital ridges, which allowed the brain to remold the forehead while a more normally shaped bony calvarium was formed. Histologic section through the dense metopic ridge of the patient shows complete replacement of the normal sutural ligament with dense thickened bone (D) compared with control suture material from a deceased infant of the same age (E).

with an endocranial bony spur, but premature metopic synostosis is associated with an endocranial metopic notch in 93% of cases.[13] The synostotic metopic suture is markedly thickened on histologic sections when compared with age-matched neonates who died from other causes (see Fig. 32.4). Milder degrees of metopic ridging occur fairly frequently at birth, but unless there is progressive distortion of the orbits, such mild ridging usually resolves spontaneously without treatment. This mild metopic ridging without synostosis is very common (occurring in 10–25% of normal neonates), and it should not be misdiagnosed as metopic synostosis.[17]

MANAGEMENT AND PROGNOSIS

Generally, no treatment is required in mild cases without associated orbital deformity. Yee et al. summarized the various anthropometric cranial measurements

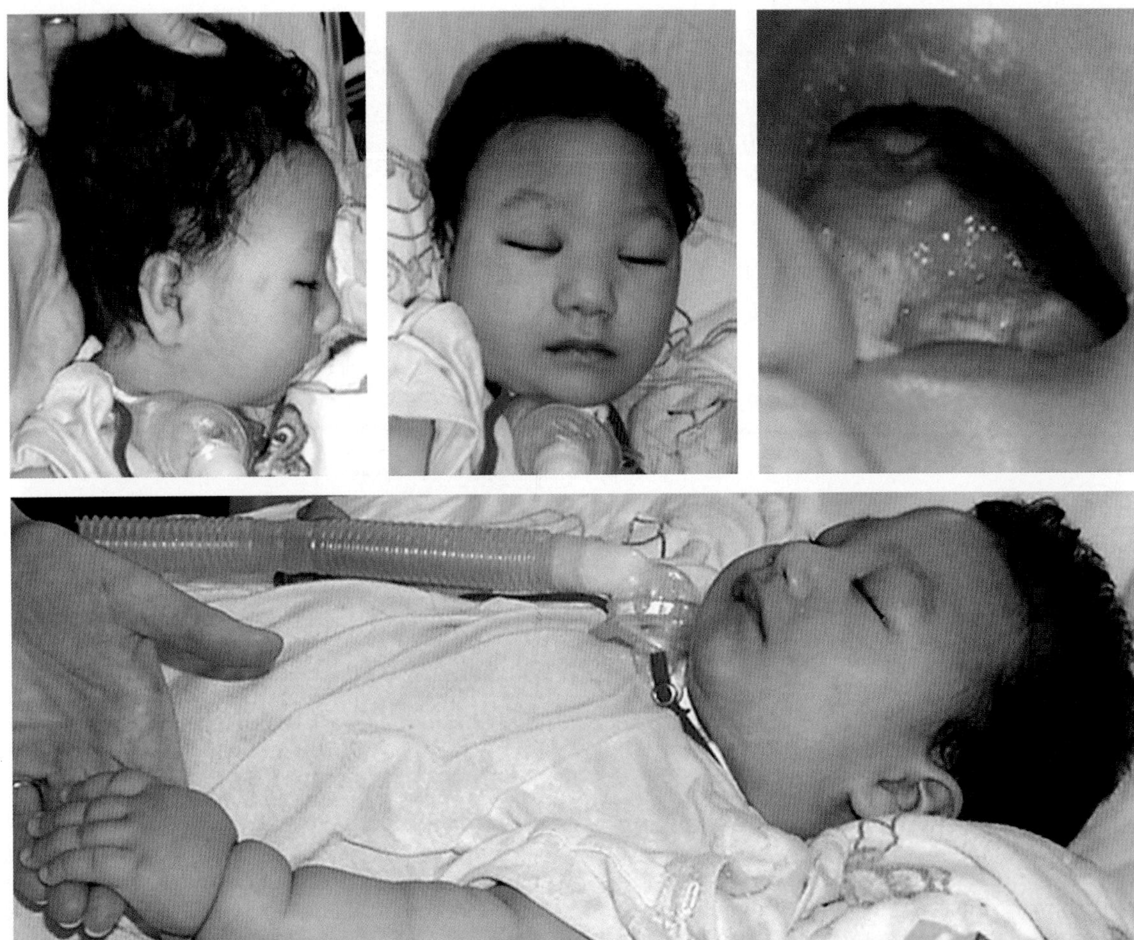

FIGURE 32.5 This patient with Opitz C trigonocephaly syndrome was one of three infants born into a family with this autosomal recessive syndrome and normal chromosomes via comparative genomic hybridization.

and classification systems were described for metopic craniosynostosis.[21] Endoscopic-assisted metopic synostosis correction should be performed on patients under 12 weeks, although 8 weeks is ideal (Fig. 32.7) Good results are still seen between 3 and 6 months. Patients older than 6 months are not ideal candidates unless the presenting condition is very mild.[22] Moderate to severe metopic synostosis often warrants active forehead reshaping with recontouring of the fronto-orbital bar down to and including the supraorbital ridges via a frontal calvarectomy (Fig. 32.8). In the more severe cases with ocular hypotelorism, the brows and orbital roofs are removed and relocated. These procedures are usually undertaken between 3 and 9 months of age. When surgery is restricted to just the forehead and supraorbital rims, the hypotelorism remains uncorrected and narrowness of the forehead also persists, so most surgeons prefer more extended fronto-orbital procedures that correct both the trigonocephaly and the hypotelorism by inserting an interpositional bone graft into the middle of the supraorbital bar, thus providing additional fullness in the temporal regions.[22,23] In some hospitals, hypotelorism is treated with spring-assisted surgery in children below 6 months of age and with fronto-orbital advancement with the interposition of a bone graft in the fronto-orbital region at an older age.[14,24]

Of 1713 patients treated for craniosynostosis in Paris, 237 (14%) were trigonocephalic and 76 patients over 3 years of age were studied for long-term neurodevelopmental outcome (at a mean age of 6.5 years) and associated malformations (patients with

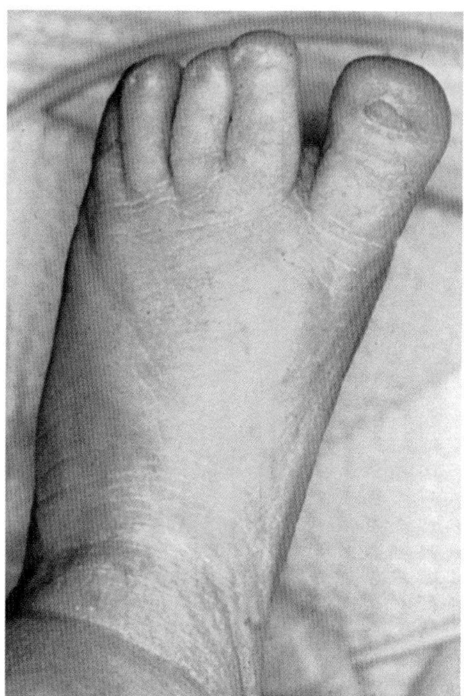

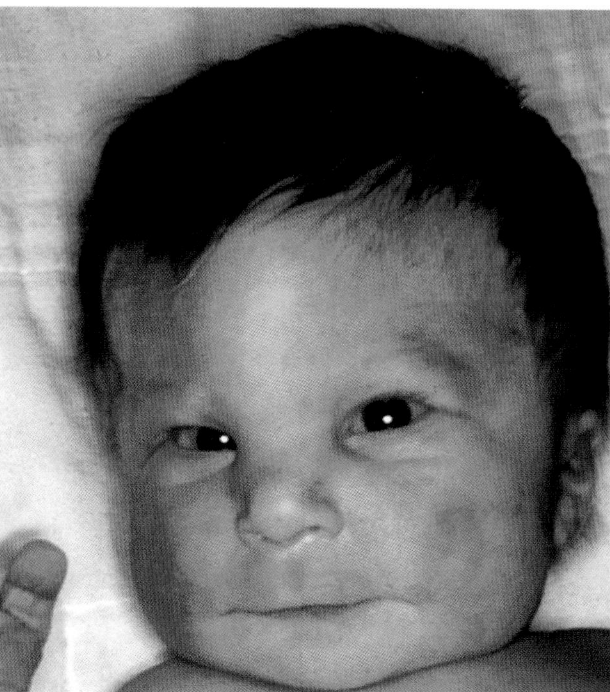

FIGURE 32.6 This patient with trigonocephaly, developmental delay, and broad thumbs and great toes has Jacobsen syndrome due to chromosomal deletion of 11q23-q24.

known syndromes and chromosomal alterations were excluded). The mean age of surgery was 11.5 months, and 22.6% of those surgically treated before 12 months of age showed impaired mental development versus 52.2% in those surgically treated after 12 months of age. Children with brain malformations such as hydrocephalus or hypoplastic corpus callosum had poorer cognitive outcomes, and 18.4% had associated extracranial malformations. Children with associated malformations were more often delayed in development (57%) than children with isolated trigonocephaly (26%). Overall, 31% of trigonocephaly patients had delayed development; this appeared to be related to the severity of the problem and the presence of associated malformations. Isolated patients who were operated on at an early age had the best cognitive outcomes.[25] Among 91 children with isolated metopic craniosynostosis, 19 (20.9%) had astigmatism, 8 (8.8%) had amblyopia, 8 (8.8%) had strabismus, 5 had myopia (5.5%), 5 had hyperopia (5.5%), and 5 had anisometropia (5.5%).[26] In children surgically treated for trigonocephaly, the incidence of ocular disorders increased with age at the time of corrective surgery and the later the reconstructive surgery was performed, the more pronounced the astigmatism.[27]

Wes et al. reported on the outcome of 147 patients who underwent surgical correction of isolated metopic craniosynostosis. Their average age at surgery was 0.83 years (range, 0.3 to 4.7 years), and there were 13 surgical complications (8.8%), 3 major (2.0%). Patients with greater than 5 years' follow-up ($n = 57$) were more likely to have temporal hollowing (odds ratio, 2.9; 95% confidence interval, 1.2–7.3), lateral orbital retrusion (odds ratio, 4.9; 95% confidence interval, 1.9–12.7), and more severe Whitaker class III or IV classification compared with those with less than 5 years' follow-up.[28]

DIFFERENTIAL DIAGNOSIS

It is important to exclude primary defects of the brain such as the holoprosencephaly malformation sequence and syndromes such as CADASIL syndrome (cerebral autosomal dominant arteriopathy with subcortical infarcts and leukoencephalopathy) or Opitz C trigonocephaly syndrome (see Fig. 32.5).[29] The latter condition includes unusual facial features, hypotonia, multiple frenula, limb defects, visceral anomalies, and mental deficiency, and it is inherited in an autosomal recessive fashion. Single-gene disorders that have abnormal

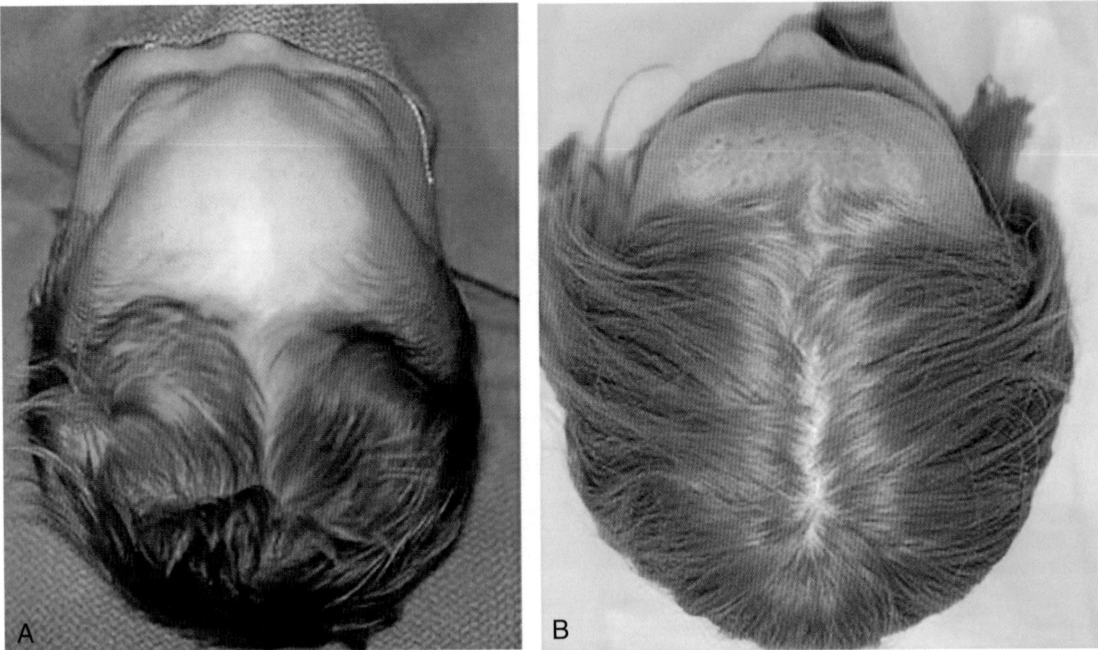

FIGURE 32.7 A, Top preoperative view of 3-month-old with metopic craniosynostosis and trigonocephaly. B, Top view of same patient 9 years after endoscopic craniectomy shows complete correction of forehead deformity. (From Jimenez DF, Moon HS. Endoscopic approaches to craniosynostosis. *Atlas Oral Maxillofac Surg Clin North Am*. 2022;30(1):63–73.)

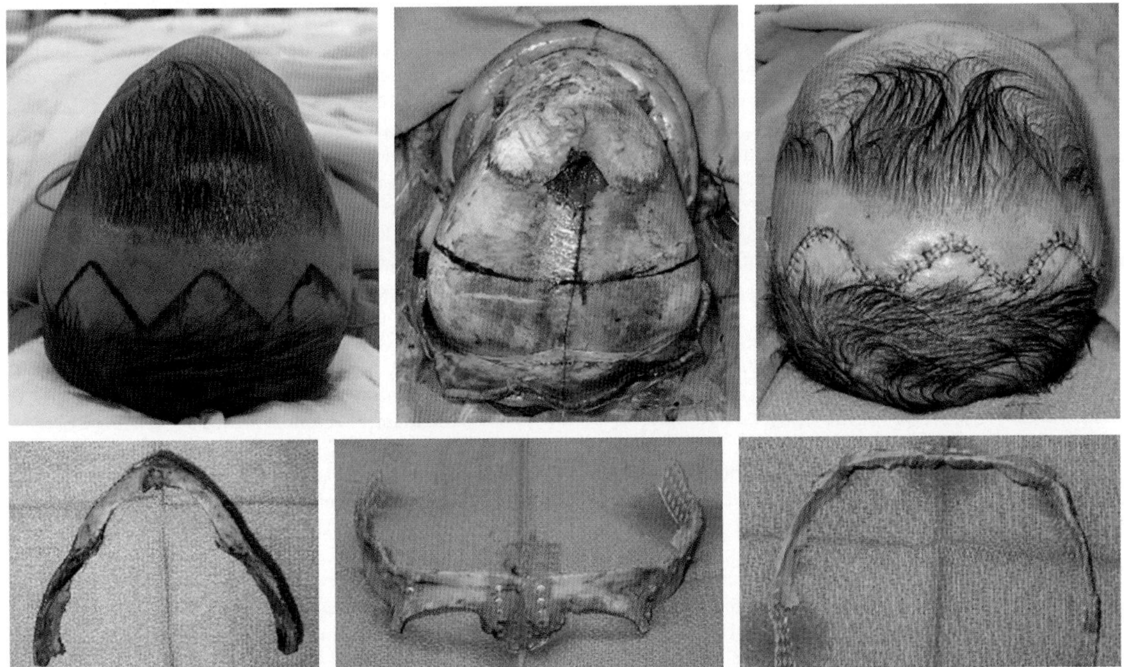

FIGURE 32.8 Before and after pictures of a patient with trigonocephaly who underwent open frontal calvarectomy with frontal reshaping and recontouring of the fronto-orbital bar down to and including the supraorbital ridges.

brain growth may develop secondary metopic synostosis.[30-32] Metopic craniosynostosis can also result from various chromosomal abnormalities, such as deletions of chromosome 9p22-p24 and 11q23-q24 (Jacobsen syndrome), as demonstrated in Fig. 32.6.[17,19,33] Because some of these chromosomal abnormalities can be quite subtle, high-resolution chromosomal studies or comparative genomic hybridization studies are indicated in children with associated malformations and neurodevelopmental problems.

References

1. Kweldam CF, van der Vlugt JJ, van der Meulen JJ. The incidence of craniosynostosis in The Netherlands, 1997-2007. *J Plast Reconstr Aesthet Surg*. 2011;64(5):583–588.
2. Blum JD, Beiriger J, Kalmar C, et al. Relating metopic craniosynostosis severity to intracranial pressure. *J Craniofac Surg*. 2022;33(8):2372–2378.
3. Ezaldein HH, Metzler P, Persing JA, Steinbacher DM. Three-dimensional orbital dysmorphology in metopic synostosis. *J Plast Reconstr Aesthet Surg*. 2014; 67(7):900–905.
4. van der Meulen J. Metopic synostosis. In. Vol 28: Childs Nerv Syst; 2012:1359–1367.
5. Lajeunie E, Le Merrer M, Marchac D, Renier D. Syndromal and nonsyndromal primary trigonocephaly: analysis of a series of 237 patients. *Am J Med Genet*. 1998;75(2):211–215.
6. Sanchez-Lara PA, Carmichael SL, Graham JM Jr, et al. Fetal constraint as a potential risk factor for craniosynostosis. *Am J Med Genet A*. 2010;152A(2):394–400.
7. Graham JM Jr, Smith DW. Metopic craniostenosis as a consequence of fetal head constraint: two interesting experiments of nature. *Pediatrics*. 1980;65(5):1000–1002.
8. Hunenko O, Karmacharya J, Ong G, Kirschner RE. Toward an understanding of nonsyndromic craniosynostosis: altered patterns of TGF-beta receptor and FGF receptor expression induced by intrauterine head constraint. *Ann Plast Surg*. 2001;46(5):546–553; discussion 553-544.
9. Smartt JM Jr, Karmacharya J, Gannon FH, et al. Intrauterine fetal constraint induces chondrocyte apoptosis and premature ossification of the cranial base. *Plast Reconstr Surg*. 2005;116(5):1363–1369.
10. Bajwa M, Srinivasan D, Nishikawa H, Rodrigues D, Solanki G, White N. Normal fusion of the metopic suture. *J Craniofac Surg*. 2013;24(4):1201–1205.
11. Guerram A, Le Minor JM, Renger S, Bierry G. Brief communication: the size of the human frontal sinuses in adults presenting complete persistence of the metopic suture. *Am J Phys Anthropol*. 2014;154(4):621–627.
12. Vu HL, Panchal J, Parker EE, Levine NS, Francel P. The timing of physiologic closure of the metopic suture: a review of 159 patients using reconstructed 3D CT scans of the craniofacial region. *J Craniofac Surg*. 2001;12(6):527–532.
13. Weinzweig J, Kirschner RE, Farley A, et al. Metopic synostosis: defining the temporal sequence of normal suture fusion and differentiating it from synostosis on the basis of computed tomography images. *Plastic and Reconstructive Surgery*. 2003;112(5):1211–1218.
14. Massenburg BB, Tolley PD, Lee A, Susarla SM. Fronto-orbital advancement for metopic and unilateral coronal craniosynostoses. *Oral Maxillofac Surg Clin North Am*. 2022;34(3):367–380.
15. van der Meulen J. Metopic synostosis. *Childs Nerv Syst*. 2012;28(9):1359–1367.
16. Lattanzi W, Bukvic N, Barba M, et al. Genetic basis of single-suture synostoses: genes, chromosomes and clinical implications. *Childs Nerv Syst*. 2012;28(9):1301–1310.
17. Azimi C, Kennedy SJ, Chitayat D, et al. Clinical and genetic aspects of trigonocephaly: a study of 25 cases. *American Journal of Medical Genetics Part A*. 2003;117A(2):127–135.
18. Cohen MM, MacLean RE. *Craniosynostosis: Diagnosis. Evaluation, and Management*. 2nd ed. New York: Oxford University Press; 2000.
19. Jehee FS, Johnson D, Alonso LG, et al. Molecular screening for microdeletions at 9p22-p24 and 11q23-q24 in a large cohort of patients with trigonocephaly. *Clinical Genetics*. 2005;67(6):503–510.
20. Lajeunie E, Barcik U, Thorne JA, El Ghouzzi V, Bourgeois M, Renier D. Craniosynostosis and fetal exposure to sodium valproate. *Journal of Neurosurgery*. 2001;95(5):778–782.
21. Yee ST, Fearon JA, Gosain AK, Timbang MR, Papay FA, Doumit G. Classification and management of metopic craniosynostosis. *J Craniofac Surg*. 2015;26(6):1812–1817.
22. Havlik RJ, Azurin DJ, Bartlett SP, Whitaker LA. Analysis and treatment of severe trigonocephaly. *Plast Reconstr Surg*. 1999;103(2):381–390.
23. Collmann H, Sorensen N, Krauss J. Consensus: trigonocephaly. *Childs Nerv Syst*. 1996;12(11):664–668.
24. Maltese G, Tarnow P, Tovetjarn R, Kolby L. Correction of hypotelorism in isolated metopic synostosis. *J Plast Surg Hand Surg*. 2014;48(1):63–66.
25. Bottero L, Lajeunie E, Arnaud E, Marchac D, Renier D. Functional outcome after surgery for trigonocephaly. *Plast Reconstr Surg*. 1998;102(4):952–958; discussion 959-960.
26. Nguyen TB, Shock LA, Missoi TG, Muzaffar AR. Incidence of amblyopia and its risk factors in children with isolated metopic craniosynostosis. *Cleft Palate Craniofac J*. 2016;53(1):e14–17.
27. Denis D, Genitori L, Conrath J, Lena G, Choux M. Ocular findings in children operated on for plagiocephaly and trigonocephaly. *Childs Nerv Syst*. 1996;12(11):683–689.
28. Wes AM, Paliga JT, Goldstein JA, Whitaker LA, Bartlett SP, Taylor JA. An evaluation of complications, revisions, and long-term aesthetic outcomes in nonsyndromic metopic craniosynostosis. *Plastic and Reconstructive Surgery*. 2014;133(6):1453–1464.
29. Riordan CP, Lyon HN, McIntyre JK. Craniosynostosis of the metopic suture in a patient with CADASIL/Lehman syndrome. *J Craniofac Surg*. 2021;32(8):e737–e739.

30. Brasil AS, Malaquias AC, Kim CA, et al. KRAS gene mutations in Noonan syndrome familial cases cluster in the vicinity of the switch II region of the G-domain: report of another family with metopic craniosynostosis. *Am J Med Genet A*. 2012;158a(5):1178–1184.
31. Adiyapatham S, Murugesan A. Novel mutation causing Zellweger syndrome. *BMJ Case Rep*. 2023;16(3):e252014.
32. Wu RT, Timberlake AT, Abraham PF, et al. *SMAD6* genotype predicts neurodevelopment in nonsyndromic craniosynostosis. *Plast Reconstr Surg*. 2020;145(1): 117e–125e.
33. Penny LA, Dell'Aquila M, Jones MC, et al. Clinical and molecular characterization of patients with distal 11q deletions. *Am J Hum Genet*. 1995;56(3):676–683.

CHAPTER 33

Lambdoidal Craniosynostosis

KEY POINTS

- Lambdoidal craniosynostosis is often an isolated anomaly but can be associated with muscular torticollis or an abnormal fetal lie/birth presentation.
- Differential diagnosis includes nonsynostotic deformational posterior plagiocephaly, synostotic anterior plagiocephaly, and other forms of craniosynostosis.
- Unilateral lambdoidal craniosynostosis results in the protrusion of the ipsilateral mastoid bone, palpable sutural ridging, occipital flattening, downward displacement of the auricle, and trapezoidal cranial asymmetry.
- Early recognition and appropriate management, such as repositioning, physical therapy, and helmet therapy, can successfully treat deformational plagiocephaly, while lambdoidal craniosynostosis should be evaluated by a craniofacial team and may require surgical intervention.
- Surgical intervention involves posterior calvarectomy to prevent facial scoliosis and reshape the occipital bones, allowing for full expansion of the skull.

GENESIS

Lambdoidal craniosynostosis occurs in approximately 1 in 33,000–40,000 births and is the least common form of craniosynostosis, accounting for only 2% to 5% of all cases.[1-4] Misdiagnosis of nonsynostotic deformational posterior plagiocephaly with occipital flattening as lambdoidal craniosynostosis has resulted in apparent epidemics of craniosynostosis, in which the proportion of lambdoidal craniosynostosis cases was reported as more than 40% of total craniosynostosis cases in Colorado, United States, and more than 70% in York-Selby, England.[5-11] Both of these "epidemics" of craniosynostosis arose during the time when Western cultures were shifting their infant sleeping position from prone to supine in an effort to reduce the incidence of sudden infant death syndrome (SIDS).[12] With this change, infants no longer move their heads from one side to the other as they do in the prone sleeping position; thus placing infants on their backs quickly magnified any inequity in resting position such that asymmetric occipital flattening developed in infants with positional torticollis. Because the lambdoid sutures are not readily visualized on skull radiographs, nonvisualization of these sutures in an asymmetrically flattened occiput was interpreted as lambdoidal craniosynostosis. Further complicating this diagnosis is the fact that most lambdoidal craniosynostosis occurs as an isolated anomaly in an otherwise normal child and is frequently associated with muscular torticollis, which suggests that many cases of lambdoidal craniosynostosis are a consequence of fetal compression. Lambdoidal craniosynostosis can result from constraint of the posterior cranium associated with abnormal fetal lie or presentation. Lambdoidal synostosis has no clear genetic etiology. Discordant synostosis has been reported in one monozygotic twin; there is also an unsubstantiated report of concordance in dizygotic twins and a single report of dizygotic twins concordant for contralateral lambdoidal synostosis.[13] There are also reports of children with rare de novo single-gene mutations and chromosome abnormalities who manifest lambdoidal craniosynostosis as one component of a broader pattern of altered morphogenesis.[7,14-17]

FEATURES

Unilateral lambdoidal craniosynostosis results in plagiocephaly, which differs from that seen in deformational posterior plagiocephaly. Lambdoidal synostotic can be either isolated, associated with posterior sagittal synostosis ("Mercedes-Benz" syndrome), or oxycephalic form anterior plagiocephaly due to unicoronal craniosynostosis.[18,19] Parents and physicians may note

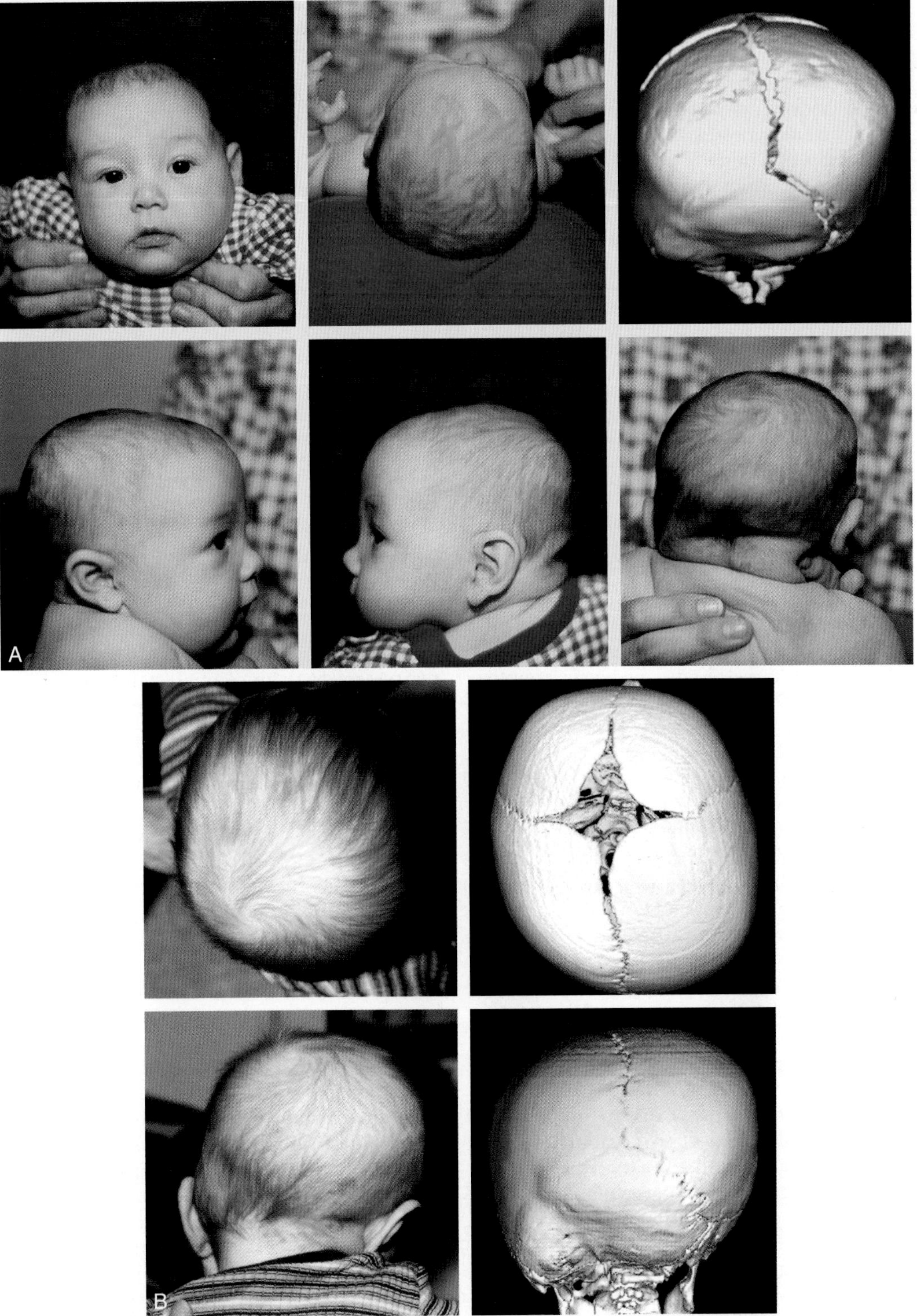

FIGURE 33.1 **A** and **B** Two infants with left lambdoid synostosis. Note ridging of the involved lambdoid suture, downward displacement of the auricle, trapezoidal cranial asymmetry when viewed from the vertex position, downward canting of the posterior cranial base with a small posterior fossa, and peaking of the contralateral parietooccipital area. The girl shown in (**A**) is demonstrated radiographically in Fig. 33.2, and she is shown before and after surgery in Fig. 33.3.

apparent protrusion of the mastoid bone on the involved side, as well as palpable sutural ridging. Unlike coronal craniosynostosis, facial structures and orbits are usually not initially affected by lambdoidal craniosynostosis, although unilateral involvement results in ipsilateral occipital flattening with ridging of the involved lambdoid suture and downward vertical displacement of the auricle (Fig. 33.1).[5,10,20] Radiographic and clinical signs include trapezoidal cranial asymmetry when viewed from the vertex position, small posterior fossa, and sutural sclerosis, but sole reliance on skull radiographs and clinical signs alone has led to misdiagnosis, so it is best to confirm the diagnosis of suspected lambdoidal craniosynostosis with three-dimensional computed tomography scans, which clearly image the involved suture(s) and allow a secure diagnosis to be made (Fig. 33.2).[21] There is a growing interest in using alternative technologies such as ultrasound screening. In a blinded study comparing the concordance of diagnosis between computed tomography and ultrasound of 41 children, Sze et al. found the mean sensitivity and specificity of ultrasound in distinguishing a patent from fused lambdoid suture by three blinded pediatric radiologists was 100% and 89%, respectively.[22]

During the 4-year period between 1991 and 1994, a multidisciplinary team consisting of a dysmorphologist, a pediatric neurosurgeon, and a craniofacial surgeon assessed 102 patients with posterior plagiocephaly. During this same period, the team also assessed 130 patients with craniosynostosis who required surgery.[5] Only four patients (3.1%) manifested clinical, imaging, and operative features of true unilambdoidal craniosynostosis. These features included a thick bony ridge over the fused suture with contralateral parietal and frontal bulging and an ipsilateral occipitomastoid bulge, leading to tilting of the ipsilateral skull base and a downward/posterior displacement of the ear on the synostotic side.[5,10,20] These changes resulted in a trapezoidal head shape when viewed from above, which must be distinguished from more complex forms of synostosis, combinations of excessive brachycephaly with deformational posterior plagiocephaly (see Fig. 25.1), and combined ipsilateral deformational posterior and anterior plagiocephaly. In contrast, children with deformational, nonsynostotic posterior plagiocephaly have a parallelogram-shaped head with forward displacement of the ear and frontal bossing on the side ipsilateral to the occipitoparietal flattening, accompanied by contralateral occipital bossing.[10,20] Although the majority of ears are forward displaced, in a review of ear position in 37 cases of unilateral lambdoid synostosis, 16% of ears were not displaced, 32% were anteriorly displaced, 16% were nondisplaced, 11% anteroinferiorly, 19% posteriorly, 19% posteroinferiorly, and 3% inferiorly.[23] Of the 98 patients with positional head deformation, only 3 had severe, progressive deformation that required surgery; the remainder were successfully managed with changes in sleeping position or helmet therapy.[10] Occasionally, mendosal craniosynostosis accompanies lambdoidal craniosynostosis on the same side.[24,25]

MANAGEMENT AND PROGNOSIS

There are a growing number of centers and advocates for endoscopic strip craniectomy with postoperative helmeting for patients who present with Unilateral lambdoidal craniosynostosis before 3 months of age.

Because isolated lambdoidal craniosynostosis is usually not associated with elevations in intracranial pressure, posterior calvarec to prevent facial scoliosis due to restricted posterior cranial expansion over the long term (Fig. 33.3).[26] Similar to the facial yaw or twist seen with unicoronal craniosynostosis, earlier intervention does seem to stop progression of the deformity.[26] Fig. 33.4 shows improvement of cranial distortion after early surgical reconstruction of the left lambdoid synostosis in the infant shown in Figs. 33.1A and 33.2. Fig. 33.5 shows a 9-year-old girl with untreated left lambdoid craniosynostosis and secondarily distorted facial features. The timing for lambdoidal craniosynostosis surgery can be later than for other types of craniosynostosis, and the response to surgery may be more variable, particularly with very late surgery. Surgery consists of removal of the synostotic lambdoid suture with reshaping of the occipital bones to allow full expansion of the skull in all directions. Both open and microscopic spring-mediated cranioplasty has been used in the surgical correction of craniosynostosis.[11,27,28] One small study found that traditional cranioplasty of patients with lambdoid synostosis effectively restores calvarial shape, but if done after 6 months of age, it does not significantly alter the dysmorphic features seen in the endocranium.[29] If associated torticollis is present, it should be treated vigorously with neck physical therapy targeting the affected sternocleidomastoid muscle. As shown in Fig. 25.6, the combination of positional molding with lambdoidal craniosynostosis can have an additional effect on craniofacial structures, requiring long-term treatment. Occasionally, postoperative helmet molding can help optimize results, and the possibility of

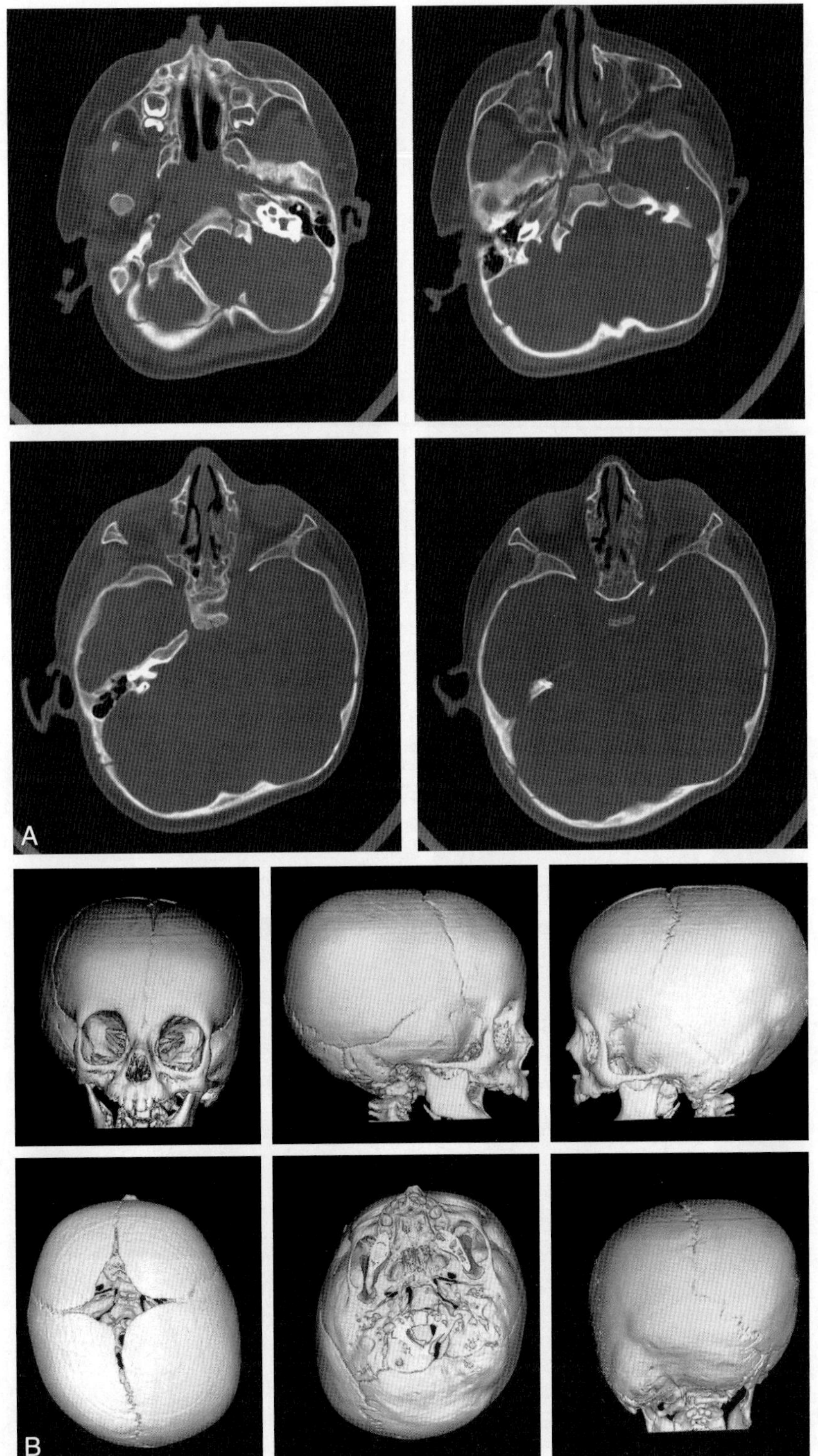

FIGURE 33.2 Computed tomography images with bone windows (A) and 3D reformatting (B) demonstrate left lambdoid synostosis with ridging, bulging of the mastoid bone, and a small posterior fossa.

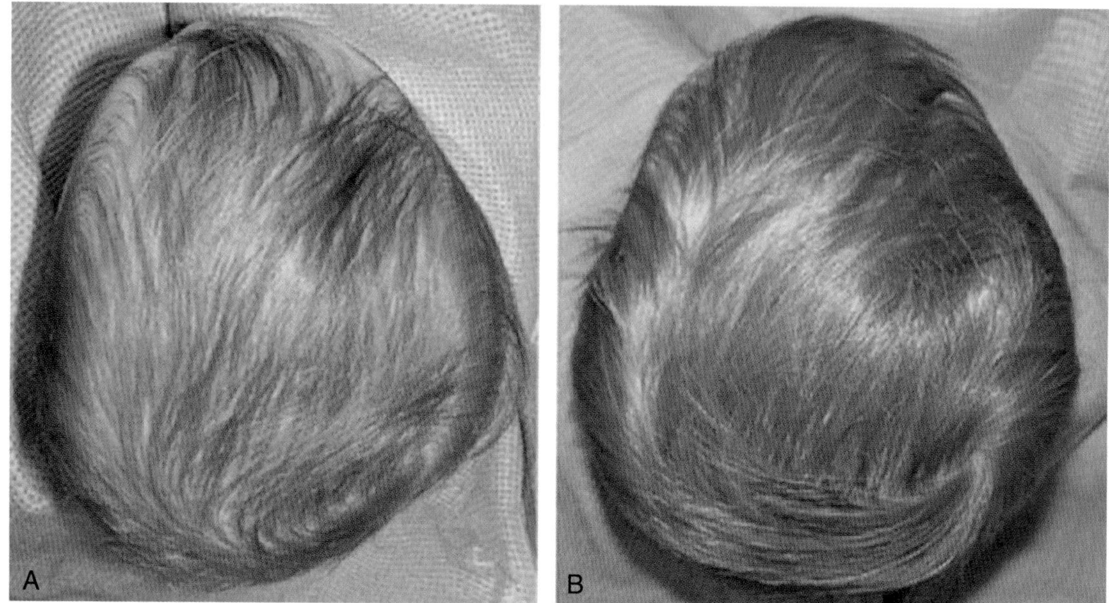

FIGURE 33.3 A, Top view of 4-month old male with right lambdoid craniosynostosis. B, Top view 2 years after endoscopic craniectomy shows complete normalization of the head. (From Jimenez DF, Moon HW. Endoscopic approaches to craniosynostosis. *Atlas Oral Maxillofac Surg Clin North Am.* 2022; 30(1): 63–73.)

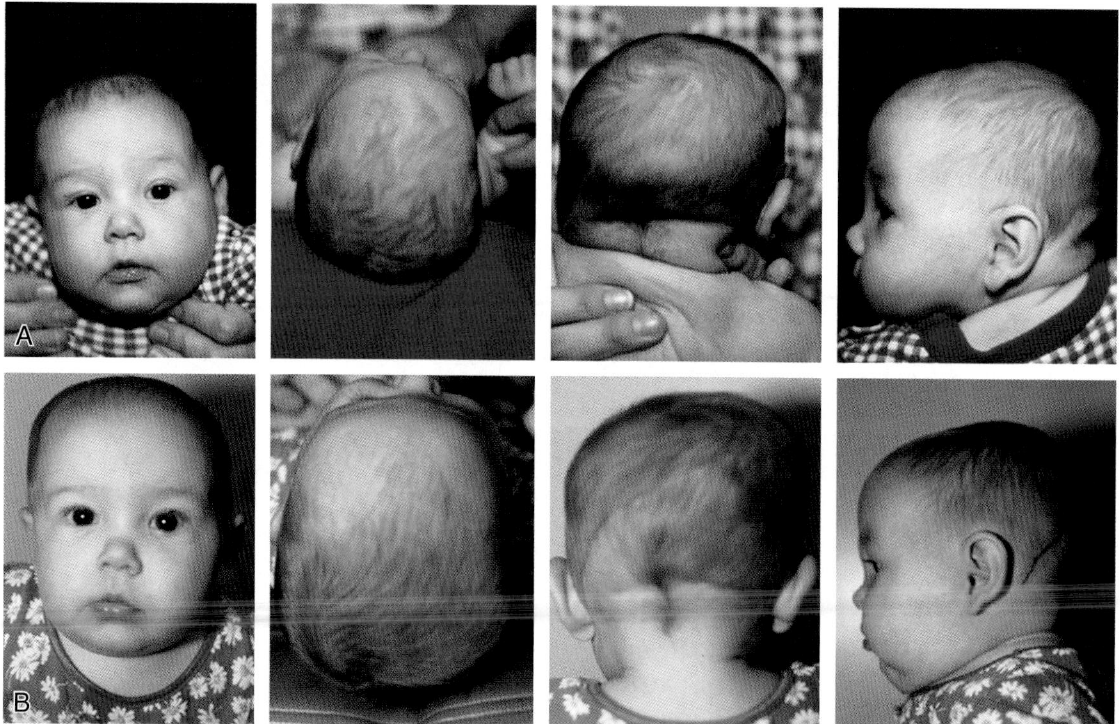

FIGURE 33.4 Three-dimensional computed tomography scans of a child with unilateral left lambdoid synostosis, before (A) and after (B) surgery.

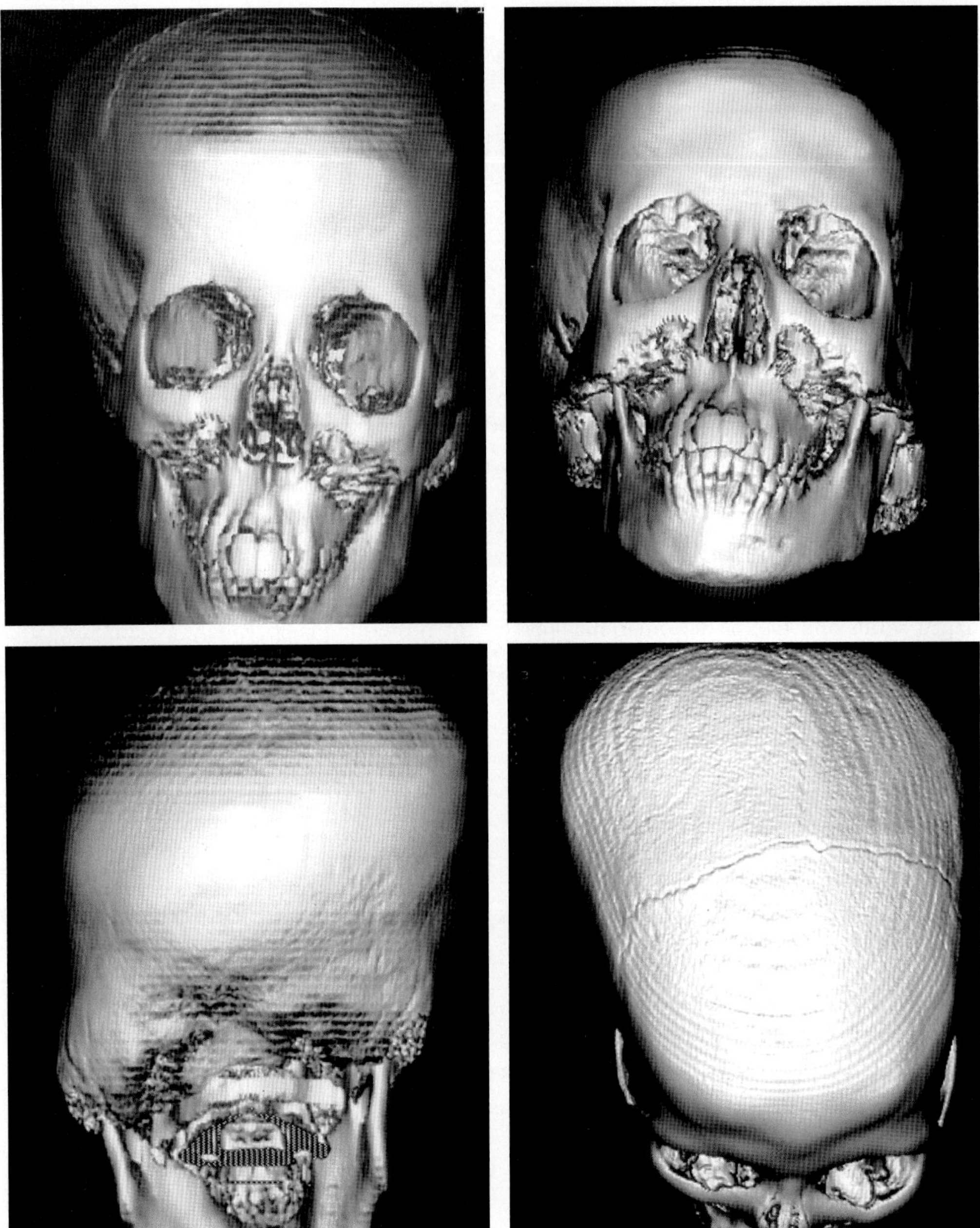

FIGURE 33.5 Three-dimensional computed tomography scan of a 9-year-old girl with marked craniofacial asymmetry due to untreated left lambdoid synostosis.

lambdoidal craniosynostosis should be kept in mind when deformational plagiocephaly fails to respond to neck physical therapy and cranial orthotic therapy. In 2022, Chiang et al. summarized the meta-analysis of three studies and described the general cognition of children with lambdoid craniosynostosis, which showed that cases scored significantly lower than their peers, but within 1 standard deviation (verbal and psychomotor development showed no significant differences).[30]

DIFFERENTIAL DIAGNOSIS

The primary differential diagnosis is between nonsynostotic deformational posterior plagiocephaly and unilambdoidal craniosynostosis. Unicoronal craniosynostosis gives rise to synostotic anterior plagiocephaly with a raised and retruded supraorbital ridge on the involved side and deviation of the nasal root toward the involved side.[31] Ipsilateral coronal and lambdoidal synostosis creates a strikingly trapezoidal head shape, and unicoronal craniosynostosis with ipsilateral posterior deformation can also create a trapezoidal head shape. Both require complex and diverse treatment planning.[32] Most of the confusion in the neurosurgical and craniofacial literature prior to 1996 is about deformational posterior plagiocephaly and lambdoidal craniosynostosis; seminal papers in the plastic surgery literature have helped distinguish between these conditions.[8,20,31-33] Interestingly, one report of "recurrent lambdoid synostosis within two families" mentions two sets of siblings with parallelogram-shaped skulls and typical deformational posterior plagiocephaly in that histology of the lambdoid suture showed no bony ridging but rather only a fibrous zone between the two adjacent lambdoid bone fronts,[34] yet true familial lambdoidal synostosis is exceedingly rare.[1] Reports such as this provide reason for caution regarding the many incorrect reports of occipital plagiocephaly attributed to lambdoidal craniosynostosis that exist in the literature prior to late 1996 (i.e., large operative series of cases with obvious deformational plagiocephaly treated by lambdoid craniectomies when repositioning efforts failed to correct the asymmetry).[9,11,35,36]

By 1997, most craniofacial centers had become aware of these distinctions and emphasized that deformational plagiocephaly was more common in males, more frequently right-sided, and usually delayed in presentation due to persistent head turning, which is usually not true of lambdoid synostosis.[37] Lambdoidal craniosynostosis manifests a trapezoidal head shape from birth and shows ipsilateral lambdoid ridging with occipitomastoid bossing and downward ear displacement on the involved side, as well as contralateral parietal bossing.[8,20,31,32,38] Huang et al. noted slight posterior displacement of the ear on the involved side, while Menard and David noted anterior displacement on the involved side.[32,38] The cases shown in Fig. 33.1 reveal some anterior and downward displacement of the ear on the involved side, but these cases also had ipsilateral torticollis along with lambdoidal craniosynostosis. This association of torticollis with lambdoidal craniosynostosis may suggest that an unusual fetal position is a predisposition to lambdoidal craniosynostosis. Normally, the head flexes anteriorly when it descends into the birth canal; hence most cases of torticollis have ipsilateral jaw compression and canting due to this flexion; however, if the head were to retroflex instead (which is uncommon), it could compress the lambdoid suture on that side and lead to the association of lambdoidal craniosynostosis and ipsilateral torticollis, with the combined effects of torticollis-related plagiocephaly and synostosis leading to extensive craniofacial deformation (see Fig. 25.6).

Among cases of posterior plagiocephaly, unilambdoidal craniosynostosis is quite uncommon; it accounts for only 2% to 4% of cases.[5,33] In a Seattle series from 1991 to 2001, there were 1537 cases of posterior deformational plagiocephaly, and 690 cases of craniosynostosis required surgery; 17 of the latter cases had true lambdoidal craniosynostosis (2.5%).[5] The 15% to 20% occurrence of lambdoidal craniosynostosis in earlier surgical series clearly represents overdiagnosis of posterior plagiocephaly as lambdoidal craniosynostosis before its clinical picture was fully described and documented.[35,39] The misdiagnosis of posterior deformation as unilambdoidal craniosynostosis serves to emphasize that deformational nonsynostotic posterior plagiocephaly due to muscular torticollis should be treated promptly with neck physical therapy in early infancy so as to allow effective repositioning. When neck physical therapy and repositioning are not effective by 6 months of age, helmet therapy may be required to correct head asymmetry, along with neck physical therapy for torticollis through age 12 months. Thus the primary mode of treatment for infants with torticollis-plagiocephaly deformation sequence is neck physical therapy, not surgery. If there is clinical concern regarding the possibility of lambdoid synostosis, a three-dimensional computed tomography scan will usually help clarify the diagnosis.

References

1. Watson CC, Griessenauer CJ, Tubbs RS, Johnston JM. Lambdoidal synostosis in dizygotic twins with a family history of an undiagnosed connective tissue disorder. *Childs Nerv Syst.* 2014;30(6):1117–1120.
2. Lattanzi W, Bukvic N, Barba M, et al. Genetic basis of single-suture synostoses: genes, chromosomes and clinical implications. *Childs Nerv Syst.* 2012;28(9):1301–1310.
3. Borad V, Cordes EJ, Liljeberg KM, Sylvanus TS, Lim PK, Wood RJ. Isolated lambdoid craniosynostosis. *J Craniofac Surg.* 2019;30(8):2390–2392.
4. Chiang SN, Fotouhi AR, Doering MM, et al. Cognitive development in lambdoid craniosynostosis: a systematic

review and meta-analysis. *The Cleft Palate Craniofacial Journal*. 0(0):10556656221129978.
5. Huang MH, Gruss JS, Clarren SK, et al. The differential diagnosis of posterior plagiocephaly: true lambdoid synostosis versus positional molding. *Plast Reconstr Surg*. 1996;98(5):765–774; discussion 775-766.
6. Graham JM Jr. Craniofacial deformation. *Ballier Clin Pediatr*. 1998;6:293–315.
7. Cohen MM, MacLean RE. *Craniosynostosis: Diagnosis. Evaluation, and Management*. 2nd ed. New York: Oxford University Press; 2000.
8. Dias MS, Klein DM. Occipital plagiocephaly: deformation or lambdoid synostosis? II. A unifying theory regarding pathogenesis. *Pediatr Neurosurg*. 1996;24(2):69–73.
9. Alderman BW, Fernbach SK, Greene C, Mangione EJ, Ferguson SW. Diagnostic practice and the estimated prevalence of craniosynostosis in Colorado. *Arch Pediatr Adolesc Med*. 1997;151(2):159–164.
10. Ellenbogen RG, Gruss JS, Cunningham ML. Update on craniofacial surgery: the differential diagnosis of lambdoid synostosis/posterior plagiocephaly. *Clin Neurosurg*. 2000;47:303–318.
11. Al-Jabri T, Eccles S. Surgical correction for unilateral lambdoid synostosis: a systematic review. *J Craniofac Surg*. 2014;25(4):1266–1272.
12. Santiago GS, Santiago CN, Chwa ES, Purnell CA. Positional plagiocephaly and craniosynostosis. *Pediatr Ann*. 2023;52(1):e10–e17.
13. Rogers GF, Edwards PD, Robson CD, Mulliken JB. Concordant contralateral lambdoidal synostosis in dizygotic twins. *J Craniofac Surg*. 2005;16(3):435–439.
14. Park JP, Graham JM Jr, Berg SZ, Wurster-Hill DH. A de novo interstitial deletion of chromosome 6 (q22.2q23.1). *Clin Genet*. 1988;33(2):65–68.
15. Timberlake AT, Kiziltug E, Jin SC, et al. De novo mutations in the BMP signaling pathway in lambdoid craniosynostosis. *Hum Genet*. 2023;142(1):21–32.
16. Lemyre E, Lemieux N, Décarie JC, Lambert M. Del(14)(q22.1q23.2) in a patient with anophthalmia and pituitary hypoplasia. *Am J Med Genet*. 1998;77(2):162–165.
17. Poot M. Structural genome variations related to craniosynostosis. *Mol Syndromol*. 2019;10(1-2):24–39.
18. Vinchon M, Guerreschi P, Karnoub MA, Wolber A. Synostosis of the lambdoid suture: a spectrum. *Childs Nerv Syst*. 2021;37(6):1991–2000.
19. Balestrino A, Secci F, Piatelli G, et al. Pure bilateral lambdoid and posterior sagittal synostosis (Mercedes-Benz syndrome): case report and literature review. *World Neurosurg*. 2019;128:77–82.
20. Ehret FW, Whelan MF, Ellenbogen RG, Cunningham ML, Gruss JS. Differential diagnosis of the trapezoid-shaped head. *Cleft Palate-Craniofacial Journal*. 2004;41(1):13–19.
21. Haas-Lude K, Wolff M, Will B, Bender B, Krimmel M. Clinical and imaging findings in children with non-syndromic lambdoid synostosis. *Eur J Pediatr*. 2014;173(4):435–440.
22. Sze RW, Parisi MT, Sidhu M, et al. Ultrasound screening of the lambdoid suture in the child with posterior plagiocephaly. *Pediatr Radiol*. 2003;33(9):630–636.
23. Koshy JC, Chike-Obi CJ, Hatef DA, et al. The variable position of the ear in lambdoid synostosis. *Ann Plast Surg*. 2011;66(1):65–68.
24. Muroi A, Enomoto T, Ihara S, Ishikawa E, Inagaki T, Matsumura A. Developmental changes in the occipital cranial sutures of children less than 2 years of age. *Childs Nerv Syst*. 2021;37(2):567–572.
25. Rogers GF, Edwards PD, Robson CD, Mulliken JB. Concordant contralateral lambdoidal synostosis in dizygotic twins. *J Craniofac Surg*. 2005;16(3):435–439.
26. Dempsey RF, Monson LA, Maricevich RS, et al. Nonsyndromic craniosynostosis. *Clin Plast Surg*. 2019;46(2):123–139.
27. Teichgraeber JF, Baumgartner JE, Viviano SL, Gateno J, Xia JJ. Microscopic versus open approach to craniosynostosis: a long-term outcomes comparison. *J Craniofac Surg*. 2014;25(4):1245–1248.
28. Shakir S, Roy M, Lee A, Birgfeld CB. Management of sagittal and lambdoid craniosynostosis: minimally invasive approaches. *Oral Maxillofac Surg Clin North Am*. 2022;34(3):421–433.
29. Elliott RM, Smartt JM, Taylor JA, Bartlett SP. Does conventional posterior vault remodeling alter endocranial morphology in patients with true lambdoid synostosis? *J Craniofac Surg*. 2013;24(1):115–119.
30. Chiang SN, Fotouhi AR, Doering MM, et al. Cognitive development in lambdoid craniosynostosis: a systematic review and meta-analysis. *Cleft Palate Craniofac J*. 20221055665622129978.
31. Bruneteau RJ, Mulliken JB. Frontal plagiocephaly: synostotic, compensational, or deformational. *Plastic and Reconstructive Surgery*. 1992;89(1):21–31.
32. Menard RM, David DJ. Unilateral lambdoid synostosis: morphological characteristics. *J Craniofac Surg*. 1998;9(3):240–246.
33. Jones BM, Hayward R, Evans R, Britto J. Occipital plagiocephaly: an epidemic of craniosynostosis? Craniosynostosis needs to be distinguished from more common postural asymmetry. *Br Med J*. 1997;315(7110):693–694.
34. Fryburg JS, Hwang V, Lin KY. Recurrent lambdoid synostosis within 2 families. *Am J Med Genet*. 1995;58(3):262–266.
35. Muakkassa KF, Hoffman HJ, Hinton DR, Hendrick EB, Humphreys RP, Ash J. Lambdoid synostosis. Part 2: Review of cases managed at The Hospital for Sick Children, 1972-1982. *J Neurosurg*. 1984;61(2):340–347.
36. Levy ML, McComb JG, Wells K, Gans W, Raffel C, Sloan G. Comparison of operative versus nonoperative treatment of functional lambdoid synostosis. *Journal of Neurosurgery*. 1995;82(2):A362–A363.
37. Kuo AA, Tritasavit S, Graham JM Jr. Congenital muscular torticollis and positional plagiocephaly. *Pediatr Rev*. 2014;35(2):79–87; quiz 87.
38. Huang MH, Mouradian WE, Cohen SR, Gruss JS. The differential diagnosis of abnormal head shapes: separating craniosynostosis from positional deformities and normal variants. *Cleft Palate Craniofac J*. 1998;35(3):204–211.
39. McComb JG. Treatment of functional lambdoid synostosis. *Neurosurg Clin N Am*. 1991;2(3):665–672.

CHAPTER 34

Multiple Sutural Craniosynostosis

KEY POINTS

- Multiple sutural synostosis can result from a profound degree of prenatal head constraint or genetic mutations in genes associated with a syndromic form of craniosynostosis.
- Differential diagnosis is important considering the natural history and prognosis of different syndromes.
- Elevated intracranial pressure is more common in multiple sutural synostosis compared to single suture synostosis.
- Symptoms include a cloverleaf-shaped head, increased intracranial pressure signs, optic atrophy, proptosis, and loss of vision.
- Treatment involves early extensive calvarectomy, posterior skull release, fronto-orbital advancement, and possible ventriculoperitoneal shunt insertion.

GENESIS

Constraint as the cause of multiple sutural synostosis (sagittal, metopic, coronal, and/or lambdoid) is unusual and usually results from a profound degree of prenatal head constraint.[1,2] The complete restoration of normal form after early and effective surgery is much more likely when constraint is the cause of the problem (Figs. 34.1 and 34.2).[3] Multiple sutural synostosis can also result from genetic mutations in one of several genes (*ERF*, *FGFR1*, *FGFR2*, *FGFR3*, *MEGF8*, *MSX2*, *POR*, *RAB23*, *RECQL4*, *TWIST1*, *WDR35*), all of which result in syndromes that may present with cloverleaf skull.[4-8] The cloverleaf skull shape is caused by multiple suture synostosis that involves the coronal, lambdoid, and metopic sutures with bulging of the cerebrum through the open sagittal suture or through open squamosal sutures (Figs. 34.3 and 34.4). There may also be synostosis of the sagittal and squamosal sutures with eventration through a widely patent anterior fontanel. One common syndrome associated with cloverleaf skull is thanatophoric dysplasia type 2, which is due to mutations in *FGFR3*. Type 2 Pfeiffer syndrome is usually due to mutations in *FGFR2* and can result in cloverleaf skull, as can Crouzon syndrome and Apert syndrome, which are also due to mutations in *FGFR2*. Some rare syndromes, such as Crouzon syndrome with acanthosis nigricans (see Fig. 34.3B, C), Baller-Gerold syndrome, and Boston craniosynostosis syndrome, sometimes manifest cloverleaf skull.[9] Baller-Gerold syndrome is a rare autosomal recessive condition with radial aplasia/hypoplasia and craniosynostosis caused by *RECQL4* mutations.[10] In Boston craniosynostosis syndrome, the mutant *MSX2* product has enhanced affinity for binding to its deoxyribonucleic acid (DNA) target sequence, resulting in activated osteoblastic activity and aggressive cranial ossification.[11-13] In Crouzon syndrome with acanthosis nigricans (also called Crouzonoid craniosynostosis with acanthosis nigricans), a specific *FGFR3* gain-of-function mutation (p.A1a391Glu) leads to early-onset acanthosis nigricans during childhood, often with associated choanal atresia and hydrocephalus. The association of choanal atresia with hydrocephalus in an individual with Crouzon syndrome–like facial features should suggest molecular analysis for this particular mutation, and the combination of hydrocephalus with craniosynostosis may predispose a person toward a cloverleaf skull.[14] It is believed that premature closure of the spheno-occipital synchondrosis is associated with the midface hypoplasia in patients with Crouzon syndrome.[15] Bilateral lambdoid and posterior sagittal synostosis is another rare disorder characterized by invagination of the occipital squame resulting in a step-like deformity of the occiput, and a typical head shape described as anterior turricephaly with mild brachycephaly.[16]

FEATURES

In multiple sutural craniosynostosis, the limitations of calvarial expansion are so extreme that there is

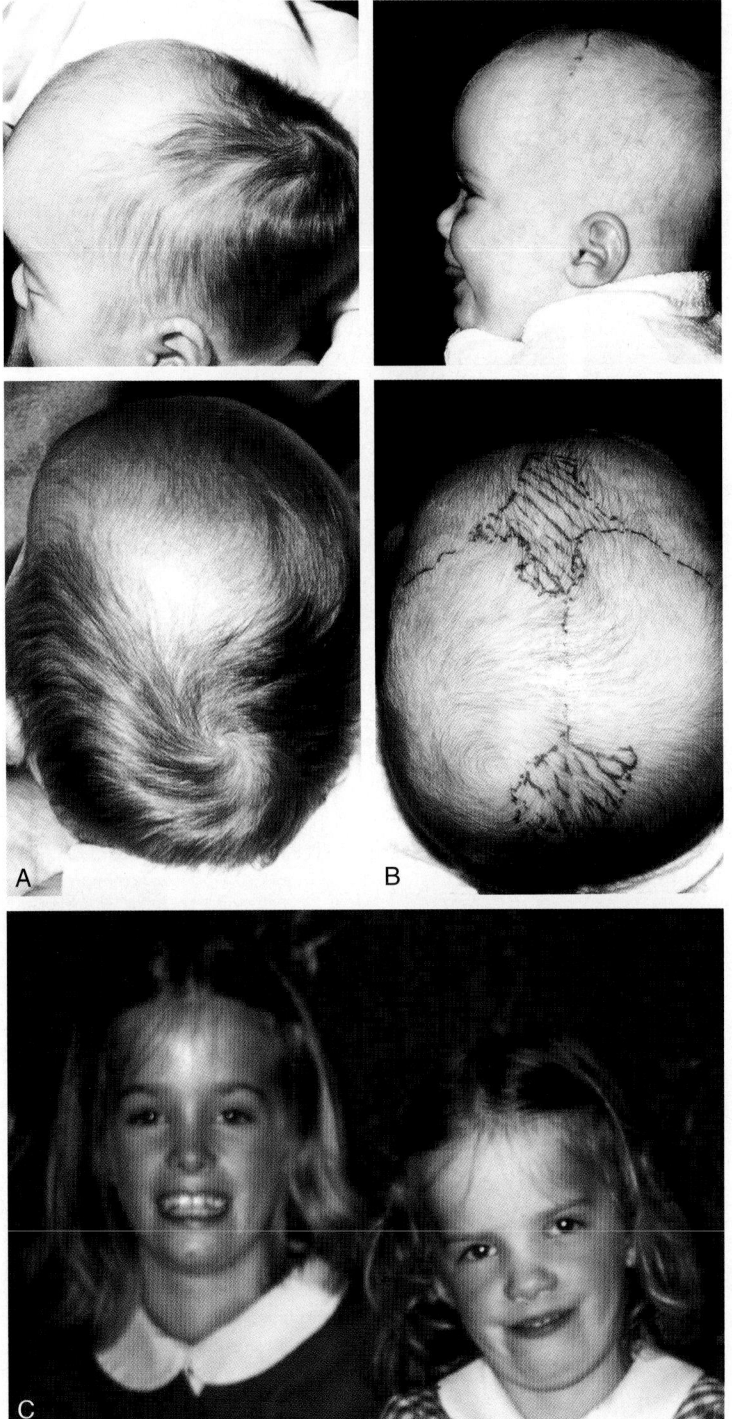

FIGURE 34.1 **A,** This infant has a cloverleaf skull appearance due to sagittal, coronal, and lambdoidal craniosynostosis. Only the metopic suture was open, and the brain growth ballooned out into this region. The coronal synostosis in addition to the bulging forehead region had distorted the mid- and upper face. A calvarectomy was performed from the supraorbital ridge to below the coronal suture, above the mastoid and the foramen magnum. The aberrant calvarium was discarded, and within several weeks a new calvarium began to form from the remaining dura mater. **B,** Two months after calvarectomy, the new calvarium had formed functional sutures at the sites of dural reflection and fontanelles, where the sutures join. **C,** At age 5 years, the patient had not required any additional surgical procedures, and she resembled her older sister in appearance. (From Hanson JW, Sayer MP, Knopp LM, et al. Subtotal neonatal calvariectomy for severe craniosynostosis. *J Pediatr.* 1977;91:257–269.)

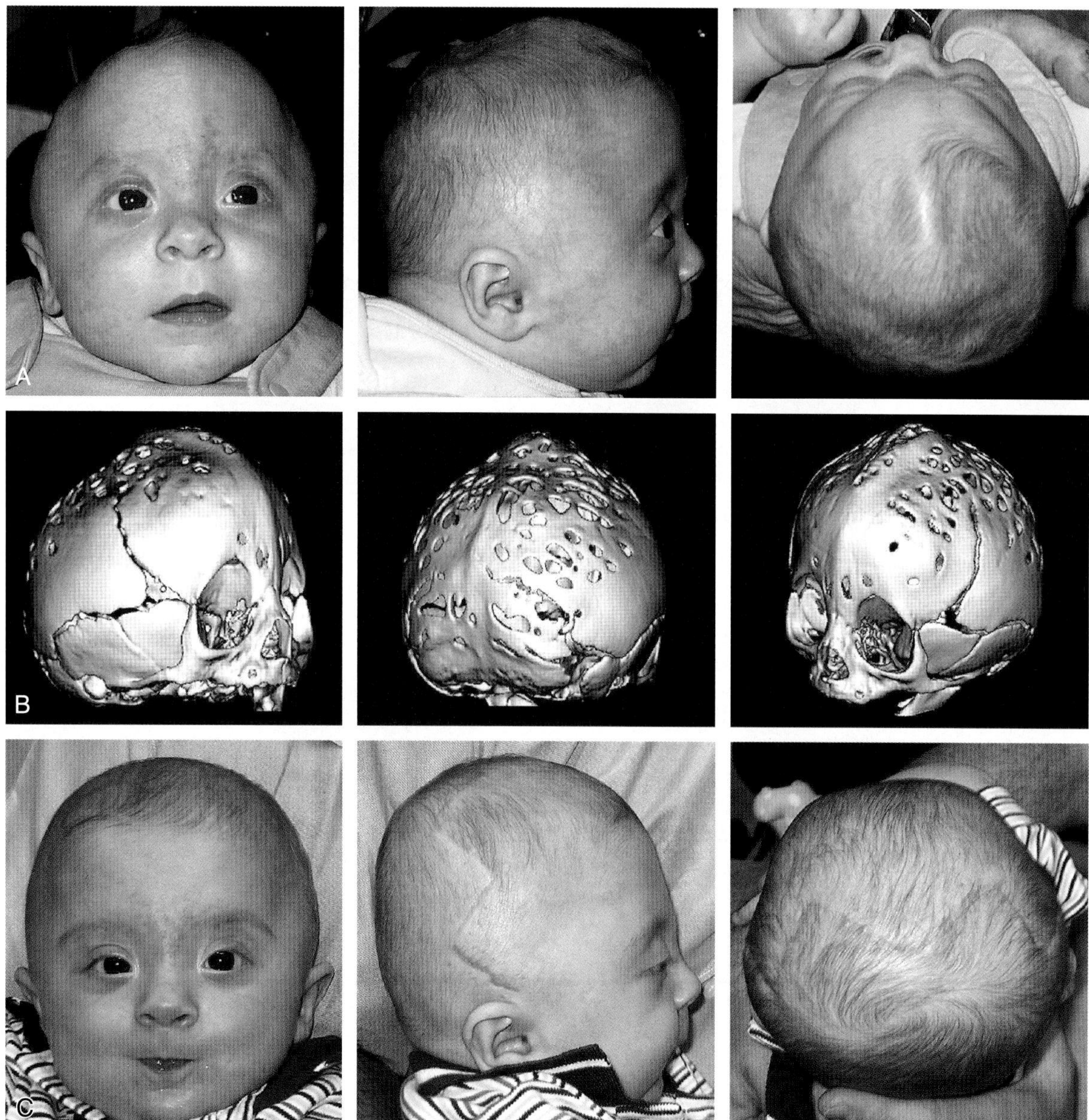

FIGURE 34.2 This neonate was born with synostosis of all midline sutures, as well as the superior coronal sutures and medial portions of the lambdoid sutures. He was part of a twin pregnancy in which prenatal ultrasounds showed that he was in a breech position, with his cranium pinched between the legs of his twin brother. The diagnosis of craniosynostosis was suspected prenatally, and the twins were delivered by cesarean section at 29 weeks of gestation. An extensive calvarectomy was performed at age 4 months. The patient is 3 months old in the preoperative photographs (A) and 12 months old in photographs taken after cranial orthotic therapy (C). His postoperative cephalic index of 103% was reduced to 92% after 5 months of orthotic therapy. B, Note prominent convolutional markings over the superior portions of the skull in the three-dimensional computed tomography scans. Such findings suggest increased intracranial pressure.

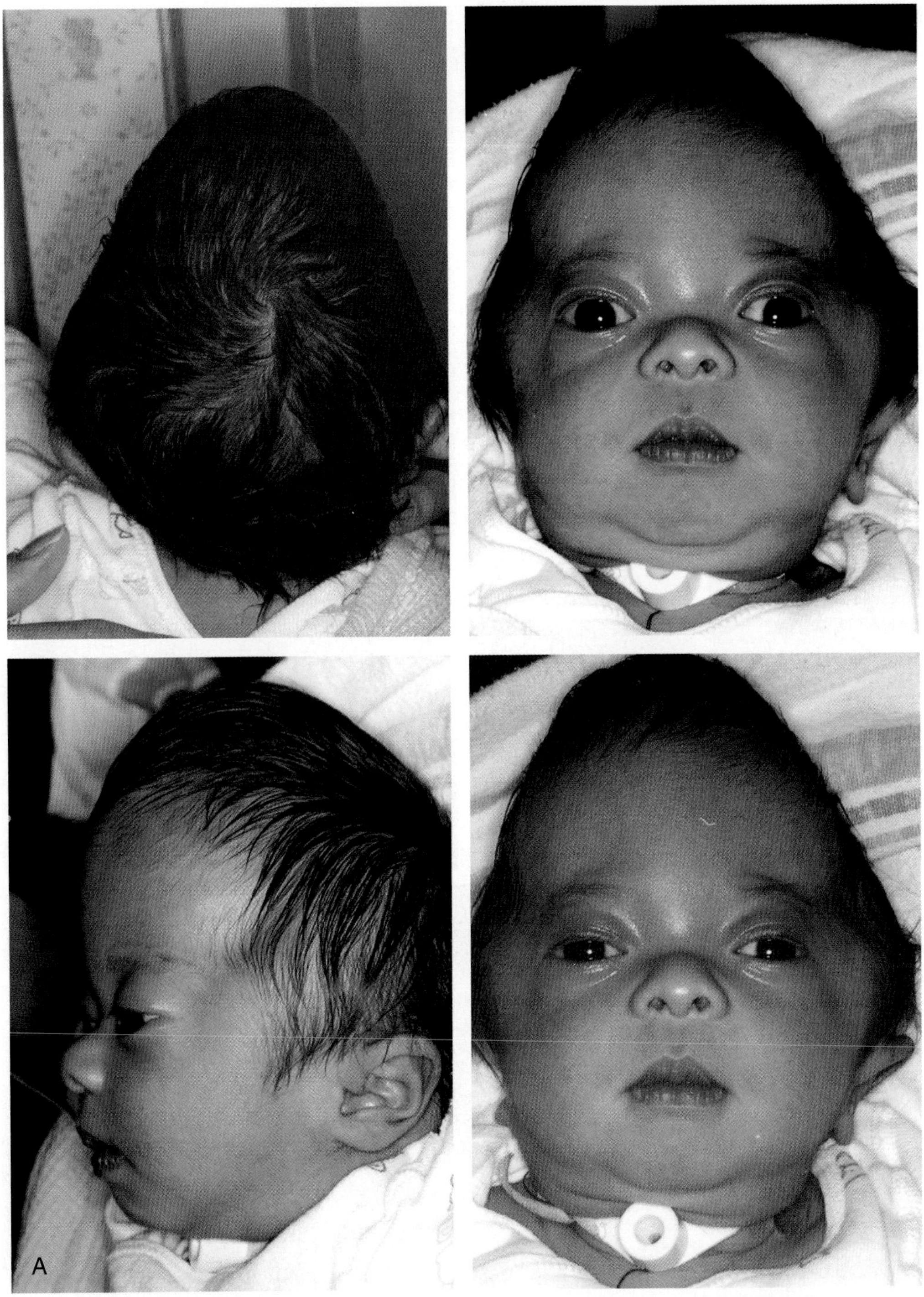

FIGURE 34.3 **A,** This patient has Crouzonoid craniosynostosis with acanthosis nigricans due to an Ala391Glu substitution in *FGFR3*, resulting in multiple suture synostosis and a cloverleaf skull at age 9 days. He had associated hydrocephalus and choanal atresia, and required early posterior and anterior cranial reconstruction in addition to shunting for hydrocephalus and tracheostomy for choanal atresia.

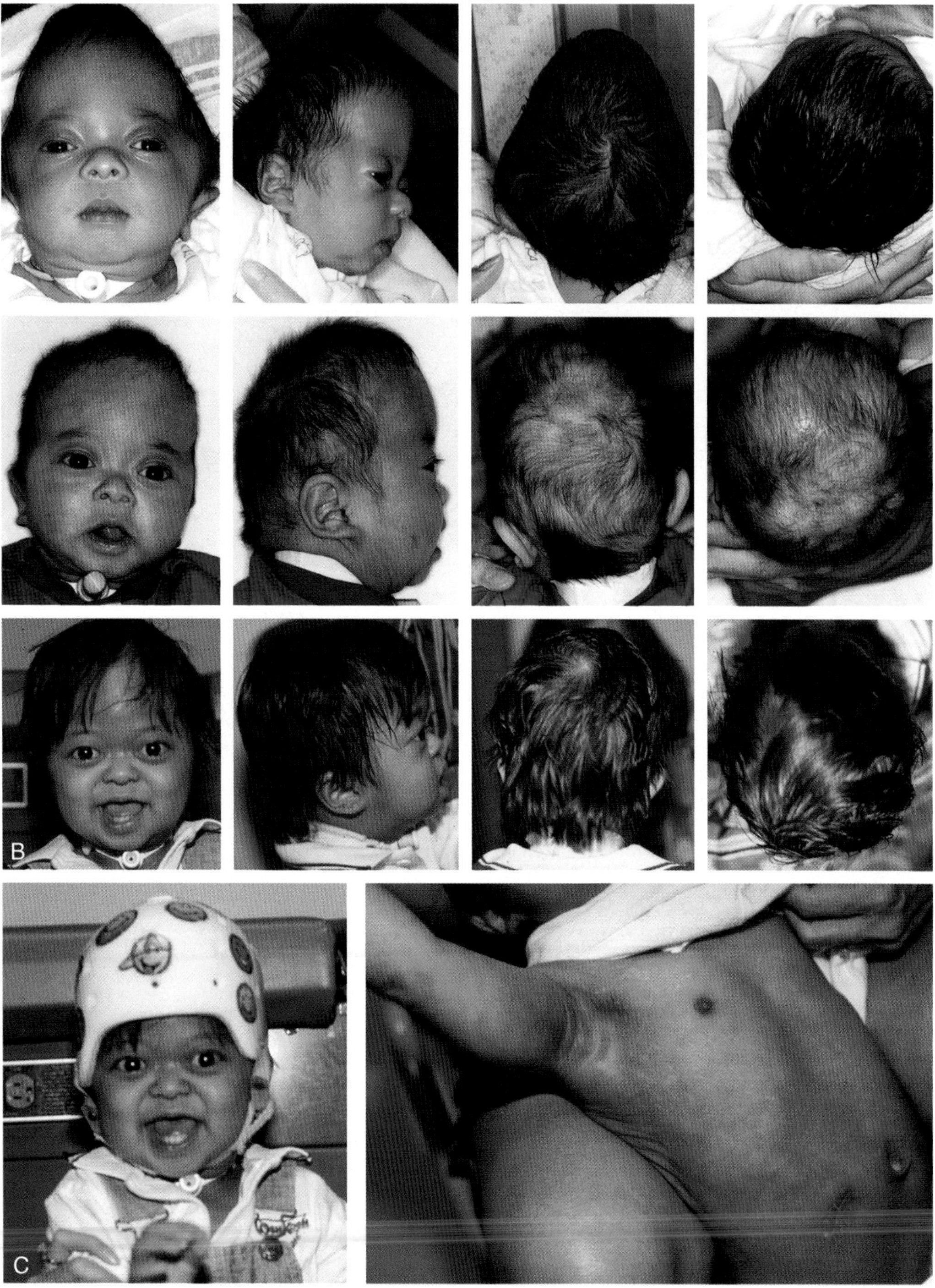

FIGURE 34.3, cont'd **B,** The same patient after posterior remodeling and shunting for hydrocephalus at age 9 days and anterior remodeling at age 9 months. **C,** From ages 2 to 24 months, the patient received cranial orthotic therapy after both surgical procedures to channel brain growth into a symmetric cranial shape. By the end of this treatment period, striking acanthosis nigricans was apparent, leading to the diagnosis of Crouzonoid craniosynostosis with acanthosis nigricans due to an Ala391Glu substitution in *FGFR3*. The use of two consecutive postoperative orthotics facilitated optimal correction after each subtotal calvarectomy and prevented excessive molding after each surgery.

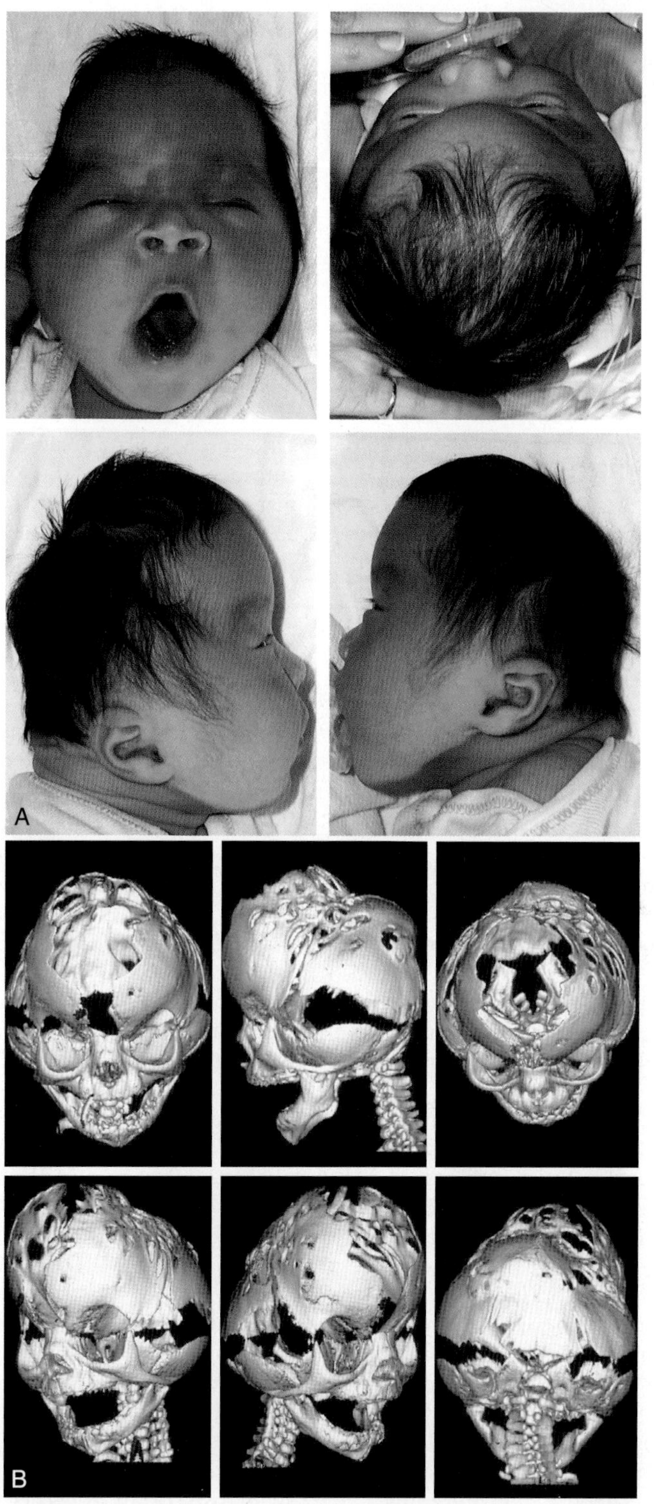

FIGURE 34.4 **A,** This patient also has multiple suture synostosis resulting in a cloverleaf skull *(top)*, but no mutation could be found in *FGFR1*, *FGFR2*, *FGFR3*, *TWIST*, *MSX2*, or *ALX4*. **B,** Three-dimensional computed tomography scans show multiple sutural synostosis with multiple areas of cranial thinning.

limited room for brain growth. This condition is more likely to result in elevated intracranial pressure than is single suture synostosis.[17] Besides the cloverleaf head shape caused by multiple suture synostosis, there are usually signs of increased intracranial pressure, with prominent convolutional markings and a "beaten copper" or lacunae radiographic appearance over the inner table of the skull (Fig. 34.4B), and may result in soft tissue herniation.[18,19] Papilledema, optic atrophy, proptosis, and loss of vision may occur.[20] Combinations of sutural synostosis, such as sagittal with coronal, are also referred to as *compound craniosynostosis*.

MANAGEMENT AND PROGNOSIS

Several unique considerations must be taken into account when managing patients with multiple suture craniosynostosis. The timing, progression, and clinical course vary from patient to patient and are influenced by multiple factors, acting at different steps of the child's growth. Consequently, the protocols, evaluations, and management require a tailored approach.[21] The multidisciplinary care team should include ophthalmologic follow-up to help minimize the risk to vision posed by such entities as papilledema and amblyopia.[20,22] Early extensive calvarectomy is usually merited to preserve brain function and development, as well as to allow for reformation of more normal craniofacial features. Syndromic craniosynostosis has a high rate of hydrocephaly, and therefore early treatment may also help prevent the development of associated macrocephaly, ventriculomegaly, and Chiari I malformation. One center summarized their experience with 33 patients with syndromic craniosynostosis where 18 (54.5%) developed ventriculomegaly and 13 (39.4%) required ventriculoperitoneal shunt placement. Six patients (18.2%) required shunt placement previous to craniofacial surgery. Seven patients (21.2%) required a shunt after craniofacial surgery.[23] Many craniofacial surgeons prefer to begin with a posterior skull release in the early months of life (mean age, 4 months), followed by fronto-orbital advancement around the end of the first year (mean age, 14 months); a ventriculoperitoneal shunt may be inserted at the time of the first procedure if associated hydrocephalus is present.[15,23] The advances of implantable surgical springs, distraction osteogenesis, and external distraction devices used with frontofacial monobloc advancement have increased the safety of the procedure.[24,25] Distraction osteogenesis has been used in patients with cloverleaf skull and multiple suture synostosis, and in one study showed improvement of severe cranial lacunae and signs of increased intracranial pressure.[21] Endoscopy-assisted surgery for complex craniosynostosis has been assessed in children under 4 months of age and is thought to represent a rare alternative management option,[26] yet endoscope-assisted craniectomy combined with helmet therapy may be a viable single-stage treatment option for combined metopic-sagittal synostosis.[27] The use of postoperative orthotic molding can help channel brain growth into a more normal form, leading to improved postoperative results compared with those obtained via surgery alone (see Fig. 34.3C).[14,28] When lambdoid synostosis occurs as part of a syndrome with multiple suture involvement, there is often bilateral involvement, and early posterior release may alleviate some associated increased intracranial pressure. Rarely, in some instances of syndromic coronal craniosynostosis, the combination of sagittal synostosis with underlying coronal synostosis has a corrective effect, and delayed sagittal synostosis repair can prevent the need for a second operation as effectively as a postsurgical cranial orthotic device (Fig. 34.5).

Patients with craniofacial dysostosis syndromes need to be followed carefully for hydrocephalus, which is often part of the syndrome rather than a result of the multiple suture synostosis.[29] Restricted growth of the posterior fossa is particularly common in severe craniofacial dysostosis syndromes. Hanson et al.[30] considered the case shown in Fig. 34.1A, B to be an early example of the efficacy of a neonatal subtotal neonatal calvarectomy at 13 days for severe nonsyndromic craniosynostosis without any associated hydrocephalus. This child was clinically normal and closely resembled her older sister at 5 years of age, and subsequent procedures were not needed. Future studies that follow neurodevelopmental progress and serial head circumference and other clinical outcomes will help guide further treatment guidelines.[31]

DIFFERENTIAL DIAGNOSIS

As emphasized previously, this severe degree of multiple suture craniosynostosis may be more common in genetically determined disorders, such as Crouzon syndrome, Apert syndrome, Pfeiffer syndrome, or Saethre-Chotzen syndrome, than in fetal head constraint. In Crouzon syndrome, sagittal and coronal synostosis occur together in 19% of patients, and involvement of the sagittal, coronal, and lambdoid

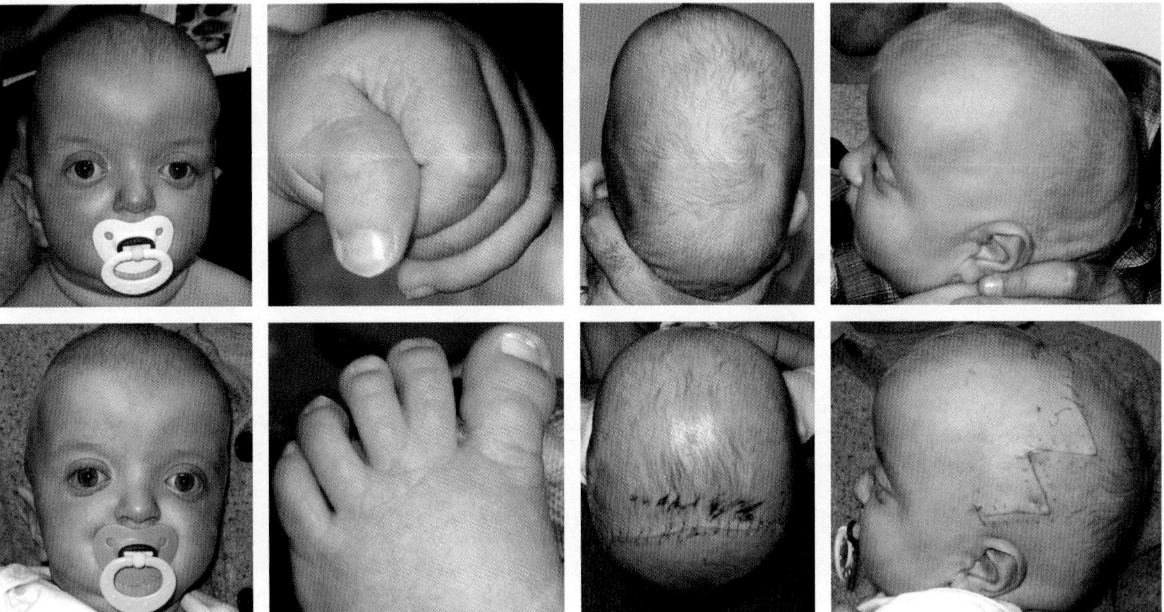

FIGURE 34.5 This boy with Pfeiffer syndrome experienced early fetal head descent and developed sagittal synostosis, which counteracted the normal tendency of his coronal sutures to fuse. Consequently, the repair of sagittal synostosis was delayed from ages 4 to 6 months. No postoperative orthotic was used, and by 9 months of age his coronal synostosis had progressed.

sutures is even more common.[32,33] It is critically important to understand the natural history of the disorder being treated, because thanatophoric dysplasia and Pfeiffer syndrome type 2 have significant early lethality, whereas other syndromes may be much more amenable to successful early treatment without a high incidence of long-term morbidity or mortality.

References

1. Kajdic N, Spazzapan P, Velnar T. Craniosynostosis: recognition, clinical characteristics, and treatment. *Bosn J Basic Med Sci*. 2018;18(2):110–116.
2. Al-Shaqsi S, Forrest CR. Multi-suture craniosynostosis in Sotos syndrome: a case report. *Craniomaxillofacial Research & Innovation*. 2023;827528464231166828.
3. Metzler P, Zemann W, Jacobsen C, Lubbers HT, Gratz KW, Obwegeser JA. Cranial vault growth in multiple-suture nonsyndromic and syndromic craniosynostosis: a postoperative long-term anthropometric follow-up. *J Craniofac Surg*. 2013;24(3):753–757.
4. Cohen MM Jr. Cloverleaf skulls: etiologic heterogeneity and pathogenetic variability. *J Craniofac Surg*. 2009;20(Suppl 1):652–656.
5. Bessenyei B, Nagy A, Balogh E, et al. Achondroplasia with multiple-suture craniosynostosis: a report of a new case of this rare association. *American Journal of Medical Genetics Part a*. 2013;161(10):2641–2644.
6. Albino FP, Wood BC, Oluigbo CO, Lee AC, Oh AK, Rogers GF. Achondroplasia and multiple-suture craniosynostosis. *J Craniofac Surg*. 2015;26(1):222–225.
7. Afshari FT, Gallo P, Shafi A, et al. ERF-related craniosynostosis and surgical management in the paediatric cohort. *Childs Nerv Syst*. 2023;39(4):983–988.
8. Liu T, Liu G, Jiang S, Hu Y, Zhang M, Liu X. A novel therapeutic hypothesis for craniosynostosis syndromes: clover to clever. *Med Hypotheses*. 2020;144:109837.
9. Cohen MM, MacLean RE. *Craniosynostosis: Diagnosis. Evaluation, and Management*. 2nd ed. New York: Oxford University Press; 2000.
10. Van Maldergem L, Siitonen HA, Jalkh N, et al. Revisiting the craniosynostosis-radial ray hypoplasia association: Baller-Gerold syndrome caused by mutations in the *RECQL4* gene. *J Med Genet*. 2006;43(2):148–152.
11. Warman ML, Mulliken JB, Hayward PG, Muller U. Newly recognized autosomal dominant disorder with craniosynostosis. *Am J Med Genet*. 1993;46(4):444–449.
12. Jabs EW, Muller U, Li X, et al. A mutation in the homeodomain of the human *MSX2* gene in a family affected with autosomal dominant craniosynostosis. *Cell*. 1993;75(3):443–450.
13. Ma L, Golden S, Wu L, Maxson R. The molecular basis of Boston-type craniosynostosis: the Pro148-->His mutation in the N-terminal arm of the MSX2 homeodomain stabilizes DNA binding without altering nucleotide sequence preferences. *Hum Mol Genet*. 1996;5(12):1915–1920.

14. Schweitzer DN, Graham JM Jr, Lachman RS, et al. Subtle radiographic findings of achondroplasia in patients with Crouzon syndrome with acanthosis nigricans due to an Ala391Glu substitution in *FGFR3*. *Am J Med Genet*. 2001;98(1):75–91.
15. Sgouros S, Goldin JH, Hockley AD, Wake MJ. Posterior skull surgery in craniosynostosis. *Childs Nerv Syst*. 1996;12(11):727–733.
16. Pillai S, Cochrane D, Singhal A, Steinbok P. Bilateral lambdoid and posterior sagittal craniosynostosis: management, evolution, and outcome. *Childs Nerv Syst*. 2013;29(11):2117–2121.
17. Renier D, Sainte-Rose C, Marchac D, Hirsch JF. Intracranial pressure in craniostenosis. *J Neurosurg*. 1982;57(3):370–377.
18. Mohseni M, Nejat F, Chegini P, El Khashab M. Multiple acquired encephaloceles: dramatic end point of chronic untreated intracranial hypertension in multi-suture craniosynostosis. *Pediatr Neurosurg*. 2012;48(6):397–398.
19. Poonia A, Giridhara P, Sheoran D. Copper beaten skull. *J Pediatr*. 2019;206:297–297.e291.
20. Duan M, Skoch J, Pan BS, Shah V. Neuro-ophthalmological manifestations of craniosynostosis: current perspectives. *Eye Brain*. 2021;13:29–40.
21. Tamburrini G, Caldarelli M, Massimi L, Gasparini G, Pelo S, Di Rocco C. Complex craniosynostoses: a review of the prominent clinical features and the related management strategies. *Childs Nerv Syst*. 2012;28(9):1511–1523.
22. Slavkin HC, Sanchez-Lara PA, Chai Y, Urata M. A model for interprofessional health care: lessons learned from craniofacial teams. *J Calif Dent Assoc*. 2014;42(9):637–644.
23. Tcherbbis Testa V, Jaimovich S, Argañaraz R, Mantese B. Management of ventriculomegaly in pediatric patients with syndromic craniosynostosis: a single center experience. *Acta Neurochir (Wien)*. 2021;163(11): 3083–3091.
24. Paternoster G, Haber SE, Khonsari RH, James S, Arnaud E. Craniosynostosis: monobloc distraction with internal device and its variant for infants with severe syndromic craniosynostosis. *Clin Plast Surg*. 2021;48(3):497–506.
25. Dunaway DJ, Budden C, Ong J, James G, Jeelani NUO. Monobloc distraction and facial bipartition distraction with external devices. *Clin Plast Surg*. 2021;48(3):507–519.
26. Rivero-Garvia M, Marquez-Rivas J, Rueda-Torres AB, Ollero-Ortiz A. Early endoscopy-assisted treatment of multiple-suture craniosynostosis. *Childs Nerv Syst*. 2012;28(3):427–431.
27. Zubovic E, Skolnick GB, Naidoo SD, Bellanger M, Smyth MD, Patel KB. Endoscopic treatment of combined metopic-sagittal craniosynostosis. *J Neurosurg Pediatr*. 2020;26(2):113–121.
28. Delye HHK, Borstlap WA, van Lindert EJ. Endoscopy-assisted craniosynostosis surgery followed by helmet therapy. *Surg Neurol Int*. 2018;9:59.
29. Hersh DS, Hughes CD. Syndromic craniosynostosis: unique management considerations. *Neurosurg Clin N Am*. 2022;33(1):105–112.
30. Hanson JW, Sayers MP, Knopp LM, Macdonald C, Smith DW. Subtotal neonatal calvariectomy for severe craniosynostosis. *J Pediatr*. 1977;91(2):257–260.
31. Carlisle MP, Mehta ST, Sykes KJ, Singhal VK. Serial head circumference and neurodevelopmental screening after surgical correction for single- and multiple-suture craniosynostosis. *Cleft Palate-Craniofacial Journal*. 2012;49(2):177–184.
32. Lajeunie E, Le Merrer M, Bonaiti-Pellie C, Marchac D, Renier D. Genetic study of scaphocephaly. *Am J Med Genet*. 1996;62(3):282–285.
33. Mulliken JB, Gripp KW, Stolle CA, Steinberger D, Muller U. Molecular analysis of patients with synostotic frontal plagiocephaly (unilateral coronal synostosis). *Plast Reconstr Surg*. 2004;113(7):1899–1909.

Section IX
Cranial Bone Variations

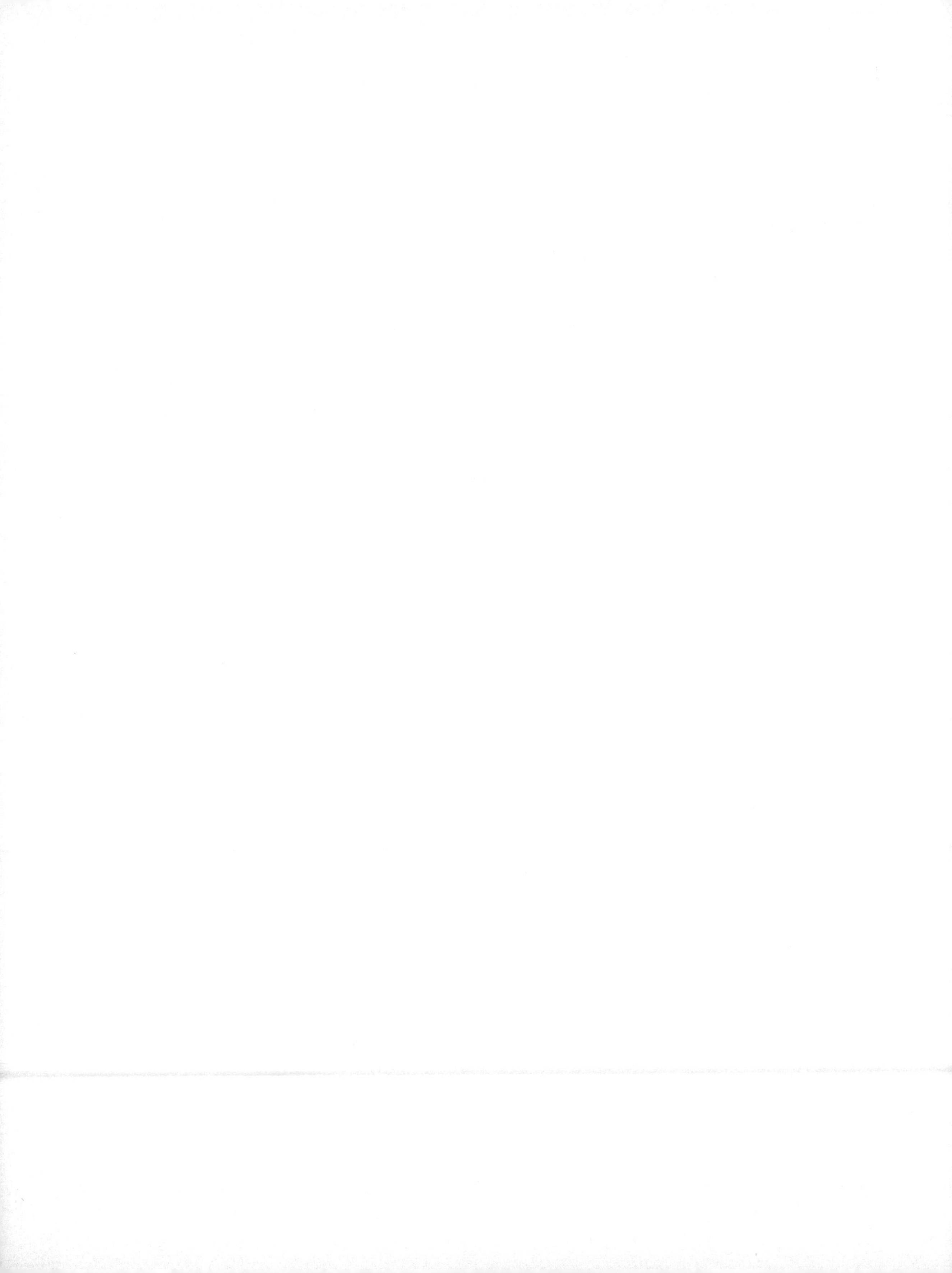

CHAPTER 35

Vertex Birth Molding

KEY POINTS

- Vertex birth molding is the bony adjustments within the cranial vault and soft tissue swelling due to external fetal head compression during delivery.
- Factors such as fetal head position and size, gestational age, maternal pelvic shape, and uterine contractions influence the degree of molding.
- During vertex molding, the frontal and occipital bones slide under the parietal bones, elongating the occipitofrontal diameter and reducing the vertical diameter of the fetal head.
- Recovery from molding occurs in two phases: acute elastic recovery before delivery and slower viscoelastic recovery in the postpartum period.
- Spontaneous resolution of normal vertex birth molding is generally excellent, and no treatment is usually necessary.

GENESIS

Vertex birth molding describes the mechanical changes in fetal head shape due to external compression on the cranium from bony adjustments within the cranial vault that occur as the neonate in vertex presentation passes through the birth canal. Additional soft tissue swelling can significantly alter the shape of the neonatal head, and pressure against the fetal cranium can delay normal ossification in the vertex region, resulting in benign vertex craniotabes. Humans have an unusual pelvis, a large fetal head, and a complicated mechanism of labor. One major feature of human evolution is marked delay in neural development, such that our brains continue to grow slowly over a much longer period than do the brains of other primates. The modern human brain is only 25% of its adult size at birth and continues to grow at a rapid rate throughout the first year of life, when it reaches 50% of its adult size.[1] Human brains are 95% of adult size by 10 years of age. In comparison, a chimpanzee brain is already 40% of its adult size by birth and reaches 80% of the adult volume by the end of the first year. A 1-year-old *Homo erectus* brain was closer to that of apes in its growth pattern and measured 72% to 84% of adult size at that age, which implies differences in the development of cognitive abilities in *Homo erectus* compared with modern humans.[1] The early delivery of the human head appears to leave the cranium much more vulnerable to mechanic forces than in other species. The birth canal is a deep curved tube through which a mature fetal head can only pass by rotating as it descends. A number of factors influence the individual fetal cranial response to the normal forces of labor around the time of delivery, such as fetal head position and size, gestational age, maternal pelvic shape and dimensions, and the quality of uterine contractions.[2–4]

During normal vertex molding, anteroposterior compression causes the frontal and occipital bones to slide under the parietal bones along the entire length of the coronal and lambdoid sutures. This elongates the occipitofrontal diameter to its greatest possible extent so as to diminish the vertical diameter of the fetal head to its smallest dimensions (Fig. 35.1). The fetal pathologist John Ballantyne noted that during vertex molding, the occipital bone rotated in an anteroposterior direction on an "occipital hinge," with a range of motion that is much greater in a 7-month fetus than in a term infant. He also noted that an infant's head recovered to its unmolded state within 6 days after delivery.[5] Holland studied the impact of mechanical stress on the fetal head and noted that the dura mater underlying the cranial bones acted as a protective mechanism to reduce the stress transmitted to the cranial contents.[6] Decreases in dural growth-stretch tension across a suture can trigger synostosis, whereas excessive dural pressure can decrease ossification, leading to craniotabes and increased cranial flexibility. Holland described the fetal skull as a pliable shell composed of loosely jointed plates attached to

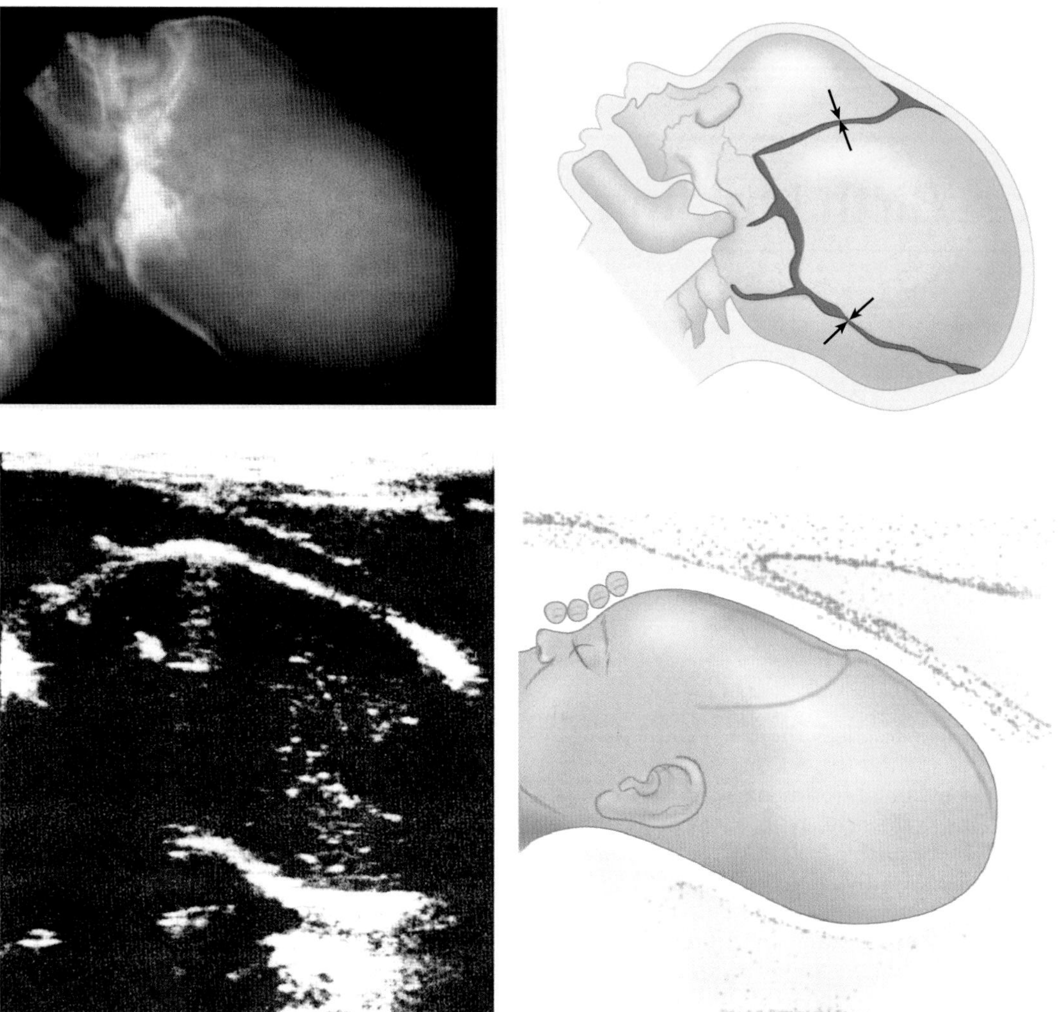

FIGURE 35.1 During normal vertex molding, anteroposterior compression causes the frontal and occipital bones to slide under the parietal bones along the entire length of the coronal and lambdoid sutures. This elongates the occipitofrontal diameter to its greatest possible extent in order to diminish the vertical diameter of the fetal head to its smallest dimensions. This is shown in the illustration and radiograph in the top frames; the bottom frames show an ultrasound view and illustration.

a rigid cranial base, suggesting that the frontal and parietal bones bend under pressure in relation to movement at the occipital hinge.

Moloy examined the hinge action of occipital and frontal bones radiographically in stillborn infants and noted that the cranial base was capable of bending slightly to allow elevation of the occipital plates, and that biparietal pressure decreased the transverse diameter enough to prevent the frontal and occipital bones from overriding the parietal bones when longitudinal pressure was applied.[7] Borell and Fernstrom used radiographs to assess molding as the fetal head passed through the birth canal, and they confirmed that vertex molding was characterized by an elevation of the vertex, an increase in the biparietal diameter, and an inward displacement of the occipital and frontal bones, which caused an overall reduction in the occipitofrontal diameter (see Fig. 35.1). They noted an association between the amount of molding and the length of labor, and they attributed normal vertex molding to pressures from the soft tissues rather than the bony pelvis.[8,9] They noted that a contracted pelvis resulted in more severe fetal head molding than seen in normal deliveries, and that excessive muscular contraction in the lower uterine

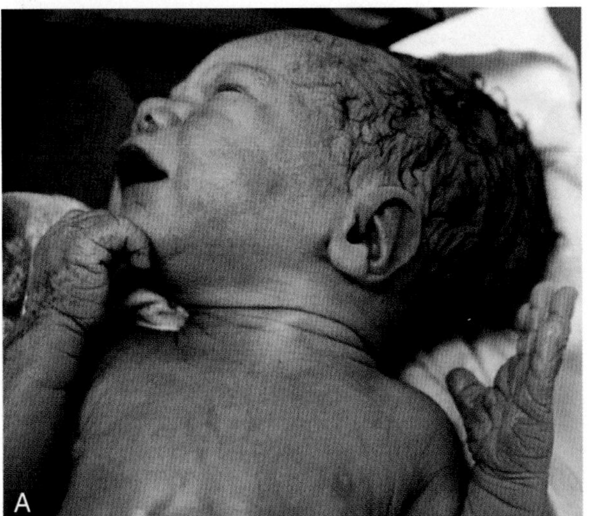

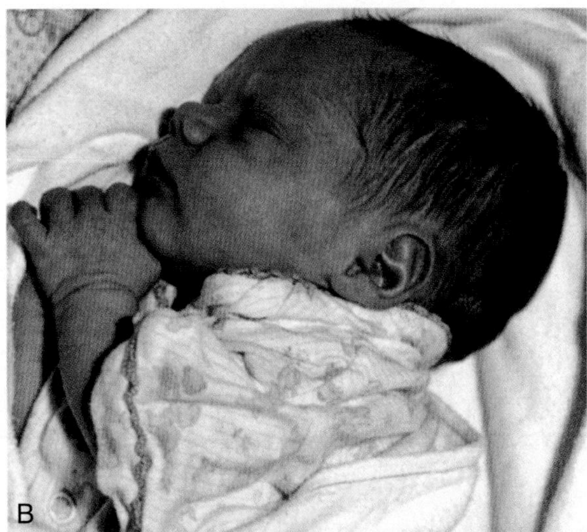

FIGURE 35.2 This small-for-gestational-age infant with rapid postnatal catch-up growth showed marked molding immediately after being born (**A**) to a small primigravida woman. By age 4 days (**B**), the molding had resolved.

segment resulted in excessive vertex molding, with increased elevation of the fetal vertex (Figs. 35.2–35.4).

In 1980, McPherson and Kriewall[10] used engineering structural analysis techniques to investigate the biomechanics of fetal head molding. They observed that fetal cranial bone is capable of deforming under load distributions typical of normal labor, with preterm parietal bone capable of undergoing two to four times the amount of deformation than term parietal bone for the same load distribution. Although this may not result in more obvious extensive cranial molding, the transmission of pressure may be a contributing factor to the increased incidence of birth trauma and intracranial bleeds in preterm infants. In a photographic and anthropometric study of vertex molding in 319 term infants delivered vaginally, several factors influenced the degree of molding. Infants born to primiparous women, after oxytocin-stimulated labors, and via vacuum extraction showed significantly more molding. The duration of the first stage of labor did not influence the degree of molding, but a prolonged second stage in primiparous mothers was associated with more extensive molding. Infants born in the occipitoposterior and in breech presentation showed significantly less molding than those born in occipitoanterior presentations. Some degree of molding does occur within the uterus prior to labor, and repetitive Braxton-Hicks contractions throughout pregnancy were also a factor that influenced the head shape of infants before the onset of labor.[11] Extreme fetal head elongation due to vertex molding from fetal cephalic fixation with persistent uterine contractions has been noted via prenatal ultrasonography as early as 30 weeks of gestation.[12] More recently sutures and fontanels can be modeled, characterized, and studied in silico to simulate the second stage of labor in the vertex presentation and assess a time-dependent response and effects of a prolonged second stage of labor on head molding.[13]

FEATURES

During initial cervical dilatation, pressure is greatest on the upper portion of the parietal bones, which leads to a decrease in biparietal diameter and a slight increase in the height and curvature of the vertex (see Figs. 35.1–35.5). At complete dilatation, the biparietal diameter decreases to its smallest dimension, with continued elevation and curvature of the vertex in addition to inward bending of both the frontal and occipital bones. As the fetus descends, pressure shifts to the lower portions of the parietal bones, causing them to rotate inward and move upward, thereby increasing the biparietal diameter as well as progressively widening the temporosquamosal and sagittal sutures. Recovery from this molded state takes place in two phases: an acute elastic recovery before the head is actually delivered; and a second, slower viscoelastic recovery during the postpartum period, which is usually completed 3 to 7 days after delivery.[10]

In the normal fetus presenting in the vertex position, there may be appreciable molding of the head at birth.

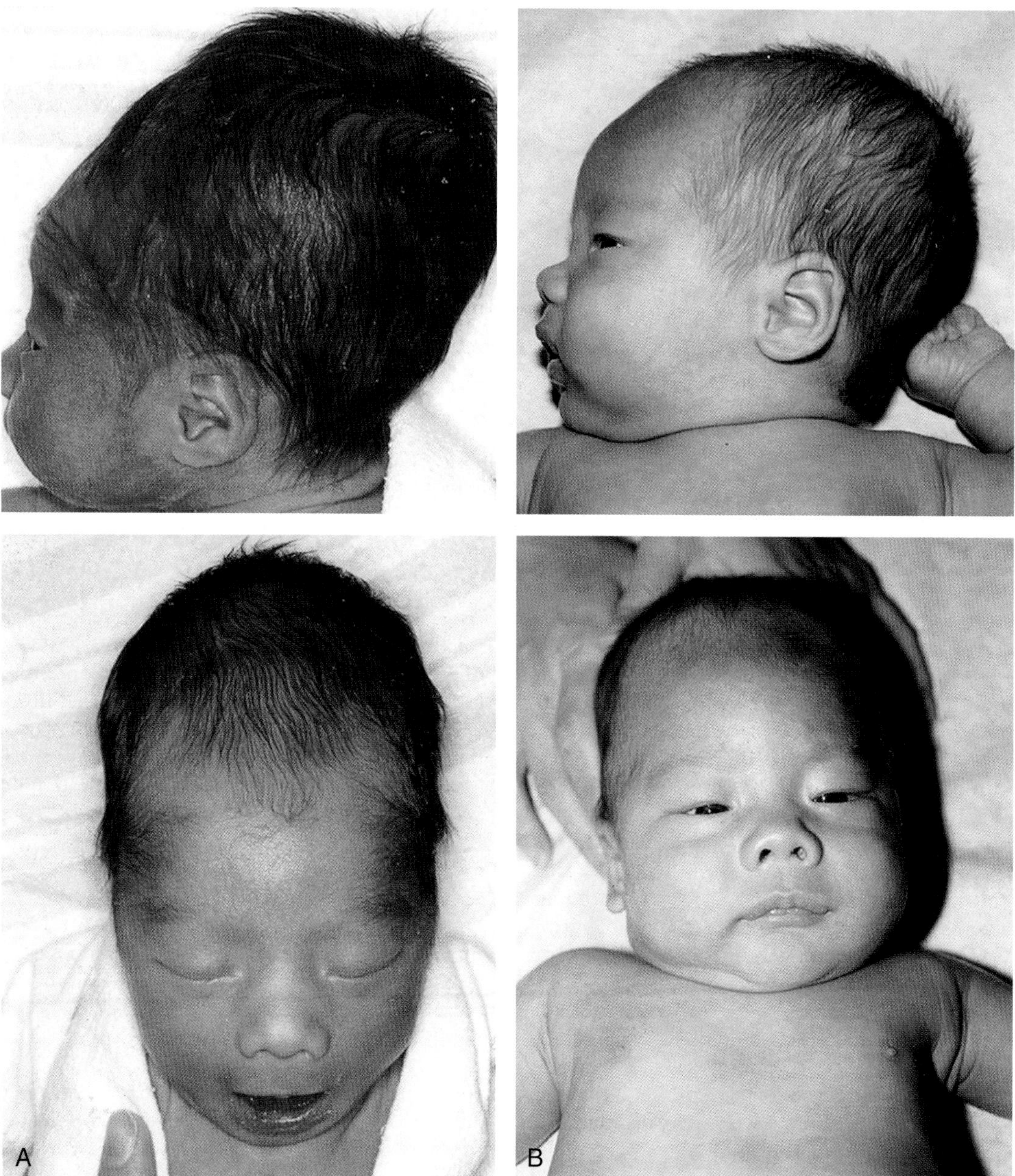

FIGURE 35.3 **A,** At birth, this infant had been in prolonged vertex. **B,** By 2 months of age, the molding had only partially resolved.

This is especially likely if the infant is the first born, if the fetal head was located deep in the uterine outlet for a prolonged time, or if the mother has a prolonged second stage of labor and/or an incompletely dilated rigid cervix. The typical vertex-molded newborn head is elongated and cylindrical, and resumes a rounded shape within the first week of life (see Figs. 35.1 and 35.2).[14] The forehead tends to slope, and the parietooccipital region is prominent. Head circumference measurements may be spuriously low owing to the impact of normal vertex molding. The head circumference usually shifts upward by 1 to 3 days after birth as the head remolds in relation to the true brain shape (see Fig. 35.2). Persistent vertex molding usually reflects prolonged molding during the second stage of labor due to prolonged entrapment of the fetal head.

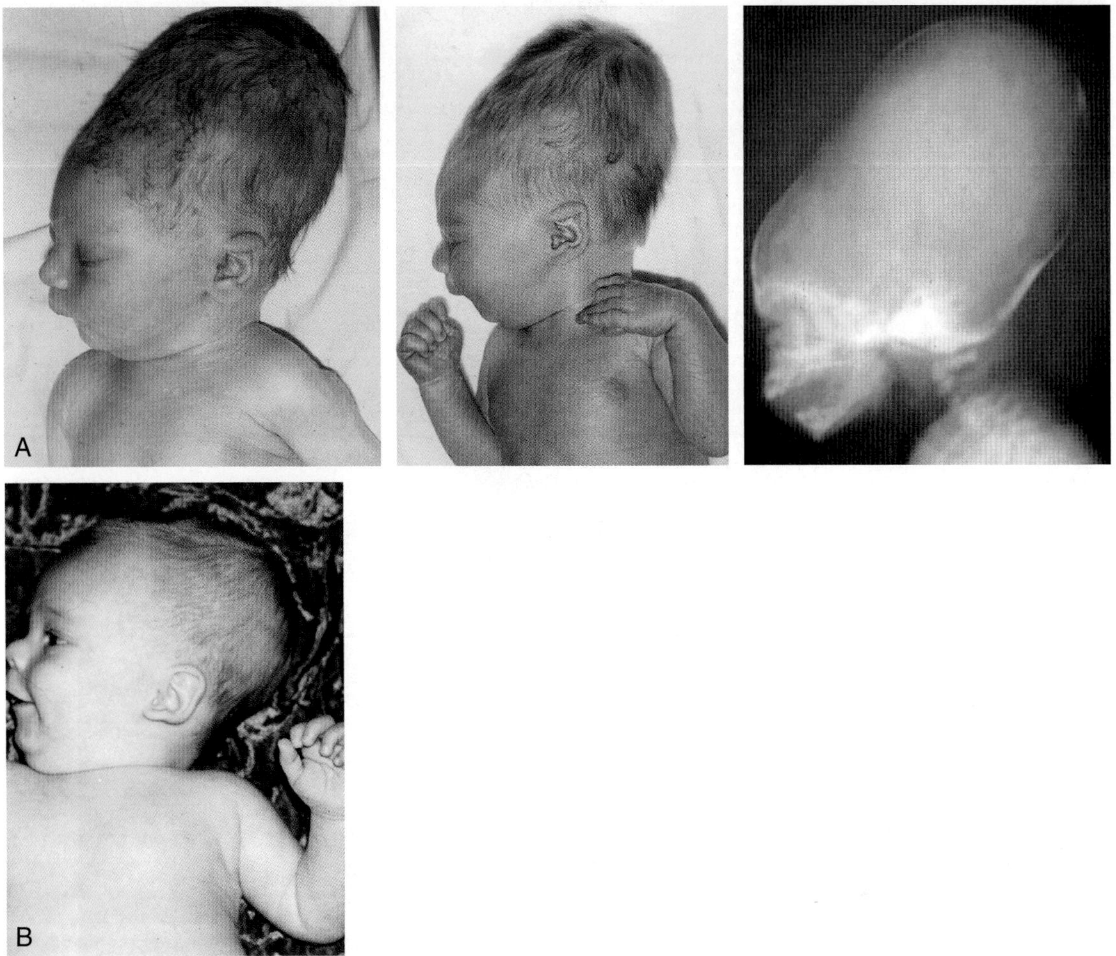

FIGURE 35.4 **A,** Extreme molding was associated with a prolonged second stage of labor due to a tight cervix that did not fully dilate prior to the delivery of this large infant. The cone-shaped vertex was palpably softened (craniotabes). **B,** The same infant at age 3 months. The craniotabes resolved, but vertex molding persists.

MANAGEMENT AND PROGNOSIS

The prognosis for spontaneous resolution of normal vertex birth molding and any accompanying traumatic components is generally excellent, and usually no treatment is necessary other than reassuring the parents that the baby is normal (see Figs. 35.2 and 35.3). With extensive vertex molding, management of the infant's resting position will usually facilitate a complete return to normal form (see Fig. 35.5).[14] It is important to observe the infant during the first week after birth to monitor resolution. During this period, the use of several procedures is worthwhile. The surface on which the baby's head rests should be relatively soft, and care should be taken to position the baby's head on the prominent vertex region during sleep. A rolled diaper or receiving blanket can be placed under the neck and shoulders in the supine resting position to provide support and maintain head position (see Fig. 35.5).[14] Another measure that may be used when the baby is upright in a car seat or infant swing is to place a silk or nylon stocking (sized to fit snugly but not tightly) over the baby's calvarium. This stocking can be filled with a 2- to 3-oz beanbag. The weight should be placed directly over the occipital prominence in an effort to collapse the cone. The cone-shaped cranium may foster a tendency for the infant to lie on one side of the head and face, so it is important to try to minimize postnatal plagiocephaly by alternating the side on which the baby is placed to sleep. If the baby is

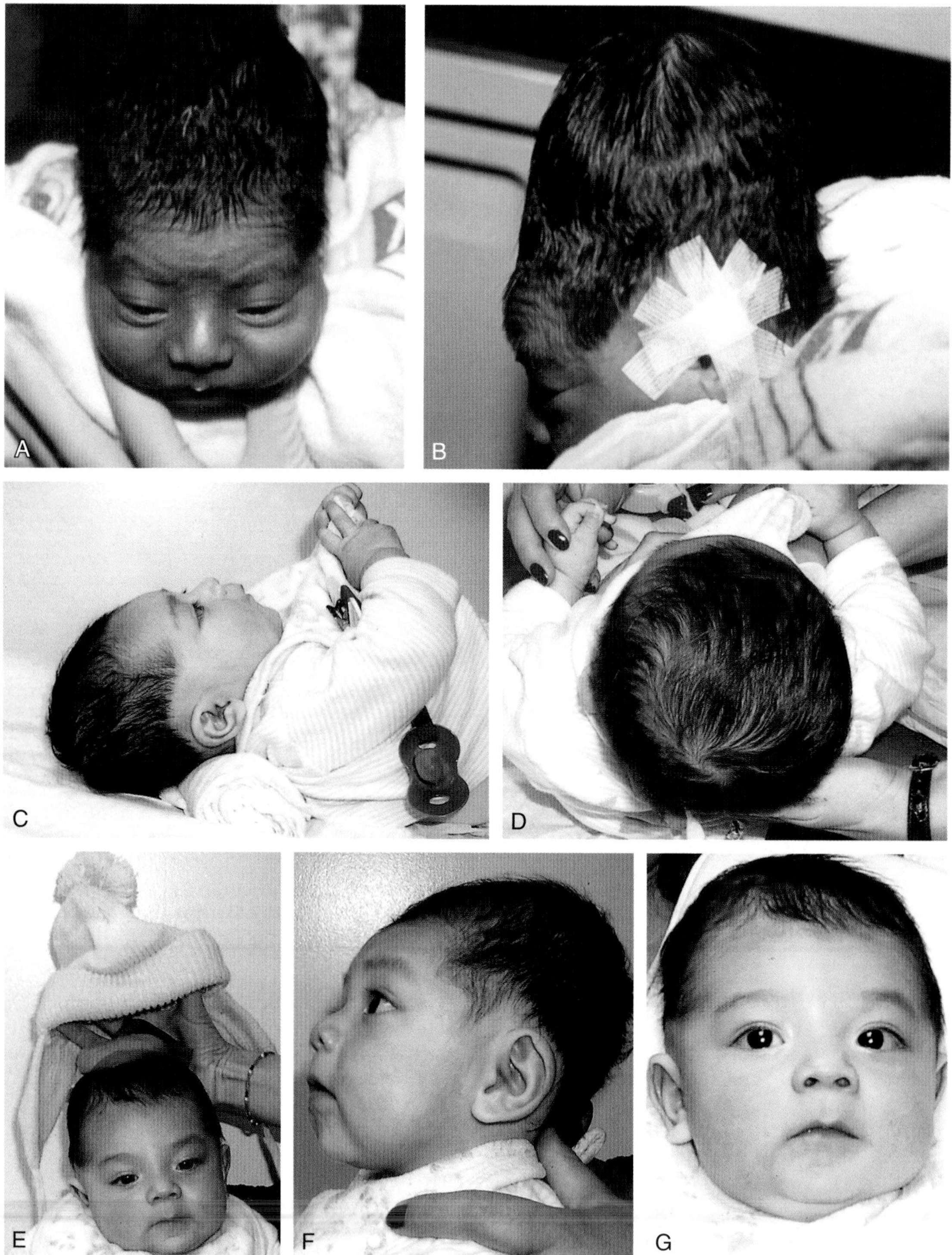

FIGURE 35.5 This male infant is shown at birth with a conic head shape and marked craniotabes (**A, B**) and at 2 and 3 months of age (**C–G**) after active management to resolve his extensive vertex molding and deformed auricle. He was positioned on his prominent vertex during sleep, with a rolled blanket under his neck and shoulders in the supine resting position to provide support and maintain head position. **E,** Another measure used when the baby was upright involved placing a 2- to 3-oz beanbag over the vertex and holding it in place with a knit cap. The weight was placed directly over the occipital prominence in an effort to collapse the cone.

allowed to rest exclusively on the sides of the head, the deformation may become stabilized and the elongated, conic head shape will persist; thus it is important to apply pressure to the vertex to help collapse the conic head shape (see Fig. 35.4).[14]

DIFFERENTIAL DIAGNOSIS

Occasionally, vertex molding is so extensive that the possibility of craniosynostosis, encephalocele, or other causes of aberrant head shape becomes a concern. In addition, persistent fetal vertex molding can lead to permanent deformation of head shape if corrective postnatal positioning interventions are not undertaken. The differential diagnosis may include microcephaly, isolated or syndromic craniosynostosis, and various soft tissue deformities. A spuriously small occipitofrontal head circumference may give a mistaken impression of microcephaly, as may the sloping forehead. Clinical judgment of the apparent overall brain size, in addition to follow-up head circumference measurements as the calvarium returns toward a more normal shape, will usually resolve any questions in this regard. At the leading part of the parietooccipital region, edema of the skin and subcutaneous tissues may be present (the so-called *caput succedaneum*). Craniotabes may also be extensive in the vertex region (see Figs. 35.4 and 35.5). Hemorrhages may occasionally be evident in the sclera and in the retina, and a traumatic subperiosteal hemorrhage may also be present, most commonly in the outer table of the parietal bone, which will give rise to a soft, fluctuant mass. With time, its borders will become elevated and craterlike as the raised periosteum begins to deposit bone at its borders. The subperiosteal hemorrhage, with a subsequent "crater rim" of bone at its outer borders, may give the impression of a depressed skull fracture, but it is actually a benign lesion. Rarely, posterior fossa hemorrhage in the term neonate can lead to severe molding with elongation of the head. Such cases are readily distinguished from benign vertex molding by abnormal neurologic examination. Finally, other calvarial deformations can result when a hand or arm is caught across the skull for a prolonged period of time (Fig. 35.6).

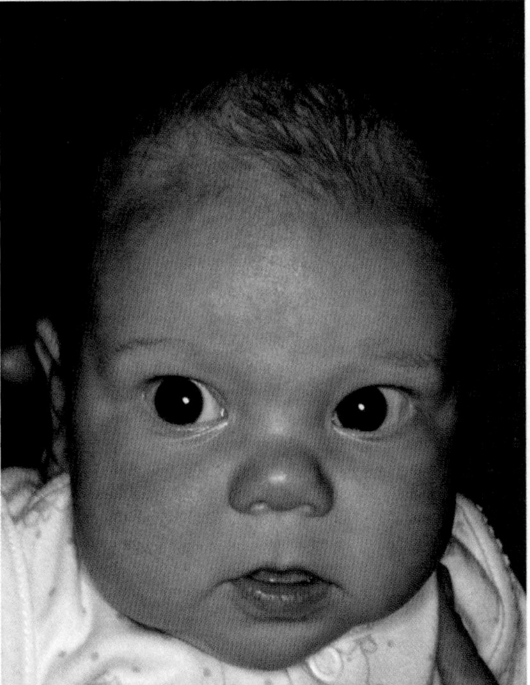

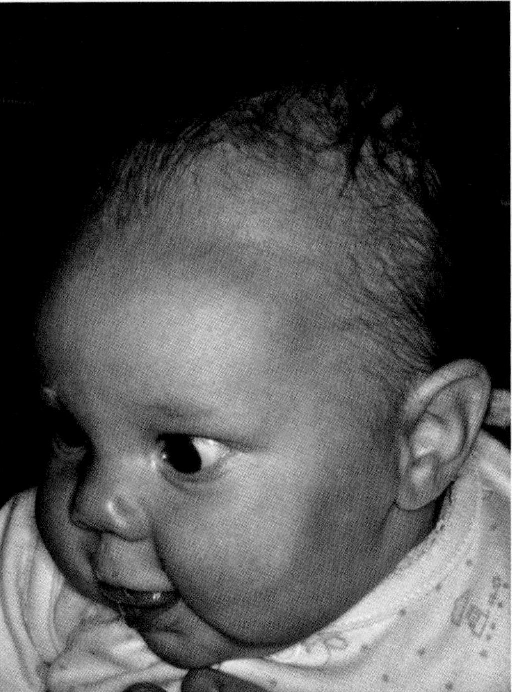

FIGURE 35.6 This infant with a prominent calvarial indentation above the frontal bones was born with her arm across her forehead. The indentation persisted during early infancy but was expected to resolve with subsequent calvarial remodeling. The frontal skull shape resembled that seen in vertex molding, but review of the birth history revealed the true cause.

References

1. Coqueugniot H, Hublin J-J, Vellon F, et al. Early brain growth in *Homo erectus* and implications for cognitive ability. *Nature.* 2004;431:299–302.
2. Compton AA. Soft tissue and pelvic dystocia. *Clin Obstet Gynecol.* 1987;30:69–76.
3. Graham JM Jr. Craniofacial deformation. *Balliere Clin Pediatr.* 1998;6:293–315.
4. Moura R, Borges M, Oliveira D, et al. A biomechanical study of the birth position: a natural struggle between mother and fetus. *Biomech Model Mechanobiol.* 2022 Jun;21(3):937-951.
5. Ballantyne JW. The head of the infant at birth. *Edin Med J.* 1890;36:97–111.
6. Holland E. Cranial stress in the foetus during labour and the effects of excessive stress on the intracranial contents, with an analysis of 81 cases of torn tentorium cerebelli and subdural cerebral hemorrhage. *J Obstet Gynaecol Br Emp.* 1922;29:549–571.
7. Moloy HC. Studies of head molding during labor. *Am J Obstet Gynecol.* 1942;44:762–782.
8. Borell U, Fernstrom I. X-ray diagnosis of muscular spasm in the lower part of the uterus from the degree of moulding of the fetal head. *Acta Obstet Gynecol Scand.* 1959;38:188–189.
9. Borell U, Fernstrom I. The mechanisms of labor in face and brow presentation. *Acta Obstet Gynecol Scand.* 1960;39:626–644.
10. McPherson GK, Kriewall TJ. The elastic modulus of fetal cranial bone: a first step towards an understanding of the biomechanics of fetal head molding. *J Biomechanics.* 1980;13:9–16.
11. Sorbe B, Dahlgren SS. Some important factors in the molding of the fetal head during vaginal delivery: a photographic study. *Int J Gynaecol Obstet.* 1983;21:205–212.
12. Carla SJ, Wyble L, Lense J, et al. Fetal head molding: diagnosis by ultrasound and a review of the literature. *J Perinatol.* 1991;11:105–111.
13. Moura R, Borges M, Vila Pouca MCP, et al. A numerical study on fetal head molding during labor. *Int J Numer Method Biomed Eng.* 2021;37(1):e3411.
14. Graham JM Jr, Kumar A. Diagnosis and management of extensive vertex birth molding. *Clin Pediatr.* 2006;45:672–678.

CHAPTER 3 6

Vertex Craniotabes

KEY POINTS

- Vertex craniotabes is characterized by diminished mineralization in the superior portions of the parietal bones, caused by prolonged forceful pressure on vertex during birth.
- The affected region of the calvarium feels soft to palpation and may exhibit a "ping-pong" sensation on compression.
- The sides of the calvarium and other skeletal regions are typically unaffected, helping to differentiate it from generalized mineralization problems.
- The condition is more likely to occur in first born infants who have experienced early fetal head descent and prolonged vertex presentation.
- Studies have investigated a possible link between craniotabes and neonatal rickets owing to maternal vitamin D deficiency, but the correlations are not consistent.
- The prognosis for postnatal recovery is excellent, and no special precautions or tests are needed unless there is suspicion of generalized craniotabes or osteomalacia associated with vitamin D deficiency.

GENESIS

Prolonged forceful pressure on the presenting part, usually at the vertex affecting the superior portions of the parietal bones, may result in diminished mineralization within the compressed region. The calvarium is generated from the underlying dura mater, and persistent growth-stretch tensile forces restrain cranial ossification and maintain sutural patency. Persistent cranial pressure mimics the mechanical impact of growth-stretch forces and results in temporarily restrained, localized calvarial ossification. Craniotabes is more likely to occur in first born infants, and elicited history often shows that the fetus has experienced early fetal head descent and has been in the vertex position deep within the maternal pelvis for an unusually long period of time. Because this is usually the mother's first pregnancy, she may not be aware of anything unusual other than symptoms of urinary frequency and pressure. The frequency of reported cases of craniotabes has varied over time, with congenital infection thought to be a common underlying cause in the past.[1] Today, craniotabes can be a fairly common finding and may be found in up to 20–30% of normal neonates.[2,3] Mild degrees of compression-related craniotabes occur in about 2% of newborns, whereas more extensive degrees of craniotabes are less common.[2,4]

Since the theory of a compression-related pathogenesis for benign vertex craniotabes was first advanced in 1979,[4,5] several reports have investigated whether craniotabes might be a useful sign for the detection of subclinical rickets due to vitamin D deficiency.[6–11] Most studies failed to demonstrate any significant correlations among maternal and infant serum vitamin D, calcium, phosphorus, and alkaline phosphatase levels; craniotabes; and skeletal mineralization. However, one study showed small but statistically significant decreases in serum calcium and phosphate in mothers of infants with craniotabes compared with mothers of infants with a normal calvarium.[8] There has been a number of reports of newborns being born with severe craniotabes owing to insufficient maternal sunlight exposure during the COVID-19 pandemic.[12] Another study showed that the mean serum 25-hydroxyvitamin D level by radio assay was significantly lower in newborns with craniotabes and in their mothers compared with control mother-infant pairs without craniotabes.[13] Two papers each presenting four cases of neonatal rickets were reported in infants with craniotabes who were born to mothers with florid osteomalacia due to vitamin D–deficiency rickets (causing these mothers hip and back pain and an impaired waddling gait).[10,14] Both the infants and their mothers had low serum concentrations of 25-hydroxyvitamin D, elevated alkaline phosphatase, and borderline or low serum calcium and phosphorous, and they responded to treatment with vitamin D. In one population-based study, nutritional rickets was associated with Black race, breast-feeding, low birth weight, and stunted growth. Four of 13 patients (31%) who underwent 25-hydroxyvitamin D testing had values less than 10 ng/mL.[15] These studies indicate that deficient maternal vitamin D intake can lead to neonatal rickets in which craniotabes may be a presenting feature, and this diagnosis should be considered in any infant without signs of fetal head compression whose mother may be at risk for nutritional deficiency; however in these cases, the infant usually manifests generalized craniotabes and osteomalacia. There have been genetic syndromes such as Noonan syndrome described with craniotabes, but these have all been linked to vitamin D–deficiency rickets.[16]

FEATURES

The superior parietooccipital region tends to be soft to palpation by the examining fingers, and often there is a "ping-pong" sensation on finger compression. This tactile sensation resembles the indentation and snapping rebound felt when pressing on a ping-pong ball. In extreme cases, the entire top of the head can be involved (Figs. 36.1 and 36.2). The presence of a normally firm bony calvarium along the sides of the calvarium and in the mastoid regions readily differentiates this benign type of craniotabes from other forms caused by a generalized mineralization problem such as hypophosphatasia, osteogenesis imperfecta, or infantile rickets. Within the affected region of the calvarium, the sutures and fontanelles may feel wider than usual. Accentuated vertex molding and other features noted in Chapter 35 are also common associated features. The fetus with vertex craniotabes has often been more constrained than usual in late gestation and experienced prolonged vertex presentation, and there may be mild-to-moderate limitation of full movement in some joints, especially those of the lower limbs. Benign vertex craniotabes has not been reported in infants who presented in breech position, and radiolucency of the parietal bones in the vertex of the skull is considered to be a normal anatomic variant on neonatal head computed tomography scans.[17]

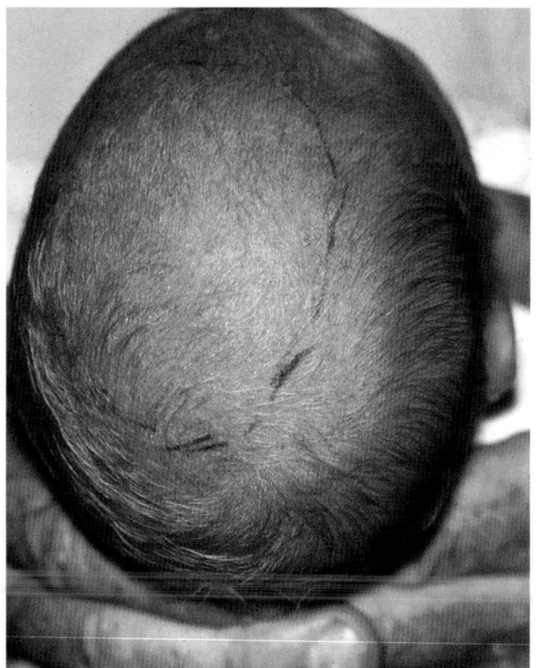

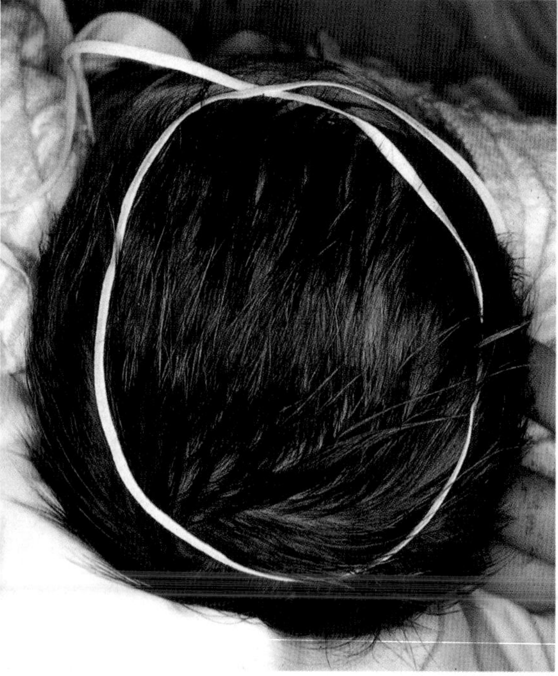

FIGURE 36.1 These newborn infants were in prolonged vertex presentation with the head engaged. Relatively forceful pressure by the examiner over the tops of the heads of the babies did not cause discomfort, this having been the normal situation for the infant in utero. Areas of soft "ping-pong" craniotabes are outlined in the vertex region.

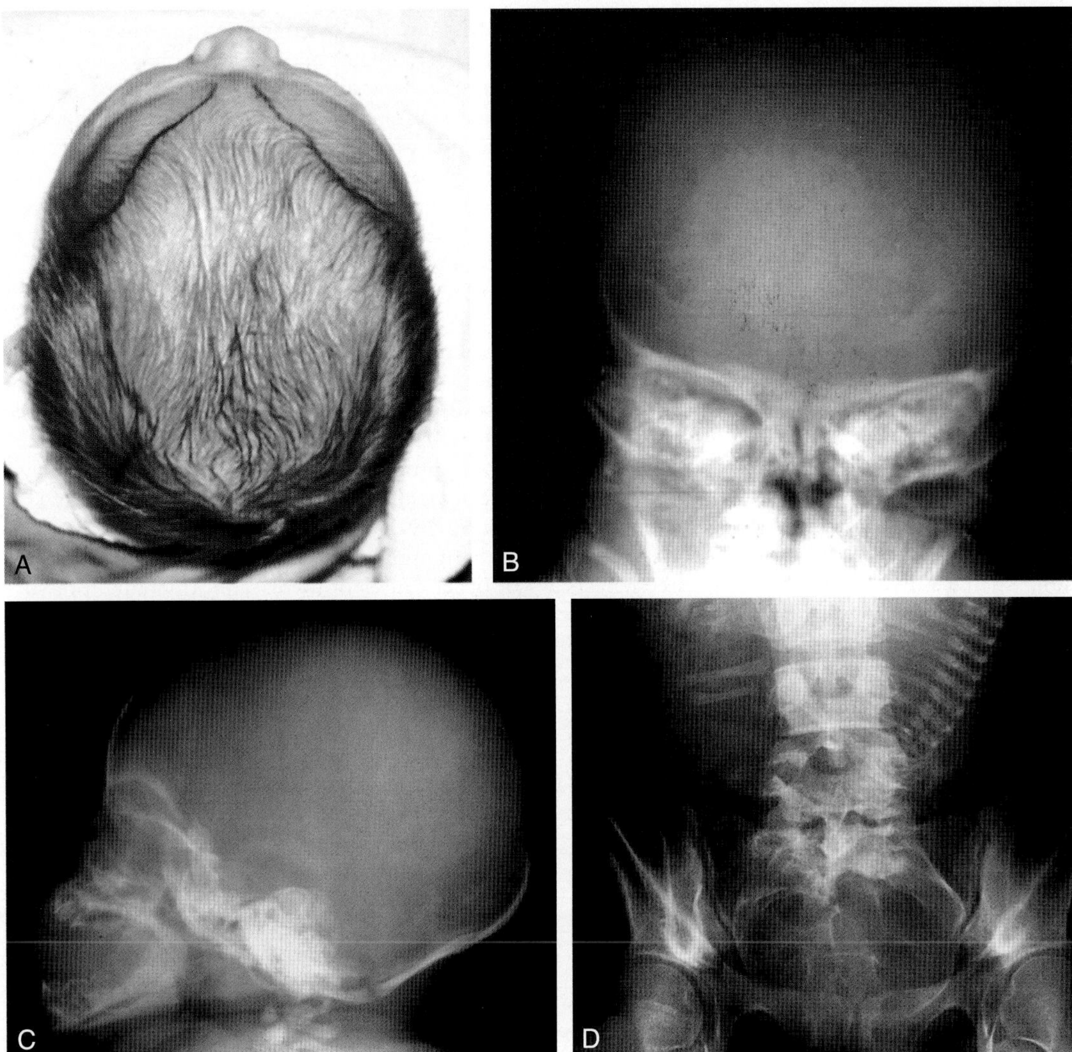

FIGURE 36.2 Vertex craniotabes (**A**), with skull radiographs (**B** and **C**) demonstrating diminished mineralization over the vertex. The infant's primigravida mother noted early lightening and felt the baby's head rubbing against the rim of her pelvis as she walked 3 miles to and from her college classes. **D,** A pelvic radiograph of the mother taken 2 weeks before delivery, when her obstetrician documented fetal head engagement, demonstrates the position of the fetal head in the pelvis. Such early lightening in a primiparous mother is unusual.

MANAGEMENT, PROGNOSIS, AND COUNSEL

The prognosis for postnatal recovery is excellent, and the parents should be reassured that there is no risk in handling the "soft head," and that generally no special precautions or studies are merited.[18] They should also be counseled that the infant's calvarium will likely mineralize in a normal fashion within 1–2 months. In fact, Medline Plus of the US National Library of Medicine and the National Institute of Health recommends no tests or treatment for craniotabes in normal neonates (http://www.nlm.nih.gov/medlineplus/ency/article/001591.htm).

If the mother has vitamin D–deficient rickets and the infant has generalized craniotabes and osteomalacia, this condition generally responds promptly to vitamin D therapy over the next few months. Some authors have suggested treating breast-fed infants with craniotabes with vitamin D or, preferably, treating all pregnant women with vitamin D.[18,19] Although there is modest evidence to support a relationship between maternal 25(OH)D status and offspring birth weight, bone mass and serum calcium concentrations, these findings are limited by their observational nature (birth weight, bone mass) or risk of bias.[20] As with other defects of skeletal mineralization, such as osteogenesis imperfecta and hypophosphatasia, care must be taken initially to avoid fractures.

DIFFERENTIAL DIAGNOSIS

Initial concern may be generated regarding the possibility of a generalized problem of bone mineralization, such as hypophosphatasia, osteogenesis imperfecta, congenital syphilis, or rickets. The clinical examination of the entire calvarium should help resolve such concerns. The sides of the calvarium should be of normal firmness with benign vertex craniotabes, and no other skeletal developmental problems should be present. Craniotabes may be one of the earliest signs of vitamin D-deficient rickets; however, it usually takes several months to deplete vitamin D stores and manifest this deficiency (unless the mother is severely deficient in vitamin D and has signs of rickets herself). One study from Japan found a seasonal pattern of presentation that correlated with serum parathyroid hormone and alkaline phosphatase. Of 1120 consecutive infants born in Japan, craniotabes was present in 246 (22.0%) neonates, and the incidence had obvious seasonal variations, highest in April-May and lowest in November, and breast-fed infants had a significantly higher serum parathyroid hormone and alkaline phosphatase compared with formula-fed infants.[18]

Vitamin D-deficiency rickets is generally accompanied by metaphyseal changes at the wrist and low 25-hydroxyvitamin D concentrations (<12 ng/mL), with a variably elevated alkaline phosphatase level. The isolated compression-related type of vertex craniotabes is usually not an indication for radiographs or measurement of serum vitamin D, calcium phosphorus, or alkaline phosphatase. If there is concern about a systemic problem, then close clinical follow-up should resolve this situation without excessive laboratory or radiographic studies, because the "soft head" due to compression quickly normalizes postnatally.

Infants with osteogenesis imperfecta show generalized osteomalacia, often with blue sclera and brittle bones that fracture during delivery. The calvarium may demonstrate interspersed islands of palpable bones (Wormian bones, see Chapter 41). Extensive calvarial defects consisting of absence or severe hypoplasia of the parietal bones can occur in cleidocranial dysplasia with C-terminal mutations in RUNX2 that preserve the runt domain.[21] Classically, cleidocranial dysplasia consists of large fontanelles, wide sutures, clavicular hypoplasia, supernumerary teeth, and short stature. Parietal foramina occur laterally to the midline and have well-demarcated edges, and these inherited skull ossification defects can be caused by mutations in either *MSX2* or *ALX4*.[22] Because they are inherited in an autosomal dominant fashion, there may be an affected parent and a positive family history. The "soft head" may also convey the impression of open sutures and fontanelles, and the question of hydrocephalus or other causes of increased intracranial pressure may be raised. Such concerns may be fostered by increased transillumination in the vertex region when a strong light is held against the soft portion of the calvarium. The infant's head circumference, head shape, and general clinical status, in addition to palpation of the firm portion of the calvarium around the sides of the skull, should resolve these concerns without the need to resort to any other studies.

References

1. Evans C, Michie C. British Society for the History of Paediatrics and Child Health G03(P) Craniotabes: time for an old physical sign to be put to use? *Arch Dis Child.* 2013;98(Suppl 1):A7.
2. Fox GN, Maier MK. Neonatal craniotabes. *Am Fam Physician.* 1984;30(6):149–151.
3. Wada Y, Kubo K, Tsubata S. Craniotabes in a newborn. *Cmaj.* 2020;192(40):E1163.
4. Graham JM Jr, Smith DW. Parietal craniotabes in the neonate: its origin and significance. *J Pediatr.* 1979;95(1):114–116.
5. Aase JM. Structural defects as consequence of late intrauterine constraint: craniotabes, loose skin, and asymmetric ear size. *Semin Perinatol.* 1983;7(4):270–273.
6. Pettifor JM, Isdale JM, Sahakian J, Hansen JD. Diagnosis of subclinical rickets. *Arch Dis Child.* 1980;55(2):155–157.
7. Pettifor JM, Pentopoulos M, Moodley GP, Isdale JM, Ross FP. Is craniotabes a pathognomonic sign of rickets in 3-month-old infants? *S Afr Med J.* 1984;65(14):549–551.
8. Kokkonen J, Koivisto M, Lautala P, Kirkinen P. Serum calcium and 25-OH-D3 in mothers of newborns with craniotabes. *J Perinat Med.* 1983;11(2):127–131.
9. Congdon P, Horsman A, Kirby PA, Dibble J, Bashir T. Mineral content of the forearms of babies born to

Asian and white mothers. *Br Med J (Clin Res Ed).* 1983;286(6373):1233–1235.
10. Park W, Paust H, Kaufmann HJ, Offermann G. Osteomalacia of the mother: rickets of the newborn. *Eur J Pediatr.* 1987;146(3):292–293.
11. Reif S, Katzir Y, Eisenberg Z, Weisman Y. Serum 25-hydroxyvitamin D levels in congenital craniotabes. *Acta Paediatr Scand.* 1988;77(1):167–168.
12. Arai N, Matsunami N, Yamamoto N, Li J. A case of a full-term newborn with severe craniotabes due to insufficient maternal sunlight exposure during the COVID-19 pandemic. *Pediatr Neonatol.* 2023 https://doi.org/10.1016/j.pedneo.2023.04.002. (Epub ahead of print).
13. Alzahrani AA. Perception of rickets disease among parents in Al-Baha Province, Saudi Arabia. *Int J Gen Med.* 2022;15:5043–5049.
14. Innes AM, Seshia MM, Prasad C, et al. Congenital rickets caused by maternal vitamin D deficiency. *Paediatr Child Health.* 2002;7(7):455–458.
15. Thacher TD, Fischer PR, Tebben PJ, et al. Increasing incidence of nutritional rickets: a population-based study in Olmsted County, Minnesota. *Mayo Clin Proc.* 2013;88(2):176–183.
16. Nagara S, Usui S, Kawashiri M, Kondo M, Yamagishi A. A case of Noonan syndrome with skull defect due to vitamin D deficiency rickets. *Clin Pediatr Endocrinol.* 2021;30(1):71–73.
17. Pastakia B, Herdt JR. Radiolucent "zones" in parietal bones seen on computed tomography: a normal anatomic variant. *J Comput Assist Tomogr.* 1984;8(1):108–109.
18. Yorifuji J, Yorifuji T, Tachibana K, et al. Craniotabes in normal newborns: the earliest sign of subclinical vitamin D deficiency. *J Clin Endocrinol Metab.* 2008;93(5):1784–1788.
19. Heo JS, Ahn YM, Kim AE, Shin SM. Breastfeeding and vitamin D. *Clin Exp Pediatr.* 2022;65(9):418–429.
20. Harvey NC, Holroyd C, Ntani G, et al. Vitamin D supplementation in pregnancy: a systematic review. *Health Technol Assess.* 2014;18(45):1–190.
21. Cunningham ML, Seto ML, Hing AV, Bull MJ, Hopkin RJ, Leppig KA. Cleidocranial dysplasia with severe parietal bone dysplasia: C-terminal RUNX2 mutations. *Birth Defects Res A Clin Mol Teratol.* 2006;76(2):78–85.
22. Mavrogiannis LA, Taylor IB, Davies SJ, Ramos FJ, Olivares JL, Wilkie AO. Enlarged parietal foramina caused by mutations in the homeobox genes ALX4 and MSX2: from genotype to phenotype. *Eur J Hum Genet.* 2006;14(2):151–158.

CHAPTER 37

Anterior Fontanel Bone

KEY POINTS

- The anterior fontanel on rare occasions ossifies and forms a bony plate.
- An anterior frontal bone can be seen in normal infants as a variant or in association with craniosynostosis.
- The anterior fontanelle is an integral part of the pediatric exam, and any abnormalities such as delayed closure can be associated with various pathologic conditions.
- Diagnosis is important to differentiate it from craniosynostosis or skull fractures.
- Radiographic examination can help confirm the presence of an anterior fontanel bone.

GENESIS

On very rare occasions, the anterior fontanel will ossify into a bony plate that may be slightly elevated in relation to the rest of the cranium. It is believed that they arise from the formation of abnormal cranial ossification centers.[1] This may occur due to decreased growth-stretch tensile forces across the anterior fontanel, and can be present at birth or appear later in infancy.[2] It is sometimes seen with multiple suture synostosis and can also occur in otherwise normal infants (similar to Wormian bones, see Chapter 41), in which case it is considered a normal variant.[3] It is thought to be associated with other anatomical anomalies such as osteogenesis imperfecta, rickets, and other bone dysplasias, with only one report in the literature where there was a recurrence in siblings.[4] The anterior fontanel normally closes between 4 and 26 months, with 90% closing between 7 and 19 months and 42% closing before 12 months.[5-7] The area of the anterior fontanel can be calculated and compared to published standards of infant groups based on gestational age at birth or chronological age.[8-10] Delayed closure of the fontanel has been associated with a variety of pathologic conditions such as osteogenesis imperfecta, hypophosphatasia, cleidocranial dysplasia, and various other skeletal dysplasias. An ossified anterior fontanel does not carry the same significance.[11] In one cohort of 11 patients with anterior fontanel bones referred to a craniofacial center, 5 had craniosynostosis (1 sagittal, 3 metopic, 1 bicoronal), 1 had acrocallosal syndrome, and 5 were isolated. All patients in the surgical cohort had good postoperative results, and the others were followed and had normal development.[12] This can also be referred to as a bregmatic Wormian bone and has been reported with metopic synostosis.[13-15] According to Oostra et al., supernumerary bones that result from normal, nonfused ossification centers are likely to be different from bones deriving from additional centers within the sutures and fontanels.[16]

FEATURES

Instead of the usual flat, uncalcified, diamond-shaped anterior fontanel, there is a slightly raised, diamond-shaped plate of bone in its place (Figs. 37.1 and 37.2).

MANAGEMENT AND PROGNOSIS

If the child is otherwise normal with no signs of craniosynostosis or osteogenesis imperfecta, then parents can be reassured that this is a normal variant (see Fig. 37.1A).[11] Occasionally the anterior fontanel bone is associated with early closure of the sagittal suture (see Fig. 37.1B). The shape of the anterior fontanel bone often remains visible on skull radiographs throughout childhood and into adulthood, with a characteristic appearance on Towne skull radiographic projection.[2]

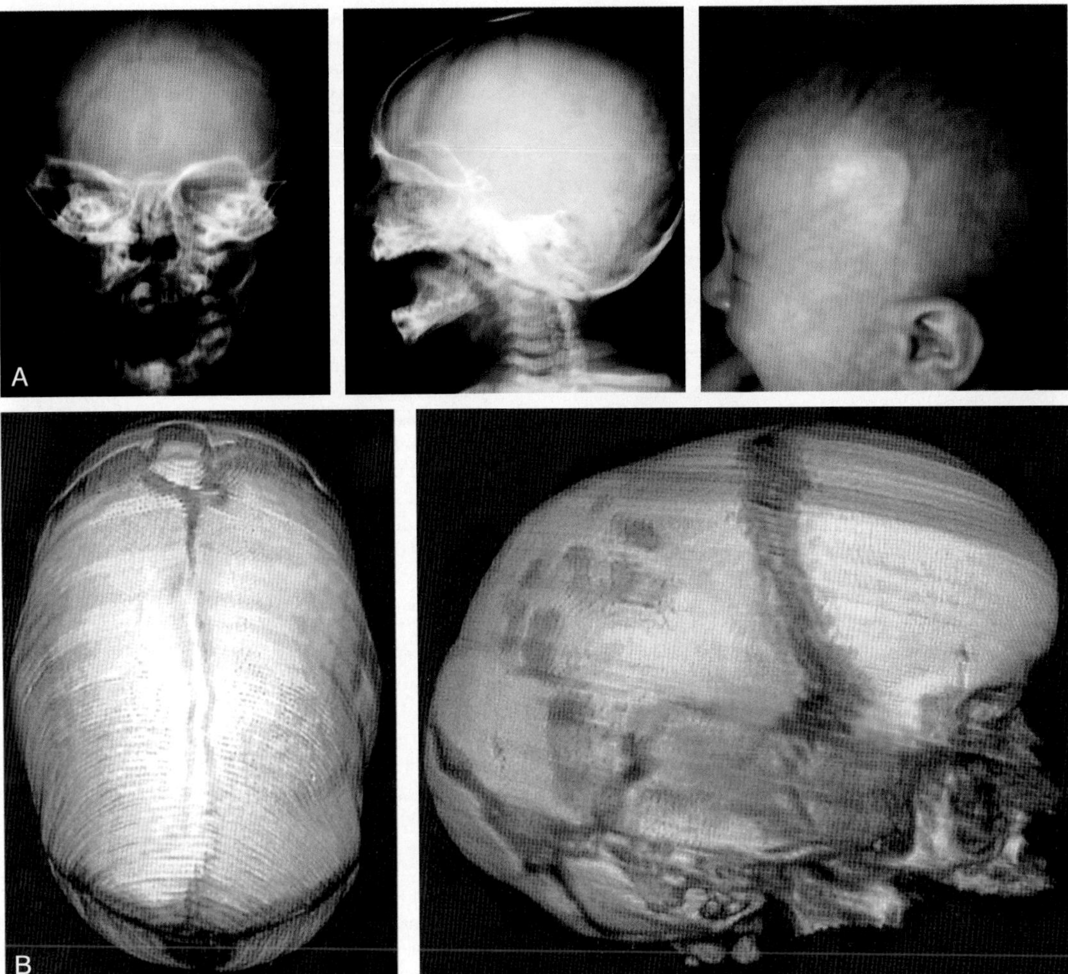

FIGURE 37.1 **A,** This otherwise normal infant demonstrated ossification of the anterior fontanel bone. **B,** In this infant with the sagittal suture closely approximated on 3D cranial computed tomography, there is an anterior fontanel bone with other sutures widely patent and an open posterior fontanel.

DIFFERENTIAL DIAGNOSIS

The correct diagnosis of anterior fontanel bone is especially important in those babies suspected to have craniosynostosis because of a "closed fontanel." After X-ray examination of the skull following head trauma, the roentgenographic appearance may lead the unaware observer into a misdiagnosis of skull fracture.[2] If multiple suture synostosis is present (Fig. 37.2), it should be evident from examination of the head shape and demonstrable on radiographs and three-dimensional computed tomography scans. A careful search for associated anomalies should be undertaken to assist in identification of any underlying syndrome. Infants with osteogenesis imperfecta show generalized osteomalacia with blue sclerae and brittle bones that may fracture during delivery. The calvarium may also demonstrate interspersed islands of palpable bones (Wormian bones). The appearance of the fusing anterior fontanel bone can be confused with a depressed skull fracture in the lateral radiographic projection.[17]

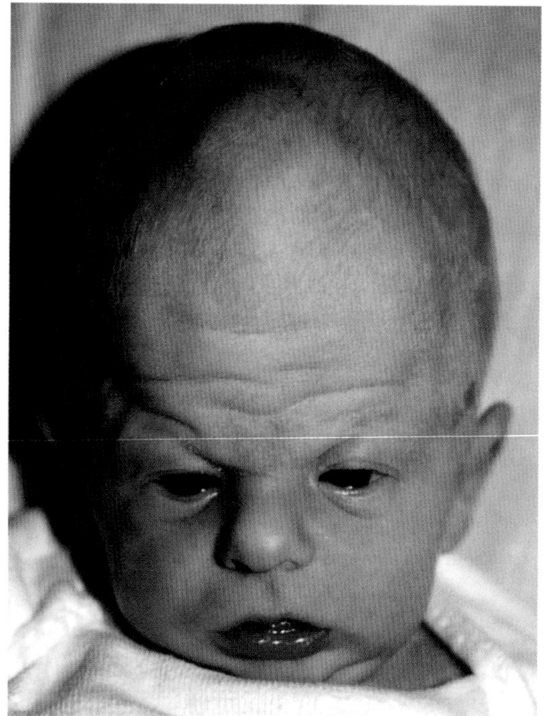

FIGURE 37.2 This child with craniotelencephalic dysplasia was born with multiple sutural synostosis and an obvious anterior fontanel bone.

References

1. Johal J, Iwanaga J, Loukas M, Tubbs RS. Anterior fontanelle Wormian bone / fontanellar bone: a review of this rare anomaly with case illustration. *Cureus*. 2017;9(7):e1443.
2. Berant M, Shrem M, Wagner Y. Anterior fontanel bone: a reminder to pediatricians and radiologists. *Clin Pediatr (Phila)*. 1977;16(9):795–796.
3. Keats TE. *Atlas of Normal Roentgen Variants That May Simulate Disease*. St Louis: Mosby; 1992:13–15.
4. Boroian TV, Attwood CR, Jaconette JR. Anterior fontanel bone in siblings. *Am J Dis Child*. 1964;108:625–626.
5. Kiesler J, Ricer R. The abnormal fontanel. *Am Fam Physician*. 2003;67(12):2547–2552.
6. Aisenson MR. Closing of the anterior fontanelle. *Pediatrics*. 1950;6(2):223–226.
7. Popich GA, Smith DW. Fontanels: range of normal size. *J Pediatr*. 1972;80(5):749–752.
8. Duc G, Largo RH. Anterior fontanel: size and closure in term and preterm infants. *Pediatrics*. 1986;78(5): 904–908.
9. Jackson GL, Hoyer A, Longenecker L, Engle WD. Anterior fontanel size in term and late preterm hispanic neonates: description of normative values and an alternative measurement method. *Am J Perinatol*. 2010;27(4):307–312.
10. Davies DP, Ansari BM, Cooke TJH. Anterior fontanelle size in neonate. *Arch Dis Child*. 1975;50(1):81–83.
11. Berant M, Shrem M, Wagner Y. Anterior fontanel bone: reminder to pediatricians and radiologists. *Clin Pediatr*. 1977;16(9):795–796.
12. Woods RH, Johnson D. Absence of the anterior fontanelle due to a fontanellar bone. *J Craniofac Surg*. 2010;21(2):448–449.
13. Stotland MA, Do NK, Knapik TJ. Bregmatic Wormian bone and metopic synostosis. *J Craniofac Surg*. 2012;23(7 Suppl 1):2015–2018.
14. Barberini F, Bruner E, Cartolari R, et al. An unusually-wide human bregmatic Wormian bone: anatomy, tomographic description, and possible significance. *Surg Radiol Anat*. 2008;30(8):683–687.
15. Pickett AT, Montes MA. Wormian bone in the anterior fontanelle of an otherwise well neonate. *Cureus*. 2019;11(5):e4741.
16. Oostra R-J, van der Wolk S, Maas M, Hennekam RCM. Malformations of the axial skeleton in the museum Vrolik: II: craniosynostoses and suture-related conditions. *American Journal of Medical Genetics Part a*. 2005;136A(4):327–342.
17. Girdany BR, Blank E. Anterior fontanel bones. *Am J Roentgenol Radium Ther Nucl Med*. 1965;95:148–153.

CHAPTER 38

Parietal Foramina

KEY POINTS

- Parietal foramina are symmetric oval calvarial defects located near the parietal eminences, separated by a narrow bridge of bone.
- Diagnosis is aided by palpation, radiography, antenatal sonography, and magnetic resonance imaging.
- Parietal foramina can occur in isolation or as part of multiple congenital anomaly syndromes with autosomal dominant inheritance with variable expression and intrafamilial variability observed.
- Parietal foramina can manifest as cranium bifidum in early life and develop into parietal foramina later.
- Care must be taken during delivery to avoid trauma to the brain, and complications such as scalp defects, seizures, headaches, and structural brain abnormalities can occur in some cases.
- Surgery is generally unnecessary as the defects tend to ossify on their own.

GENESIS

Parietal foramina are rare calvarial defects estimated to occur in fewer than 1 in 25,000 births.[1] They present as symmetric oval defects situated on either side of the sagittal suture near the parietal eminences and are separated from each other by a narrow bridge of bone (Fig. 38.1). They represent defects of calvarial ossification, with their size decreasing with advancing age. They manifest via autosomal dominant inheritance with variable expression with considerable intrafamilial variability.[2,3] Goldsmith initially called this condition "Catlin marks" after observing the condition in 16 members of a five-generation family with the surname Catlin.[4] This condition can present as cranium bifidum in early life and develop into parietal foramina by later childhood. Cranium bifidum means literally "cleft skull" and it presents as a wide opening between the frontal and parietal bones. In normal fetuses, the frontal, parietal, and squamous parts of the temporal bones undergo intramembranous ossification, which is a direct ossification of the vascularized membrane. These parts are usually ossified in the fifth month of gestation.[5] When there is insufficient ossification around the parietal notch, they end up as large parietal foramina. Wilkie et al.[6] described heterozygous *MSX2* mutations in three unrelated families with enlarged parietal foramina, which suggests that loss of *MSX2* activity results in calvarial defects. A second gene has been implicated in those families who do not link to 5q34-q35 (the location of *MSX2*), and mutations or deletions of *ALX4* or *TWIST1* can also result in parietal foramina.[7–11] Absence or severe hypoplasia of the parietal bones can occur in cleidocranial dysplasia with mutations in *RUNX2*.[12] Cleidocranial dysplasia consists of large fontanels, wide sutures, clavicular hypoplasia, supernumerary teeth, and short stature. Parietal foramina occur laterally to the midline and have well-demarcated edges. Because of the availability of high-resolution antenatal sonography and magnetic resonance imaging, as well as neonatal magnetic resonance imaging, early detection of cranial and intracranial anomalies and the developmental features of this condition can be recognized.[13,14]

FEATURES

Usually, parietal foramina present as symmetric oval bony defects situated on each side of the sagittal suture and separated from each other by a narrow bridge of bone, and their size diminishes with age (Fig. 38.2). They are covered with scalp tissue and hair, and are detected through palpation and radiography. Occasionally, brain covered by dura and intact scalp can bulge through extensive lesions, suggesting the possibility of an encephalocele, but the location of these lesions off the midline differentiates them from

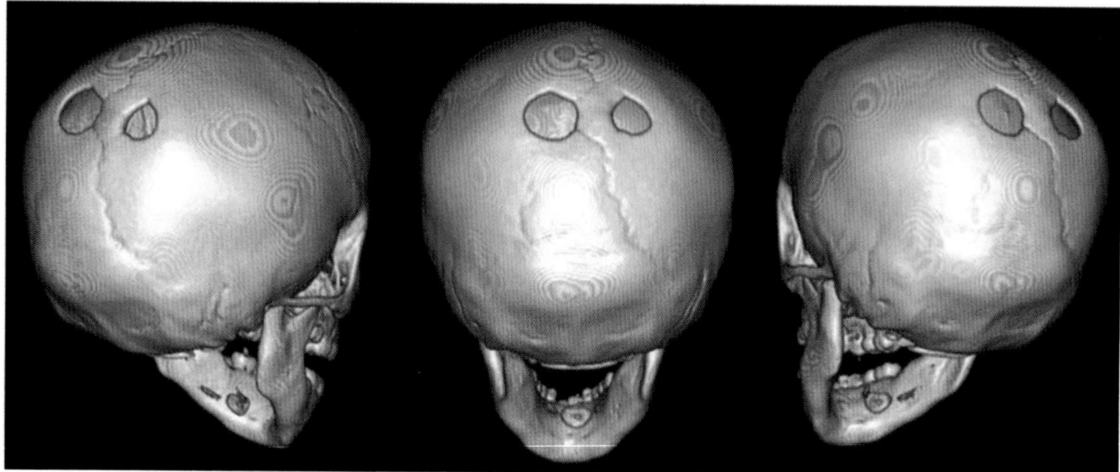

FIGURE 38.1 Three-dimensional computed tomography reconstruction images of a 6-year-old child with bilateral parietal calvarial defects.

neural tube closure defects. Sometimes the entire sagittal suture remains widely patent from the frontal to the parietal bones (cranium bifidum), with the defect subsequently ossifying inward to resemble parietal foramina during mid-childhood or adulthood.[5] Parietal foramina may occur as an isolated trait due to mutations in or haploinsufficiency of either *MSX2* or *ALX4*,[6,8,15] or it may be a component of a multiple congenital anomaly syndrome such as frontonasal dysplasia type 2, Saethre-Chotzen syndrome, cleidocranial dysplasia, or Rubinstein-Taybi syndrome.[16] The combination of parietal foramina with multiple exostoses is now known to be a contiguous gene deletion of *ALX4* and *EXT2* on chromosome 11p11-p12 (also termed Potocki-Shaffer syndrome).[17,18]

MANAGEMENT, PROGNOSIS, AND COUNSEL

Surgery is usually unnecessary because the lesions tend to ossify inward on their own, but occasionally a protective helmet is used for extensive defects. Although most remain asymptomatic, they may be associated with other pathologies and occasionally become symptomatic.[19] There are few reports on the surgical management of persistent enlarged biparietal foramina.[20] Care must be exercised during delivery to avoid trauma to the brain, which underlies such extensive parietal foraminal defects. Although generally believed to be a benign variant, scalp defects, seizures, headaches, and structural brain abnormalities have been reported in a small percentage of affected patients.[21] Skull fractures between the foramina have been reported in the literature and thus may increase the risk of skull fracture after trauma.[22]

DIFFERENTIAL DIAGNOSIS

Location and intact scalp tissue help differentiate parietal foramina from an encephalocele. In addition, this lesion must be differentiated from scalp vertex aplasia (see Chapter 39), which is also inherited in an autosomal dominant fashion when it occurs as an isolated trait. There is usually denuded scalp over such lesions, which can include both scalp and calvarium, but their location in the midline near the hair whorl sets these lesions apart from parietal foramina. Scalp vertex cutis aplasia usually heals with some degree of scarring, which results in the absence of scalp hair; therefore the scalps of both parents should be examined for these bald spots. Occasionally, areas of scalp vertex aplasia can be part of a syndrome such as trisomy 13, or they can result from vascular disruption in utero. When scalp vertex aplasia occurs with absence of digits, the possibility of Adams-Oliver syndrome needs to be considered. Finally, vertex craniotabes may present as an extensive area of incomplete calvarial ossification over the vertex in the midline, but the edges are not sharp and demarcated as in parietal foramina, and vertex craniotabes resolves quite rapidly within the first few months after birth.

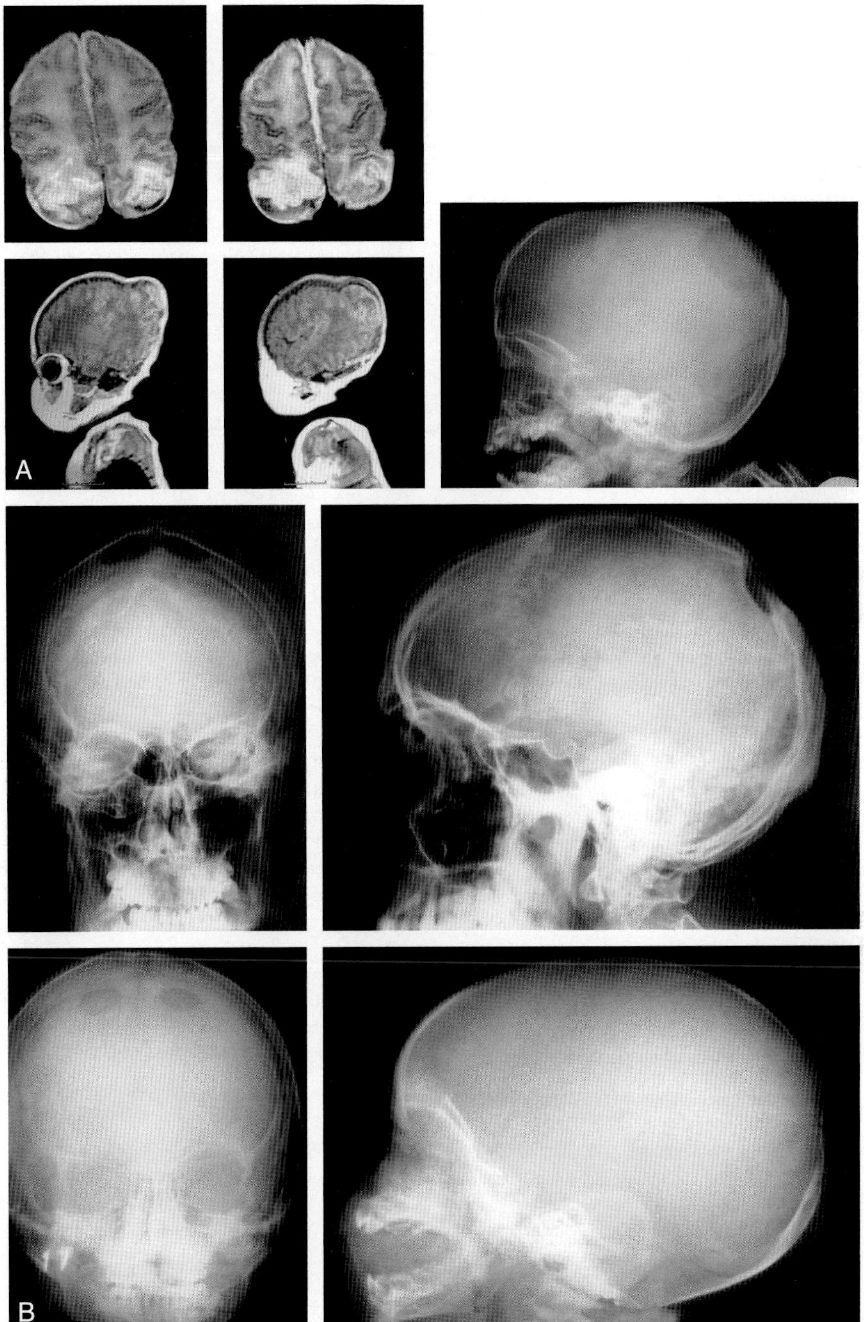

FIGURE 38.2 Familial parietal foramina. **A,** Large parietal defects at birth detected by magnetic resonance imaging *(top and center)*, with partial closure demonstrated by 16 months of age on skull radiographs *(bottom)*. **B,** Parietal foramina in other members of this four-generation family with isolated parietal foramina. (Courtesy of Mark Stefan, Madigan Army Hospital, Tacoma, WA.)

References

1. Dharwal K. Foramina parietalia permagna: the ins and outs. *Folia Morphol.* 2012;71(2):78–81.
2. Griessenauer CJ, Veith P, Mortazavi MM, et al. Enlarged parietal foramina: a review of genetics, prognosis, radiology, and treatment. *Childs Nerv Syst.* 2013;29(4):543–547.
3. Preis S, Engelbrecht V, Lenard HG. Aplasia-cutis-congenita and enlarged parietal foramina (Catlin marks) in a family. *Acta Paediatr.* 1995;84(6):701–702.
4. Goldsmith WM. The 'Catlin mark': the inheritance of an unusual opening in the parietal bones. *J Hered.* 1922;13:69–71.
5. Little BB, Knoll KA, Klein VR, Heller KB. Hereditary cranium bifidum and symmetric parietal foramina are the same entity. *Am J Med Genet.* 1990;35(4):453–458.
6. Wilkie AO, Tang Z, Elanko N, et al. Functional haploinsufficiency of the human homeobox gene *MSX2* causes defects in skull ossification. *Nat Genet.* 2000;24(4):387–390.
7. Bertola DR, Rodrigues MG, Quaio CR, Kim CA, Passos-Bueno MR. Vertical transmission of a frontonasal phenotype caused by a novel *ALX4* mutation. *Am J Med Genet A.* 2013;161A(3):600–604.
8. Wu YQ, Badano JL, McCaskill C, Vogel H, Potocki L, Shaffer LG. Haploinsufficiency of *ALX4* as a potential cause of parietal foramina in the 11p11.2 contiguous gene-deletion syndrome. *Am J Hum Genet.* 2000;67(5):1327–1332.
9. Mavrogiannis LA, Taylor IB, Davies SJ, Ramos FJ, Olivares JL, Wilkie AO. Enlarged parietal foramina caused by mutations in the homeobox genes *ALX4* and *MSX2*: from genotype to phenotype. *Eur J Hum Genet.* 2006;14(2):151–158.
10. Bote Gascón M, Martínez Del Río C, García Ron A. Foramina parietalia permagna: clinical radiological evaluation of a Spanish family with an undescribed mutation in the *ALX4* gene. *An Pediatr (Engl Ed).* 2021;95(2):121–122.
11. Walters ME, Lacassie Y, Azamian M, et al. Vertical transmission of a large calvarial ossification defect due to heterozygous variants of *ALX4* and *TWIST1*. *Am J Med Genet A.* 2021;185(3):916–922.
12. Cunningham ML, Seto ML, Hing AV, Bull MJ, Hopkin RJ, Leppig KA. Cleidocranial dysplasia with severe parietal bone dysplasia: C-terminal *RUNX2* mutations. *Birth Defects Res A Clin Mol Teratol.* 2006;76(2):78–85.
13. Fink AM, Maixner W. Enlarged parietal foramina: MR imaging features in the fetus and neonate. *Am J Neuroradiol.* 2006;27(6):1379–1381.
14. Nemec SF, Nemec U, Brugger PC, et al. MR imaging of the fetal musculoskeletal system. *Prenat Diagn.* 2012;32(3):205–213.
15. Mavrogiannis LA, Antonopoulou I, Baxova A, et al. Haploinsufficiency of the human homeobox gene *ALX4* causes skull ossification defects. *Nat Genet.* 2001;27(1):17–18.
16. Altunoglu U, Satkin B, Uyguner ZO, Kayserili H. Mild nasal clefting may be predictive for *ALX4* heterozygotes. *Am J Med Genet A.* 2014;164A(8):2054–2058.
17. Ferrarini A, Gaillard M, Guerry F, et al. Potocki-Shaffer deletion encompassing *ALX4* in a patient with frontonasal dysplasia phenotype. *Am J Med Genet A.* 2014;164A(2):346–352.
18. Trajkova S, Di Gregorio E, Ferrero GB, et al. New insights into Potocki-Shaffer syndrome: report of two novel cases and literature review. *Brain Sci.* 2020;10(11):788. https://doi.org/10.3390/brainsci10110788.
19. Griessenauer CJ, Veith P, Mortazavi MM, et al. Enlarged parietal foramina: a review of genetics, prognosis, radiology, and treatment. *Childs Nerv Syst.* 2013;29(4):543–547.
20. Wallace RD, Uygur S, Konofaos P, Klimo P Jr. Repair of congenital enlarged parietal foramina with porous polyethylene implants. *J Craniofac Surg.* 2023; https://doi.org/10.1097/SCS.0000000000009311. (Epub ahead of print).
21. Pang D, Lin A. Symptomatic large parietal foramina. *Neurosurgery.* 1982;11(1):33–37.
22. Edwards LS, Sachs JR, Elster AD. Skull fractures through parietal foramina: report of two cases. *J Comput Assist Tomogr.* 2012;36(3):308–309.

CHAPTER 39

Aplasia Cutis Congenita

Scalp Vertex Cutis Aplasia, Temporal Triangular Alopecia

KEY POINTS

- Aplasia cutis congenita (ACC) is a congenital absence of skin, most commonly affecting the scalp and characterized by raw areas that mature into atrophic scars devoid of hair.
- ACC can occur in isolation or associated with other abnormalities and malformations, such as spinal dysraphism, encephaloceles, epidermal nevus, or nevus sebaceous syndrome.
- The cause of ACC is heterogeneous and can include vascular disruption, infection, trauma, teratogens, and a range of genetic factors.
- Treatment of ACC depends on the size and depth of the lesion and may involve wound care, excision, and reconstruction.
- Early closure of extensive scalp defects is important to prevent complications such as hemorrhage or meningitis.

GENESIS

Aplasia cutis congenita (ACC) is a congenital, localized absence of skin that most commonly affects the scalp. The frequency is 1 per 3000 live births and can occur in isolation or as part of a heterogeneous group of syndromes. Frieden's classification system divides ACC into nine subtypes (Table 39.1 and Figs. 39.1–39.8).[1] ACC begins as multiple or solitary, sharply marginated raw areas with absence of skin (resembling ulceration); these areas mature into atrophic scars devoid of hair, usually in the scalp vertex area or midline superior occipital region.[2] Although most defects are small and superficial, approximately 20% involve absence of the skull, exposing the brain and sagittal sinus and increasing the risk for hemorrhage or infection.[3,4] When associated dura is absent, there is usually no bony regeneration.[4] The cause of these ACC lesions is heterogeneous and includes incomplete closure of the neural tube, vascular disruption of watershed areas of necrosis (from placental insufficiency), intrauterine infection, amniotic adhesions, trauma, teratogens, and genetic factors.[5-7] Because vascular disruption and placental infarcts are seen in antiphospholipid antibody syndrome, some cases of extensive ACC may be related to this maternal disease state or other genetic causes of thrombophilia during pregnancy.[8,9]

FEATURES

Lesions may be ulcerated, bullous, cicatricial, or covered with a tough, translucent membrane, and occasionally they extend to the bone or dura.[2] They may be circular, elongated, stellate, or triangular in shape and of variable depth.[10] Approximately 86% of the solitary lesions occur on the scalp, with most near the parietal hair whorl.[11,12] ACC type 1 manifests scalp involvement without other abnormalities (see Figs. 39.1 and 39.6), and when familial, it manifests autosomal dominant inheritance.[13,14] Less frequently, other parts of the body may be involved, with or without associated defects. When the lesions are midline and overlie the spine or midcranium, they can be associated with occult spinal dysraphism or tiny encephaloceles (ACC type 4). When there are multiple areas of ACC involving primarily the lower extremities, particularly the flank, thighs, and knees, a careful examination of the placenta may reveal a fetus papyraceus, which occurs in 1 in 12,000 live births and affects 1 in 200 twin pregnancies (see Fig. 39.2).[15-19] Larger defects can present with complications such as hemorrhage, venous thrombosis, and (rarely) meningitis (see Fig. 39.3). With extensive ACC and other vascular disruptive defects, survival in the neonatal period can be severely compromised.[19,20] ACC can be associated with teratogenic

Table 39.1 FREIDEN'S CLASSIFICATION OF APLASIA CUTIS CONGENITA

Group	Definition	Inheritance
1	Isolated scalp involvement; may be associated with single defects	AD (***BMS1***)/sporadic
2	Scalp ACC with limb-reduction defects (Adams-Oliver syndrome); may be associated with encephalocele	AD (***ARHGAP31***, ***DLL4***, ***NOTCH1***, ***RBPJ***)/AR (***DOCK6***, ***EOGT***)
3	Scalp ACC with epidermal nevus	Sporadic
4	ACC overlying occult spinal dysraphism, spina bifida, or meningoencephalocele	Sporadic
5	ACC with placental infarcts	Sporadic
6	ACC with epidermolysis bullosa	AD/AR or sporadic
7	ACC localized to extremities without blistering; usually affecting pretibial areas and dorsum of hands and feet	AD or AR
8	ACC caused by teratogens (e.g., varicella, herpes, methimazole)	Sporadic
9	ACC associated with malformation syndromes (e.g., trisomy 13, deletion 4p-, deletion Xp22.1, ectodermal dysplasia, Johanson-Blizzard syndrome, Adams-Oliver syndrome, amniotic band disruption complex)	Variable

ACC, Aplasia cutis congenita; *AD*, autosomal dominant; *AR*, autosomal recessive.
From Frieden IJ. Aplasia cutis congenita: a clinical review and proposal for classification. *J Am Acad Dermatol*. 1986;14:646–660.

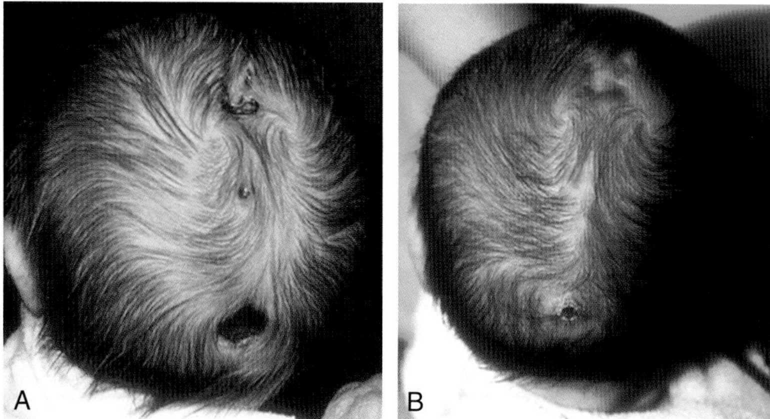

FIGURE 39.1 Scalp aplasia cutis congenita type 1 in an infant at birth (**A**) and several weeks later (**B**). There were no associated anomalies, and the father had a similar scalp lesion.

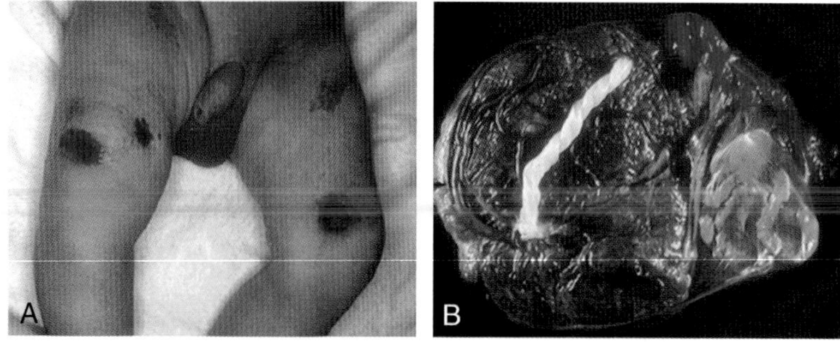

FIGURE 39.2 Aplasia cutis congenita type 5 (**A**) in association with a deceased monozygous fetus papyraceus (**B**). Note the lesions in the inguinal region and over the knees, which are typical for this type of aplasia cutis congenita and should prompt a thorough placental evaluation.

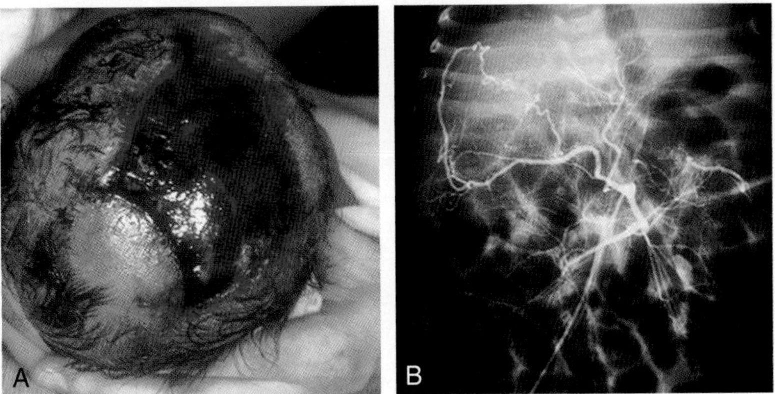

FIGURE 39.3 Extensive scalp aplasia cutis congenita type 5 (**A**) in association with single umbilical artery and congenital infarction of liver and gallbladder (as demonstrated by angiography) (**B**). This type of defect should prompt an evaluation for thrombophilia and other types of vascular disruptive defects.

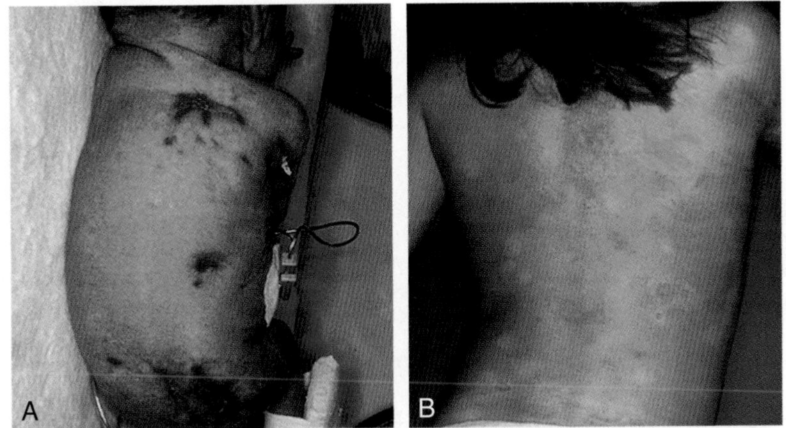

FIGURE 39.4 Aplasia cutis congenita type 8 in association with congenital herpes simplex infection. **A,** Appearance at birth. **B,** Appearance several years later, after lesions healed with scarring.

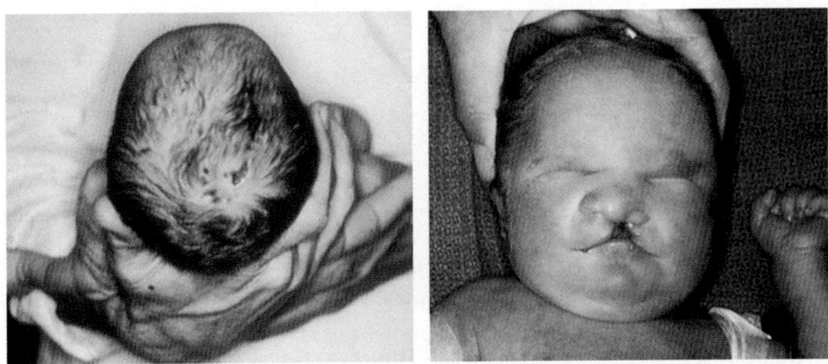

FIGURE 39.5 Aplasia cutis congenita type 9 in association with trisomy 13.

exposures (e.g., Methimazole)[21,22] or genetic disorders (see Figs. 39.4–39.7), and it is important to search for associated malformations in order to counsel parents concerning prognosis and recurrence risks in relation to the underlying disorder. ACC associated with epidermal nevus or nevus sebaceous syndrome (or ACC type 3) is the association of a sebaceous nevus (a linear, yellow verrucose nevus) on the head and neck with variable ocular, cerebral, neurologic, skeletal, cardiac, and other abnormalities, usually occurring sporadically.[23]

Epidermolysis bullosa (EB) is a term applied to a group of hereditary skin disorders that result in the formation of blisters after minor skin trauma. The three subtypes are based on the histopathologic location of the bullae: (1) dystrophic EB with subepidermal bullae below the periodic acid-Schiff (PAS)–staining basement membrane; (2) junctional EB with subepidermal bullae above the PAS-staining membrane; and (3) simplex EB with intraepidermal bullae in the suprabasal area.[24] Dystrophic and simplex EB can be either autosomal recessive or dominant, but junctional EB is always autosomal recessive. EB can be associated with pyloric atresia and/or ACC and manifest autosomal recessive inheritance, and histopathology is usually of the junctional type.[24] These findings suggest that when ACC occurs with EB, it is most likely to be autosomal recessive, and some cases of junctional EB with pyloric atresia have demonstrated mutations in integrin beta 4.[24]

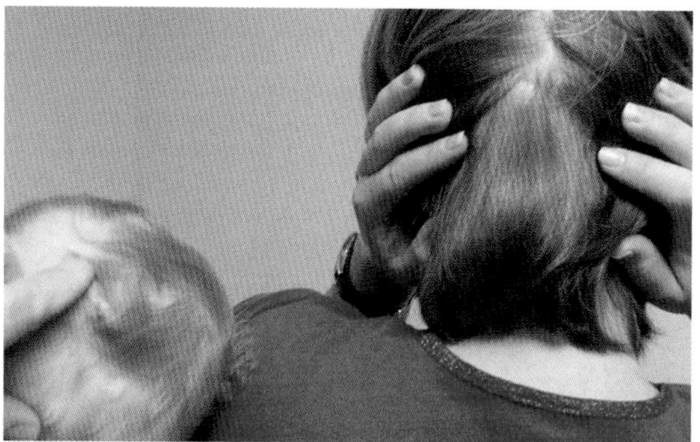

FIGURE 39.6 Aplasia cutis congenita type 1 in a mother and child after small lesions (<1 cm in diameter) healed spontaneously.

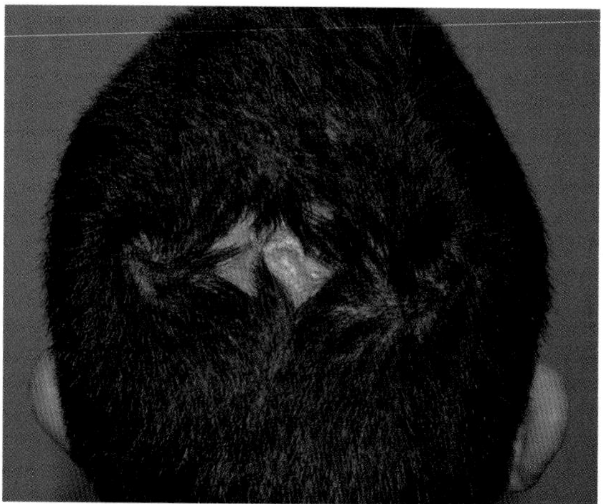

FIGURE 39.8 Healed scalp in a 16-year-old with aplasia cutis congenita type 9 who was found to have an 825 Kb deletion on chromosome 19p13.3.

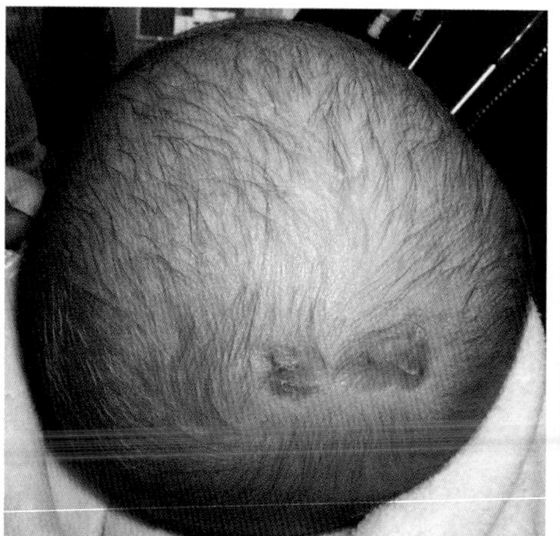

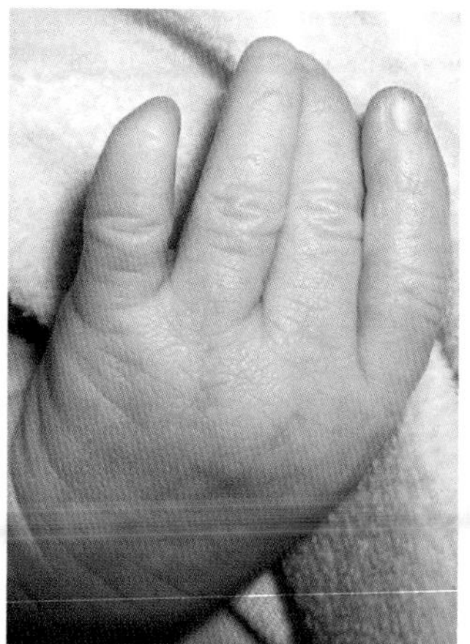

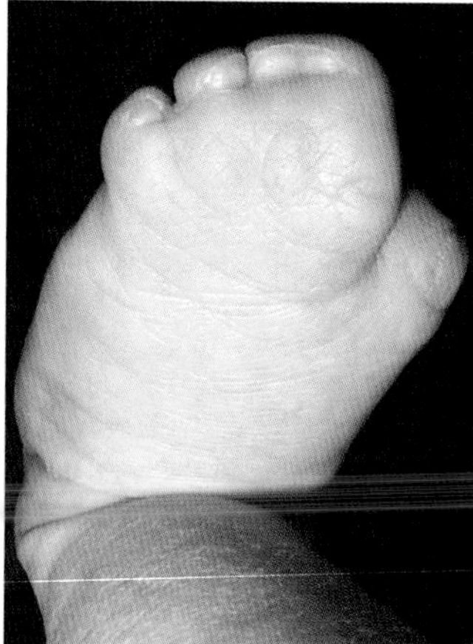

FIGURE 39.7 Adams-Oliver syndrome showing typical scalp aplasia cutis congenita associated with digital hypoplasia/syndactyly in a hand and foot. (From Verdyck P, Holder-Espinasse M, Van Hul W, et al. Clinical and molecular analysis of nine families with Adams-Oliver syndrome. *Eur J Hum Genet.* 2003;11:457–463.)

Finally, ACC has been associated with numerous cytogenetic and genetic malformation syndromes, some of which are listed in Table 39.1 under ACC type 9 (see Figs. 39.5 and 39.7).[5,9,14,25–29]

MANAGEMENT, PROGNOSIS, AND COUNSEL

Wound treatment in 1-cm lesions with superficial ulceration is conservative with application of antibacterial dressings, but more extensive or deep lesions may require reconstruction of the scalp. Small hairless areas can be excised and covered with a neighboring flap from the scalp.[30] This approach works for most common scalp ACC type 1 lesions, which are most frequently round, punched-out lesions in the vertex region or, less frequently, triangular lesions in the temporal region (termed *temporal triangular alopecia*).[30] With extensive scalp lesions (i.e., >6 cm in diameter), it is especially important to avoid eschar formation immediately after birth by covering exposed dura with split-thickness skin grafts from adjacent healthy scalp and with moist dressings.[31] Prompt closure is important because of the high risk of fatal hemorrhage from the sagittal sinus when the eschar becomes dry and separated, which causes the underlying dura to become damaged and tear.[4,20,32] Once the superficial defect is completely healed, the subsequent scar alopecia can be treated by tissue-expanded local flaps, pericranial flaps, or free vascularized flaps when the child is older.[33] Also, with prompt and early closure and healthy underlying dura, cranial bone growth will occur, and the risk of fatal hemorrhage or meningitis is greatly lessened.[4,20,32] For the treatment of extensive scalp defects, some surgeons have used engineered skin consisting of an initial graft of autologous cultured fibroblasts (that lay down type IV collagen, fibronectin, and laminin), followed by a graft of cultured keratinocytes.[34] The combination of dermal and epithelial characteristics in such grafts is thought to reduce scar formation.[35] An underlying bone defect is found in approximately 20% of patients. Most skull defects close spontaneously. However when there are no signs of ossification, closure is recommended. The split rib graft procedure has been used with good cosmetic and functional results.[36,37] Patients with Adams-Oliver syndrome (characterized by ACC and transverse terminal limb defects) may require extra care with split-thickness skin grafts because of abnormal vascularity in the scalp skin.[28,38] This syndrome is inherited in a markedly variable autosomal dominant fashion and often results in associated dural and skull defects, and is caused by mutations in *ARHGAP31*, *DLL4*, *DOCK6*, *EOGT*, *NOTCH1*, or *RBPJ*.[39–42] No mutations in *ALX4*, *MSX1*, *MSX2*, *CART1*, *P63*, *RUNX2*, and *HOXD13* reported.[12,43] When there are extensive associated dural defects (as may occur in Adams-Oliver syndrome), autologous full-thickness cranial bone grafts may be required to close the skull defects prior to skin grafting.[4,44]

DIFFERENTIAL DIAGNOSIS

Differential diagnosis is extensive and includes the initial distinction between ACC and occult spina bifida or meningoencephalocele and the determination of whether ACC is isolated or part of a broader pattern of altered morphogenesis, as delineated in Table 39.1.

References

1. Frieden IJ. Aplasia cutis congenita: a clinical review and proposal for classification. *J Am Acad Dermatol.* 1986;14(4):646–660.
2. Tan HH, Tay YK. Familial aplasia cutis congenita of the scalp: a case report and review. *Ann Acad Med Singapore.* 1997;26(4):500–502.
3. Nichols DD, Bottini AG. Aplasia cutis congenita. Case report. *J Neurosurg.* 1996;85(1):170–173.
4. Ploplys EA, Muzaffar AR, Gruss JS, Ellenbogen RG. Early composite cranioplasty in infants with severe aplasia cutis congenita: a report of two cases. *Cleft Palate Craniofac J.* 2005;42(4):442–447.
5. Evers ME, Steijlen PM, Hamel BC. Aplasia cutis congenita and associated disorders: an update. *Clin Genet.* 1995;47(6):295–301.
6. Higgins C, Price A, Craig S. Aplasia cutis congenita. *BMJ Case Rep.* 2022;15(9).
7. Jiang Y, Yu X, Deng MG, et al. Maternal SARS-CoV-2 infection and aplasia cutis congenita in a newborn. *J Eur Acad Dermatol Venereol.* 2022;36(11):e868–e870.
8. Roll C, Hanssler L, Voit T, Gillessen-Kaesbach G. Aplasia cutis congenita: etiological relationship to antiphospholipid syndrome? *Clin Dysmorphol.* 1999;8(3):215–217.
9. Schierz IAM, Giuffrè M, Del Vecchio A, Antona V, Corsello G, Piro E. Recognizable neonatal clinical features of aplasia cutis congenita. *Ital J Pediatr.* 2020;46(1):25.
10. Rudolph RI, Schwartz W, Leyden JJ. Bitemporal aplasia cutis congenita. Occurrence with other cutaneous abnormalities. *Arch Dermatol.* 1974;110(4):615–618.
11. Demmel U. Clinical aspects of congenital skin defects. I. Congenital skin defects on the head of the newborn. *Eur J Pediatr.* 1975;121(1):21–50.
12. Stephan MJ, Smith DW, Ponzi JW, Alden ER. Origin of scalp vertex aplasia cutis. *J Pediatr.* 1982;101(5):850–853.
13. Itin P, Pletscher M. Familial aplasia cutis congenita of the scalp without other defects in 6

members of three successive generations. *Dermatologica.* 1988;177(2):123–125.
14. Fimiani M, Seri M, Rubegni P, et al. Autosomal dominant aplasia cutis congenita: report of a large Italian family and no hint for candidate chromosomal regions. *Arch Dermatol Res.* 1999;291(12):637–642.
15. Mannino FL, Jones KL, Benirschke K. Congenital skin defects and fetus papyraceus. *J Pediatr.* 1977;91(4):559–564.
16. Daw E. Fetus papyraceus—11 cases. *Postgrad Med J.* 1983;59(695):598–600.
17. Leaute-Labreze C, Depaire-Duclos F, Sarlangue J, et al. Congenital cutaneous defects as complications in surviving co-twins: aplasia cutis congenita and neonatal volkmann ischemic contracture of the forearm. *Arch Dermatol.* 1998;134(9):1121–1124.
18. Ustuner P, Dilek N, Saral Y, Ustuner I. Coexistence of aplasia cutis congenita, faun tail nevus and fetus papyraceus. *J Dermatol Case Rep.* 2013;7(3):93–96.
19. Lane W, Zanol K. Duodenal atresia, biliary atresia, and intestinal infarct in truncal aplasia cutis congenita. *Pediatr Dermatol.* 2000;17(4):290–292.
20. Kantor J, Yan AC, Hivnor CM, Honig PJ, Kirschner R. Extensive aplasia cutis congenita and the risk of sagittal sinus thrombosis. *Arch Dermatol.* 2005;141(5):554–556.
21. Karg E, Bereg E, Gaspar L, Katona M, Turi S. Aplasia cutis congenita after methimazole exposure in utero. *Pediatr Dermatol.* 2004;21(4):491–494.
22. Arai M, Tsuno T, Konishi H, et al. A disproportionality analysis of the adverse effect profiles of methimazole and propylthiouracil in patients with hyperthyroidism using the Japanese adverse drug event report database. *Thyroid.* 2023;33(7):804–816. https://doi.org/10.1089/thy.2023.0030.
23. Hogler W, Sidoroff A, Weber F, Baldissera I, Heinz-Erian P. Aplasia cutis congenita, uvula bifida and bilateral retinal dystrophy in a girl with naevus sebaceous syndrome. *Br J Dermatol.* 1999;140(3):542–543.
24. Maman E, Maor E, Kachko L, Carmi R. Epidermolysis bullosa, pyloric atresia, aplasia cutis congenita: histopathological delineation of an autosomal recessive disease. *Am J Med Genet.* 1998;78(2):127–133.
25. Zvulunov A, Kachko L, Manor E, Shinwell E, Carmi R. Reticulolinear aplasia cutis congenita of the face and neck: a distinctive cutaneous manifestation in several syndromes linked to Xp22. *Br J Dermatol.* 1998;138(6):1046–1052.
26. Edwards MJ, McDonald D, Moore P, Rae J. Scalp-ear-nipple syndrome: additional manifestations. *Am J Med Genet.* 1994;50(3):247–250.
27. Baris H, Tan WH, Kimonis VE. Hypothelia, syndactyly, and ear malformation--a variant of the scalp-ear-nipple syndrome? Case report and review of the literature. *Am J Med Genet A.* 2005;134A(2):220–222.
28. Beekmans SJ, Wiebe MJ. Surgical treatment of aplasia cutis in the Adams-Oliver syndrome. *J Craniofac Surg.* 2001;12(6):569–572.
29. Verdyck P, Holder-Espinasse M, Hul WV, Wuyts W. Clinical and molecular analysis of nine families with Adams-Oliver syndrome. *Eur J Hum Genet.* 2003;11(6):457–463.
30. Kruk-Jeromin J, Janik J, Rykala J. Aplasia cutis congenita of the scalp: report of 16 cases. *Dermatol Surg.* 1998;24(5):549–553.
31. Schnabl SM, Horch RE, Ganslandt O, et al. Aplasia cutis congenita: plastic reconstruction of three scalp and skull defects with two opposed scalp rotation flaps and split thickness skin grafting. *Neuropediatrics.* 2009;40(3):134–136.
32. Yang JY, Yang WG. Large scalp and skull defect in aplasia cutis congenita. *Br J Plast Surg.* 2000;53(7):619–622.
33. Maillet-Declerck M, Vinchon M, Guerreschi P, et al. Aplasia cutis congenita: review of 29 cases and proposal of a therapeutic strategy. *Eur J Pediatr Surg.* 2013;23(2):89–93.
34. Donati V, Arena S, Capilli G, Carrera G, Ciralli F, Liberatore A. Reparation of a severe case of aplasia cutis congenita with engineered skin. *Biol Neonate.* 2001;80(4):273–276.
35. Hui CLY, Ngeow AJH, Ang DSY, Ong YS. A rare case of extensive aplasia cutis congenita: our surgical approach. *J Plast Reconstr Aesthet Surg.* 2023;80:193–199.
36. Beekmans SJ, Don Griot JP, Mulder JW. Split rib cranioplasty for aplasia cutis congenita and traumatic skull defects: more than 30 years of follow-up. *J Craniofac Surg.* 2007;18(3):594–597.
37. Burkhead A, Poindexter G, Morrell DS. A case of extensive aplasia cutis congenita with underlying skull defect and central nervous system malformation: discussion of large skin defects, complications, treatment and outcome. *J Perinatol.* 2009;29(8):582–584.
38. Udayakumaran S, Mathew J, Panikar D. Dilemmas and challenges in the management of a neonate with Adams-Oliver syndrome with infected giant aplasia cutis lesion and exsanguination: a case-based update. *Childs Nerv Syst.* 2013;29(4):535–541.
39. Hassed SJ, Wiley GB, Wang S, et al. *RBPJ* mutations identified in two families affected by Adams-Oliver syndrome. *Am J Hum Genet.* 2012;91(2):391–395.
40. Del Gaudio F, Liu D, Lendahl U. Notch signalling in healthy and diseased vasculature. *Open Biol.* 2022;12(4):220004.
41. Yang XF, Shi SW, Chen K. Case report: recombinant human epidermal growth factor gel plus kangfuxin solution in the treatment of aplasia cutis congenita in a case with Adams-Oliver syndrome. *Front Surg.* 2022;9:1072021.
42. Tian H, Chu F, Li Y, Xu M, Li W, Li C. Synergistic effects of rare variants of *ARHGAP31* and *FBLN1* in vitro in terminal transverse limb defects. *Front Genet.* 2022;13:946854.
43. Verdyck P, Blaumeiser B, Holder-Espinasse M, Van Hul W, Wuyts W. Adams-Oliver syndrome: clinical description of a four-generation family and exclusion of five candidate genes. *Clin Genet.* 2006;69(1):86–92.
44. Nieto-Benito LM, Suárez-Fernández R, Campos-Domínguez M. A novel pathogenic variation of *DOCK6* gene: the genotype-phenotype correlation in Adams-Oliver syndrome. *Mol Biol Rep.* 2023;50(6):5519–5521.

CHAPTER 40

Cephalohematoma

KEY POINTS

- Cephalohematoma is a subperiosteal extracranial hemorrhage often from an injury to the cranial periosteum during labor or a traumatic delivery.
- Risk factors include vacuum extraction, forceps delivery, fetal scalp monitors, instrumentation, and increased birth weight.
- Complications of cephalohematoma can include underlying skull fracture, anemia, hyperbilirubinemia, calcification, or infection.
- Cephalohematomas are usually localized and may resolve spontaneously within a few weeks or months.
- In rare cases, cephalohematomas can become infected, requiring incision, drainage, and antibiotic treatment.
- Calcified cephalohematomas may persist and can be managed with aspiration or, if necessary, surgical intervention to correct skull deformity.

GENESIS

Cephalohematoma is a common problem occurring in about 2.5% of newborns.[1] It is a subperiosteal extracranial hemorrhage that may enlarge after delivery, sometimes taking weeks to resolve. This condition contrasts with the scalp edema of caput succedaneum, which reaches its maximal size at birth and usually resolves within a few days.[2] Both lesions are believed to result from an injury to the cranial periosteum during labor or during a traumatic delivery, but they have also been detected as echogenic bulges on the cranium during prenatal ultrasound evaluations, which suggests that they can also arise in utero.[3,4] Among 16,292 fetuses undergoing comprehensive ultrasound examinations between 1993 and 1996, seven cephalohematomas were detected on exams performed between 23 and 38 weeks of gestation (five occipital and two temporal). A diagnosis of cephalohematoma was confirmed by the neonatologist in two cases, and caput succedaneum was diagnosed in the remaining five cases. It was not possible to distinguish between cephalohematoma and caput succedaneum prenatally. None of these affected neonates were delivered by vacuum extraction or forceps, or had any signs of intracranial hemorrhage or skull fracture by ultrasound, and none required any treatment. Five of these seven cases had associated premature rupture of membranes, with oligohydramnios noted in four cases, suggesting oligohydramnios might have played a role.[5] In 2014, Kim et al. reported that 25 out of 46 of their patients with cephalohematomas had some amount of intracranial hemorrhage on neuroimaging with no significant difference in the clinical manifestations between those with and those without intracranial hemorrhage.[1] In 10 cases of cephalohematomas with a lineal skull facture, 9 had intracranial hemorrhage.[1] In 2021, Ulma et al. reported on their 25-year experience and described their treatment and outcomes of 72 infants diagnosed with cephalohematomas.[6] Thirty required surgery with a mean age at the time of surgery of 8.6 months. Twenty-one surgical patients (70%) required inlay bone grafting. All surgery patients had improvement in calvarial shape, with eight having enough blood loss to require a transfusion.

Cephalohematoma (adjusted odds ratio [aOR], 5.5; $P<.001$), subdural hematoma (aOR, 2.4; $P<.001$), and caput succedaneum (aOR 1.13; $P=0.006$) have all been found more frequently in infants delivered by vacuum extraction than in infants delivered without intervention "spontaneously."[7-10] Cephalohematoma occurs in 1–2% of spontaneous deliveries compared with 4% of vacuum or forceps deliveries.[11] In a prospective randomized trial of 322 cases involving continuous versus intermittent vacuum extractions, cephalohematomas were associated with the station of the presenting part, asynclitism, and increasing application-to-delivery time. None of the infants with cephalohematomas experienced any long-term complications or needed blood transfusions,[12] but fetal death and stillbirth have been reported after prenatal diagnosis of a fetal subdural hematoma following suspected or confirmed trauma.[13-16] Thus cephalohematomas can occur prior to the onset of labor, especially with premature rupture of membranes and prolonged oligohydramnios. Maternal abdominal trauma can result in more serious subdural hematomas that can be seen by prenatal ultrasound, and this type of intracranial hemorrhage may threaten fetal survival.

Because vacuum extraction has been associated with cephalohematomas, there are concerns about whether this mode of delivery may result in more serious intracranial vascular injuries (subdural, cerebral, intraventricular, or subarachnoid hemorrhages). Among 583,340 live-born singleton infants weighing 2500–4000 g who were born to nulliparous women between 1992 and 1994 in California, the rate of intracranial hemorrhage was significantly higher among infants delivered by vacuum extraction, forceps, or cesarean section during labor than among infants delivered spontaneously.[17] Assisted vaginal delivery, which was reported to increase the rate of cephalohematoma up to 10.8%.[18] There was an incremental increase in the rate of hemorrhage if more than one method of delivery was used. Because the rate of hemorrhage was not significantly higher among infants delivered by cesarean section before labor, much of the morbidity associated with operative vaginal delivery is thought to be due to an underlying abnormality of labor rather than the specific operative procedure. The rate of intracranial hemorrhage has decreased threefold (to less than 1%) following the substitution of plastic cups for metal cups in vacuum extractors during the 1980s.[17]

Most cephalohematomas are caused by birth trauma, and documented risk factors include fetal scalp monitors, instrumentation, and increased birth weight.[19] The mechanism of injury is related to forces that lift the scalp and pericranium off the underlying bone, thus shearing vessels and causing blood to collect in this potential space.[20,21] Most cephalohematomas resolve spontaneously during the first few weeks after birth, depending on their size. Complications can include an underlying skull fracture, anemia, hyperbilirubinemia, calcification/ossification, or (rarely) infection of the hematoma.[22,23] Infants and toddlers that present to medical care with a cephalohematoma can be because of an accidental impact event or fall, but contact extra-axial hemorrhages with subdural hemorrhages are often considered indicative of abuse or major trauma.[24]

FEATURES

Traumatic subperiosteal hemorrhages occur most frequently in the outer table of the parietal bone, giving rise to a soft fluctuant mass (Fig. 40.1). Thus cephalohematomas occur beneath the periosteum, with no

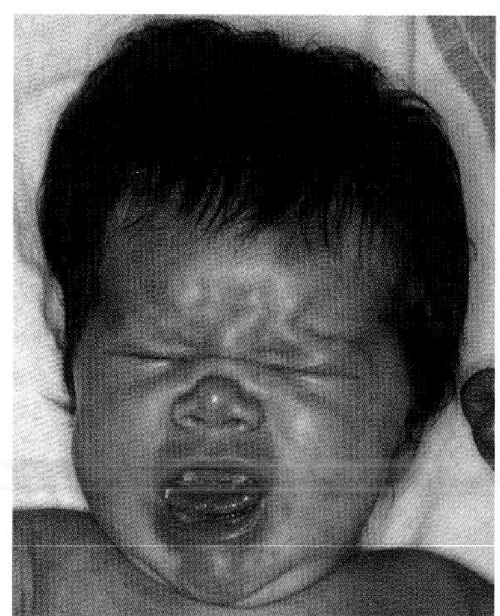

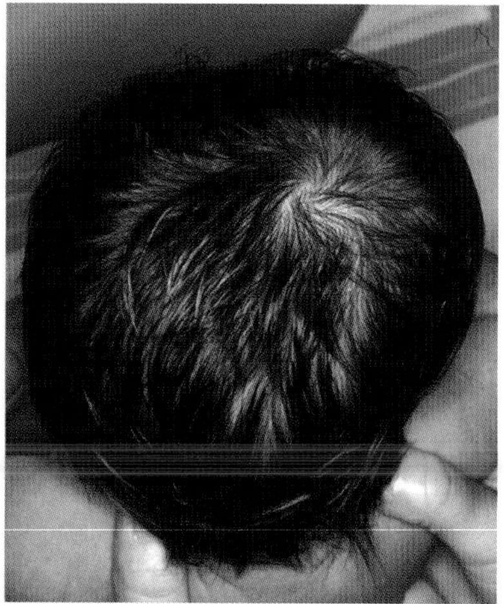

FIGURE 40.1 Right facial droop from traumatic right lower facial palsy with associated traumatic right parietal cephalohematoma. These lesions occur most frequently in the right superior parietal region.

extension over a sutural margin, and definite palpable edges are usually evident. Collections of blood within the superficial subcutaneous tissues are termed *caput succedaneum*. Cephalohematomas may become apparent or enlarge after delivery, sometimes taking weeks to resolve, whereas the edema of caput succedaneum usually reaches maximal size at birth and resolves within a few days, even when it is extensive in size. Subgaleal hematomas are located between the galea aponeurotica and pericranium, and because they are not restricted to the periosteal boundaries within cranial sutures, they can expand rapidly to involve the entire scalp and cause life-threatening volume loss, whereas cephalohematomas tend to remain localized.[19] Most cephalohematomas resorb within the first week, and if the clot has not resorbed by the fourth week, the clot may form fibrous tissue, with calcification beginning at the periphery of the hematoma.[20,25] With time the borders of a cephalohematoma may become elevated and craterlike as the raised periosteum begins to deposit bone at its borders. Calcified cephalohematomas usually resolve slowly over the next few years during the normal process of cranial bone remodeling with calvarial growth, but some lesions may persist and require further management (Figs. 40.2 and 40.3).

MANAGEMENT AND PROGNOSIS

Cephalohematomas are benign lesions that begin as soft fluctuant masses within the periosteum of the parietal bones. Parents should be reassured that most cephalohematomas resolve during the first month of postnatal life. In rare cases, extensive cephalohematomas may slowly calcify during the first year of life.[26] Rarely, cephalohematomas can become infected, usually in the setting of a predisposing factor such as trauma or a systemic infection that results in sepsis or meningitis.[27–30] One center in Japan reported that out of 29 newborns with infected cephalohematomas,

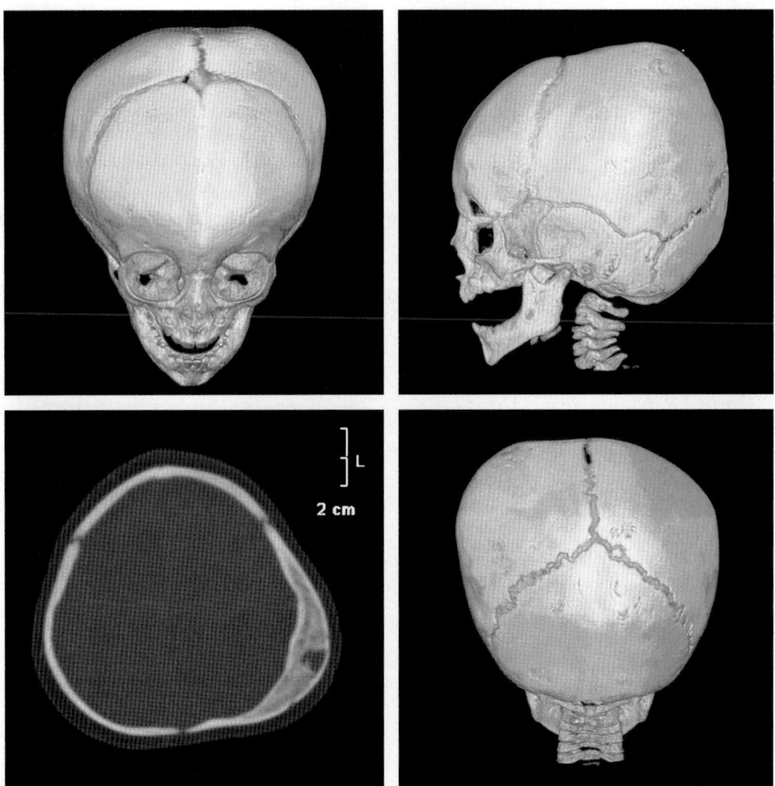

FIGURE 40.2 Persistent left calcified cephalohematoma at 7 months of age, shown by three-dimensional computed tomography scan with a cross-sectional image through the lesion. (Courtesy Dr. Michael Cunningham and Darcy King, Division of Craniofacial Medicine, Department of Pediatrics, University of Washington Medical School, Seattle, WA.)

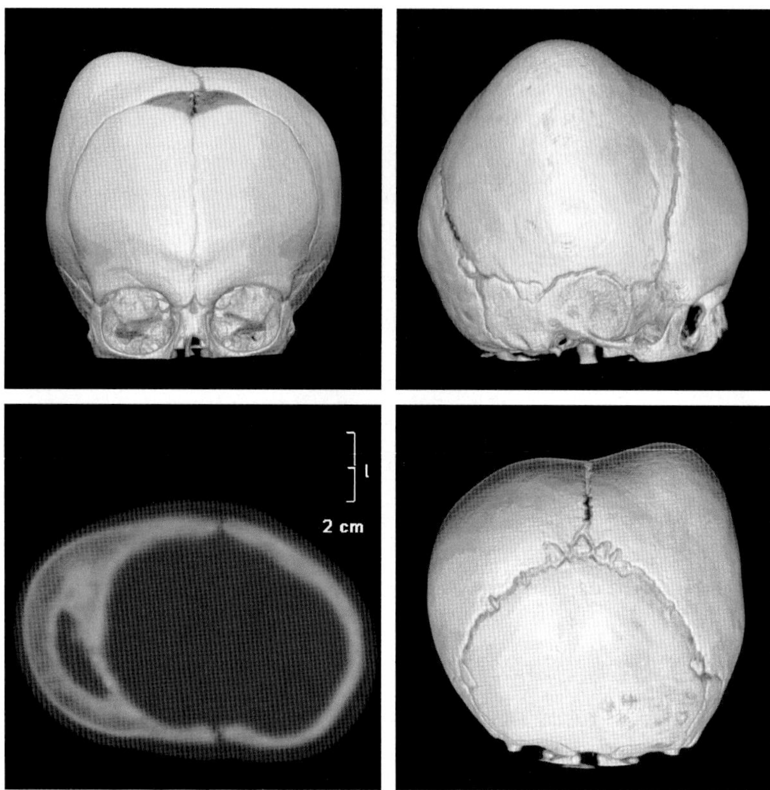

FIGURE 40.3 Persistent right calcified cephalohematoma at 11 months of age, shown by three-dimensional computed tomography scan with a cross-sectional image through the lesion. This lesion was surgically reconstructed. (Courtesy Dr. Michael Cunningham and Darcy King, Division of Craniofacial Medicine, Department of Pediatrics, University of Washington Medical School, Seattle, WA.)

8 had developed sepsis, 3 meningitis, 1 osteomyelitis, and 3 patients died.[30] An increase in the size of the cephalohematoma after 48 hours, failure to resorb, or signs of an infected wound (an enlarging, fluctuant, erythematous lesion with demineralization of the underlying bone) should prompt incision and drainage with culture for identification of the infectious agent. The most common organism (in about half the cases) is *Escherichia coli*, but a wide variety of other organisms have been reported, and it is important to determine the type of organism and its sensitivities to antibiotics.[23] Early-onset infection of cephalohematoma occurs within the first 2 weeks, usually due to bacteremic seeding from a systemic infection; delay in diagnosis or drainage can prove fatal. Late-onset cases occur after 3 weeks and are usually associated with cellulitis over the lesion and osteomyelitis in the underlying bone. In both early- and late-onset cases, the mainstay of treatment is incision and drainage with long-term antibiotic treatment, especially when osteomyelitis is present.[26,27,29] Cephalohematomas have also been found with cranial epidural hematomas, which have been treated by needle aspiration.[31] If an extensive cephalohematoma fails to resorb after 1 month, some clinicians advocate aspiration of the lesion to prevent formation of fibrous tissue and calcification. This should only be done using sterile technique with variation in the needle trajectory to prevent formation of a straight tract through which hematoma fluid can leak or infection can be introduced.[26] There has been one report of spontaneous drainage of a neonatal cephalohematoma in an infant who presented with recurrent neonatal bacteremia.[32] In two infants with extensive calcified cephalohematomas evident at ages 3–4 months, the use of a cranial orthotic led to prompt resolution of the lesion during the next 3–5 months (Fig. 40.4).[19] If the calcified cephalohematoma leads to significant asymmetry and deformity of the skull, surgical intervention may be required to correct the resulting skull deformity.[33]

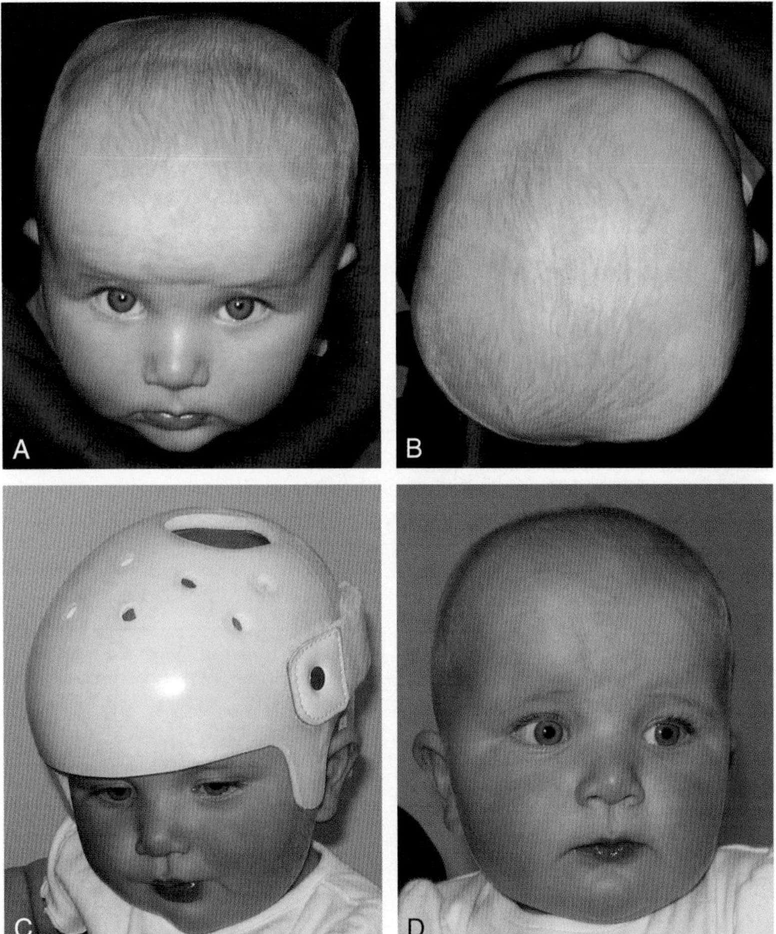

FIGURE 40.4 A, This female infant was seen at 6 months with torticollis-plagiocephaly deformation sequence resulting in right occipital flattening and a 1.2-cm diagonal difference. After a vacuum-suction delivery, she had a 4 × 6-cm calcified cephalohematoma in the right superior parietal bone, which did not change in size for 5 months after birth. **B,** When viewed from above, the calcified cephalohematoma obscured the view of her occipital flattening, which was sufficient to merit orthotic therapy. She wore a cranial orthotic with an off-centered opening in the top (**C**) so as to apply pressure to the calcified cephalohematoma, which resolved over the next 4 months, as did the plagiocephaly (**D**).

DIFFERENTIAL DIAGNOSIS

At the cranial vertex, edema of the skin and subcutaneous tissues may occur, the so-called *caput succedaneum*. Caput succedaneum can cross suture lines and is maximal in size at birth; it resolves in just a few days. The subperiosteal hemorrhage associated with a cephalohematoma may manifest a subsequent "crater rim" of bone at its outer borders, which sometimes gives the impression of a depressed skull fracture, but a cephalohematoma is a benign lesion. Epidural hematoma is extremely rare in the neonate and usually due to postnatal head trauma resulting from a fall and skull fracture; however, it can also be associated with an overlying cephalohematoma. When a skull fracture is suspected beneath a cephalohematoma, a computed tomography scan will clarify the clinical picture, and a craniotomy can be performed to relieve pressure on the brain through the prompt evacuation of the epidural hematoma that may result from tearing of a meningeal artery or venous bleeding.[34] Posterior encephaloceles can mimic occipital cephalohematomas and can be differentiated by magnetic resonance imaging.[35]

References

1. Kim HM, Kwon SH, Park SH, Kim YS, Oh KW. Intracranial hemorrhage in infants with cephalohematoma. *Pediatr Int.* 2014;56(3):378–381.
2. Meng A, Purohith A, Huang A, Litvinchuk T. Traumatic birth injury in a term neonate. *Cureus.* 2022;14(12):e32737.
3. Parker LA. Part 1: Early recognition and treatment of birth trauma: injuries to the head and face. *Adv Neonatal Care.* 2005;5(6):288–297; quiz 298-300.
4. Parker LA. Part 2: Birth trauma: injuries to the intraabdominal organs, peripheral nerves, and skeletal system. *Adv Neonatal Care.* 2006;6(1):7–14.
5. Petrikovsky BM, Schneider E, Smith-Levitin M, Gross B. Cephalhematoma and caput succedaneum: do they always occur in labor? *Am J Obstet Gynecol.* 1998;179(4):906–908.
6. Ulma RM, Sacks G, Rodoni BM, et al. Management of calcified cephalohematoma of infancy: the University of Michigan 25-year experience. *Plast Reconstr Surg.* 2021;148(2):409–417.
7. Fall O, Ryden G, Finnstrom K, Finnstrom O, Leijon I. Forceps or vacuum extraction? A comparison of effects on the newborn infant. *Acta Obstet Gynecol Scand.* 1986;65(1):75–80.
8. Teng FY, Sayre JW. Vacuum extraction: does duration predict scalp injury? *Obstet Gynecol.* 1997;89(2):281–285.
9. Ferraz A, Nunes F, Resende C, Almeida MC, Taborda A. [Short-term neonatal outcomes of vacuum-assisted delivery. A case-control study]. *An Pediatr (Engl Ed).* 2019;91(6):378–385.
10. Levin G, Elchalal U, Yagel S, et al. Risk factors associated with subgaleal hemorrhage in neonates exposed to vacuum extraction. *Acta Obstet Gynecol Scand.* 2019;98(11):1464–1472.
11. Broekhuizen FF, Washington JM, Johnson F, Hamilton PR. Vacuum extraction versus forceps delivery: indications and complications, 1979 to 1984. *Obstet Gynecol.* 1987;69(3 Pt 1):338–342.
12. Bofill JA, Rust OA, Devidas M, Roberts WE, Morrison JC, Martin JN Jr. Neonatal cephalohematoma from vacuum extraction. *J Reprod Med.* 1997;42(9): 565–569.
13. Demir RH, Gleicher N, Myers SA. Atraumatic antepartum subdural hematoma causing fetal death. *Am J Obstet Gynecol.* 1989;160(3):619–620.
14. Gunn TR, Becroft DM. Unexplained intracranial haemorrhage in utero: the battered fetus? *Aus & NZ J Obstet Gynaecol.* 1984;24(1):17–22.
15. Winter 3rd TC, Mack LA, Cyr DR. Prenatal sonographic diagnosis of scalp edema/cephalohematoma mimicking an encephalocele. *AJR.* 1993;161(6):1247–1248.
16. Grylack L. Prenatal sonographic diagnosis of cephalohematoma due to pre-labor trauma. *Pediatr Radiol.* 1982;12(3):145–147.
17. Towner D, Castro MA, Eby-Wilkens E, Gilbert WM. Effect of mode of delivery in nulliparous women on neonatal intracranial injury. *N Engl J Med.* 1999;341(23):1709–1714.
18. Simonson C, Barlow P, Dehennin N, et al. Neonatal complications of vacuum-assisted delivery. *Obstet Gynecol.* 2007;109(3):626–633.
19. Petersen JD, Becker DB, Fundakowski CE, Marsh JL, Kane AA. A novel management for calcifying cephalohematoma. *Plast Reconstr Surg.* 2004;113(5):1404–1409.
20. Kaufman HH, Hochberg J, Anderson RP, Schochet SS Jr, Simmons GM Jr. Treatment of calcified cephalohematoma. *Neurosurgery.* 1993;32(6):1037–1039; discussion 1039-1040.
21. Wong CH, Foo CL, Seow WT. Calcified cephalohematoma: classification, indications for surgery and techniques. *J Craniofac Surg.* 2006;17(5):970–979.
22. Watchko JF. Identification of neonates at risk for hazardous hyperbilirubinemia: emerging clinical insights. *Pediatric clinics of North America.* 2009;56(3):671–687. Table of Contents.
23. Li D, Tsiang JT, Mackey KA, Bonwit A, Pappu S. Cephalohematomas, an occult nidus for infection and inflammation: a case report and review of the literature. *Surg Neurol Int.* 2023;14:38.
24. Jordan W, James Benson M, Jeffrey O, et al. Extra-axial haemorrhages in young children with skull fractures: abuse or accident? *Archiv Dis Childhood.* 2022;107(7):650.
25. Kandemirli SG, Cingoz M, Bilgin C, Olmaz B. Temporal evolution of imaging findings in ossified cephalohematoma. *J Craniofac Surg.* 2020;31(4):e375–e378.
26. Firlik KS, Adelson PD. Large chronic cephalohematoma without calcification. *Pediatr Neurosurg.* 1999;30(1):39–42.
27. Goodwin MD, Persing JA, Duncan CC, Shin JH. Spontaneously infected cephalohematoma: case report and review of the literature. *J Craniofac Surg.* 2000;11(4):371–375; discussion.
28. Kao HC, Huang YC, Lin TY. Infected cephalohematoma associated with sepsis and skull osteomyelitis: report of one case. *Am J Perinatol.* 1999;16(9):459–462.
29. Weiss KJ, Edwards MS, Hay LM, Allen CH. *Escherichia coli*–infected cephalohematoma in an infant. *Clin Pediatr (Phila).* 2009;48(7):763–766.
30. Chang HY, Chiu NC, Huang FY, Kao HA, Hsu CH, Hung HY. Infected cephalohematoma of newborns: experience in a medical center in Taiwan. *Pediatr Int.* 2005;47(3):274–277.
31. Smets KJ, Vanhauwaert D. Treatment of cranial epidural hematoma in a neonate by needle aspiration of a communicating cephalhematoma. *Eur J Pediatr.* 2010;169(5):617–619.
32. Kersten CM, Moellering CM, Mato S. Spontaneous drainage of neonatal cephalohematoma: a delayed complication of scalp abscess. *Clin Pediatr (Phila).* 2008;47(2):183–185.
33. Kortesis BG, Pyle JW, Sanger C, Knowles M, Glazier SS, David LR. Surgical treatment for scaphocephaly

and a calcified cephalohematoma. *J Craniofac Surg.* 2009;20(2):410–413.
34. Lieu AS, Sun ZM, Howng SL. Bilateral epidural hematoma in a neonate. *Kaohsiung J Med Sciences.* 1996;12(7):434–436.
35. van Tellingen V, Obihara CC, van Tilborg GF, van Dijken PJ. MRI diagnosis of occipital cephalohematoma mimicking an encephalocele. *Am J Perinatol.* 2008;25(3):153–155.

CHAPTER 41

Wormian Bones

KEY POINTS

- Wormian bones are accessory bones found within cranial suture lines that vary in size and quantity, with few and small bones being common and many large bones being extremely rare.
- A majority of children with an excessive number of Wormian bones have some abnormality of the central nervous system.
- They occur most commonly in the lambdoid sutures and within fontanels.
- Wormian bones are thought to result from variations in dural growth stretch along open sutures and within fontanels, causing ossification defects.
- Wormian bones may form in relation to changes in pressure along the lambdoid sutures, such as in fronto-occipital head binding and craniosynostosis.

GENESIS

Wormian bones are accessory bones that occur within cranial suture lines and are often considered to be a simple anatomical variant. Although they themselves do not cause any impairment, their significance as a clinical finding is variable.[1-3] The prevalence varies by size and quantity. In a 2019 Greek study of 124 dry adult skulls, 74.7% had Wormian bones, most commonly located in the lambdoid suture (44.6%), followed in order of frequency by the coronal suture (39.8%), asterion (21% on the left and 15.3% on the right side), and parietomastoid suture (15.1% on the left and 13.9% on the right side).[4] Individuals with few and small (<4 mm) Wormian bones are fairly common and individuals with many large (greater than 10 mm) Wormian bones (Fig. 41.1) are extremely rare.[5] To be considered pathologically significant, they must number more than 10 in number, be larger than 6 mm by 4 mm, and be arranged in a general mosaic pattern.[2] In one study, the majority of children with an "excessive" number of Wormian bones had some abnormality of the central nervous system.[6] Reported abnormalities ranged from gross malformations to minimal brain dysfunction, although this study may have been biased because it used a hospital-based population. Thus some individuals with many Wormian bones may have other anomalies and/or central nervous system dysfunction. The name *Wormian bones* is derived from a Danish anatomist named Olaus Worm who described these small irregular ossicles located within cranial sutures in a letter to Thomas Bartholin in 1643.[6,7] They occur most commonly in the lambdoid sutures and within fontanels, and the pathogenesis of Wormian bones is thought to be related to variations in dural growth stretch along open sutures and within fontanels, causing ossification defects.[8,9] Such sutural bones persist and are not incorporated into the adjacent bone during mineralization and maturation. Although the prevalence of Wormian bones in the general population varies from 8% to 15%, the true prevalence is around 14%.[6,7] Males are more often affected than females, and differences among ethnic groups have been noted, with the highest incidence in Chinese individuals (80%).[7] Ethnic variation in Wormian bones may suggest a possible genetic influence, but environmental influences could also play a role.

A positive correlation has been noted between the frequency of lambdoid Wormian bones and the degree of deformation observed in primitive cultures that practice fronto-occipital head binding, which suggests that these bones form in relation to changes in pressure along the lambdoid sutures.[10,11] Note that the term "Inca bone" was initially used as a synonym for *Wormian bones* in deformed Peruvian skulls, which were mistakenly considered to be a racial trait.[7] In rabbits with premature coronal synostosis, Wormian bones

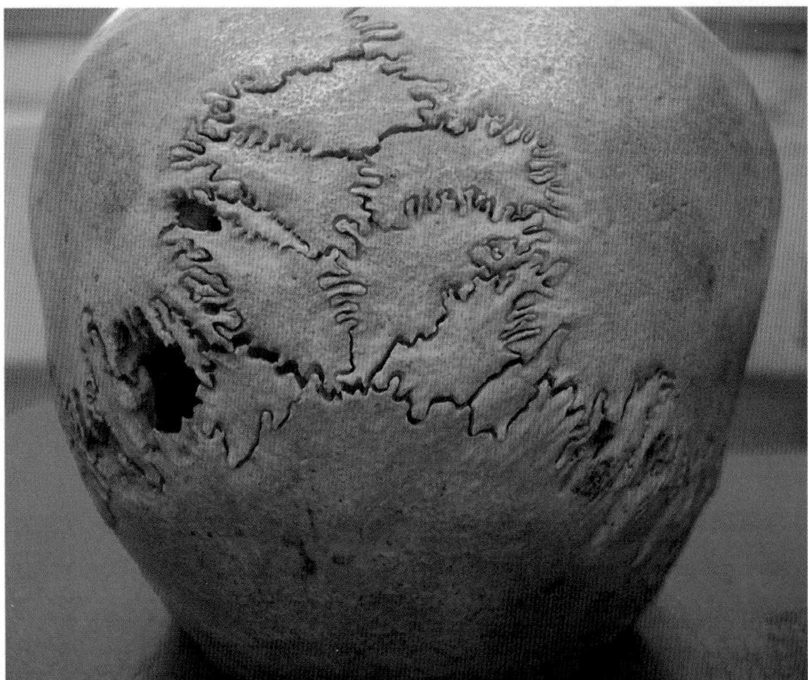

FIGURE 41.1 Image of a dry human skull with many large Wormian bones along the lambdoidal sutures and their junction with the sagittal suture.

appeared in the coronal and sagittal sutures after the onset of cranial growth alterations induced by premature coronal synostosis, which suggests that Wormian bones form in relation to external factors.[12] One study tabulated the frequency and location of large Wormian bones (>1 cm) in three-dimensional computed tomography scans from 207 cases of craniosynostosis and compared this data to control. Among cases of craniosynostosis, large Wormian bones were significantly more frequent (117 out of 207 three-dimensional computed tomography scans) than in control skulls (131 out of 485), with a 3.5-times greater odds of developing a Wormian bone with premature suture closure ($P < .001$) (Fig. 41.2).[3] Several others have also since reported Wormian bones in craniosynostosis and other head shape deformities.[13-16] Nondeformed crania have more Wormian bones than circumferentially deformed crania but have fewer Wormian bones than anteroposteriorly deformed crania.[17] This may relate to variations in tension across the sutures, a hypothesis tested by O'Loughlin, who demonstrated that the frequency and location of Wormian bones vary depending on the type and degree of cranial deformation, with posteriorly placed Wormian bones appearing in greater numbers in deformed crania and with sagittal synostosis.[18]

The increased frequency of Wormian bones noted in Chinese infants might be related to their traditional supine infant sleeping position and the resultant pressure against their occiput. If so, an increased frequency of Wormian bones may soon be noted in other cultures that have adopted the supine sleep positioning to prevent sudden infant death syndrome (SIDS), and it might be expected that more Wormian bones will be associated with a higher Cephalic Index (biparietal diameter divided by the anteroposterior diameter multiplied by 100). One study in fact measured the Cephalic Index and counted the number of Worman bones in pre-Colombian purposefully deformed skulls and compared them to control skulls from a medical school anatomy course. They found that the higher the Cephalic Index (i.e., more brachycephalic), the more Wormian bones were found within the skull sutures.[3]

FEATURES

Wormian bones are accessory bones that occur within cranial suture lines or fontanelles.[6,7] They occur singly or in large numbers and are diagnosed radiographically. They appear as intramembranous ossifications and, in

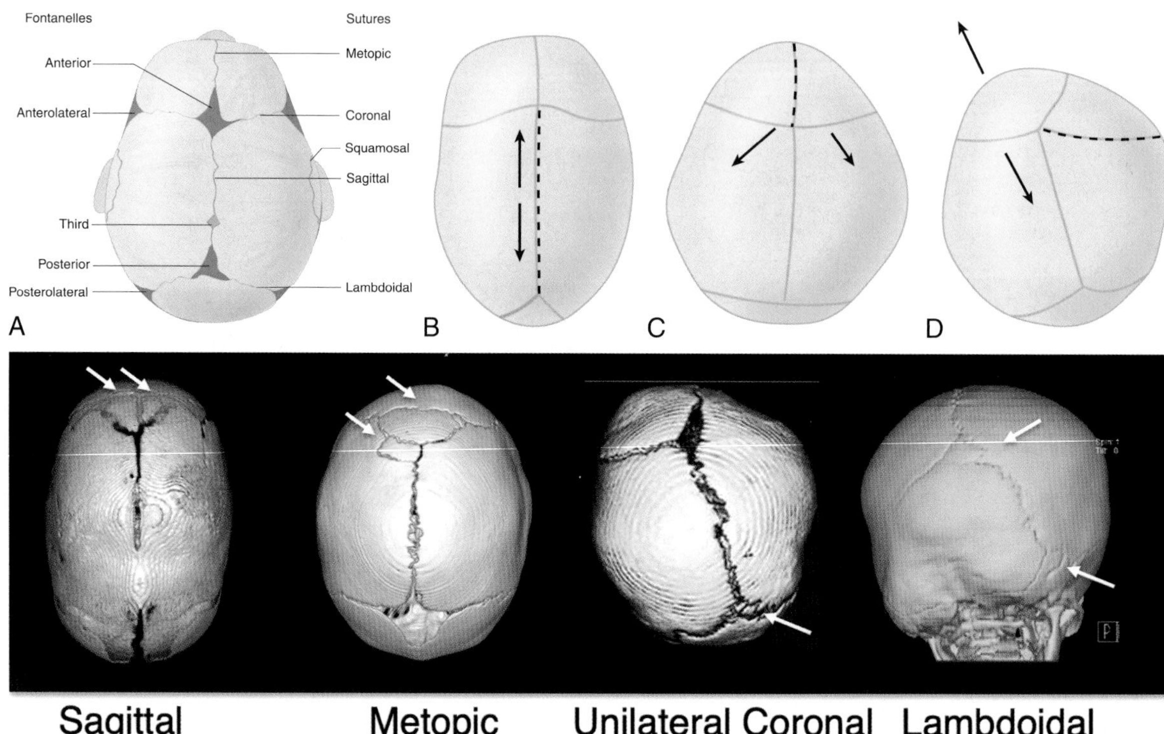

FIGURE 41.2 Diagrams and three-dimensional computed tomography scan reconstructions depicting (**A**) sagittal synostosis, (**B**) metopic synostosis, (**C**) right unilateral coronal synostosis, and (**D**) left lambdoidal synostosis. Arrows point to accessory or Wormian bones noted in open sutures or fontanels.

the fetus, are composed of a single layer of compact bone on the dural side.[10] Although they can occur within any suture, they are rare in coronal or sagittal sutures and appear most frequently in the lambdoid sutures and other posterior sutures. Wormian bones are usually normal variants that can be detected prenatally. Given the large number of associated syndromes for which they are an associated finding, the prenatal detection of Wormian bones should prompt a search for other associated anomalies involving the brain and for metabolic abnormalities affecting skull ossification.[10,19]

MANAGEMENT AND PROGNOSIS

Wormian bones require no management other than the recognition of their significance as possibly being associated with an underlying disorder that may require diagnosis and management (e.g., craniosynostosis).[2,3] Wormian bones are commonly seen in osteogenesis imperfecta (Fig. 41.3) and other disorders that result in defective cranial bone mineralization, such as cleidocranial dysplasia (Fig. 41.4), hypophosphatasia, pycnodysostosis, Hajdu-Cheney syndrome (Fig. 41.5), Grant syndrome, and multicentric carpotarsal osteolysis syndrome (*MFAB* gene).[1] Such infants also become quite brachycephalic as a consequence of occipital pressure from postnatal supine positioning with soft cranial bones, which may increase the propensity to form Wormian bones.[19] Wormian bones are also associated with conditions with hypotonia as well as disorders of premature aging such as progeria, acrogeria, and mandibular dysplasia, as well as with Menkes syndrome.

DIFFERENTIAL DIAGNOSIS

Wormian bones could be mistaken for a skull fracture, but experienced radiographic interpretation should resolve this error.

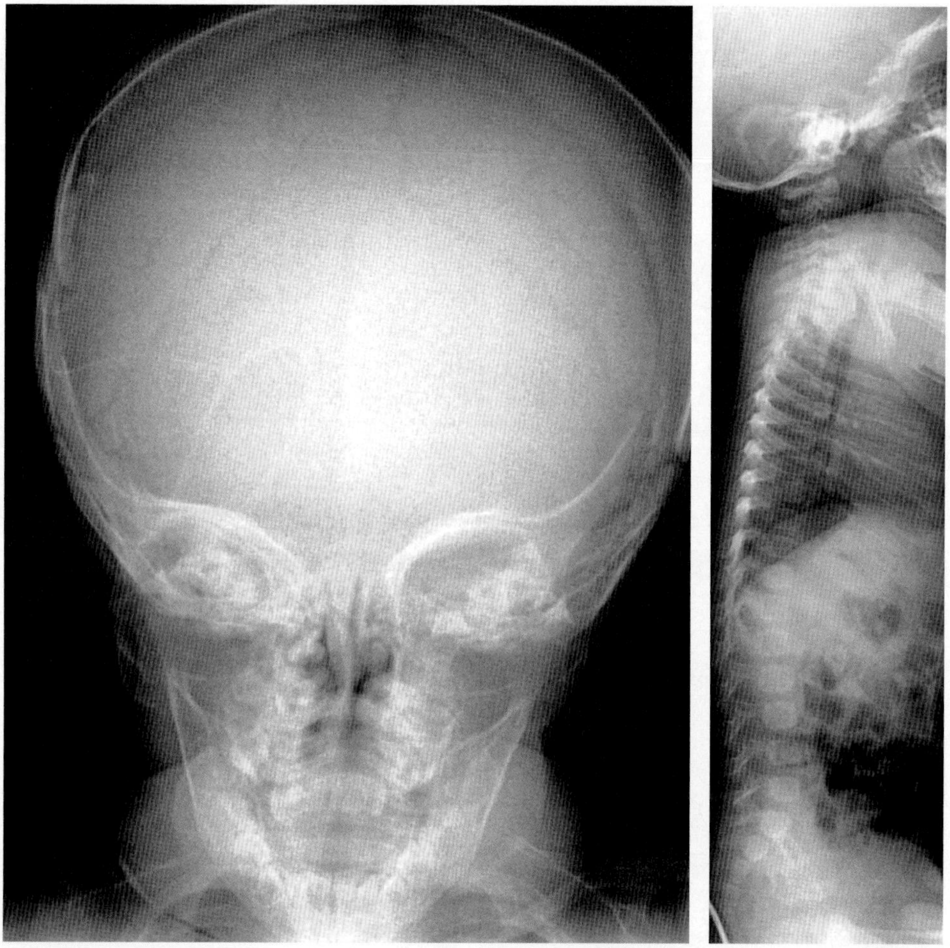

FIGURE 41.3 This child with osteogenesis type IV due to defective collagen type 1 has marked osteopenia of the skull and spine with multiple Wormian bones, as well as a history of multiple fractures with minimal trauma.

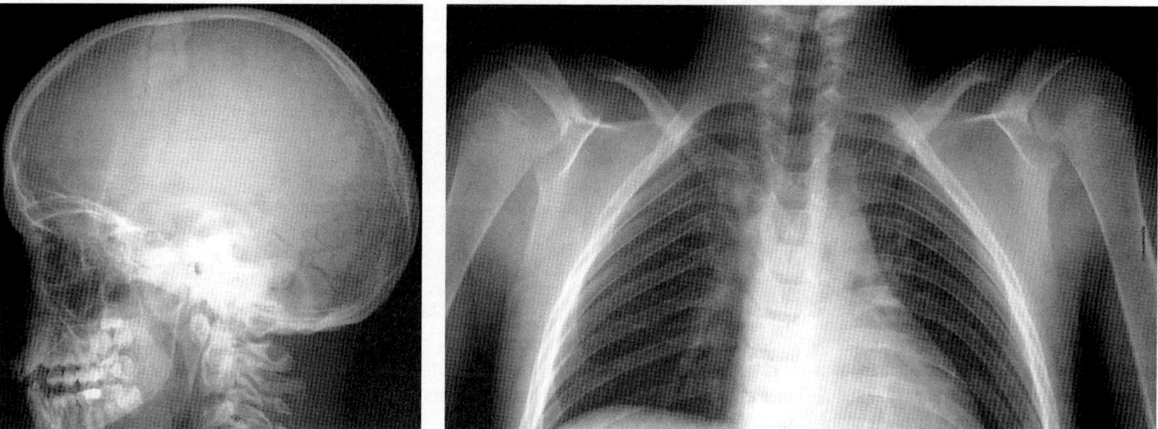

FIGURE 41.4 This child with cleidocranial dysplasia has multiple Wormian bones and clavicular hypoplasia, with delayed eruption of teeth and delayed closure of the anterior fontanelle due to a mutation in *CBFA1* (RUNX2).

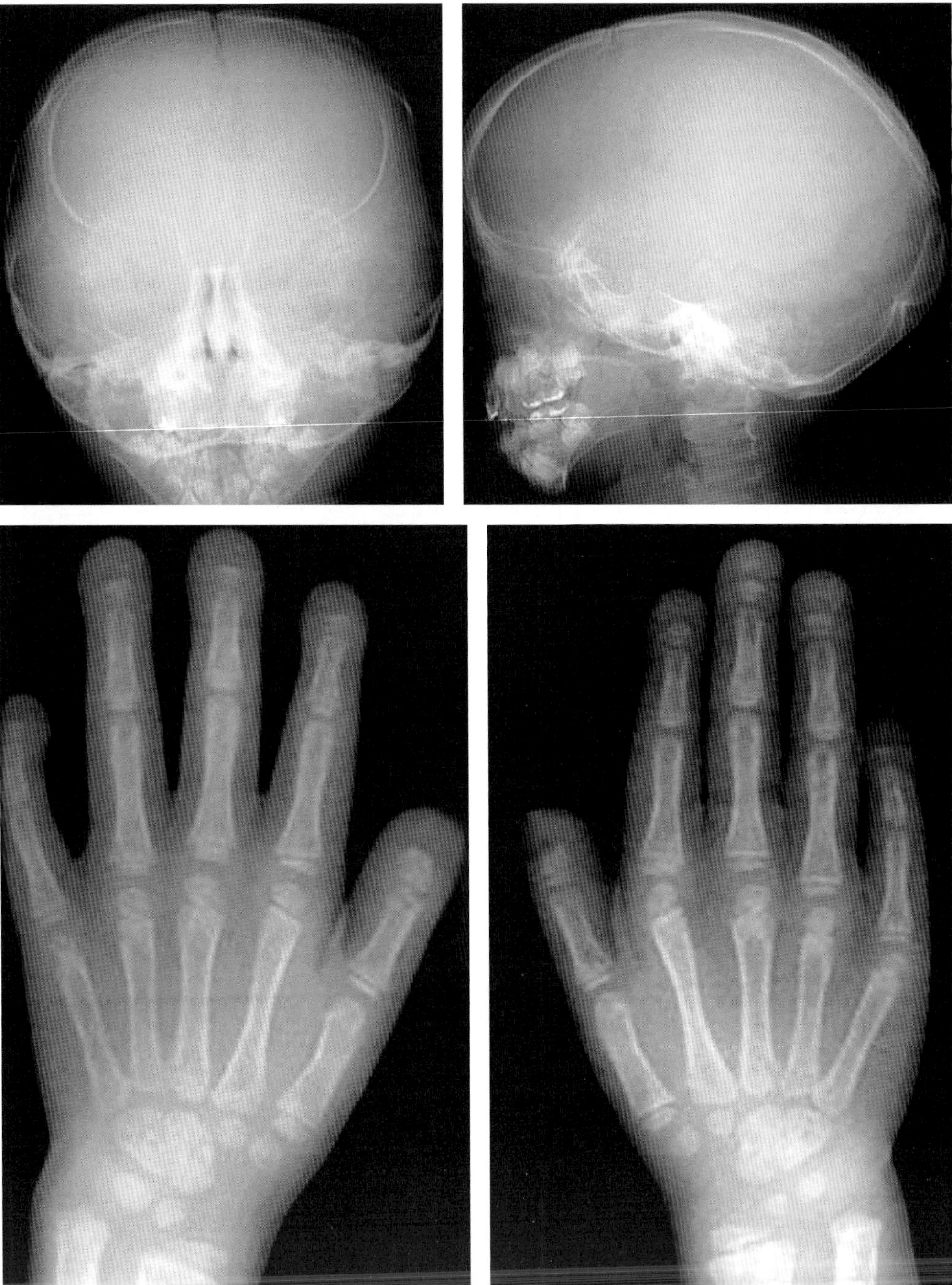

FIGURE 41.5 This person with Hajdu-Cheney syndrome has an autosomal dominant condition resulting in generalized osteoporosis with frequent fractures and acro-osteolysis resulting in short stature, micrognathia, premature loss of teeth, joint hypermobility, and open cranial sutures with multiple Wormian bones. Note that the underdeveloped distal phalanges are due to defective bone development rather than loss of normally formed bone; thus this is actually pseudo–acro-osteolysis, similar to what is seen in pycnodysostosis.

References

1. Al Kaissi A, Ryabykh S, Ben Chehida F, et al. The tomographic study and the phenotype of Wormian bones. *Diagnostics (Basel)*. 2023(5):13.
2. Bellary SS, Steinberg A, Mirzayan N, et al. Wormian bones: a review. *Clin Anat*. 2013;26(8):922–927.
3. Sanchez-Lara PA, Graham JM. Jr, Hing AV, Lee J, Cunningham M. The morphogenesis of wormian bones: a study of craniosynostosis and purposeful cranial deformation. *Am J Med Genet A*. 2007;143a(24):3243–3251.
4. Natsis K, Piagkou M, Lazaridis N, et al. Incidence, number and topography of Wormian bones in Greek adult dry skulls. *Folia Morphologica*. 2019;78(2):359–370.
5. Marti B, Sirinelli D, Maurin L, Carpentier E. Wormian bones in a general paediatric population. *Diagn Interv Imaging*. 2013;94(4):428–432.
6. Pryles CV, Khan AJ. Wormian bones. A marker of CNS abnormality? *Am J Dis Child*. 1979;133(4):380–382.
7. Jeanty P, Silva SR, Turner C. Prenatal diagnosis of wormian bones. *J Ultrasound Med*. 2000;19(12):863–869.
8. Khan AA, Asari MA, Hassan A. Unusual presence of Wormian (sutural) bones in human skulls. *Folia Morphol (Warsz)*. 2011;70(4):291–294.
9. Pickett AT, Montes MA. Wormian bone in the anterior fontanelle of an otherwise well neonate. *Cureus*. 2019;11(5):e4741.
10. Bennett KA. The etiology and genetics of wormian bones. *Am J Phys Anthropol*. 1965;23(3):255–260.
11. White CD. Sutural effects of fronto-occipital cranial modification. *Am J Phys Anthropol*. 1996;100(3):397–410.
12. Burrows AM, Caruso KA, Mooney MP, Smith TD, Losken HW, Siegel MI. Sutural bone frequency in synostotic rabbit crania. *Am J Phys Anthropol*. 1997;102(4):555–563.
13. Stotland MA, Do NK, Knapik TJ. Bregmatic wormian bone and metopic synostosis. *J Craniofac Surg*. 2012;23(7 Suppl 1):2015–2018.
14. Tonni G, Lituania M, Rosignoli L. Craniosynostosis with wormian bone, bowing of the long bones, unilateral short femur, and focal fibula deficiency: a prenatal diagnostic dilemma. *JCU*. 2013;41(7):448–452.
15. Samson TD, Beals SP, Rekate HL. Massive Wormian bone at the cranial apex: identification, correction and outcome. *J Craniofac Surg*. 2008;19(1):96–100.
16. Agrawal D, Steinbok P, Cochrane DD. Pseudoclosure of anterior fontanelle by wormian bone in isolated sagittal craniosynostosis. *Pediatr Neurosurg*. 2006;42(3):135–137.
17. Anton SC, Jaslow CR, Swartz SM. Sutural complexity in artificially deformed human (*Homo sapiens*) crania. *J Morphology*. 1992;214(3):321–332.
18. O'Loughlin VD. Effects of different kinds of cranial deformation on the incidence of wormian bones. *Am J Phys Anthropol*. 2004;123(2):146–155.
19. Graham JM. Jr, Kreutzman J, Earl D, Halberg A, Samayoa C, Guo X. Deformational brachycephaly in supine-sleeping infants. *J Pediatr*. 2005;146(2):253–257.

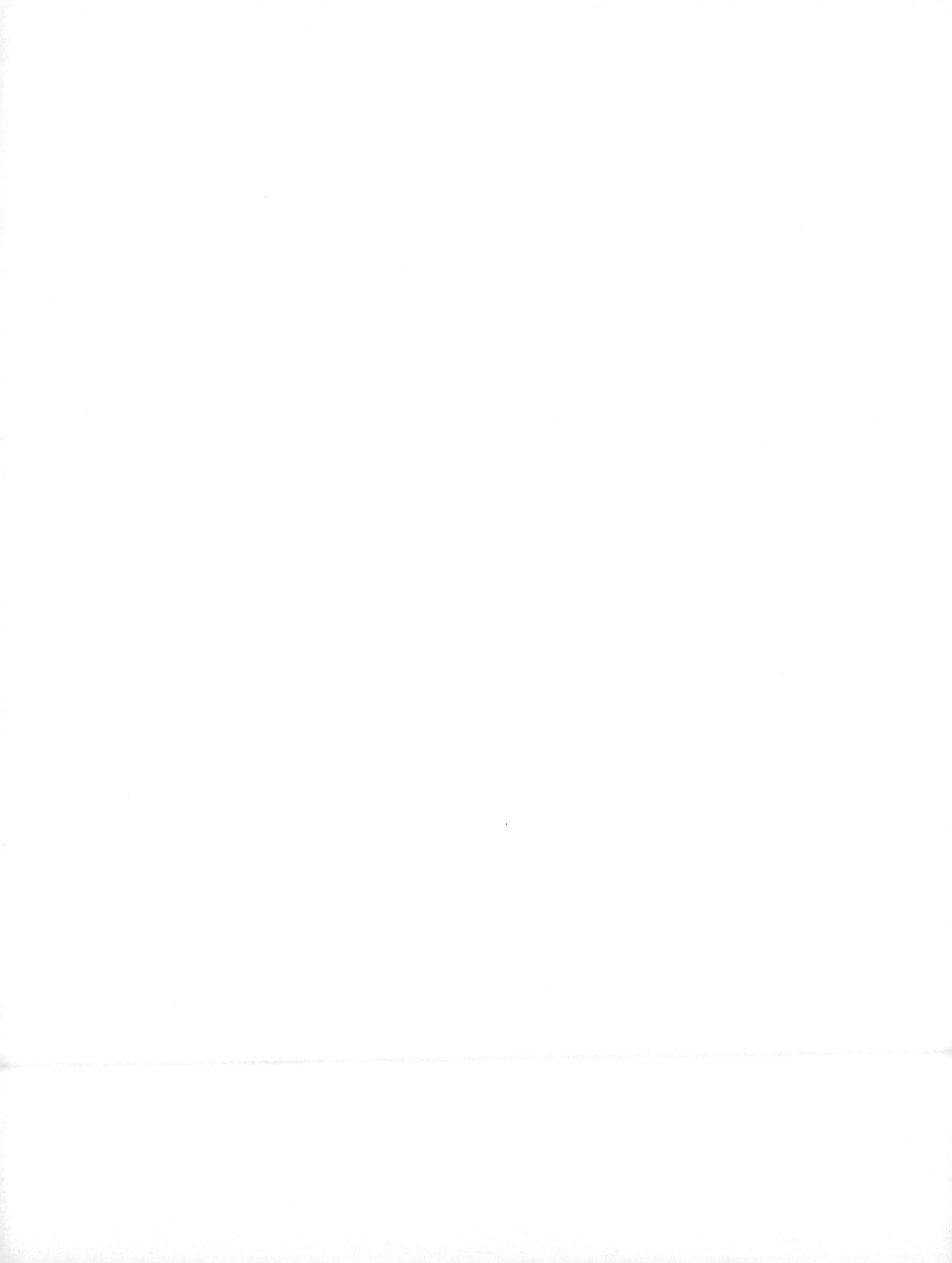

Section X
Abnormal Birth Presentation

CHAPTER 42

Breech Presentation Deformation

KEY POINTS

- Breech presentation is considered normal in premature fetuses before 32 weeks of gestation but is responsible for one-third of all deformations in term newborns.
- Factors leading to breech presentation include prematurity, twinning, chronic amniotic fluid leakage, uterine malformations, placenta previa, maternal hypertension, and fetal malformations.
- Primigravida women, especially older primigravida women, are more likely to have breech presentation due to uterine shape and limited space.
- Traumatic injuries following vaginal breech delivery can include fractures, dislocations, nerve injuries, cerebral hemorrhages, bruising, cord prolapse, birth asphyxia, and testicular trauma.
- The type of breech presentation (frank, complete, or footling) does not significantly affect adverse outcomes associated with the mode of delivery.

GENESIS

The frequency of singleton breech presentation at term is 3.1% and rises to 6.2% when multiple births are included.[1–3] Breech presentation is an important cause of deformation, and fully one-third of all deformations occur in babies who have been in breech presentation (Fig. 42.1).[2,4,5] Because 2% of newborns have deformations, this indicates that 0.6% of neonates have one or more deformations due to breech presentation; therefore this topic will be given extensive coverage. Among infants born with deformations, 32% were in breech presentation (vs. 5–6% of normally formed infants), and 23% of malformed infants were also in breech presentation.[6] Among 142 infants with spina bifida, 38% were in breech presentation and 68% of these infants had lower extremity weakness or paralysis. Among those infants with paralyzed legs, 93% manifested breech presentation; thus breech presentation becomes more likely with fetal inability to power the legs.[6] Numerous fetal and maternal factors can lead to breech presentation and thereby increase the risk for adverse outcomes. Some of these factors include prematurity (25% breech), twinning (34% breech), oligohydramnios due to chronic leakage (64% breech), uterine malformations, placenta previa, maternal hypertension, and fetal malformations.

Breech presentation is more common in primigravida women, especially older primigravida women, presumably because of the shape of the uterus and the reduced space for fetal and uterine growth. The spatial restrictions associated with twinning also increase the likelihood of breech presentation, especially for the second-born. In a 2023 study of over 355,990 singleton pregnancies, breech presentation occurred 20% more often in singleton pregnancies conceived via both assisted reproductive technology (adjusted odds ratio: 1.20, 95% confidence interval: 1.10–1.30, $P < .001$) and ovulation induction (adjusted odds ratio: 1.21, 95% confidence interval (CI): 1.04–1.39, $P < .05$) than naturally conceived pregnancies. No significant associations were observed between the three modes of conception and transverse/shoulder or face/brow presentations.[7] The prematurely born baby is also less likely to have shifted into the vertex birth position, and prematurity is more common with multiple births. Unless there is oligohydramnios or twinning, the premature fetus in breech presentation generally does not have associated deformations because there has not been sufficient constraint to cause molding. Furthermore, breech presentation can be considered normal with prematurity because at 32 weeks of gestation, 25% of all fetuses are in breech presentation; after this time, the majority of fetuses shift into vertex presentation. Any situation that causes oligohydramnios,

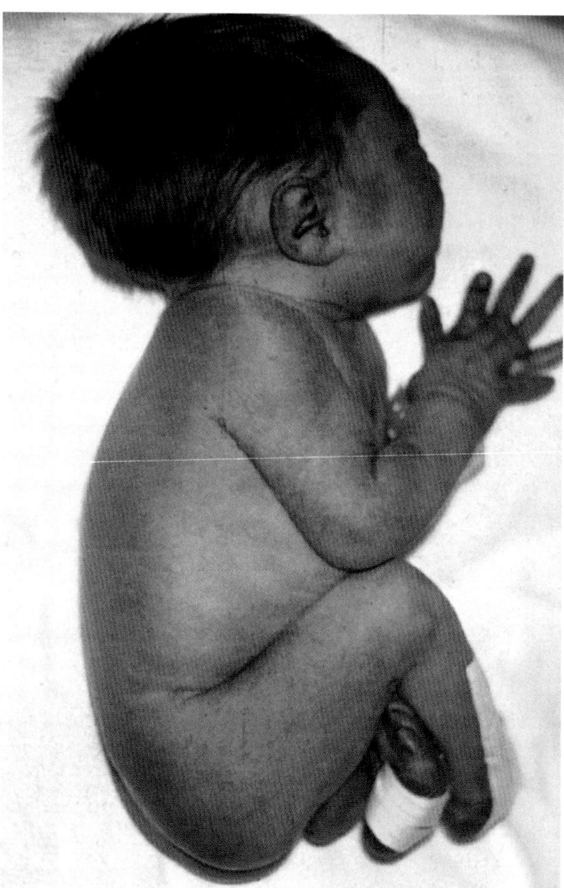

FIGURE 42.1 This term infant was delivered from a complete breech presentation and is shown in their position of comfort with a breech head, prominent occipital shelf, and equinovarus foot deformations.

whether it be chronic leakage of amniotic fluid or lack of urine flow into the amniotic space, will restrict movement and greatly increase the chance of the fetus being in breech presentation. Alterations in the size and shape of the uterine cavity may also increase the frequency of breech presentation. This may be secondary to uterine structural anomalies or myomas. The implantation and placement of the placenta may also be a factor, as 66% of placentas in breech delivery implant in the cornual-fundal region (vs. 4% of vertex presentations), whereas in 76% of vertex presentations, the placenta implants on the midwall of the uterus (vs. 4% of breech presentations).[3]

Although the best mode of delivery for infants in breech presentation is controversial, most studies suggest that the risk for neonatal morbidity and mortality is increased when infants in breech presentation are delivered vaginally as opposed to via cesarean section.[3,6,8-10] Delivery-related neonatal injury during cesarean delivery is more frequent in the reverse breech extraction method compared with standard vertex extraction.[11] Traumatic injuries following vaginal delivery of breech infants can include fractures (clavicle, femur, humerus) dislocations, brachial plexus injuries, facial nerve injuries, cephalic hematomas, cerebral hemorrhages, bruising with hyperbilirubinemia, cervical cord injuries, cord prolapse, birth asphyxia, and testicular trauma.[12,13] In most large series, these types of injuries occur less frequently with cesarean delivery, but in some recent series using modern delivery methods, the rate of such injuries is similar in planned vaginal breech delivery compared with elective cesarean section. In 2009, a study of 1345 term breech deliveries found no statistical difference in low 5-minute Apgar scores and arterial cord blood pH between vaginal delivery and cesarean section, although there were higher rates of severe plexus injuries and two neonatal deaths after a trial of labor whereas no perinatal deaths of a term breech infant in the cesarean group.[14] In a 2005 study of 1433 breech infants, Pradhan et al. compared the outcome of infants born by prelabor cesarean section with those delivered vaginally or by cesarean section in labor and found that those in labor were significantly more likely to have low 5-minute Apgar scores (0.9% vs. 5.9%, $P < .0001$) and require admission to the neonatal unit (1.6% vs. 4%, $P = .0119$). Despite the these differences, there was no significant difference in long-term morbidity between the two groups and no difference in rates of cerebral palsy.[15] These and many other studies have led some authors to suggest that with a normal pelvis and normal term birth weight, assisted vaginal breech delivery by an experienced obstetrician may be as safe as cesarean section delivery.[16-18] However, a 2022 metaanalysis assessing the maternal and fetal risks of planned vaginal breech delivery versus planned cesarean of 94,285 births found that the relative risk of perinatal mortality was 5.48 (95% CI: 2.61–11.51) times higher in the vaginal delivery group, 4.12 (95% CI: 2.46–6.89) for birth trauma, and 3.33 (95% CI: 1.95–5.67) for Apgar results. Maternal morbidity showed a relative risk 0.30 (95% CI: 0.13–0.67) times higher in the planned cesarean group.[19] Clinical practice guidelines for vaginal delivery of a breech presentation were published in 2006 by the American College of Obstetricians and Gynecologists and in 2009 by the Society of Obstetricians and Gynaecologists of Canada.[20,21]

Because of the risk of cervical cord injuries with vaginal delivery, most studies have relegated breech infants with hyperextended heads for automatic cesarean section.[6] Trials of vaginal delivery have succeeded in 60% to 70% of patients, without significant differences in outcome measures for primiparas versus multiparas or for frank versus non-frank breech presentations.[16] In North America, 70% to 80% of all women with breech presentation deliver by cesarean section (with similar trends observed in other parts of the world), so obstetric resident training experience with vaginal breech deliveries may be insufficient to guarantee sufficient expertise.[22]

Breech presentation shows a familial tendency, and 22% of multiparous women delivering a breech infant had previously experienced a breech delivery. If the first infant in a family is breech-born, there is a 9.4% chance the second child will be breech-born; whereas if the first child is vertex, there is only a 2.4% chance the second will be breech (this being the background risk for breech delivery).[23] Women with recurring breech presentation have a lower risk of adverse perinatal outcome, possibly due to increased attention to perinatal care.[10] The familial tendency toward breech deliveries may be related to inherited uterine structural characteristics (see Chapter 45), or it may be a consequence of a genetic neuromuscular or fetal malformation syndrome such as myotonic dystrophy. Presumably, the lower risk of adverse perinatal outcome relates to detection of maternal anatomic abnormalities (or fetal genetic abnormalities) that might result in closer follow-up during subsequent pregnancies.

In about 70% of fetuses in breech presentation, the legs are extended in front of the abdomen (Fig. 42.2). Once the movements of the fetus become limited by extension of the legs in front of the abdomen, the fetus has less chance of extricating itself from the breech presentation,[23] and Dunn has used the analogy of the "folding body press" wrestling hold.[3] Once a wrestler has an opponent in a position with the legs in front of the abdomen, there is little the opponent can do to escape. Breech presentation with the hips flexed and

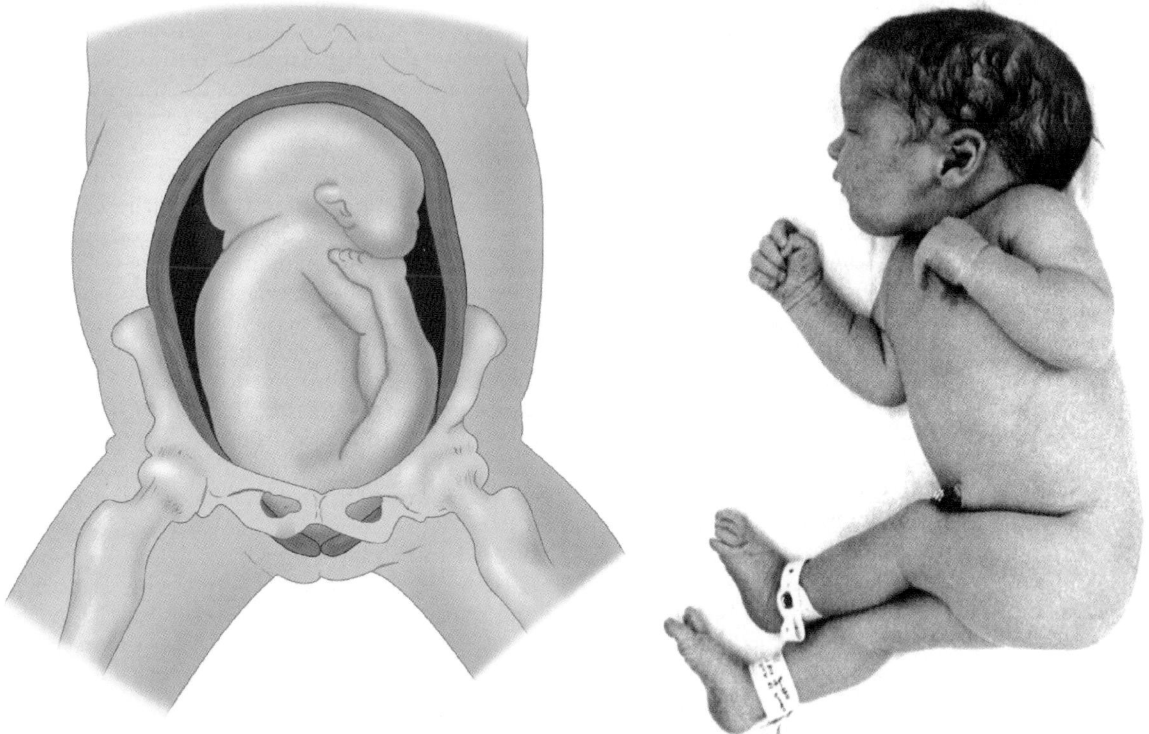

FIGURE 42.2 Frank breech presentation in a term infant. Note their extended legs with flexed thighs and shoulders thrust up beneath the occipital shelf in their position of comfort.

knees extended is termed *frank breech* (see Figs. 42.2 and 42.3A and D). When the hips and knees are flexed, it is called *complete breech* (Fig. 42.3C), and when the hips and knees are extended, it is referred to as to *the footling breech*, as depicted in Fig. 42.3B. With modern methods of delivery, the particular type of breech presentation appears to have no significant effect on adverse outcomes associated with the mode of delivery, despite that cord prolapse occurs much less frequently with frank breech presentation (0.4%) versus complete breech (4–10.5%) or footling breech presentation (15–28.5%).[24,25]

FEATURES

Prolonged breech position in late fetal life gives rise to increased uterine fundal pressure and molding of the fetal head, which may become retroflexed. This type of constraint results in anteroposterior elongation of the head (dolichocephaly) with a prominent occipital shelf, the so-called "breech head" (Fig. 42.4).[26] In cases of ultrasonographic biometric discrepancy between biparietal diameter and femur length, the fetal position should be taken into account.[27] The shoulders are often thrust under the lower auricle, and the mandible may be distorted. The legs may be caught in front of the fetus, which tends to dislocate the hips and, occasionally, causes genu recurvatum of the knee and often calcaneovalgus position of the feet.[28,29] In the frank breech position, with the legs flexed across the abdomen, the feet are likely to be compressed into a calcaneovalgus position, whereas in the complete breech position with the knees flexed, equinovarus foot deformation may develop.[30] The genital region, as the presenting part, may be molded and edematous (Fig. 42.5). Dunn noted that 32% of all deformations in the neonate were related to breech presentation.[3] In his series of more than 6000 babies, 100% of genu recurvatum cases related to breech presentation, as did 50% of hip dislocation cases and 20% to 25% each for cases of mandibular asymmetry, torticollis, and talipes equinovarus (Fig. 42.6). Traction to the brachial plexus or phrenic nerve during difficult deliveries or vaginal breech deliveries may occur, and 75% of cases of diaphragmatic paralysis caused by birth injury have associated brachial plexus palsy.[31–33]

Craniofacial

The head is elongated into a dolichocephalic form, often with a prominent occipital shelf.[27] There may be redundant folds of skin in the posterior neck as a result of compression due to retroflexion of the head (Fig. 42.7). The lambdoid sutures may appear to be overlapping because of the fetal head constraint. The lower auricle may be forced upward into the location where the shoulder has been, and the manubrial region of the mandible may have a "hollow" appearance. The shoulder compression is often asymmetric; hence there may be asymmetry of the mandible with an upward "tilt" on the more compressed side. Torticollis may occur secondary to asymmetric stretching or frank tearing of the sternocleidomastoid muscle, or due to clavicular fracture during a traumatic breech vaginal delivery, and 20% of torticollis cases occur in babies who were in breech presentation.[2,3,5] A study of 224 term infants in breech presentation compared with 3107 term infants in vertex presentation revealed the following anomalies to be associated with breech presentation: frontal bossing, prominent occiput, upward-slanting palpebral fissures, low-set ears, torticollis, and congenital hip dislocation.[34] Dolichocephaly was confirmed by caliper measurements on 100 term infants in breech presentation and compared with 100 term infants in vertex presentation. Third-trimester biparietal diameters were smaller than expected in the breech infants, and the birth cephalic index was less than 76%.[35]

Limbs

All gradations of hip dislocation occur in breech presentation, which is considered to be a consequence of the constrained position in utero forcing the hip from its usual socket. The legs have generally been hyperflexed in front of the fetus, and this is often the "position of comfort" in the early neonatal period (see Figs. 42.2 and 42.3). As a consequence, it may be difficult to fully extend and abduct the hips into the position that is usually used to detect dislocation of the hips. Full movement at the knees may also be somewhat limited. Frank breech presentation is the most common cause of genu recurvatum. The extended leg position may lead to calcaneovalgus foot deformity, whereas the flexed leg position more commonly leads to an equinovarus foot deformity. Traction to the brachial plexus, especially the upper plexus, occurs during delivery when the angle between the neck and shoulder is suddenly and forcibly increased with the arms in an adducted position. This can also occur during breech deliveries when the adducted arm is pulled forcefully downward to free the after-coming head, which accounts for 9% to 24% of brachial plexus palsies.[31,33]

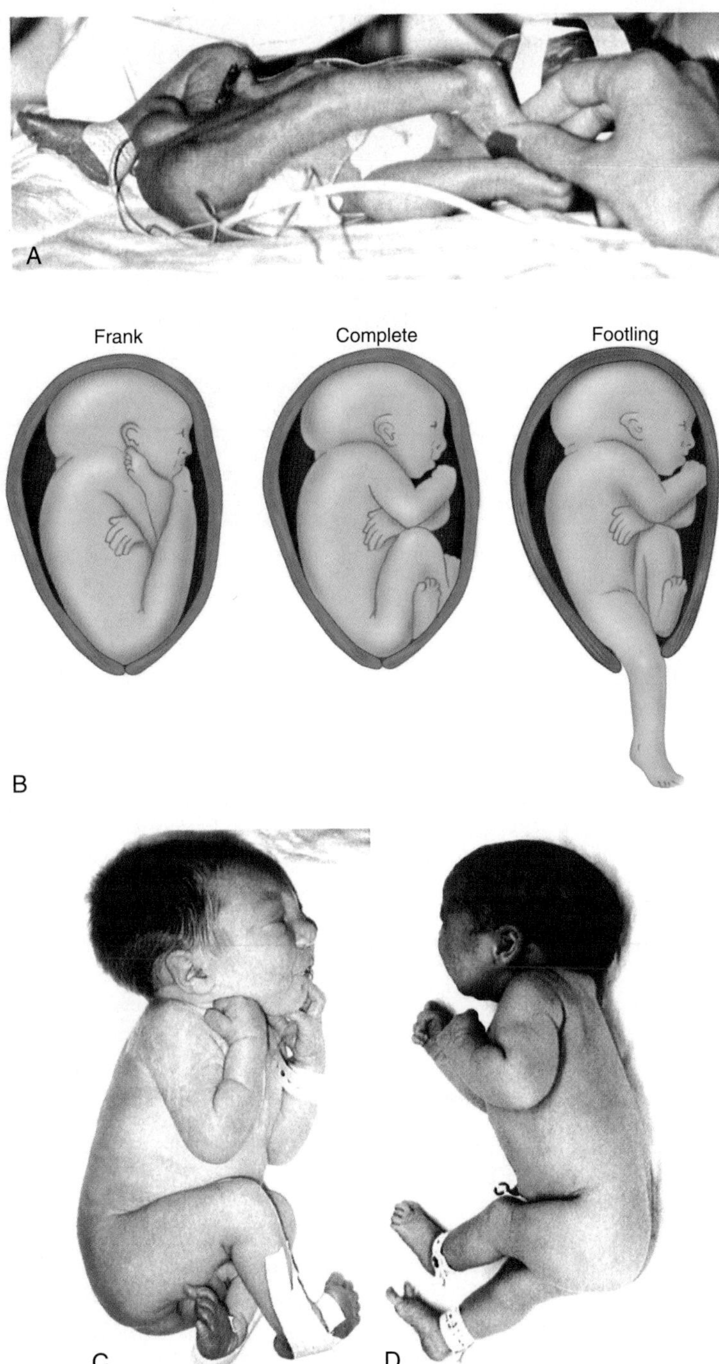

FIGURE 42.3 A, This infant was born prematurely from a frank breech presentation with genu recurvatum as a consequence. B, Diagrams of types of breech presentation. C, This infant had been in complete breech presentation with flexed thighs and knees. Taping treated the equinovarus foot deformations, and a breech head is clearly evident. D, This infant with extended knees and flexed thighs had been in prolonged frank breech presentation with dislocated hips and a breech head. Note the characteristic position of comfort. When the thighs were extended, the result was great discomfort.

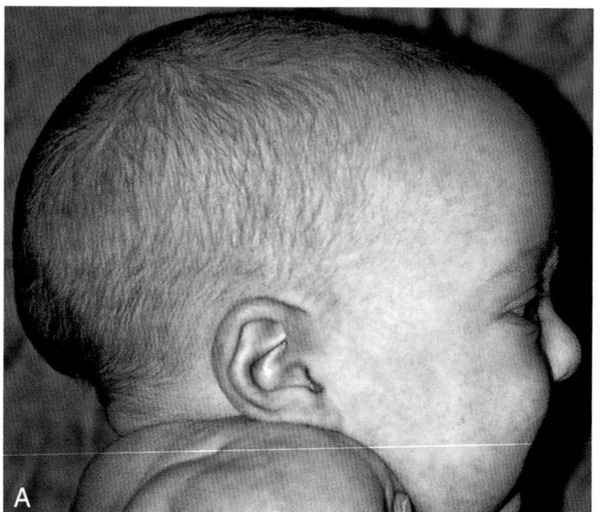

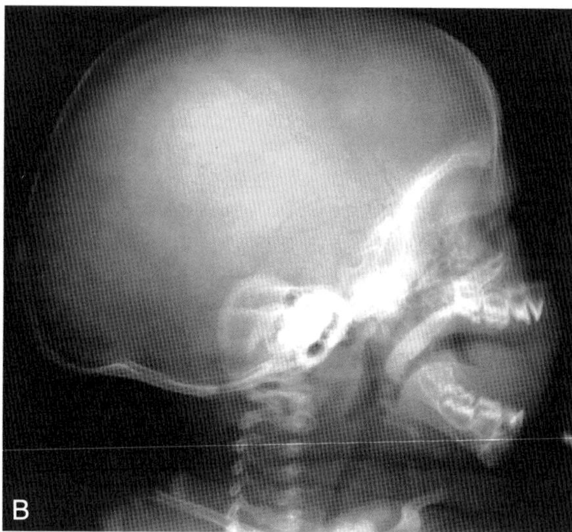

FIGURE 42.4 A, This dolichocephalic breech head demonstrates the tendency for the lower auricle to be uplifted by pressure from the shoulder in utero. B, The prominent occipital shelf is evident on a lateral skull radiograph.

The lower plexus is most susceptible to injury when traction is exerted on an abducted arm, such as occurs during breech deliveries when traction is applied to the trunk or legs while the after-coming arm is fixed in abduction.[26] When traction is particularly rapid and forceful, then diffuse multifocal injury occurs, including avulsion of the roots from the cord in the most severe injuries. Fractures of the femur, humerus, and clavicle are more common in breech babies, as is bruising with secondary hyperbilirubinemia.[3,6]

Genitalia

The buttocks and genitalia tend to be the leading parts at delivery and may show edema and/or bruising (Fig. 42.5). Hydrocele of the testicle is also frequent.[36,37]

OTHER COMPLICATIONS OF BREECH PRESENTATION

Complications presented in this section result primarily from vaginal delivery of a baby in breech presentation. The risk of vaginal delivery must be weighed in each case against the risk of cesarean section. Because more cesarean sections are being performed for breech presentation, especially in the primigravida, the frequency of serious complications has decreased. In 2014, Velmmix et al. summarized data from a large Dutch population-based cohort (1999–2007) that included 58,320 breech deliveries, comparing outcome data before and after 2000. They found an increase in the elective cesarean rate (from 24–60%) and, as a consequence, overall perinatal morbidity and mortality decreased. Neonatal trauma decreased from 4.8% to 2.2% and perinatal deaths decreased from 1.3% to 0.7%.[38] Previously perinatal mortality was 13% for breech presentation, and prematurely born infants, twins, and babies with malformations accounted for much of this mortality rate.[3] It is important to appreciate that the premature baby is more likely to be in the breech position in early gestation. However, it is also important to realize that the breech position *itself* is frequently associated with premature labor. The overall frequency of breech presentation in premature deliveries between 28 and 36 weeks of gestation was 24%.[3] For the term singleton infant in breech presentation without malformation, the perinatal mortality was 1%.[3] The breech fetus is more likely to have the head become entrapped during the second stage of labor, which tends to increase the frequency of tentorial tears and intracranial bleeding, asphyxia (five- to sixfold greater risk), and trauma relating to the attempt to "pull" out the infant during a vaginal delivery.[3] Serious consequences include trauma to the cervicothoracic nerve roots, brachial plexus, and/or compression of the vertebral artery with cerebral ischemia.

In 2022, Nordborg et al. published a metaanalysis of 32 articles published between 1990 and 2021 assessing the safety for the mother and child in 530,604 breech

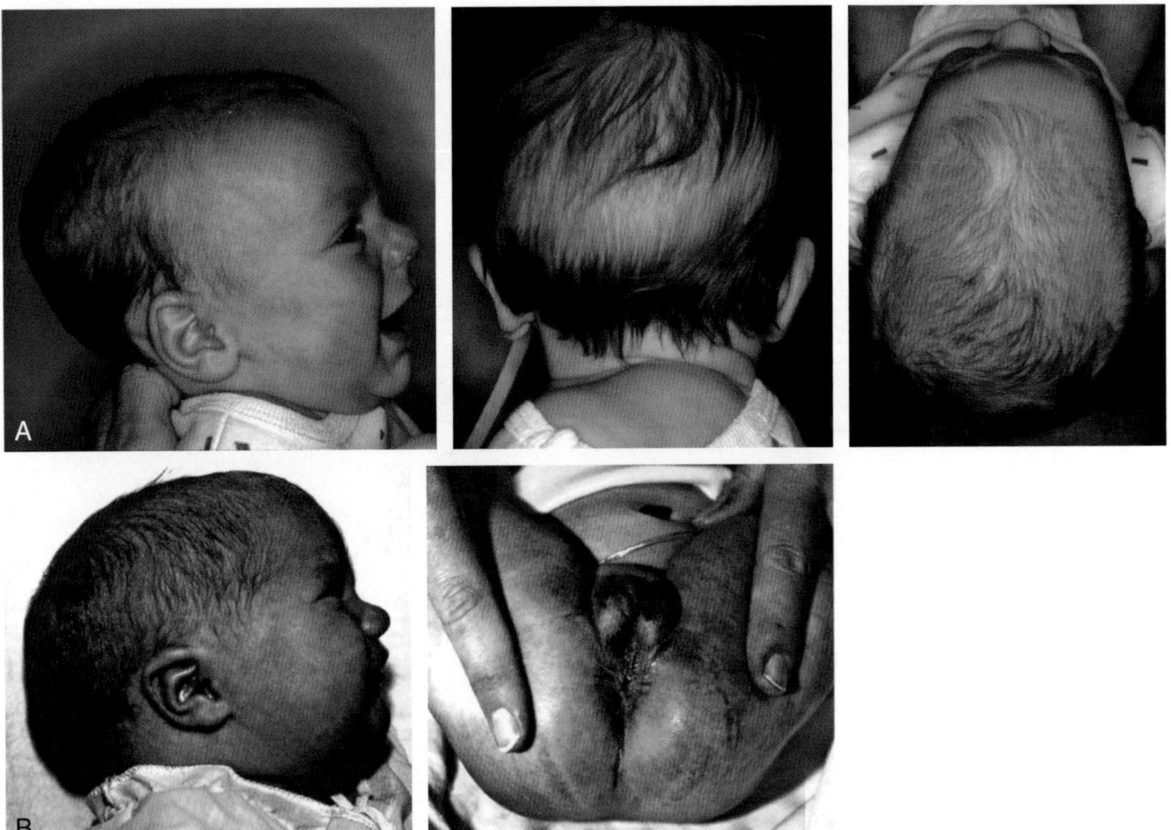

FIGURE 42.5 A, This infant exhibits breech head and overfolded superior helix. B, The edematous swelling on the labia majora and hemorrhagic edematous swelling of the labia minora and external vagina are secondary to prolonged constraint of this presenting part in the frank breech presentation. Look carefully for the ring-like zone around the buttocks and genitalia, which appears to represent the site of cervix indentation on the presenting part.

pregnancies and comparing the intended mode of delivery.[39] The only randomized trial showed reduced risk of perinatal mortality for planned cesarean section, risk ratio (RR): 0.27 (95% CI: 0.08–0.97; 2078 women; low certainty of evidence), stillbirths excluded. A metaanalysis of cohort studies resulted in a similar estimate, RR: 0.36 (95% CI: 0.25–0.51; 21 studies; 388,714 women; low certainty of evidence). They also found reduced risk for outcomes representing perinatal morbidity at 0 to 28 days: 5-min Apgar score less than 7 in one randomized controlled trial, RR: 0.27 (95% CI: 0.12–0.58; 2033 women; moderate certainty of evidence) and in a metaanalysis, RR0.1 (95% CI: 0.14–0.26; 18 studies; 217,024 women; moderate certainty of evidence); Apgar score less than 4 at 5 min, RR: 0.39 (95% CI: 0.19–0.81; 5 studies; 44,498 women; low certainty of evidence); and pH less than 7.0, RR: 0.23 (95% CI: 0.12–0.43; 4 studies; 13,440 women; low certainty of evidence). Outcomes for the mother were similar in the groups except for reduced risk for experience of urinary incontinence in the group of planned cesarean section, RR: 0.62 (95% CI: 0.41–0.93; 1 study; 1940 women; low certainty of evidence). The conversion rate from planned vaginal delivery to emergency cesarean section ranged from 16% to 51% (median: 41.8%; 10 studies; 50,763 women; moderate certainty of evidence).[39]

In a metaanalysis of 24 studies of singleton term breech deliveries published between 1966 and 1992, perinatal mortality was corrected to exclude antepartum stillbirths and infants with major congenital anomalies. The corrected perinatal mortality rate ranged from 0 to 48 per 1000 births among the 24 reports and was higher among infants in the planned

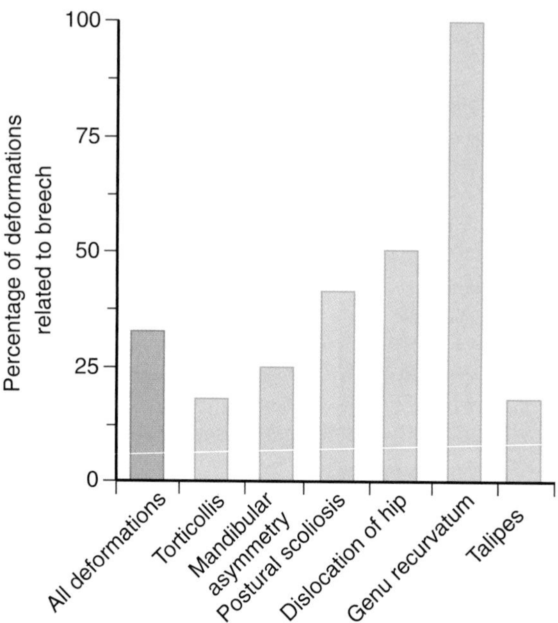

FIGURE 42.6 The percentage of particular deformations related to breech presentation in Dunn's study of more than 6000 newborn infants. (From Dunn PM. Fifth European Congress of Perinatology. *Uppsala, Sweden*, 1976:79.)

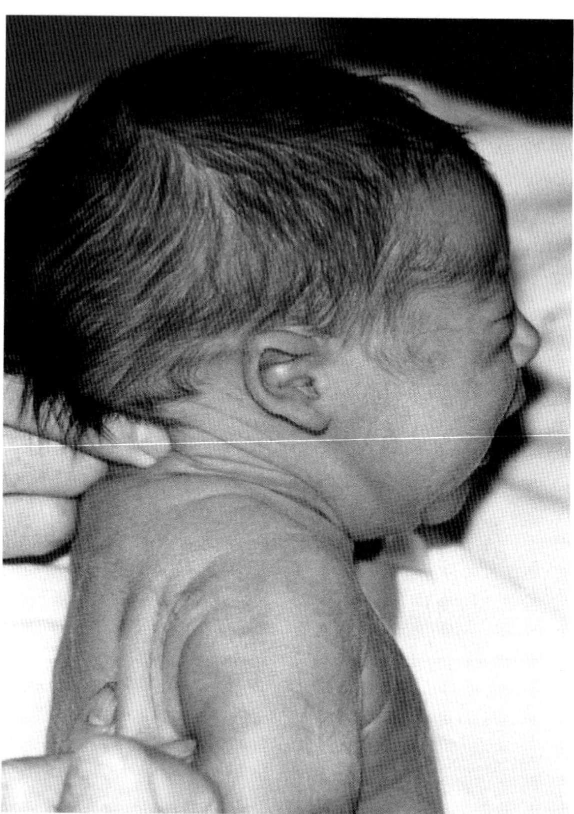

FIGURE 42.7 Breech head with overfolded superior helix and marked skin redundancy over the back from marked compression due to prolonged oligohydramnios.

vaginal delivery group than in the planned cesarean group (odds ratio [OR]: 3.86; 95% CI: 2.22–6.69).[6] The main causes of death were head entrapment, cerebral injury and hemorrhage, cord prolapse, and severe asphyxia. Cord prolapse occurred in as many as 7.4% of women who had a trial of labor, depending on the type of breech presentation (0–2% for frank breech, 5–10.5% for complete breech, 8–16% for double footling breech, and 10–28.5% for single footling breech), with cord prolapse twice as common in multiparas (6%) than in nulliparas (3%).[6] Low 5-minute Apgar scores (i.e., less than 7) occurred more frequently in the planned vaginal delivery group (OR: 1.95; 95% CI: 1.45–2.61), and the incidence of birth trauma was 0.3% to 6% among the 24 studies (OR: 3.96; 95% CI: 2.76–5.67). If all the retrospective studies were excluded, the OR for traumatic birth injuries in the prospective studies was 5.16 (95% CI: 2.63–10.13), and long-term infant morbidity occurred more frequently in the planned vaginal delivery group (OR: 2.88; 95% CI: 1.04–7.97).[6] Cerebral palsy was noted in 16 of 26 affected children and was associated with perinatal factors such as hyperextended head, cord prolapse, or difficult delivery.[6] Overall maternal morbidity was lower among women in the planned vaginal delivery group (OR: 0.61; 95% CI: 0.47–0.80).[6] In a 1999 registry-based case-control study, they found that the risk of cerebral palsy among term breech presentation infants did not seem to be related to mode of delivery.[40]

Among 371,692 singleton live births in breech presentation between 1989 and 1991 in the United States, cesarean delivery had significantly lower neonatal mortality for all birth-weight groups when compared with primary vaginal births, despite a higher prevalence of fetal malformations in the cesarean group.[1] In the group with birth weights >2500 g, neonatal mortality in the primary vaginal birth group was 5.3 per 1000 versus 3.2 per 1000 in the cesarean group.[1] In a study of 15,818 nonmalformed term singleton Swedish infants delivered from breech presentation between 1987 and 1993, infants delivered vaginally were at higher risk for infant mortality (OR: 2.5) and birth injury (OR: 12.2).[41] Infants delivered by emergency cesarean section were at increased risk for neonatal seizures (OR: 4.1), and infants delivered vaginally or by emergency cesarean section were at increased risk for low 5-minute Apgar scores. Maternal morbidity was highest among women who delivered by emergency cesarean section (2.8%) when compared with elective cesarean section (1.7%) and vaginal delivery (1.8%).[41] Among 39,353 Norwegian breech presentation births delivered between 1967 and 1994, the perinatal loss rate was 5.6% (vs. 1.3% for nonbreech presentations), and if antenatal stillbirths were excluded, the rates were 3.9% for breech versus 0.76% for vertex, suggesting that live breech infants were five times more likely to die during the perinatal period than nonbreech infants.[10] The relative risk for perinatal death was higher for vaginal delivery than for cesarean delivery (relative risk: 5.4; 95% CI: 4.7–6.2). Studies that reported no significant differences in neonatal morbidity and mortality for vaginal versus cesarean deliveries of infants in breech presentation generally involved smaller numbers (705 or 268 consecutive breech presentations) at one or two institutions.[16,24]

Of gravest concern is the vaginal delivery of a breech fetus with a hyperextended head (ultrasound-measured angle of less than 90 degrees between the cervical vertebrae and the tangent plane of the occipital bone), which occurs in 11% to 15% of breech fetuses and was associated with cervical cord damage in 8 of 11 cases delivered vaginally versus 0 of 20 fetuses delivered by cesarean section.[42] Abroms et al. reported a 21% incidence of cervical cord transection among 88 neonates born with hyperextension of the head associated with breech and transverse presentations.[43] All neonates with cord transection were delivered vaginally, whereas none of the neonates delivered by cesarean section suffered permanent spinal cord transection. These results have been confirmed in other studies demonstrating a 22% risk of long-term neurologic sequalae in association with hyperextension of the fetal head and a high risk of spinal cord injury that may be prevented by elective cesarean delivery.[44–49] The acute symptoms of cervical cord transection are usually respiratory problems, a weak cry, poor muscle tone, poor feeding, and often death with high cervical lesions.

In vaginal breech deliveries, the mechanism of injury is usually longitudinal distraction, which leaves the vertebral column intact and occurs most frequently in the lower cervical or upper thoracic region, resulting in symptoms of diaphragmatic breathing and hypotonia with hyperreflexia that is worse in the lower extremities, with or without associated brachial plexus and phrenic nerve injury.[49,50] Thus, plain radiographs are not helpful, but spinal ultrasound and magnetic resonance imaging can localize and define the extent of the lesion (Fig. 42.8).[50–53] Survivors are usually severely debilitated with spastic diplegia or quadriplegia. Lesser degrees of cord damage at C5 to C6 may produce hand and forearm weakness with flexor weakness and wrist drop. Less commonly, the damage occurs at the C8 to T1 cord level, yielding extensor weakness with the fingers and hands flexed. About 50% of infants with Erb and Klumpke pareses recover, usually by 3 to 5 months of age. Compression of the vertebral artery may occur, which yields secondary problems in the medullary area of the brain. A number of cerebral palsy cases in the past may have been related to problems engendered by vaginal breech delivery; however, one recent paper attributes the higher risk of cerebral palsy in breech versus vertex presentations (OR: 1.56; 95% CI: 0.9–2.4) to a higher rate of breech infants who are small for gestational age.[40] Breech presentation infants were more commonly classified as diplegic (77.8%) than were vertex presentation infants (42.3%).[40]

Another complication that may be secondary to vaginal breech delivery is traumatic transection of the pituitary stalk during delivery, with consequent hypopituitarism.[54–56] Among patients with ectopia of the posterior pituitary, absence or hypoplasia of the pituitary stalk, and hypoplasia of the anterior pituitary, there is a strong association with vaginal breech delivery and multiple pituitary hormone deficiency.[55,56] A traumatic cause could only explain 32% of such cases, and other cases had associated congenital midline brain anomalies.[56,57] One paper suggested that vaginal breech delivery of patients with this syndrome resulted in multiple pituitary hormone deficiencies, whereas cesarean section or normal vertex delivery was followed only by idiopathic growth hormone deficiency.[55]

MANAGEMENT, PROGNOSIS, AND COUNSEL

In the prevention and management of breech presentation, three factors must be considered. First is the prevention of deformities and complications due to vaginal delivery by moving the fetus into the vertex position before the time of delivery via a method referred to as *external cephalic version*. Second is the avoidance of complications related to vaginal delivery of the breech fetus by using cesarean section delivery, particularly when the fetal head is hyperextended. Third is the management of any deformations and complications after delivery of the breech fetus.

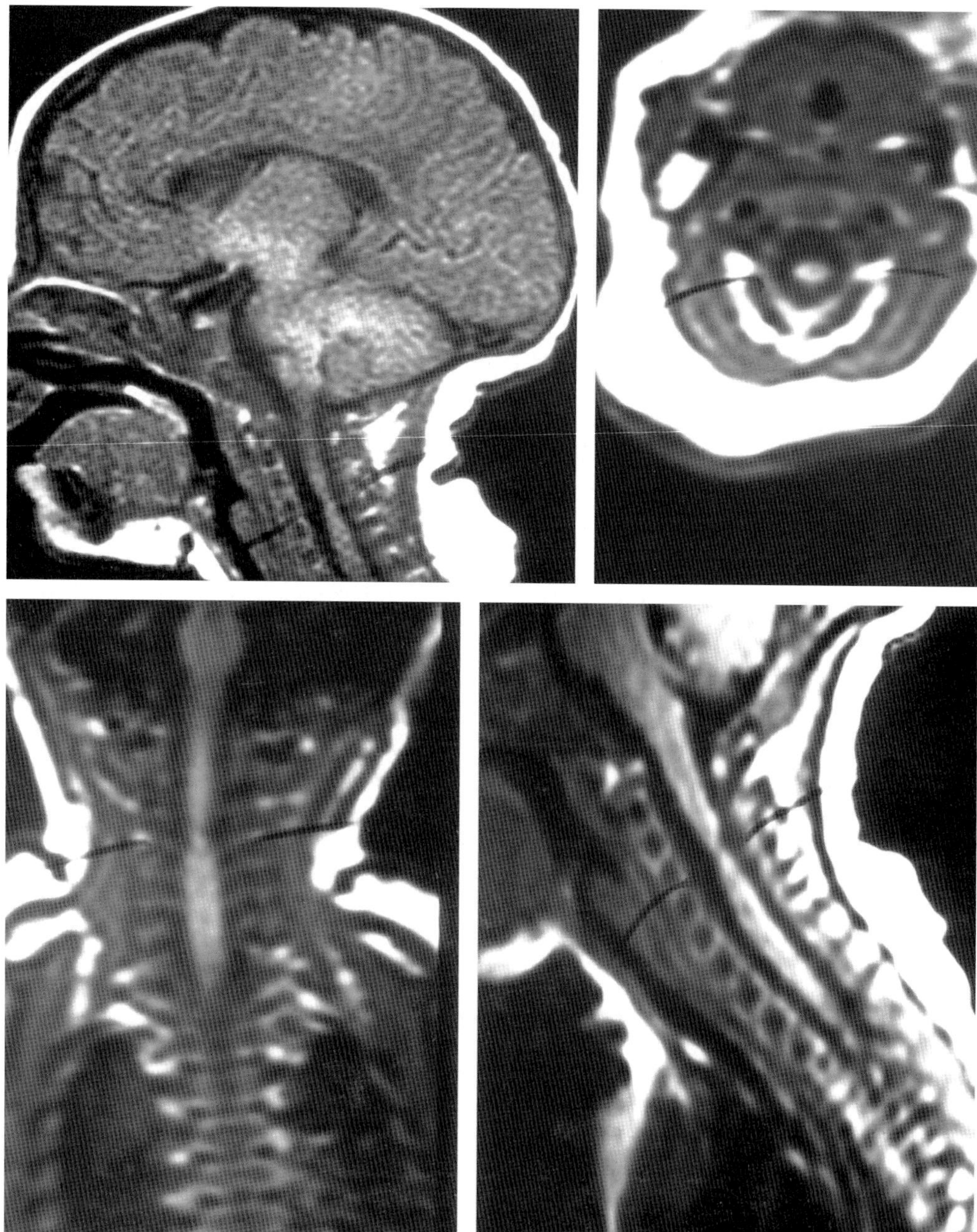

FIGURE 42.8 Cord transection caused by vaginal delivery of a fetus in breech presentation. The slash marks indicate cervical cord constriction caused by the injury.

External Cephalic Version

External cephalic version (ECV) is the external manipulation of the fetus from the breech or transverse position into the vertex position (Fig. 42.9). Current opinion holds that in late pregnancy, ECV should be offered to mothers with a singleton breech presentation, using tocolytics in nulliparous women to relax the uterus.[17] This procedure is successful in 40% of nulliparous women and 60% of multiparous women

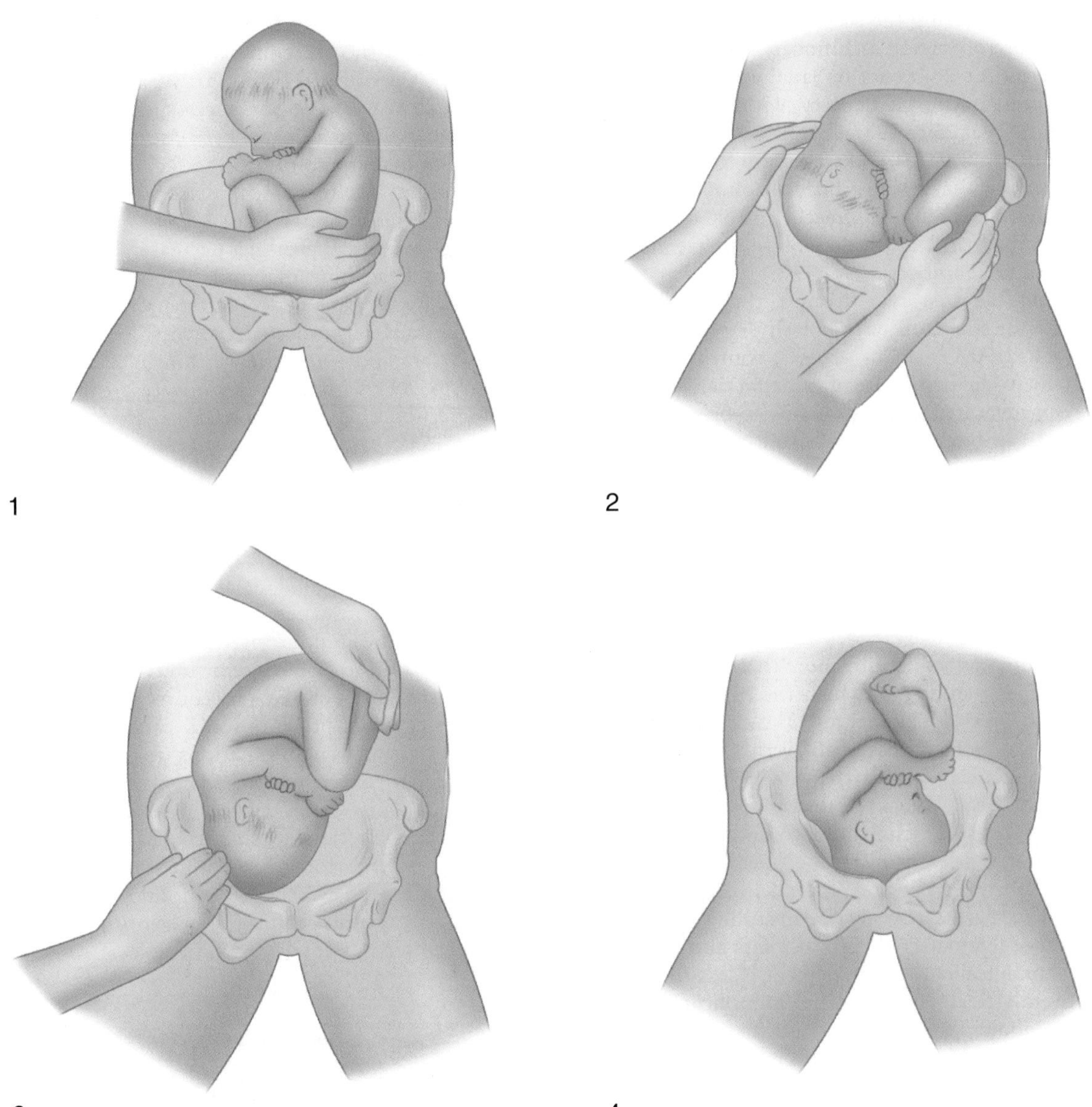

FIGURE 42.9 External cephalic version maneuvers, which are usually performed between 35 and 37 weeks of gestation, convert a breech presentation to a cephalic presentation.

when performed after 38 weeks.[10] A 2006 and 2012 Cochrane Database Review found that overall, studies of ECV were successful in 9.5% of cases and had a 7% decrease in the cesarean section rates when ECV was started early.[58] The pooled data from these studies show a statistically significant and clinically meaningful reduction in noncephalic birth (1245 women; RR: 0.46; 95% CI 0.31–0.66) and cesarean section (1245 women; RR: 0.63; 95% CI: 0.44–0.90) when ECV was attempted, although no significant differences are seen in Apgar score ratings, umbilical artery pH levels, neonatal intensive care unit admissions or perinatal deaths.[59] In a retrospective study of 157 breech deliveries and 1325 vertex deliveries followed by ultrasound examinations during the second and third trimesters (without use of version techniques), fetuses in breech presentation at 25 weeks or later were at high risk for malpresentation at delivery, with 71% of breech presentations at 25 to 29 weeks and 83% of breech presentations at 32 to 34 weeks persisting until delivery. After the 33rd week, there is little likelihood of a vertex presentation changing to breech, and 90% of fetuses in both breech and vertex presentation have assumed their final presentation.[60]

During the past two decades, the cesarean section rate for singleton term breech presentations has approached 90% in many centers, contributing substantially to the rising rate of cesarean delivery.[12] ECV has been advocated as an alternative to breech delivery and cesarean birth, and is safe and cost effective.[56,60] In a review of 12 US studies on 1339 patients undergoing external version at 35 weeks or later and using similar protocols (patient selection, tocolysis, ultrasound scanning, cardiotocographic monitoring, and Rh immunoglobulin protection), 63.3% had a vaginal delivery and 36.7% had cesarean births, whereas 83.2% of controls had cesarean delivery; thus the cesarean delivery rate was reduced by more than half.[61] Among five European studies in which external version was attempted on 541 patients at 33 weeks or later, the success rate and proportion of vertex vaginal deliveries was about 10% lower than in the United States, but the cesarean delivery rate was not significantly reduced because of the more common practice of vaginal breech delivery in Europe.[61] Fetal deaths (from placental abruption or premature delivery) in relation to ECV have been extremely rare in studies since 1980. The rate of fetomaternal transfusion is about 3%, the risk of umbilical cord entanglement is less than 1.5%, and overall fetal and maternal complication rates are each about 1%.[61] Such risks can be minimized by careful patient selection and fetal monitoring, and by using the procedure only when prompt cesarean section can be performed. ECV is generally more successful in multiparous women than nulliparous women, hence tocolysis has been advocated for nulliparous women.[17] The earlier external version is performed, the more likely it will be successful, and external version just before term is no longer encouraged because of the higher rate of spontaneous reversion and the risk of fetal distress and premature delivery.[61] Some authors who reported lower success rates of 35% for ECV attempted at 37 weeks attribute this less-than-expected rate of success to lack of experience on the part of the some operators, suggesting that the procedure be restricted to a few experienced staff members.[62] Others suggest the procedure is much safer and more successful if performed before 37 weeks (79% success rate prior to 37 weeks vs. 53% success rate if performed during or after the 37th week).[63] Use of antepartum transabdominal amnioinfusion to facilitate ECV after initial failure has met with mixed success,[64,65] and use of ECV with spinal anesthesia[66] or tocolysis at 37 weeks or later appears to decrease maternal discomfort and facilitate manipulation. There are even advocates for external version after previous cesarean section in carefully selected patients.[67,68] One study reported safe and successful version in 25 of the 38 women (65.8%) who had previous cesarean section when safety criteria were observed.[69]

Cesarean Section

When a fetus is in breech presentation, the second line of prevention is to strive to forestall the potential complications of vaginal delivery by accomplishing a cesarean section when indicated.[6,9,10,41] Box 42.1 lists some of the indications for a cesarean delivery. Cesarean section in transverse or breech presentation involves more complicated procedures than cesarean section in cephalic presentation because the former requires additional manipulations for guiding the presenting part of the fetus.[70] As concerns about the complications of vaginal delivery of the breech fetus have increased in recent years, so also has the frequency of cesarean section for breech presentation; however appropriate use of ECV has been found to be a safe and cost-effective procedure for preventing the need for cesarean section in selected patients.

BOX 42.1 FACTORS FAVORING CESAREAN SECTION DELIVERY OF A FETUS IN BREECH PRESENTATION

- Dolichocephalic breech head with prominent occipital shelf
- Hyperextended head
- Contracted pelvis
- Large baby weighing more than 4.0 kg
- Small baby weighing less than 2.5 kg
- Placenta previa
- Maternal hypertension
- Uterine dysfunction
- Primigravida, especially if ≥35 years
- Footling breech presentation
- Previous pregnancy losses

MANAGEMENT OF DEFORMATIONS AND COMPLICATIONS

After birth, the head shape and mandibular form gradually return to normal, with no management required. If the hips are dislocated, a more rigorous management is indicated (see Chapter 11). The hydrocele of the testis that may develop is considered a benign lesion that rarely merits therapy.[37] Tears of sternocleidomastoid muscles may occur, and 20% of torticollis cases occur in babies who were in breech presentation.[2] Early treatment of torticollis can prevent secondary plagiocephaly (see Chapter 24).

DIFFERENTIAL DIAGNOSIS

The most important question about infants with breech deformation complex is whether an otherwise normal infant became caught in the breech position. If so, the prognosis without birth complications is usually excellent. If the infant was in the breech presentation *because* of a fetal problem, the prognosis relates predominantly to the basic diagnosis, with the addition of secondary deformities due to breech presentation and/or the disruptive complications that may occur with vaginal delivery. The overall frequency of breech presentation in newborn babies with malformations is 23%, about eight times the general frequency.[3] These patients account for a sizable proportion of the excess mortality of babies born in breech presentation, particularly when there is intrauterine growth retardation. Certain types of malformation problems are notorious for failing to undergo normal version to a vertex presentation. The cause may be a structural defect, a neuromuscular defect, a renal defect resulting in oligohydramnios, or a problem of crowding. Table 42.1 lists some of the defects in which breech presentation is a frequent occurrence.[2,26,71]

An elongated scaphocephalic head may result from sagittal craniosynostosis. Usually, palpation of a ridged posterior sagittal suture is all that is required to clarify this diagnosis. Any doubt that might exist can usually be resolved by radiographs and follow-up examination, which usually shows progressive improvement toward normal form for the molded breech head. The shape of the breech head may yield a spuriously decreased prenatal biparietal diameter[35] or suggest an increased head circumference after birth, which raises concern about hydrocephalus or macrocephaly. Generally, this question can be resolved by simple examination of the head and sutures or cranial ultrasound.

Table 42.1 Disorders Predisposing a Fetus Toward Breech Presentation

Disorder	Breech Frequency
Lack of Leg Thrust	
Lower limb deficiency	60%
Meningomyelocele (general)	38%
Meningomyelocele with leg paralysis	93%
Neurologic Deficiency	
Anencephaly	Excess
Prader-Willi syndrome	50%
Myotonic dystrophy	Excess
Amyoplasia arthrogryposis	Excess
Smith-Lemli-Opitz syndrome	40%
Oligohydramnios with Limited Mobility	
Renal agenesis	50%
Infantile polycystic kidney disease	Excess
Urethral obstruction malformation sequence	Excess
Chronic leakage of amniotic fluid	64%
Crowding with limited mobility	
Maternal bicornuate uterus	46%
Twinning	34%

Dislocation of the hip may result from a number of causes. When there is a basic problem in the connective tissues that enhances the likelihood of mechanical dislocation, joints other than the hip are usually also affected. In the usual breech presentation patient who has developmental dysplasia of the hips, the joints are generally *less* mobile and painful when extended due to prolonged deficit in full range of movement. Finally, the multiple consequences of prolonged breech presentation may sometimes be mistakenly interpreted as a multiple malformation disorder.

References

1. Lee KS, Khoshnood B, Sriram S, Hsieh HL, Singh J, Mittendorf R. Relationship of cesarean delivery to lower birth weight-specific neonatal mortality in singleton breech infants in the United States. *Obstet Gynecol.* 1998;92(5):769–774.
2. Dunn PM. Congenital postural deformities. *Br Med Bull.* 1976;32(1):71–76.

3. Dunn PM. Breech delivery: perinatal morbidity and mortality. Presented at the 5th European Congress of Perinatal Medicine, Uppsala, Sweden, pp 76–81, 1976.
4. Moh W, Graham Jr. JM, Wadhawan I, Sanchez-Lara PA. Extrinsic factors influencing fetal deformations and intrauterine growth restriction. *J Pregnancy*. 2012;2012:750485.
5. van Cruchten C, Feijen MMW, van der Hulst R. Demographics of positional plagiocephaly and brachycephaly; risk factors and treatment. *J Craniofac Surg*. 2021;32(8):2736–2740.
6. Cheng M, Hannah M. Breech delivery at term: a critical review of the literature. *Obstet Gynecol*. 1993;82(4 Pt 1): 605–618.
7. Chen AX, Hunt RW, Palmer KR, Bull CF, Callander EJ. The impact of assisted reproductive technology and ovulation induction on breech presentation: a whole of population-based cohort study. *Aust N Z J Obstet Gynaecol*. 2023.
8. Herbst A, Thorngren-Jerneck K. Mode of delivery in breech presentation at term: increased neonatal morbidity with vaginal delivery. *Acta Obstet Gynecol Scand*. 2001;80(8):731–737.
9. Thorpe-Beeston JG, Banfield PJ, Saunders NJ. Outcome of breech delivery at term. *BMJ*. 1992;305(6856):746–747.
10. Albrechtsen S, Rasmussen S, Dalaker K, Irgens LM. Perinatal mortality in breech presentation sibships. *Obstet Gynecol*. 1998;92(5):775–780.
11. Krispin E, Fischer O, Kneller M, et al. Fetal extraction maneuvers during cesarean delivery in the second stage of labor. *J Matern Fetal Neonatal Med*. 2022;35(11):2070–2076.
12. Gunay T, Turgut A, Demircivi Bor E, Hocaoglu M. Comparison of maternal and fetal complications in pregnant women with breech presentation undergoing spontaneous or induced vaginal delivery, or cesarean delivery. *Taiwan J Obstet Gynecol*. 2020;59(3):392–397.
13. Bevilacqua E, Jani JC, Meli F, et al. Pregnancy outcomes in breech presentation at term: a comparison between 2 third level birth center protocols. *AJOG Glob Rep*. 2022;2(4):100086.
14. Mailath-Pokorny M, Preyer O, Dadak C, et al. Breech presentation: a retrospective analysis of 12-years' experience at a single center. *Wien Klin Wochenschr*. 2009;121(5-6):209–215.
15. Pradhan P, Mohajer M, Deshpande S. Outcome of term breech births: 10-year experience at a district general hospital. *BJOG*. 2005;112(2):218–222.
16. Irion O, Hirsbrunner Almagbaly P, Morabia A. Planned vaginal delivery versus elective caesarean section: a study of 705 singleton term breech presentations. *Br J Obstet Gynaecol*. 1998;105(7):710–717.
17. Chamberlain G, Steer P. ABC of labour care: unusual presentations and positions and multiple pregnancy. *BMJ*. 1999;318(7192):1192–1194.
18. Fonseca A, Silva R, Rato I, et al. Breech presentation: vaginal versus cesarean delivery, which intervention leads to the best outcomes? *Acta Med Port*. 2017;30(6):479–484.
19. Fernández-Carrasco FJ, Cristóbal-Cañadas D, Gómez-Salgado J, Vázquez-Lara JM, Rodríguez-Díaz L, Parrón-Carreño T. Maternal and fetal risks of planned vaginal breech delivery vs planned caesarean section for term breech birth: a systematic review and meta-analysis. *J Glob Health*. 2022;12:04055.
20. Kotaska A, Menticoglou S, Gagnon R, et al. SOGC clinical practice guideline: vaginal delivery of breech presentation: no. 226, June 2009. *Int J Gynaecol Obstet*. 2009;107(2):169–176.
21. ACOG Committee Opinion No. 340 Mode of term singleton breech delivery. *Obstet Gynecol*. 2006;108(1):235–237.
22. Robson S, Ramsay B, Chandler K. Registrar experience in vaginal breech delivery. How much is occurring? *Aust N Z J Obstet Gynaecol*. 1999;39(2):215–217.
23. Tompkins P. An inquiry into the causes of breech presentation. *Am J Obstet Gynecol*. 1946;51:595–606.
24. de Leeuw JP, de Haan J, Derom R, Thiery M, van Maele G, Martens G. Indications for caesarean section in breech presentation. *Eur J Obstet Gynecol Reprod Biol*. 1998;79(2):131–137.
25. Ghosh MK. Breech presentation: evolution of management. *J Reprod Med*. 2005;50(2):108–116.
26. Haberkern CM, Smith DW, Jones KL. The 'breech head' and its relevance. *Am J Dis Child*. 1979;133(2):154–156.
27. Lubusky M, Prochazka M, Langova M, Vomackova K, Cizek L. Discrepancy in ultrasound biometric parameters of the head (HC--head circumference, BPD--biparietal diameter) in breech presented fetuses. *Biomed Pap Med Fac Univ Palacky Olomouc Czech Repub*. 2007;151(2):323–326.
28. Sioutis S, Kolovos S, Papakonstantinou ME, Reppas L, Koulalis D, Mavrogenis AF. Developmental dysplasia of the hip: a review. *J Long Term Eff Med Implants*. 2022;32(3):39–56.
29. Lankinen V, Helminen M, Bakti K, Välipakka J, Laivuori H, Hyvärinen A. Known risk factors of the developmental dysplasia of the hip predicting more severe clinical presentation and failure of Pavlik harness treatment. *BMC Pediatr*. 2023;23(1):148.
30. Håberg Ø, Foss OA, Lian ØB, Holen KJ. Is foot deformity associated with developmental dysplasia of the hip? *Bone Joint J*. 2020;102-b(11):1582–1586.
31. Painter MJ, Bergman I. Obstetrical trauma to the neonatal central and peripheral nervous system. *Semin Perinatol*. 1982;6(1):89–104.
32. Reichard R. Birth injury of the cranium and central nervous system. *Brain Pathol*. 2008;18(4):565–570.
33. Shiohama T, Fujii K, Hayashi M, et al. Phrenic nerve palsy associated with birth trauma--case reports and a literature review. *Brain Dev*. 2013;35(4):363–366.
34. Hsieh YY, Tsai FJ, Lin CC, Chang FC, Tsai CH. Breech deformation complex in neonates. *J Reprod Med*. 2000;45(11):933–935.

35. Kasby CB, Poll V. The breech head and its ultrasound significance. *Br J Obstet Gynaecol.* 1982;89(2):106–110.
36. Cumston CG. Remarks on the pathology of congenital hydrocele. *Buffalo Med J.* 1897;36(12):907–919.
37. Dagur G, Gandhi J, Suh Y, et al. Classifying hydroceles of the pelvis and groin: an overview of etiology, secondary complications, evaluation, and management. *Curr Urol.* 2017;10(1):1–14.
38. Vlemmix F, Bergenhenegouwen L, Schaaf JM, et al. Term breech deliveries in the Netherlands: did the increased cesarean rate affect neonatal outcome? A population-based cohort study. *Acta Obstet Gynecol Scand.* 2014;93(9):888–896.
39. Wängberg Nordborg J, Svanberg T, Strandell A, Carlsson Y. Term breech presentation-Intended cesarean section versus intended vaginal delivery: a systematic review and meta-analysis. *Acta Obstet Gynecol Scand.* 2022;101(6):564–576.
40. Krebs L, Topp M, Langhoff-Roos J. The relation of breech presentation at term to cerebral palsy. *Br J Obstet Gynaecol.* 1999;106(9):943–947.
41. Roman J, Bakos O, Cnattingius S. Pregnancy outcomes by mode of delivery among term breech births: Swedish experience 1987-1993. *Obstet Gynecol.* 1998;92(6):945–950.
42. Ballas S, Toaff R. Hyperextension of the fetal head in breech presentation: radiological evaluation and significance. *Br J Obstet Gynaecol.* 1976;83(3):201–204.
43. Abroms IF, Bresnan MJ, Zuckerman JE, Fischer EG, Strand R. Cervical cord injuries secondary to hyperextension of the head in breech presentations. *Obstet Gynecol.* 1973;41(3):369–378.
44. Westgren M, Grundsell H, Ingemarsson I, Muhlow A, Svenningsen NW. Hyperextension of the fetal head in breech presentation. A study with long-term follow-up. *Br J Obstet Gynaecol.* 1981;88(2):101–104.
45. Caterini H, Langer A, Sama JC, Devanesan M, Pelosi MA. Fetal risk in hyperextension of the fetal head in breech presentation. *Am J Obstet Gynecol.* 1975;123(6):632–636.
46. Daw E. Management of the hyperextended fetal head. *Am J Obstet Gynecol.* 1976;124(2):113–115.
47. Weinstein D, Margalioth EJ, Navot D, Mor-Yosef S, Eyal F. Neonatal fetal death following cesarean section secondary to hyperextended head in breech presentation. *Acta Obstet Gynecol Scand.* 1983;62(6):629–631.
48. Bhagwanani SG, Price HV, Laurence KM, Ginz B. Risks and prevention of cervical cord injury in the management of breech presentation with hyperextension of the fetal head. *Am J Obstet Gynecol.* 1973;115(8):1159–1161.
49. Ballas S, Toaff R, Jaffa AJ. Deflexion of the fetal head in breech presentation. Incidence, management, and outcome. *Obstet Gynecol.* 1978;52(6):653–655.
50. de Vries E, Robben SG, van den Anker JN. Radiologic imaging of severe cervical spinal cord birth trauma. *Eur J Pediatr.* 1995;154(3):230–232.
51. Morota N, Sakamoto K, Kobayashi N. Traumatic cervical syringomyelia related to birth injury. *Childs Nerv Syst.* 1992;8(4):234–236.
52. Rossitch Jr. E, Oakes WJ. Perinatal spinal cord injury: clinical, radiographic and pathologic features. *Pediatr Neurosurg.* 1992;18(3):149–152.
53. Vialle R, Pietin-Vialle C, Ilharreborde B, Dauger S, Vinchon M, Glorion C. Spinal cord injuries at birth: a multicenter review of nine cases. *J Maternal-Fetal & Neonatal Med.* 2007;20(6):435–440.
54. Fujita K, Matsuo N, Mori O, et al. The association of hypopituitarism with small pituitary, invisible pituitary stalk, type 1 Arnold-Chiari malformation, and syringomyelia in seven patients born in breech position: a further proof of birth injury theory on the pathogenesis of "idiopathic hypopituitarism". *Eur J Pediatr.* 1992;151(4):266–270.
55. Maghnie M, Larizza D, Triulzi F, Sampaolo P, Scotti G, Severi F. Hypopituitarism and stalk agenesis: a congenital syndrome worsened by breech delivery? *Horm Res.* 1991;35(3-4):104–108.
56. Triulzi F, Scotti G, di Natale B, et al. Evidence of a congenital midline brain anomaly in pituitary dwarfs: a magnetic resonance imaging study in 101 patients. *Pediatrics.* 1994;93(3):409–416.
57. Binder G, Nagel BH, Ranke MB, Mullis PE. Isolated GH deficiency (IGHD) type II: imaging of the pituitary gland by magnetic resonance reveals characteristic differences in comparison with severe IGHD of unknown origin. *Europ J Endocrin.* 2002;147(6):755–760.
58. Hutton EK, Hofmeyr GJ, Dowswell T. External cephalic version for breech presentation before term. *Cochrane Database Syst Rev.* 2015;7:CD000084.
59. Hofmeyr GJ, Kulier R. External cephalic version for breech presentation at term. *Cochrane Database Syst Rev.* 2012;10:CD000083.
60. Tadmor OP, Rabinowitz R, Alon L, Mostoslavsky V, Aboulafia Y, Diamant YZ. Can breech presentation at birth be predicted from ultrasound examinations during the second or third trimesters? *Int J Gynaecol Obstet.* 1994;46(1):11–14.
61. Zhang J, Bowes Jr. WA, Fortney JA. Efficacy of external cephalic version: a review. *Obstet Gynecol.* 1993;82(2):306–312.
62. Thunedborg P, Fischer-Rasmussen W, Tollund L. The benefit of external cephalic version with tocolysis as a routine procedure in late pregnancy. *Eur J Obstet Gynecol Reprod Biol.* 1991;42(1):23–27.
63. Kornman MT, Kimball KT, Reeves KO. Preterm external cephalic version in an outpatient environment. *Am J Obstet Gynecol.* 1995;172(6):1734–1738; discussion 1738-1741.
64. Benifla JL, Goffinet F, Darai E, Madelenat P. Antepartum transabdominal amnioinfusion to facilitate external cephalic version after initial failure. *Obstet Gynecol.* 1994;84(6):1041–1042.
65. Adama van Scheltema PN, Feitsma AH, Middeldorp JM, Vandenbussche FP, Oepkes D. Amnioinfusion to

facilitate external cephalic version after initial failure. *Obstet Gynecol.* 2006;108(3 Pt 1):591–592.

66. Dugoff L, Stamm CA, Jones 3rd OW, Mohling SI, Hawkins JL. The effect of spinal anesthesia on the success rate of external cephalic version: a randomized trial. *Obstet Gynecol.* 1999;93(3):345–349.
67. Shalev E, Battino S, Giladi Y, Edelstein S. External cephalic version at term--using tocolysis. *Acta Obstet Gynecol Scand.* 1993;72(6):455–457.
68. Schachter M, Kogan S, Blickstein I. External cephalic version after previous cesarean section: a clinical dilemma. *Int J Gynaecol Obstet.* 1994;45(1):17–20.
69. de Meeus JB, Ellia F, Magnin G. External cephalic version after previous cesarean section: a series of 38 cases. *Eur J Obstet Gynecol Reprod Biol.* 1998;81(1):65–68.
70. Takeda J, Ishikawa G, Takeda S. Clinical tips of cesarean section in case of breech, transverse presentation, and incarcerated uterus. *Surg J (N Y).* 2020;6(Suppl 2):S81–s91.
71. Braun FH, Jones KL, Smith DW. Breech presentation as an indicator of fetal abnormality. *J Pediatr.* 1975;86(3):419–421.

CHAPTER 43

Transverse Lie Deformation

KEY POINTS

- Transverse lie is the second most common nonvertex presentation during delivery, occurring in 1.2–3 per 100 deliveries.
- Multiparity, prematurity, placenta previa, polyhydramnios, uterine anomalies, and uterine myomas are associated with transverse lie.
- Laxity of abdominal musculature in multiparous women is considered the primary factor contributing to transverse lie in these women.
- Transverse lie can lead to facial flattening, limited mandibular growth, retroflexed head, prominent occipital shelf, torticollis, scoliosis, and other associated deformations.
- Management options for transverse lie at term include expectant management, external cephalic version, or elective cesarean section.
- The facial compression resulting from transverse lie can create facial features that may resemble a malformation syndrome or craniosynostosis, leading to potential differential diagnoses.

GENESIS

Transverse lie is the second most common nonvertex presentation and occurs in 1.2–3 per 100 deliveries.[1–3] It is associated with multiparity (90%), prematurity (13%), placenta previa (11%), polyhydramnios (8%), uterine anomalies (8%), and uterine myomas (3%), especially when myomas are located in the lower uterine segment.[4,5] Predisposing factors such as uterine structural anomalies, prematurity, and placenta previa are found in 66% of primiparas, but only 33% of multiparas manifest these factors.[3] Thus multiparity is the most common factor, and women delivering transverse-lying infants tend to be older than those delivering vertex-presenting infants; the other factors such as low-lying placenta, uterine anomalies, myomas, or prematurity occur more frequently in primigravidas. Laxity of abdominal musculature in multiparous women is considered the predominant factor accounting for the liability toward transverse lie in these women. The occurrence of polyhydramnios may relate to the inability of the fetus to swallow amniotic fluid because the mouth is pushed up against the side of the uterus.

FEATURES

Full frontal constraint may flatten the face, limit mandibular growth, and cause a retroflexed head with a prominent occipital shelf. There may be associated torticollis and/or scoliosis, as well as other associated deformations (Figs. 43.1–43.3).

MANAGEMENT

Management of transverse lie at term consists of expectant management, external cephalic version, or elective cesarean section.[6,7] With expectant management, the spontaneous conversion rate to a longitudinal lie before labor is as high as 83%.[6,8,9] This must be weighed against the increased risks of cord prolapse (7–14%) and birth trauma/asphyxia with persistent transverse lie and against the risks of cesarean section.[2,10] Oligohydramnios and prolonged transverse lie may harm the fetus, producing neonatal compartment syndrome.[10] For these reasons, external version followed by induction of labor has been recommended for multiparous women, but transverse

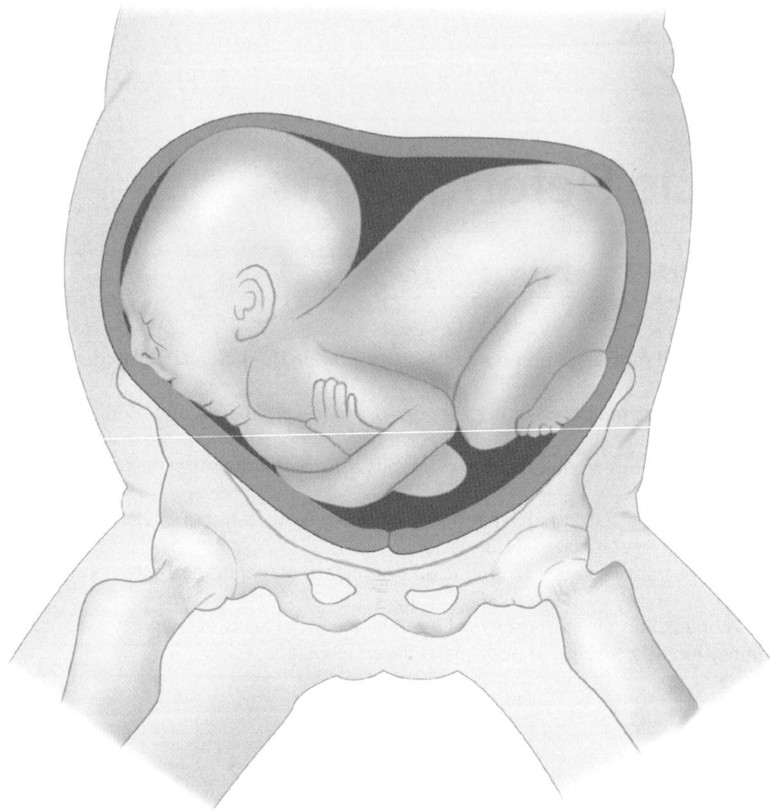

FIGURE 43.1 Transverse presentation.

lie in a primigravida should not be treated the same as in a multigravida in whom laxity of the abdomen has been the major cause for a transverse lie.[7] In a comparative study of expectant management versus external version, only 7.9% of 254 patients with an unstable lie were primiparous, and only 1 of these 11 women had spontaneous version (vs. 34% of the multiparous women). When managed by version, four (44%) primiparous women required emergency cesarean sections, whereas 94% of the multiparous women had successful vaginal deliveries.[11] Thus the rarity of transverse lie among primiparous women implies that it is likely to be accounted for by some type of underlying pathology, such as the predisposing factors listed previously. The proven value of external cephalic version in term breech deliveries and in multiparous women with a transverse lie should not be extended to primiparous women with a transverse lie, who may have some kind of underlying pathology inhibiting the normal process of version. Unresolved transverse lie is usually an indication for cesarean section using a transverse lower uterine segment incision, as neglected transverse lie can result in uterine rupture and other complications.[10,12,13] Some authors have advocated the use of intravenous nitroglycerine to induce uterine atonia and facilitate internal podalic version in cases of twins in which the second twin is in transverse lie.[14] In a study of 1039 twin pairs reviewing the indications for cesarean delivery of second twins after vaginal delivery of a first twin (combined delivery), they found the odds ratio for combined delivery for breech second twin was 2.4 compared with vertex second twins, while the odds ratio for transverse lie second twin was 182.8.[15]

DIFFERENTIAL DIAGNOSIS

The remarkable facial compression in babies born from a transverse lie can cause unusual facial features that may resemble a malformation syndrome or craniosynostosis.

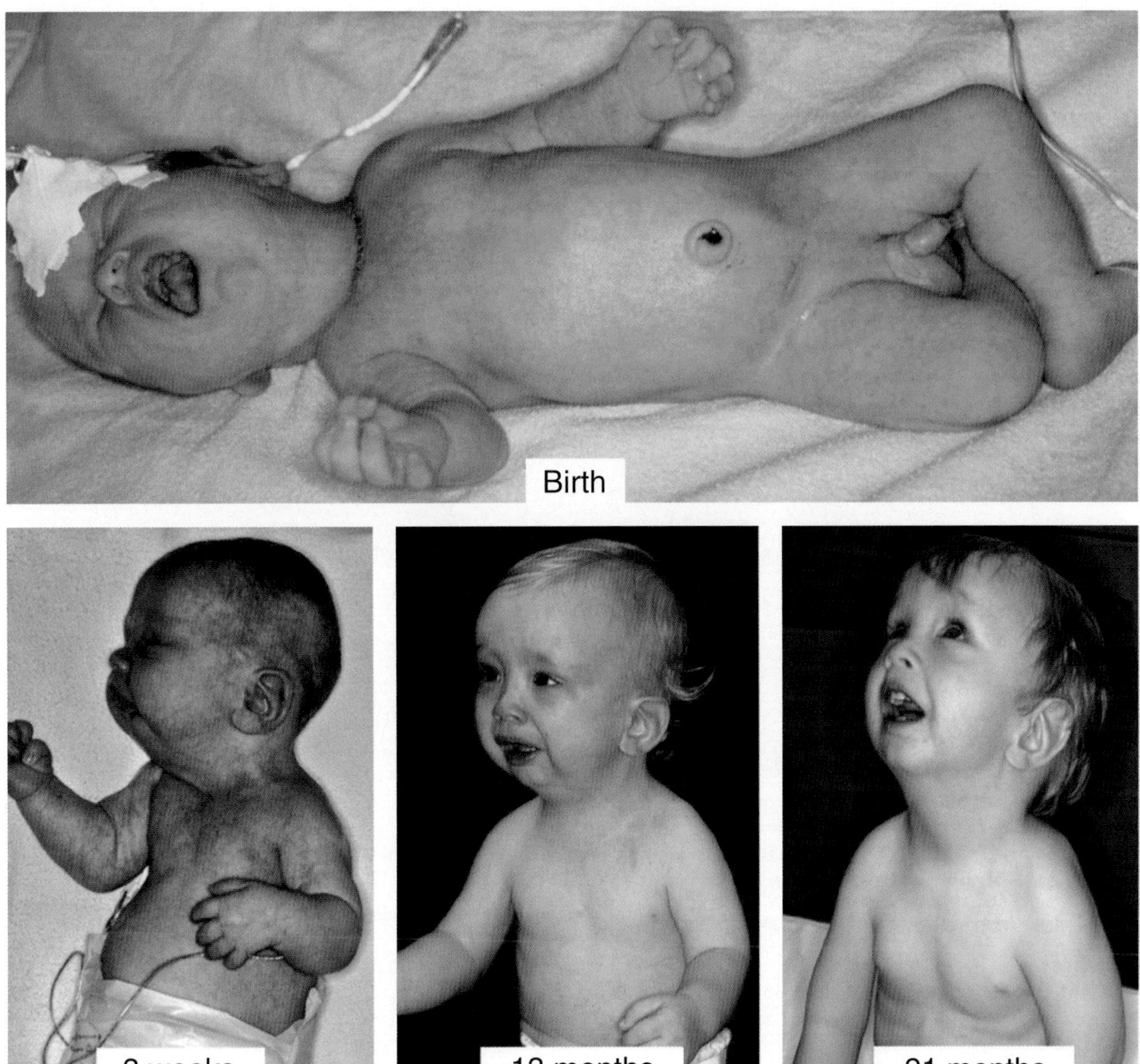

FIGURE 43.2 This infant was born at 36 weeks of gestation, having been in prolonged transverse lie since 17 weeks of gestation due to oligohydramnios that resulted from slow leakage of amniotic fluid. Despite prolonged physical therapy, the severe compression of facial structures persisted through 21 months. (See Fig. 23.1 for follow-up at age 30 months, when persistent jaw growth deficiency was still evident.)

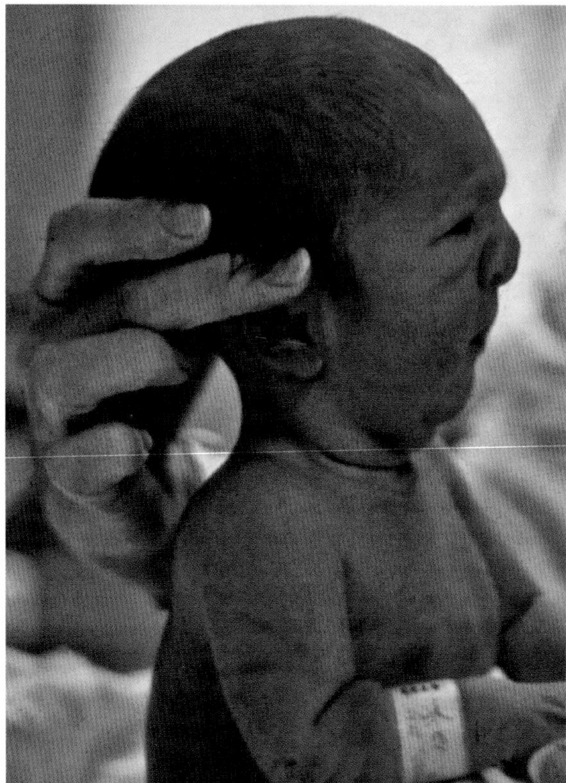
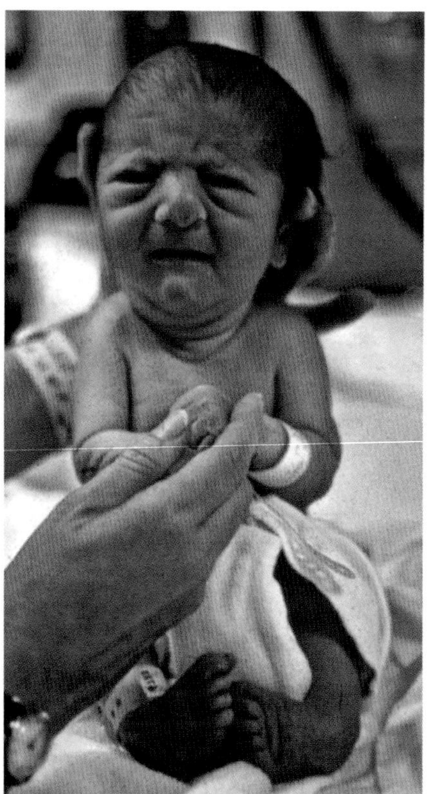

FIGURE 43.3 Flattening of the face with redundant "compression" skin folds in addition to equinovarus foot deformities in an infant who had been in prolonged transverse presentation, apparently with the head retroflexed and the face forced against the wall of the uterus. The infant's appearance progressively improved and returned to normal form. (Courtesy John Carey, University of Utah Medical School, Salt Lake City, UTh.)

References

1. Gardberg M, Leonova Y, Laakkonen E. Malpresentations: impact on mode of delivery. *Acta Obstet Gynecol Scand*. 2011;90(5):540–542.
2. Hankins GD, Hammond TL, Snyder RR, Gilstrap LC, 3rd. Transverse lie. *Am J Perinatol*. 1990;7(1):66–70.
3. Gemer O, Segal S. Incidence and contribution of predisposing factors to transverse lie presentation. *Int J Gynaecol Obstet*. 1994;44(3):219–221.
4. Moh W, Graham JM. Jr, Wadhawan I, Sanchez-Lara PA. Extrinsic factors influencing fetal deformations and intrauterine growth restriction. *J Pregnancy*. 2012;2012:750485.
5. Noor S, Fawwad A, Sultana R, et al. Pregnancy with fibroids and its and its obstetric complication. *Journal of Ayub Medical College, Abbottabad: JAMC*. 2009;21(4):37–40.
6. Phelan JP, Boucher M, Mueller E, McCart D, Horenstein J, Clark SL. The nonlaboring transverse lie: a management dilemma. *J Reprod Med*. 1986;31(3):184–186.
7. Lau WC, Fung HY, Lau TK, To KF. A benign polypoid adenomyoma: an unusual cause of persistent fetal transverse lie. *EJOGRB*. 1997;74(1):23–25.
8. Mehra S, Nguyen T, Amon E. What are the odds?: spontaneous version after preterm premature rupture of membranes. *Obstet Gynecol*. 2014;123(Suppl 1):157s–158s.
9. Oyinloye OI, Okoyomo AA. Longitudinal evaluation of foetal transverse lie using ultrasonography. *Afr J Reprod Health*. 2010;14(1):129–133.
10. Van der Kaay DC, Horsch S, Duvekot JJ. Severe neonatal complication of transverse lie after preterm premature rupture of membranes. *BMJ Case Rep.*. 2013:2013.
11. Edwards RL, Nicholson HO. The management of the unstable lie in late pregnancy. *J Obstetr Gynaec British Commonwealth*. 1969;76(8):713–718.
12. Segal S, Gemer O, Sassoon E. Transverse lower segment uterine incision in cesarean sections for transverse lie: a retrospective survey. *Arch Gynecol Obstet*. 1994;255(4):171–172.

13. Gemer O, Kopmar A, Sassoon E, Segal S. Neglected transverse lie with uterine rupture. *Arch Gynecol Obstet.* 1993;252(3):159–160.
14. Dufour P, Vinatier D, Vanderstichele S, Ducloy AS, Depret S, Monnier JC. Intravenous nitroglycerin for internal podalic version of the second twin in transverse lie. *Obstet Gynecol.* 1998;92(3):416–419.
15. Kong CW, To WWK. The predicting factors and outcomes of caesarean section of the second twin. *J Obstet Gynaecol.* 2017;37(6):709–713.

CHAPTER 44

Face and Brow Presentation Deformation

KEY POINTS

- Factors contributing to face presentation include fetal anomalies, contracted pelvis, fetopelvic disproportion, or cord around the neck.
- Face presentation is more common in large infants (>4000 g), small infants (<2300 g), and cephalopelvic disproportion.
- Cesarean section is considered if the fetus is large, the mother has a relatively small pelvis, or there is a persistent mentum posterior presentation with arrested descent.
- Manual conversion from mentum posterior to occipitoanterior presentation may be attempted in selected cases with ritodrine infusion.
- Face presentations carry an increased risk of difficult labor, and electronic fetal monitoring is recommended.
- After delivery, the restrained jaw tends to catch up toward normal, and treatment for congenital jaw subluxation is usually not required.

GENESIS

In face and brow presentations, the face is the compressed presenting part, usually with extension of the head (Fig. 44.1). *Face presentation* is an abnormal cephalic fetal presentation where the presenting part is the mentum, occurring in 1 to 2 per 1250 deliveries.[1-5] In *persistent brow presentation*, the neck is not extended as much as in face presentation, with the leading part of the face being the area between the anterior fontanelle and the orbital ridges. A brow presentation is less common and occurs in 1 in 500 to 1 in 4000 deliveries.[3,6-8] Anything that delays or prevents flexion such as fetal anomalies, contracted pelvis, fetopelvic disproportion, or cord around the neck can contribute to face presentation.[9] Face presentation is more common in large infants weighing more than 4000 g (42%), small infants weighing less than 2300 g (16%), and cephalopelvic disproportion.[1-3,10] Low birth weight and cephalopelvic disproportion have also been proposed as etiologic factors in brow presentation, with associated cephalopelvic disproportion attributed to the presenting diameters of the fetal head being greater in brow presentation than in face or vertex presentations.[3,11] High parity is a debated factor associated with face and brow presentations in some studies but not others.[4] There may actually be selection for mothers with a smaller pelvis because the fetus within a larger pelvis may convert to face or vertex before being recognized as a brow presentation. About half to two thirds of all brow presentations spontaneously convert to either face (30%) or vertex presentations (20%) if given an adequate trial of labor.[3]

When a brow converts to a face presentation, the occiput usually lodges in the maternal sacrum, and additional force on the head converts it to mentum anterior.[12] In converting from brow to vertex, the brow engages transversely and rotates to face the pubic bones, and then the head flexes to become occipitoposterior; thus many occipitoposterior presentations may have entered the pelvis as brow presentations.[12] In the era before prenatal diagnosis, the fetal mortality for face presentations was around 10%, with many deaths attributed to either attempted version, extraction, or conversion maneuvers (which are contraindicated with face or brow presentations) or to anencephaly.[1,4] When corrected to exclude anomalous infants, the mortality rate for face presentations delivered spontaneously or by low forceps is less than 2%.[3] Among all the proposing factors previously listed, high parity appears to be the most important.[3] Because increased extensor muscle tone cannot cause extension of a fetal head that is fixed in the pelvis, face presentation in a primigravida woman with an

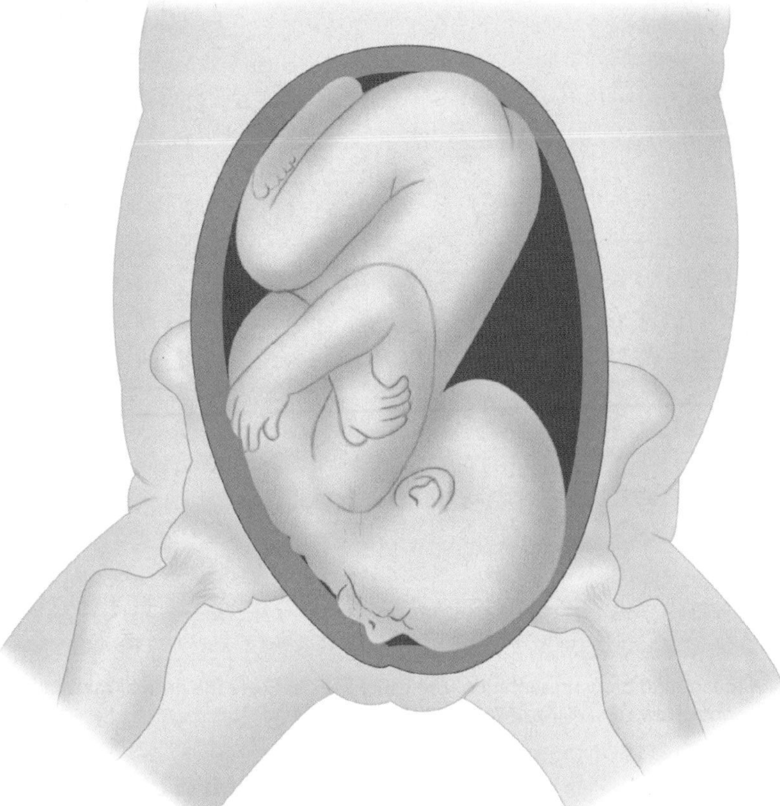

FIGURE 44.1 Face presentation with mentum transverse, emphasizing the mechanism for jaw compression and prominence of the occipital shelf.

engaged presenting part is less likely to occur during the last 2 to 3 weeks of pregnancy. On the other hand, the fetal head is often not engaged prior to the onset of labor in multiparous women, such that face presentation occurs more frequently.[3]

FEATURES

Face Presentation

In face presentation, the fetal head is hyperextended so that the occiput touches the back, and the presenting part is the fetal face between the orbital ridges and the chin (see Fig. 44.1).[3] Most cases of face presentation (97%) are diagnosed by vaginal examination during labor and delivery, with 59% of face presentations mentum anterior, 15% mentum transverse, and 27% mentum posterior.[3] The growth of the fetal mandible and nose may be restrained, and the position of comfort for the baby after birth is often with the neck retroflexed (Figs. 44.2 and 44.3). As a consequence of compression of the chin and anterior neck with retroflexion, redundant folds of skin in the anterior upper neck may be present (see Figs. 44.3–44.5), with persistent retrognathia and a prominent occipital shelf (see Figs. 44.3 and 44.4). In some instances, the prolonged facial compression causes feeding difficulties with difficulty in swallowing. There may also be jaw subluxation and a palpable/audible click as the jaw moves in and out of its socket (similar to that detected with a subluxable hip). The infant pictured in Fig. 44.4A was one such case. In another case, an infant with 24 hours of labor as a persistent mentum posterior presentation experienced significant laryngotracheal trauma, resulting in respiratory obstruction from compression against the maternal sacrum.[13]

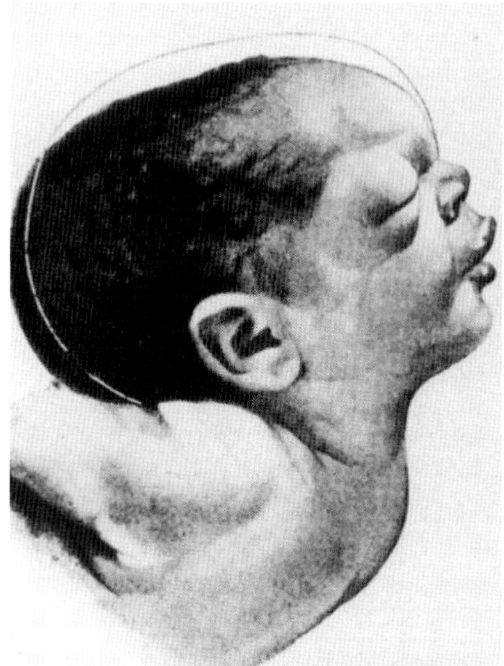
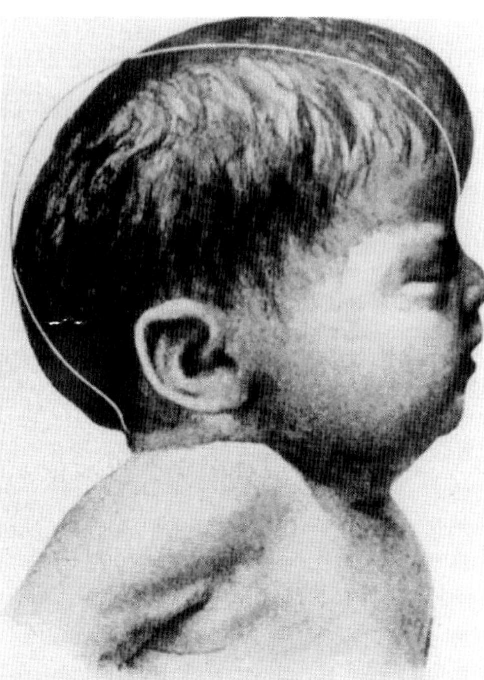

FIGURE 44.2 Examples of face and brow presentation. The white lines indicate the normal calvarial contour. (From von Ruess AR. *The Disease of the Newborn.* New York: William Wood; 1921.)

Brow Presentation

In brow presentation, the fetal head is midway between flexion and hyperextension, and the presenting part is the brow between the orbital ridges and the anterior fontanelle.[3] Most cases of brow presentation are diagnosed during labor and delivery, with cephalopelvic disproportion associated with many persistent brow presentations and resulting in prolonged dysfunctional labors. With persistent brow presentations, the fetal mouth may be forced open as the jaw is pushed against the fetal chest, thereby lengthening the presenting diameter, and one fetus, whose mouth was closed manually by the obstetrician, subsequently converted to a face presentation.[4] Such compressive forces on the chin could lead to congenital jaw subluxation, which may be detected as a palpable/audible click as the jaw moves in and out of the temporomandibular joint socket. The brow is unusually prominent, whereas the midface is less prominent than usual (see Fig. 44.1B). There may be increased molding with a large caput succedaneum in infants with persistent brow presentations in the frontoposterior position, making conversion more difficult and leading to excessively prolonged labors in 40% to 50% of cases.[3,14,15]

MANAGEMENT AND PROGNOSIS

Face and brow presentation carry an increased risk of difficult labor, with the cesarean rate being more than three times higher for face presentations than a typical vertex presentation.[9,11,16] Cesarean section merits consideration, especially if the fetus is large, the mother has a relatively small pelvis, or there is a persistent mentum posterior presentation with arrested descent.[6] One study reported higher cesarean delivery rates in women with mentum posterior face presentation and in women who did not receive oxytocin.[10] If progress is being made in dilatation and descent, the optimal management of face and brow presentations is expectant, but if progress ceases, delivery may require cesarean section.[3] Only mentum anterior face positions can be delivered vaginally because the fetal neck is not able to further extend when in the posterior position. Prolonged compression of the neck against the pubic ramus during delivery can cause trauma to the trachea or larynx.[13] The use of version and extraction in face and brow presentations is contraindicated and has been associated with high perinatal mortality in the older literature.[3] Most authors feel that it is not possible to safely deliver a term-sized fetus with a persistent

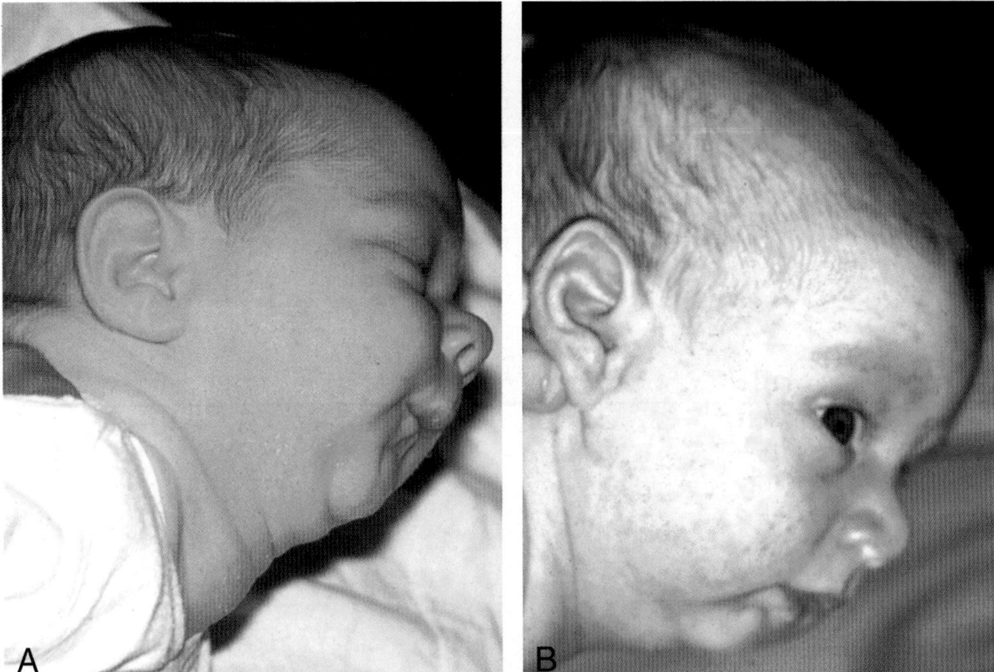

FIGURE 44.3 Newborn infant of a small primigravida mother. A, This infant was in prolonged face presentation for at least the last 2 months of gestation, leading to the extended head and restricted nasal and mandibular growth, as well as the compressive overgrowth of skin in the anterior neck. B, By 6 weeks of age, the catch-up growth of the nose and mandible is evident, and the head had settled into a more normal alignment.

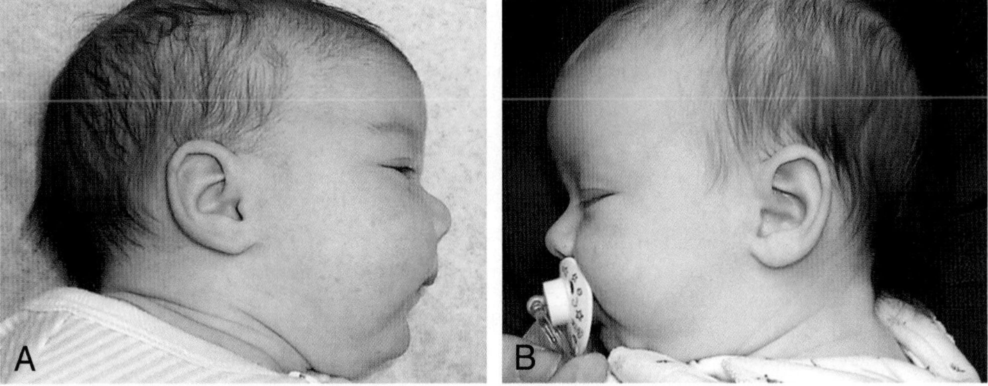

FIGURE 44.4 A, Face presentation with persistent jaw compression and prominent occipital shelf at 2 months. B, This infant presented with subluxation of the temporomandibular joint and persistent anterior neck folds.

mentum posterior presentation vaginally, but many such fetuses will spontaneously rotate and convert to mentum anterior presentation once the presenting part reaches the vaginal floor, thereby permitting vaginal delivery.[3] Fetuses with persistent brow presentations in the frontoposterior position seldom rotate and usually require cesarean delivery.[13-15] Spontaneous conversion of persistent brow presentations to allow vaginal delivery only occurs in 10% of cases, and manual conversion should only be attempted in a normal term fetus of normal size in the frontoanterior position with continual fetal monitoring under

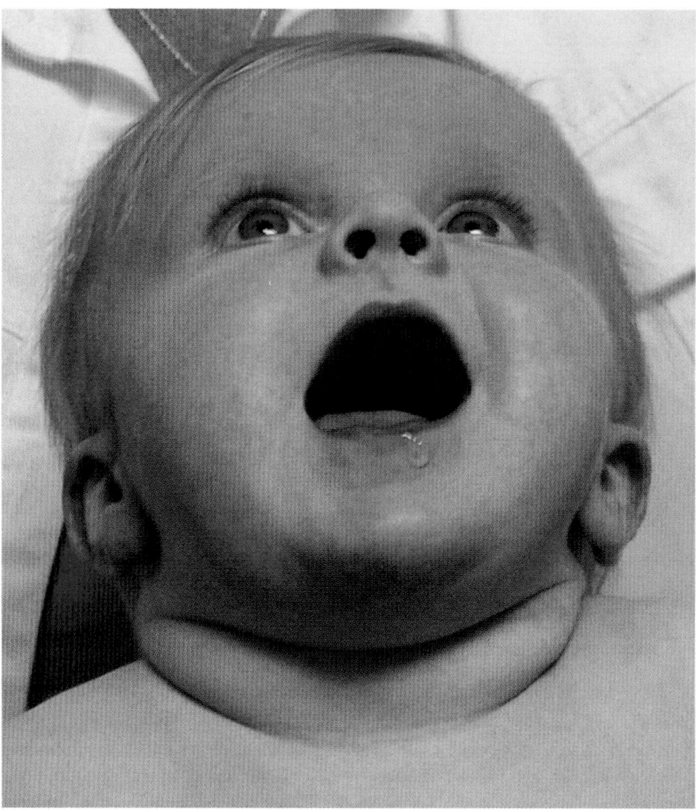

FIGURE 44.5 This 9-month-old infant had left muscular torticollis, persistent anterior neck folds, and posterior cervical retroflexion. The cervical retroflexion and feeding difficulties were initially thought to be due to gastroesophageal reflux. After brain magnetic resonance imaging and cervical spine radiographs were found to be normal, a history of mentum anterior face presentation was elicited, and physical therapy began to improve head and neck posture.

continuous lumbar anesthesia.[15] In a 2020 study of 200 woman who were beginning the second stage of labor, sonographic diagnosis of *fetal head deflexion* (measurement of the occiput-spine angle when the occiput was anterior or transverse) was diagnosed in 21.2% and was an independent risk factor for cesarean delivery both in occiput anterior (adjusted odds ratio: 5.37; 95% confidence interval: 1.819–15.869) and occiput posterior (adjusted odds ratio: 13.9; 95% confidence interval: 1.958–98.671) cases, and it was an independent risk factor for cesarean delivery regardless of the occiput position (adjusted odds ratio: 5.83; 95% confidence interval: 2.47–13.73).[17] In a 2022 study of 1002 randomized patients, prophylactic manual rotation of fetuses in occiput posterior or occiput transverse position did not increase the rate of spontaneous vaginal delivery compared with no manual rotation.[18] In many centers where manual conversion is not attempted, failure to progress often results in cesarean delivery.

In a review of fetal heart rate patterns seen in infants with face presentation, ominous patterns were seen in 59% of patients with adequate tracings (20% severe variable decelerations and 24% repetitive late decelerations), and these abnormal patterns were partly attributed to abnormal pressure on the extended head, neck, and/or eyes (similar to what has been described in occipitoposterior presentations); thus electronic fetal monitoring has been advocated for face presentation.[2,3,19,20] As long as the face is progressing through the birth canal, conversion to mentum anterior is possible, but if progress arrests or there is cephalopelvic disproportion or fetal distress, cesarean delivery may be necessary in 50% to 60% of cases.[19-21]

In a study of long-term fetal morbidity among 31 face presentations managed expectantly, 14 of 15 patients with mentum anterior presentations were delivered vaginally, with 12 of 15 not recognized as face presentations until the second stage of labor. On the other hand, 15 of 16 patients with mentum transverse or mentum posterior face presentations required cesarean delivery, and all but one were diagnosed earlier in labor (prior to 5-cm cervical dilatation) due to failed progression of labor.[21] All patients were monitored electronically, and there was an increased incidence of variable decelerations (57% vs. 32% in normal vertex deliveries), with one infant demonstrating neurologic sequelae attributable to face presentation. Other studies noted fetal distress on electronic monitoring less frequently in fetuses with a face presentation.[20,22] Even though face presentations with persistent mentoposterior presentation is an indication for cesarean section delivery, some patients refuse operative intervention. In 11 Orthodox Jewish women who refused cesarean delivery, there was intrapartum bimanual conversion from mentoposterior to occipitoanterior presentation, concomitant with ritodrine infusion in 10 of these women.[23] Safe manual flexion of the deflexed mentoposterior head into the desired occipitoanterior position was facilitated by relaxing the uterus with ritodrine infusion in these multiparous women who refused cesarean section. As a rule, cesarean section will be performed in 48% to 53% of cases of face presentation, and in most cases the diagnosis of face presentation is made during labor.[2,24,25]

After delivery of the fetus in face or brow presentation, catch-up of the restrained jaw toward normal tends to occur (see Figs. 44.4 and 44.5). Although there is hyperextension of the fetal head in vaginal face presentation, vaginal delivery does not appear to pose the same risks for spinal and cerebellar injuries as is seen with breech presentation.[21] The head gradually resumes a more normal posture, and the redundant skin that may be present on the anterior neck with face presentation usually resolves with postnatal growth. Usually, no treatment other than gentle massage is indicated for congenital jaw subluxation. The parents need to be reassured that their infant is normal. The recurrence risk is generally not significant.

DIFFERENTIAL DIAGNOSIS

Face Presentation

The diagnosis of face presentation is often delayed until late in the second stage of labor, when diagnosis is suggested by characteristic abdominal or vaginal findings. Imaging can confirm the presence of a face presentation and rule out the existence of a major anomaly (e.g., anencephaly, severe hydrocephalus with cephalomegaly, anterior neck mass, or multiple nuchal cords), which may be present in 5% to 6% of cases.[10,21] The appearance of the face at birth may raise the question of a malformation syndrome such as Treacher Collins syndrome or another syndrome with limited jaw growth. Associated malformations of the auricle, colobomas of the lower eyelid, and palpable malar gaps in Treacher Collins syndrome tends to distinguish this disorder from face presentation, as does the mode of presentation and the progressive postnatal improvement in jaw growth. Newborn infants with face presentation usually have severe facial edema, facial bruising, or ecchymosis, which usually resolve within 24 to 48 hours.[26,27]

Brow Presentation

The appearance of the face may suggest some type of craniofacial dysostosis (e.g., Crouzon syndrome). If there are additional concerns or clinical findings on examination such as hypotonia, a genetics consultation with mutation analysis should help in making this distinction.[27,28]

References

1. Fougerousse CE. Management of face presentation. *The Journal of the Arkansas Medical Society.* 1967;63(12):462–464.
2. Benedetti TJ, Lowensohn RI, Truscott AM. Face presentation at term. *Obstet Gynecol.* 1980;55(2):199–202.
3. Cruikshank DP, Cruikshank JE. Face and brow presentation: a review. *Clinical Obstetrics and Gynecology.* 1981;24(2):333–351.
4. Tapisiz OL, Aytan H, Altinbas SK, et al. Face presentation at term: a forgotten issue. *J Obstet Gynaecol Res.* 2014;40(6):1573–1577.
5. Makajeva J., Ashraf M. Delivery, Face and brow presentation. In: StatPearls. Treasure Island (FL): StatPearls Publishing Copyright © 2023, StatPearls Publishing LLC.; 2023.
6. Tapisiz OL, Aytan H, Altinbas SK, et al. Face presentation at term: a forgotten issue. *J Obstet Gynaecol Res.* 2014;40(6):1573–1577.
7. Sherer DM, Spong CY, Minior VK, Salafia CM. Increased incidence of fetal growth restriction in association with breech presentation in preterm deliveries < 32 weeks. *Am J Perinatol.* 1997;14(1):35–37.
8. Fruscalzo A, Londero AP, Salvador S, et al. New and old predictive factors for breech presentation: our experience in 14433 singleton pregnancies and a literature review. *J Matern Fetal Neonatal Med.* 2014;27(2):167–172.

9. Sharmila V, Babu TA. Unusual birth trauma involving face: a completely preventable iatrogenic injury. *Journal of Clinical Neonatology*. 2014;3(2):120–121.
10. Shaffer BL, Cheng YW, Vargas JE, Laros Jr. RK, Caughey AB. Face presentation: predictors and delivery route. *Am J Obstet Gynecol*. 2006;194(5):e10–12.
11. Bashiri A, Burstein E, Bar-David J, Levy A, Mazor M. Face and brow presentation: independent risk factors. *J Matern Fetal Neonatal Med*. 2008;21(6):357–360.
12. Borell U, Fernstrom I. The mechanism of labour in face and brow presentation. A radiological study. *Acta Obstet Gynecol Scand*. 1960;39:626–644.
13. Lansford A, Arias D, Smith BE. Respiratory obstruction associated with face presentation. *Am J Dis Children (1960)*. 1968;116(3):318–319.
14. Jennings PN. Brow presentation with vaginal delivery. *Austral & NZ J Obstet Gynaecol*. 1968;8(4):219–224.
15. Levy DL. Persistent brow presentation: a new approach to management. *Southern Med J*. 1976;69(2):191–192.
16. Arsène E, Langlois C, Clouqueur E, Deruelle P, Subtil D. Prognosis for deliveries in face presentation: a case-control study. *Arch Gynecol Obstet*. 2019;300(4):869–874.
17. Bellussi F, Livi A, Cataneo I, Salsi G, Lenzi J, Pilu G. Sonographic diagnosis of fetal head deflexion and the risk of cesarean delivery. *Am J Obstet Gynecol MFM*. 2020;2(4):100217.
18. Burd J, Gomez J, Berghella V, et al. Prophylactic rotation for malposition in the second stage of labor: a systematic review and meta-analysis of randomized controlled trials. *Am J Obstet Gynecol MFM*. 2022;4(2):100554.
19. Duff P. Diagnosis and management of face presentation. *Obstet Gynecol*. 1981;57(1):105–112.
20. Watson WJ, Read JA. Electronic fetal monitoring in face presentation at term. *Military Medicine*. 1987;152(6):324–325.
21. Westgren M, Svenningsen NW. Face presentation in modern obstetrics--a study with special reference to fetal long term morbidity. *Zeitschrift fur Geburtshilfe und Perinatologie*. 1984;188(2):87–89.
22. Schwartz Z, Dgani R, Lancet M, Kessler I. Face presentation. *Austral & NZ J Obstet Gynaecol*. 1986;26(3):172–176.
23. Neuman M, Beller U, Lavie O, Aboulafia Y, Rabinowitz R, Diamant Y. Intrapartum bimanual tocolytic-assisted reversal of face presentation: preliminary report. *Obstet Gynecol*. 1994;84(1):146–148.
24. Herabutya Y, Supakarapongkul W, Chaturachinda K. Face presentation in Ramathibodi Hospital: a 12 years study. *Journal of the Medical Association of Thailand = Chotmaihet thangphaet*. 1984;67(Suppl 2):31–35.
25. Prevedourakis CN. Face presentation. An analysis of 163 cases. *Am J Obstet Gynecol*. 1966;94(8):1092–1097.
26. Fomukong NH, Edwin N, Edgar MML, et al. Management of face presentation, face and lip edema in a primary healthcare facility case report, Mbengwi, Cameroon. *Pan Afr Med J*. 2019;33:292.
27. De Bernardo G, Svelto M, Giordano M, Sordino D. Face presentation in delivery room: what is strategy? *BMJ Case Rep*. 2017:2017.
28. Grootjen LN, Uyl NEM, van Beijsterveldt I, Damen L, Kerkhof GF, Hokken-Koelega ACS. Prenatal and neonatal characteristics of children with Prader-Willi syndrome. *J Clin Med*. 2022;11(3).

Section XI
Whole-Body Deformation or Disruption

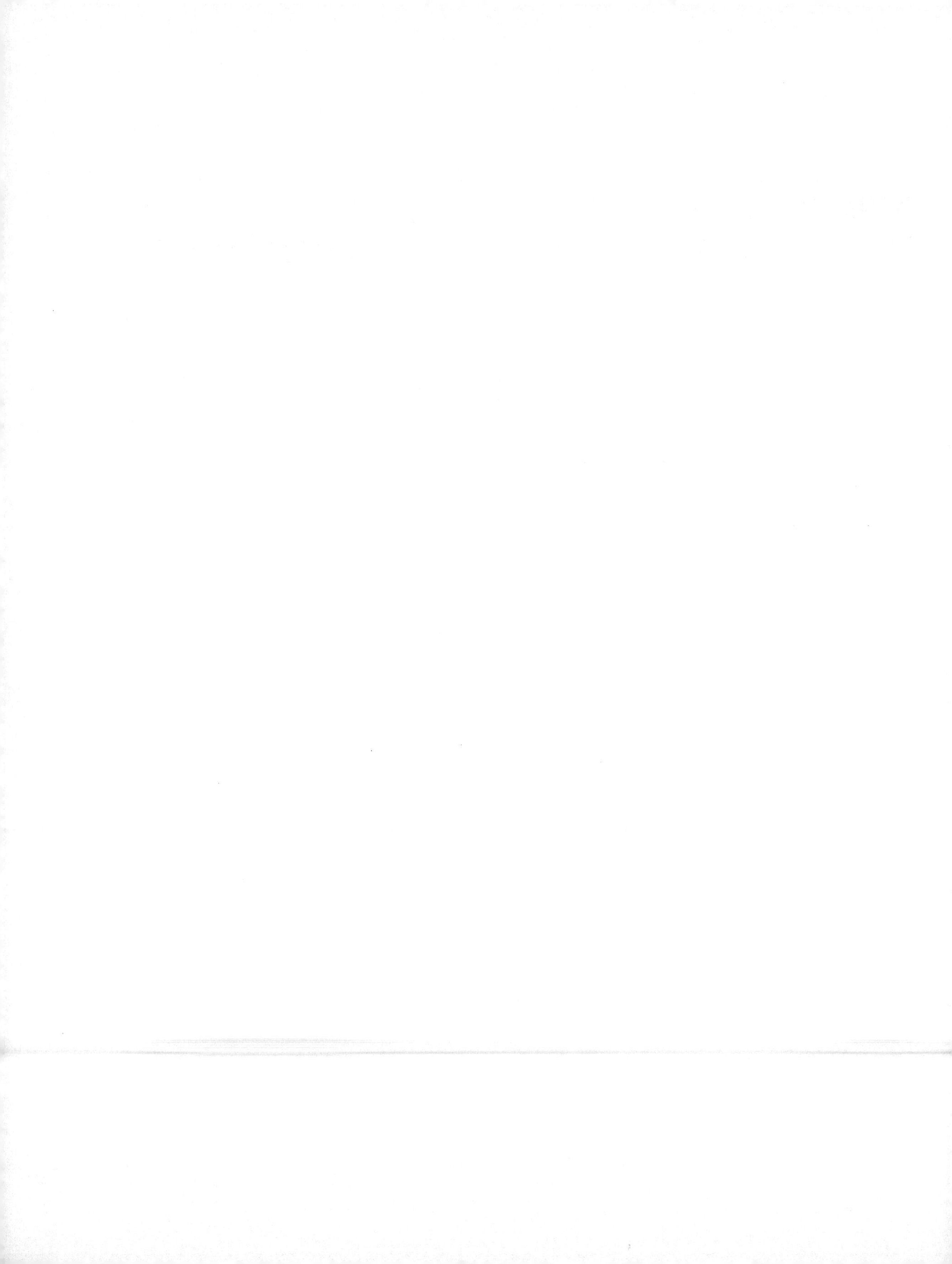

CHAPTER 45

Small Uterine Cavity Deformation

Bicornuate or Myomatous Uterus

KEY POINTS

- Various types of uterine malformations, such as bicornuate or myomatous uterus, can lead to small uterine cavity deformation, increasing the risk of fetal deformation and complications.
- Diagnostic procedures like hysterosalpingography, laparoscopy, and 3D ultrasonography are more accurate in identifying congenital uterine anomalies compared with hysterosalpingography alone.
- Different types of uterine anomalies are associated with specific reproductive outcomes, including increased rates of miscarriage, preterm birth, fetal malpresentation, and cesarean delivery.
- Uterine fibroids (leiomyomas) can cause symptoms and affect reproductive functions, leading to subfertility, early pregnancy loss, and pregnancy complications. Myomectomy may improve fertility for specific fibroid locations and sizes.
- Uterine anomalies, including bicornuate uterus, can increase the risk of congenital defects and fetal deformations, such as limb contractures and craniofacial deformations. Surgical intervention to improve uterine size and address large fibroids may enhance the chances of successful pregnancy outcomes.

GENESIS

Several different types of uterine problems can limit the size and/or shape of the uterine cavity and thus enhance the likelihood of fetal deformation.[1,2] Embryonic development of the female reproductive tract results from the fusion of Müllerian ducts and urogenital sinus. Müllerian ducts differentiate to form the uterus, fallopian tubes, cervix, and upper one-third of the vagina. Examples include a malformed uterus caused by failure of the Müllerian ducts to completely fuse during embryogenesis, resulting in either symmetric or asymmetric structural anomalies of the uterus such as didelphic uterus with duplicated cervix, bicornuate uterus, septate uterus, and arcuate uterus (Fig. 45.1). Uterine defects can be subgrouped into arcuate uteri, canalization defects (septate and subseptate uteri), and unification defects (unicornuate, bicornuate, and didelphys uteri) (Fig. 45.2). Women with a didelphic or completely septate uterus and two external uterine orifices had a significantly higher rate of cesarean delivery (91% vs. 18%) than a control group of 5763 women with normal uterine morphology. Women with a bicornuate or incomplete septate uterus and one external uterine orifice had significantly higher rates of preterm birth (27% vs. 5%) and placental abruption (14% vs. 0.7%) than the control group.[3]

Estimates of the frequency of anomalous Müllerian development vary widely based on the mode of ascertainment. Among 101 women who had routine hysterosalpingography (HSG) and 3D transvaginal sonography as part of an infertility evaluation, 6 normal uteri and 30 congenital uterine anomalies were diagnosed (3 arcuate, 1 unicornuate, 4 bicornuate, 2 didelphys, and 20 septate uteri). Congenital anomalies were correctly identified in 30 of 30 cases by 3D transvaginal sonography, but in only 10 of 30 cases by HSG. Only 7 of the 20 septi would have been surgically corrected if patients only had HSG, and 3D transvaginal sonography provided better evaluation of uterine anomalies with lower cost and morbidity.[4]

Methodologic biases affect frequency estimates because reproductive tracts are more commonly investigated in women with miscarriage and infertility, and anomalies are more prevalent in women with these problems. The most accurate diagnostic procedures are combined HSG, laparoscopy, and 3D

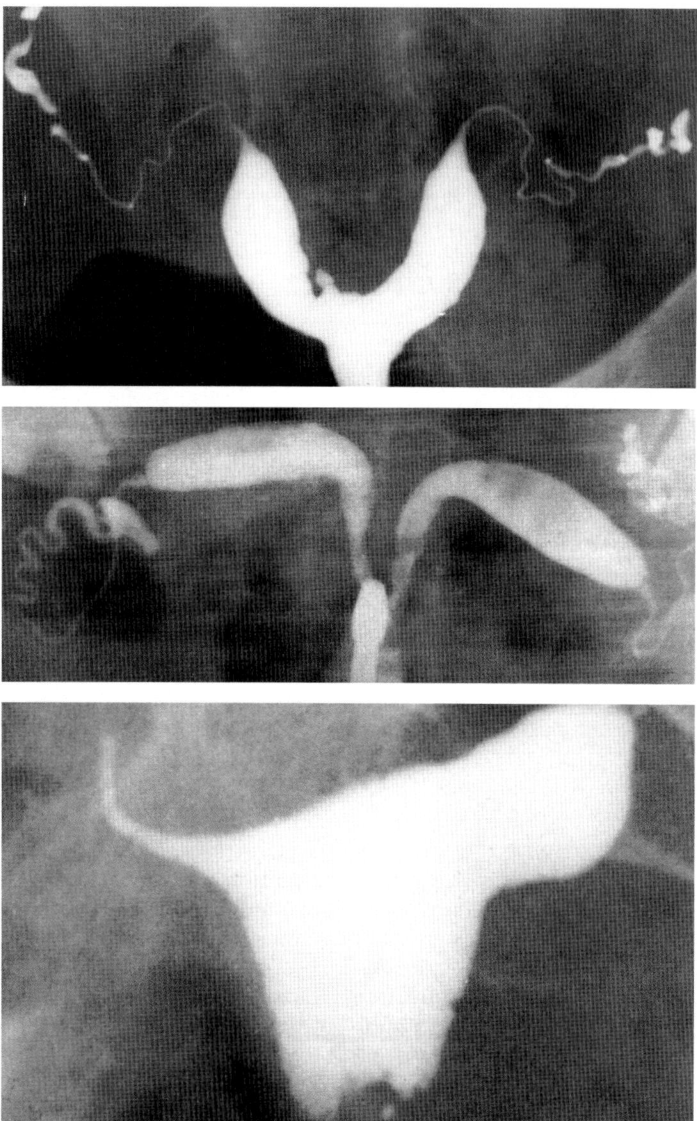

FIGURE 45.1 Three examples of a bicornuate uterus shown by hysterosalpingography, each of which was responsible for a deformational problem in the offspring.

ultrasonography.[5] The prevalence of congenital uterine anomalies is approximately 6.7% in the general population, approximately 7.3% in the infertile population, and approximately 16.7% in the recurrent miscarriage population. The arcuate uterus is the most common anomaly in the general and recurrent miscarriage population. In contrast, the septate uterus is the most common anomaly in the infertile population.[6] A systematic review of nine different studies comprising 3805 women evaluated the association between different types of congenital uterine anomalies and various reproductive outcomes.[7] Metaanalysis showed that arcuate uteri were associated with increased rates of second-trimester miscarriage and fetal malpresentation at delivery. Canalization defects reduced fertility and increased rates of miscarriage and preterm delivery. Unification defects were associated with increased rates of preterm birth and fetal malpresentation.

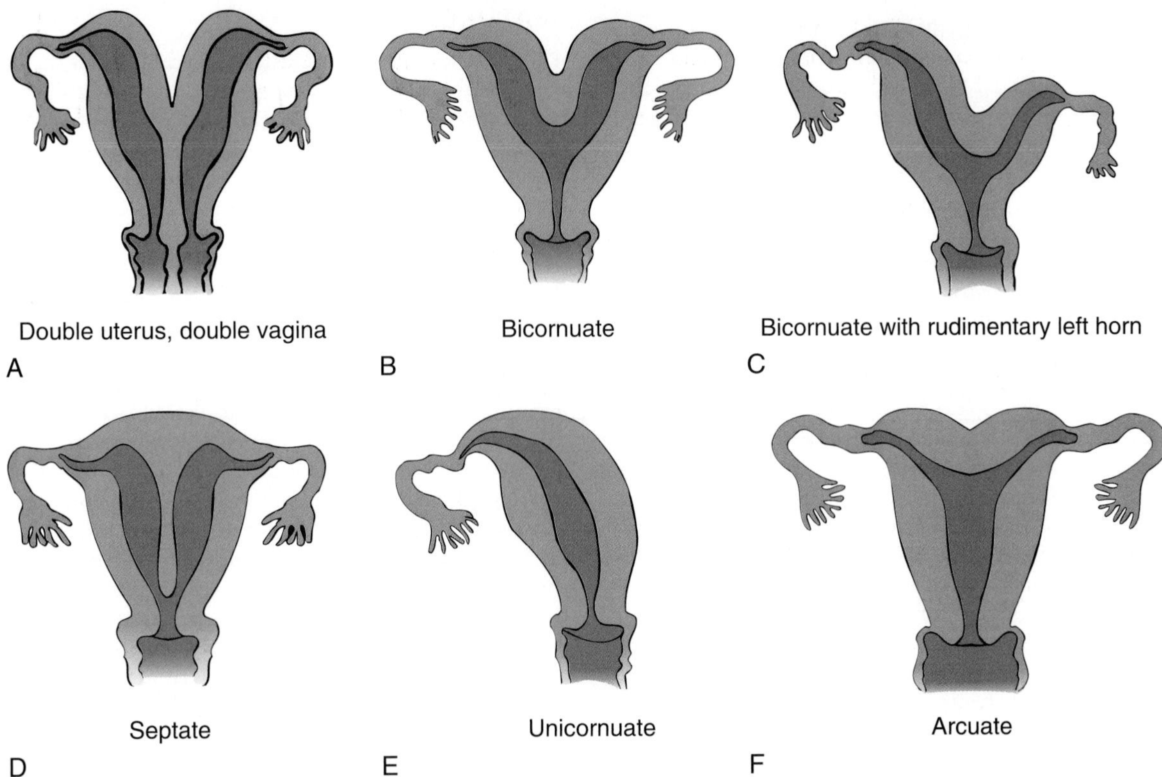

FIGURE 45.2 Congenital uterine abnormalities. **A,** Uterus didelphys: double uterus and vagina. **B,** Bicornuate uterus. **C,** Bicornuate uterus with a rudimentary left horn. **D,** Septate uterus. **E,** Unicornuate uterus. **F,** Arcuate uterus. (From The neonatal and pediatric pelvis. In: Hagen-Ansert S, ed. *Textbook of Diagnostic Sonography.* 7th ed. Mosby; 2012.)

Arcuate uteri were specifically associated with second-trimester miscarriage.[7] All uterine anomalies increase the chance of fetal malpresentation at delivery, thereby increasing the risk of craniofacial deformations and positional orthopedic defects. Among 316 women with congenital uterine malformations, 15.3% had incompetence of the cervix, so preterm delivery can result from an incompetent cervix and the malformation of the uterus.[8] Uterine rupture has also been reported, resulting in an abdominal pregnancy.[9,10] Unicornuate uterus with a rudimentary horn has a high incidence of obstetric and gynecological complications. Ruptured ectopic pregnancy in the rudimentary horn is one of the most dreaded complications that can have grave consequences for both mother and fetus.[11–13]

It is estimated that at least 1% to 2% of women have a clinically significant malformation of the uterus, and the general risk of a deformation problem for a fetus in a malformed uterus is about 30%.[2] Such deformations can include craniofacial deformations, overlapping sutures, joint contractures, limb deformations or disruptions, edema and/or grooves, and thoracic constriction resulting in pulmonary hypoplasia.[2,14–16] This would imply that 3 to 6 infants per 1000 may have a deformation problem secondary to gestation within a malformed uterus. Vascular disruption within the fetal limb can also occur with severe uterine constriction.[17] Among 556 twin pregnancies, 3.1% had a known uterine anomaly (9 septate uterus, 3 bicornuate, 3 arcuate, 1 unicornuate, and 1 didelphys). In patients with twin pregnancies, the presence of a uterine anomaly was associated with an increased risk of cerclage, preterm birth, and lower birth weights, but not fetal growth restriction.[18]

Uterine fibroids (leiomyomas) are benign tumors that become clinically apparent in many women of reproductive age. In pregnancy, many are incidentally diagnosed, and if they are large, they often require careful monitoring concerning their size, number, and location.[19] They present with a variety of symptoms including excessive menstrual bleeding, dysmenorrhea and intermenstrual bleeding, chronic pelvic pain, and pressure symptoms such as a sensation of bloatedness, increased urinary frequency, and bowel disturbance. In addition, they may affect reproductive functions, contributing to subfertility, early pregnancy loss, and later pregnancy complications. Myomectomy for submucosal fibroids greater than 2 cm and for intramural fibroids distorting the endometrial contour can improve fertility. Submucosal fibroid location and distortion of the endometrial cavity (either submucosal or deeply infiltrating intramural fibroids) are most likely to impair fertility and warrant surgical removal.[20] Nowadays, with advanced preparations, myomectomies during cesarean section are safely and frequently performed when the benefits outweigh the risks.[19] Women with prenatal exposure to diethylstilbestrol (DES) have a slightly higher incidence of fibroids compared with unexposed women.[21] The risk is strongest for women exposed to DES in the first trimester, corresponding to early stages of fetal Müllerian development. Rarely, a large uterine fibroid can also result in fetal deformation and/or disruption,[16,22] and sometimes a small fibroma will enlarge rapidly under the influence of increased levels of estrogen during late gestation. Among 121 women with 179 pregnancies and fibroids 4 cm or greater in size on ultrasonography at the dating scan, the size (4–7 cm, 7–10 cm, >10 cm), number (multiple/single), location (lower uterus/body of uterus), and type (intramural, combination of intramural/subserosal, subserosal) were ascertained. Preterm delivery was more likely in those with multiple fibroids compared with single fibroids (18% vs. 6%). There was a higher cesarean section rate for fibroids in the lower part of uterus than in the body of the uterus, as well as a higher rate of postpartum hemorrhage and increased estimated blood loss. Increasing size of fibroid was associated with greater rates of hemorrhage, increased estimated blood loss, and higher rates of admission for fibroid-related pain.[23] Women with multiple rather than large fibroids have a significantly increased risk of preterm birth and cesarean delivery, whereas large fibroids are associated with a higher risk of premature rupture of membranes.[24] There is one case report of arthrogryposis associated with the presence of a "giant" uterine fibroid.[25] When joint contractures result from space limitations within the uterus, the most common etiology is oligohydramnios, but similar constraint can occur with large fibroids.

FEATURES

All gradations of deformation of craniofacial structures, limbs, and thorax may occur, including overall constraint of fetal growth (Figs. 45.3–45.6). A deep groove in the thorax and left arm in one fetus was attributed to compression from the septum of a bicornuate uterus, whereas another fetus had marked molding of the head, which was trapped in the left uterine horn.[11] Pregnancy in a rudimentary uterine horn can lead to postdatism.[26] Prolonged constraint within a bicornuate uterus has resulted in multiple joint contractures from fetal immobility.[15,25] Another report documented prenatal detection of calvarial asymmetry in a 27-week fetus in vertex presentation due to pressure on the fetal head by a baseball-sized leiomyoma in the posterior uterine wall. At birth, there was a 3 × 4-cm depression of the left parietal bone with atrophy of the right sternocleidomastoid muscle. At age 6 months, growth and development were normal, the calvarial depression had partially resolved, and the torticollis was improved.[16] There is a significantly increased incidence of caudal dysplasia in pregnancies associated with uterine leiomyomata, possibly due to fetal leg compression (Figs. 45.7 and 45.8).[22]

Familial Müllerian duct anomalies can occur, often in association with renal and urinary tract anomalies; therefore a previous family history of Müllerian and/or renal anomalies should prompt further investigation.[27–32] Mayer-Rokitansky-Küster-Hauser (MRKH) syndrome is characterized by uterovaginal agenesis (absence of uterus, cervix, and upper part of the vagina) and can be associated with renal, skeletal, and cardiac malformations. A family with two female cousins with MRKH syndrome and unilateral renal agenesis prompted subsequent examination of healthy relatives, revealing two related males with renal agenesis and an uncle with renal cysts, suggesting hereditary renal adysplasia in these male family members.[32] A total of 67 family reports included 123 cases of MRKH syndrome and 84 non-MRKH relatives with other anomalies. These associated anomalies were dominated by renal and skeletal malformations, which are found in sporadic cases too, suggesting a possible genetic etiology. Many of these associated anomalies were asymptomatic, suggesting a need for ultrasound examinations of healthy relatives of patients with renal and/or other uterovaginal malformations.[32] Among 276 women with uterine malformations, there were 60 women with uterine malformations and unilateral renal agenesis who were compared with 216 women with uterine malformations and both kidneys

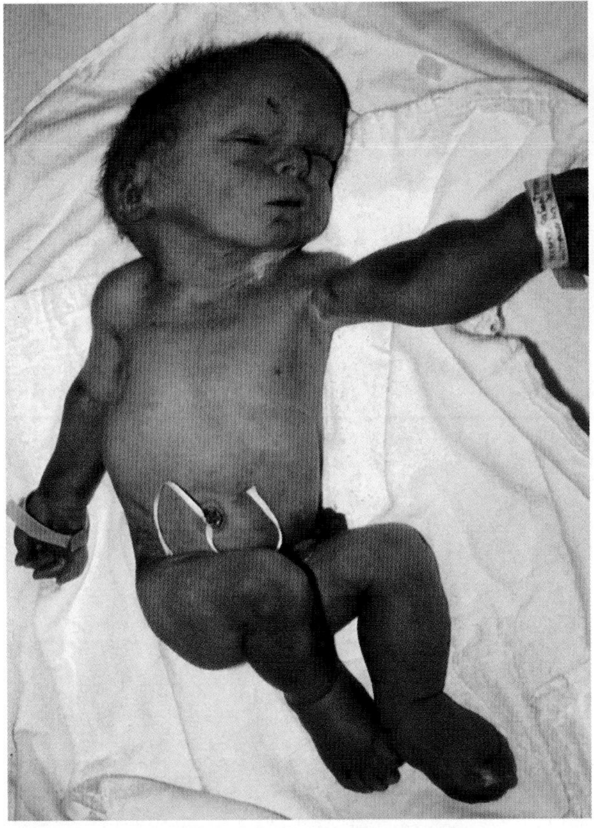

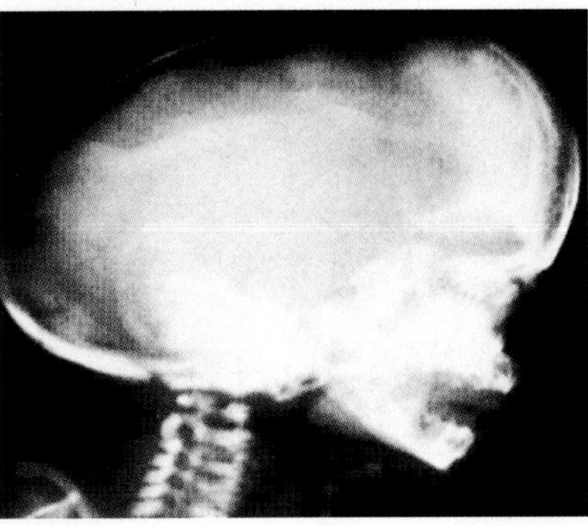

FIGURE 45.3 Severely deformed newborn infant delivered from a bicornuate uterus, who died of respiratory insufficiency owing to constraint-induced lung hypoplasia. The proximal constraint of limb has resulted in distal lymphedema, and the head has been molded out of alignment in such a manner as to give the impression of low-placed ears. The mother had a history of five previous miscarriages. (From Miller ME, Dunn PM, Smith DW. Uterine malformation and fetal deformation. *J Pediatr.* 1979;94:387.)

present. Unilateral renal agenesis was associated with either agenesis of all of the derivatives of the urogenital ridge on the same side of the body, which was usually the left side, or distal mesonephric anomalies such as a double uterus with a blind hemivagina or unilateral cervicovaginal atresia, which were most frequently on the right side. The uterine malformations that were most commonly seen in women with renal agenesis were bicornis-bicollis, didelphys, and unicornuate uteri.[33]

A small uterine cavity can result in miscarriage, stillbirth, prematurity, and fetal deformation and/or vascular disruption. Insufficient uterine space for fetal growth should be considered as one possible explanation when a history of multiple miscarriages, stillbirths, prematurity, cervical incompetence, abdominal pregnancy, and/or serious deformation problems is obtained. When pregnancies with a diagnosis of uterine anomaly (uterine septum, unicornuate uterus, bicornuate uterus, uterine didelphys) were compared with those in women with normal anatomy, the presence of a uterine anomaly was associated with preterm birth, nonbreech cesarean delivery, premature rupture of membranes, and breech presentation.[34] Patients with uterine anomalies had significantly higher rates of malpresentation (38.8%), preterm delivery (19.8%), and cesarean section (78.5%) when compared with a group of women with a normal uterus.[35] Patients with uterine anomalies had significantly lower mean birth weights and a significantly higher incidence of small-for-gestational-age neonates, and women with uterus didelphys required infertility treatment more often than patients with other uterine anomalies. The rate of malpresentation was significantly higher in patients with septate uterus in comparison to patients with uterus unicorns, and a septate uterus was associated with the poorest

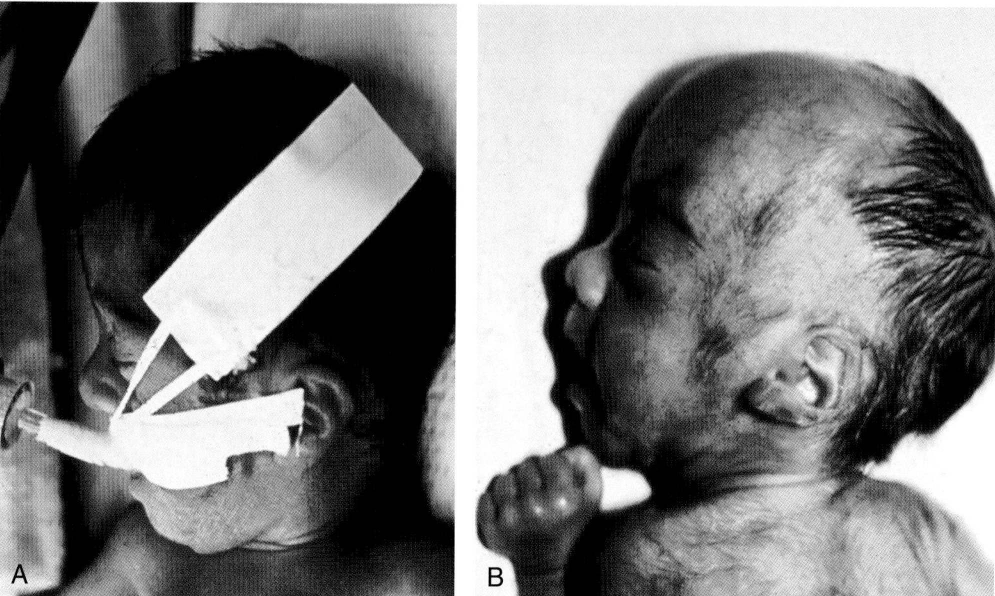

FIGURE 45.4 **A,** Infant born prematurely at 34 weeks with compressed craniofacies that initially had raised questions regarding coronal craniostenosis. **B,** Within 3 weeks, the face had grown forward and the question of craniostenosis was resolved. (Courtesy Kenneth Lyons Jones, University of California, San Diego, CA; from Miller ME, Dunn PM, Smith DW. Uterine malformation and fetal deformation. *J Pediatr.* 1979;94:387.)

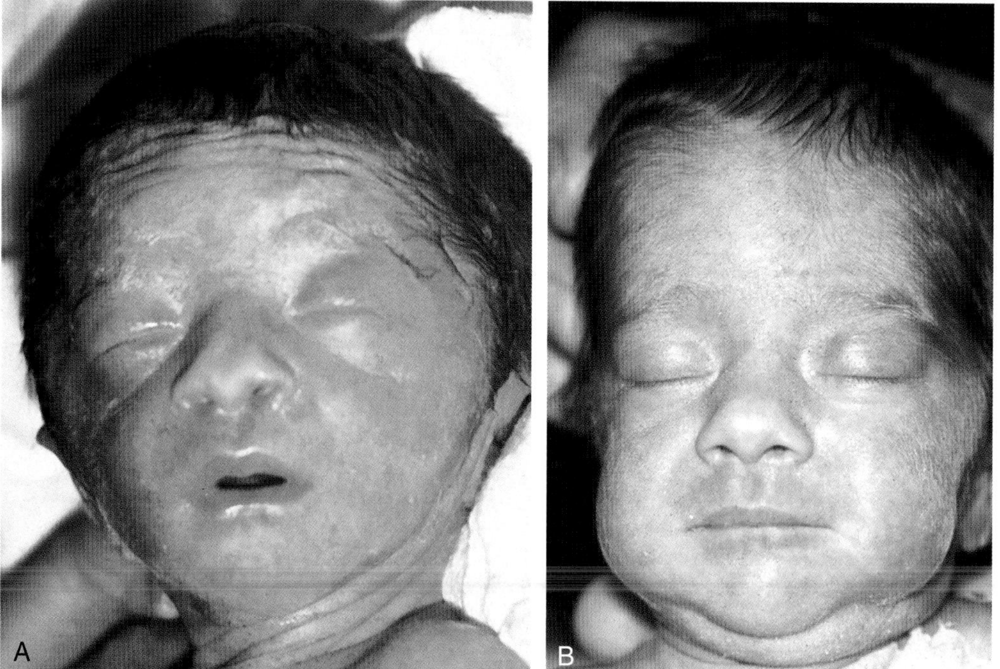

FIGURE 45.5 **A,** This infant was born at 34 weeks from a bicornuate uterus (see Fig. 45.1, *middle*), demonstrating a compressed face and nose with redundant skin. **B,** Follow-up at age 32 days showed a complete return to normal form.

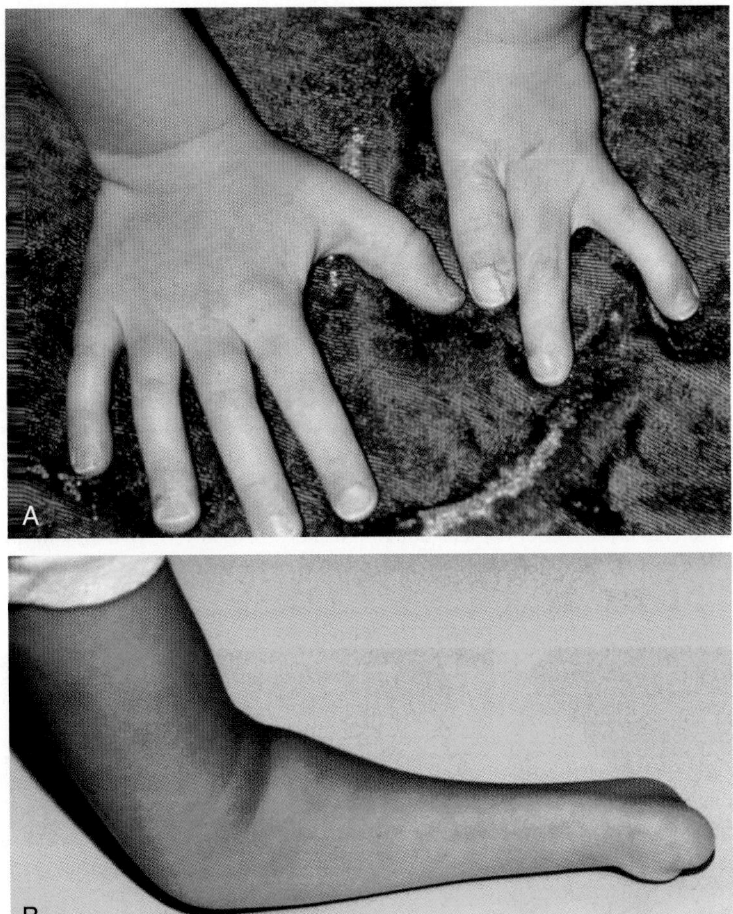

FIGURE 45.6 **A,** Ulnar longitudinal ray defect of the left hand in an infant born to a mother with a bicornuate uterus (same infant as in Fig. 45.1, *top*). **B,** Terminal transverse hemimelia of the left arm in a child born to a woman with a bicornuate uterus. (From Graham JM Jr, Miller ME, Stephan MJ, et al. Limb reduction anomalies and early in-utero limb compression. *J Pediatr.* 1980;96:1052.)

obstetric outcomes.[35] Compared with a control group of women with recurrent miscarriage and no identifiable cause, women with a septate or bicornuate uterus had more second-trimester miscarriages than controls (13–14%). Women with an arcuate, septate, or bicornuate uterus had reduced rates of biochemical pregnancy losses compared with the recurrent miscarriage control group (10–11% vs. 30.4%). Therefore pregnancies in women with recurrent pregnancy loss and uterine anomalies are not associated with early implantation failure, and these women experience their pregnancy losses at a more advanced gestational age.[36]

In a case-control study of 38 infants (32 liveborn and 6 stillborn) born to mothers with a bicornuate uterus, the risk for congenital defects was four times higher than in women with a normal uterus.[37] Five defects were significantly more common: nasal hypoplasia, omphalocele, limb deficiencies (hypoplasia or absence of metacarpals, metatarsals, phalanges), teratoma, and acardia-anencephaly. Other defects were common but did not reach statistical significance: microcephaly, microtia, esophageal atresia, syndactyly, limb contractures, scoliosis, and micrognathia. Among the 38 cases born to women with a bicornuate uterus, 34.2% had deformations (limb contractures, scoliosis, nasal hypoplasia, micrognathia, and clubfoot), which is similar to the 30% risk suggested previously.[2] Vaginal bleeding was significantly more common than in mothers with a normal uterus (54.1% vs. 14.1%), and vaginal bleeding has previously been associated with

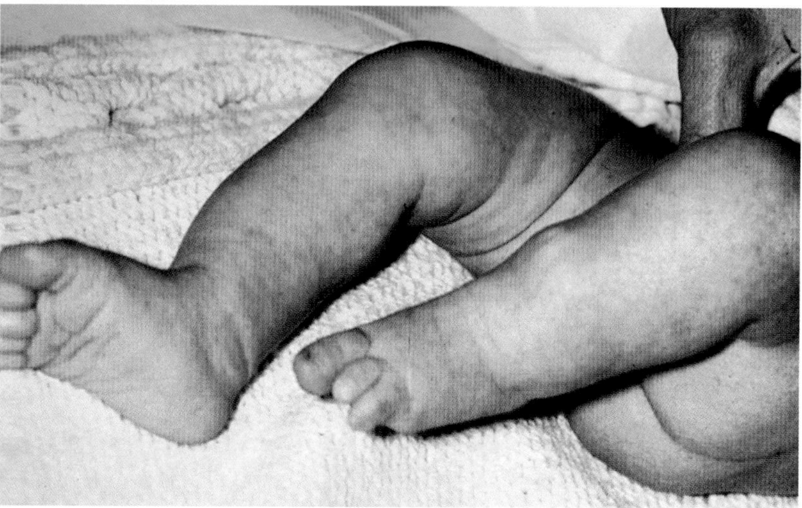

FIGURE 45.7 Fibular longitudinal ray defect of the left foot with a short, bent lower leg in an infant born to a woman with a large uterine leiomyoma.

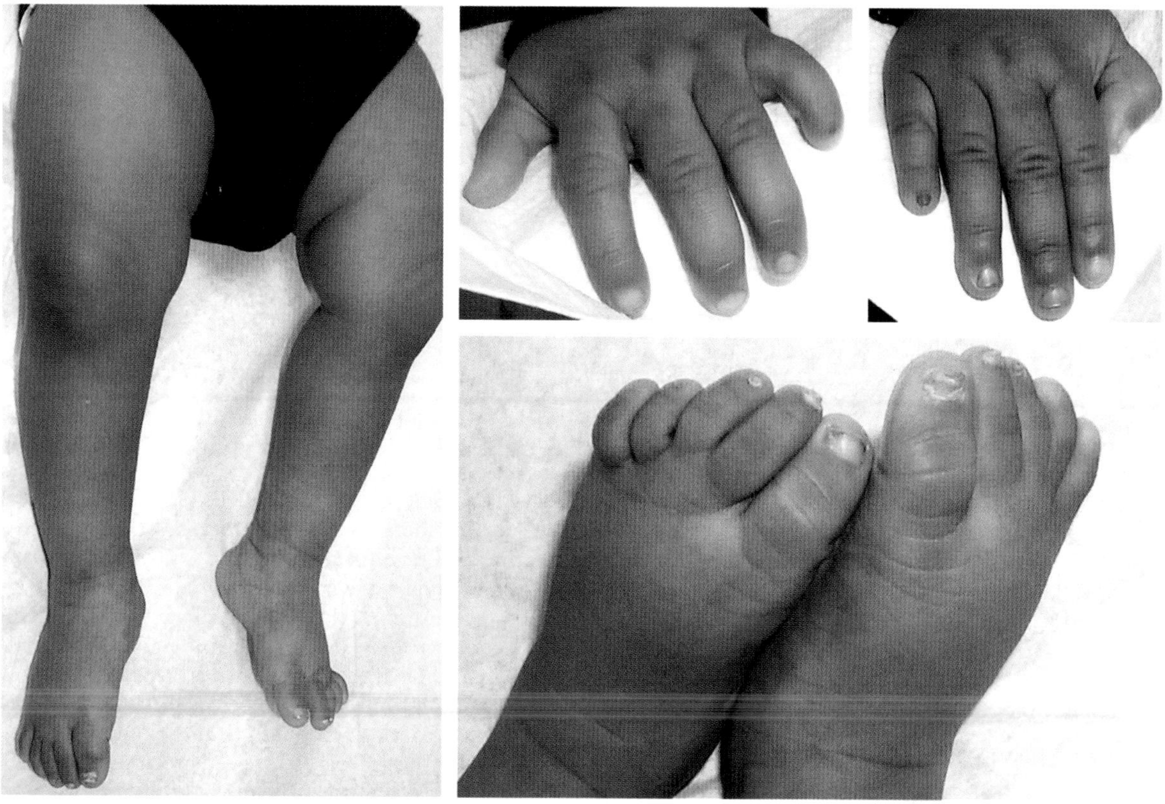

FIGURE 45.8 Hypoplastic left leg and distal digital hypoplasia in an infant delivered by cesarean section owing to extensive uterine leiomyomata, which were so enlarged that they had to be surgically resected so that the baby could be delivered.

limb reduction defects.[17,22,37] In a study of 322 women with abnormal uterine bleeding, hysteroscopy detected asymptomatic Müllerian anomalies in 10% of these women. The women with Müllerian anomalies had a significantly higher incidence of spontaneous abortion and lower cumulative live birth rates,[38,39] which suggests that some fetuses with severe defects might have been lost earlier in gestation in this case-control study of liveborn and stillborn infants.[37]

MANAGEMENT, PROGNOSIS, AND COUNSEL

Surgical improvement of the uterine size, if indicated and possible, may improve the chances of rearing a normal fetus to a term birth.[38] Large uterine fibroids may also merit consideration of surgical intervention. Among 174 patients with appropriate imaging, reproductive performance depended on the type of uterine malformation and urinary tract anomalies. The lowest percentage of women who had only live births occurred in women with bicornuate unicollis uterus (28%). Among women with uterine anomalies and unilateral renal agenesis, perinatal outcomes were much better (72% had only living children) than those with no renal agenesis (40%). The 355 pregnancies in patients with associated unilateral renal agenesis were associated with term deliveries and living children, while pregnancies in women with uterine malformation and no renal agenesis had more fetal loss, premature birth, and breech presentations. Thus if the Müllerian anomaly was the consequence of abnormal mesonephric or Wolffian morphogenesis, reproductive performance was much improved over women with an isolated Müllerian defect.[40] Among 21 women with uterine malformations and a surgically treated obstructed hemivagina and associated ipsilateral renal agenesis (12 didelphic, 6 septate, and 3 bicornuate uterus), all had surgical excision of the longitudinal vaginal septum causing the obstructed hemivagina during adolescence. Conception was attempted at a median of 13 years later in 13 of these women, who produced 22 pregnancies, with 77% of pregnancies occurring contralateral to the treated obstructed hemivagina and unilateral renal agenesis, and 91% of these pregnancies ending in delivery of a living infant. Increased rates of preeclampsia (14%), preterm delivery (36%), breech presentation (38%), and cesarean section (67%) were noted.[41] A prospective study of 170 patients with congenital uterine anomalies and two or more prior miscarriages revealed that in patients with a septate uterus, the live birth rate at the first pregnancy after ascertainment of anomalies in patients with surgery tended to be higher (81.3%) than in those without surgery (61.5%). The infertility rates were similar in both groups, whereas the cumulative live birth rate (76.1%) tended to be higher with surgery than without surgery (60.0%). Surgery showed no benefit in patients with a bicornuate uterus for having a baby, but tended to decrease the preterm birth rate and the low birth weight.[42]

Among women with fibroids diagnosed using combined transvaginal ultrasound and HSG, fibroids distorting the uterine cavity were resected via hysteroscopy in 25 women, and outcomes were compared with 54 women with fibroids not distorting the cavity who did not undergo any intervention and a second comparison group of 285 women with unexplained recurrent miscarriage.[43] The prevalence of fibroids was found to be 8.2% (79/966), and there were 264 pregnancies in women with fibroids and 936 pregnancies in women with unexplained recurrent miscarriages. In women with intracavitary distortion who underwent myomectomy, their mid-trimester miscarriage rate in subsequent pregnancies was reduced from 21.7% to 0%, resulting in a significant increase in their live birth rate from 23.3% to 52.0%. Women with fibroids not distorting the cavity had similar outcomes to women with unexplained recurrent miscarriages, achieving a 70.4% live birth rate in their subsequent pregnancies without any intervention. Fibroids were associated with increased mid-trimester losses among women with recurrent miscarriages, and resection of fibroids distorting the uterine cavity eliminated these mid-trimester losses and doubled their live birth rate in subsequent pregnancies. Women with fibroids not distorting the uterine cavity were able to achieve high live birth rates without intervention.[43] Among patients who had laparoscopic myomectomy for single and/or multiple myomas sized between 5 and 15 cm, 426 myomas were removed, and 115 (62.2%) patients had 151 pregnancies, with 38 pregnancies ending in miscarriage and 2 ectopic implantations. There were 111 successful pregnancies, with 7 preterm deliveries (6.3%), cesarean section in 69 cases (63.4%), and vaginal delivery in 42 cases (36.6%). Laparoscopic myomectomy resulted in subsequent good reproductive outcomes, both in terms of pregnancy and miscarriage rates.[44]

Regarding the surgical approach to myomectomy, current evidence from two randomized controlled trials suggests there is no significant difference between the laparoscopic and open approach regarding fertility.[45] After laparoscopic myomectomy there were 75 recurrences in 224 patients. The cumulative risk of recurrence was 4.9% at 24 months and 21.4% at 60 months after the operation. Age of 30 to 40 years and the presence of more than one fibroid at the time of initial laparoscopic myomectomy significantly increased the risk of symptomatic recurrence after laparoscopic myomectomy (31.25% and 38.71%, respectively).[46]

Uterine fibroids cause heavy prolonged bleeding, pain, pressure symptoms, and subfertility, and uterine artery embolization has been reported to be an effective and safe alternative to treat fibroids in women not desiring future fertility, with patient satisfaction rates similar to hysterectomy and myomectomy, and a shorter hospital stay and quicker return to routine activities. However, embolization is associated with a higher rate of minor complications and an increased likelihood of requiring surgical intervention within 2 to 5 years of the initial procedure.[47,48] Women with large symptomatic fibroids wishing to retain their uterus and ineligible for minimally invasive (laparoscopic or vaginal) hysterectomy are good candidates for embolization, but this procedure is controversial in younger women desiring pregnancy, mainly because of the significant risk of miscarriage (as high as 64% in some studies), as well as the increased risk of other complications of pregnancy, such as preterm delivery, abnormal placentation, and postpartum hemorrhage.[48] Genetic factors, epigenetic factors, estrogens, progesterone, growth factors, cytokines, chemokines, and extracellular matrix components have all been implicated in the pathogenesis of fibroid development and growth.[49] Gonadotropin-releasing hormone agonist therapy has been approved by the US Food and Drug Administration for reducing fibroid volume and related symptoms. Mifepristone, asoprisnil, ulipristal acetate, and epigallocatechin gallate have been shown to be effective for fibroid regression and symptomatic improvement, and they are all in clinical trials.[49]

Treatment options for symptomatic fibroids include pharmacologic, surgical, and radiologically guided interventions. The range of medical treatments allows flexible management of fibroid-related symptoms, and options include tranexamic acid, nonsteroidal anti-inflammatory drugs, contraceptive steroids, gonadotropin-releasing hormone analogs, antiprogesterone, and selective progesterone receptor modulators.[50] Medical options do not remove the fibroids, and symptoms may return when treatment is stopped. Hysterectomy is the most effective treatment, although in some cases myomectomy may be sufficient to control symptoms. Alternatives to surgery include uterine artery embolization, myolysis, and ablation by high-intensity focused ultrasound (guided with magnetic resonance imaging or ultrasound). The choice of treatment depends on fibroid size, the underlying symptoms and their severity, and the woman's desire for subsequent fertility and pregnancy, as well as the risk of recurrence.[50] Among 59 women aged 23 to 42 years with a desire to have children and who underwent laparoscopic myomectomy for symptomatic fibroids, the conception rate after the procedure was 68%, with a lower rate of miscarriages (24%) than before (43%) the procedure. Primary cesarean sections were performed in 46% because of patient preference, placental complications, and uterine rupture. Labor was successful in 62%, and uterine rupture and placental complications occurred in 10% and 13% of all pregnancies, respectively.[51]

DIFFERENTIAL DIAGNOSIS

A history of multiple miscarriages, stillbirths, and congenital anomalies may lead to a consideration of chromosomal studies in the surviving offspring and parents in search of a chromosomal alteration. Comparative genomic hybridization has sometimes detected submicroscopic cryptic chromosomal anomalies in offspring who had normal chromosome results by standard techniques. Limited uterine space should also be considered in such situations, especially when the anomalies in the offspring suggest deformation or disruption rather than malformation. This is especially important for the family because it may be possible to surgically improve the uterine situation in some women. A careful assessment of infants born from a small uterine cavity with multiple anomalies may indicate that they have multiple *deformations* rather than malformations.

References

1. Goyal LD, Dhaliwal B, Singh P, Ganjoo S, Goyal V. Management of Mullerian development anomalies: 9 years' experience of a tertiary care center. *Gynecol Minim Invasive Ther*. 2020;9(2):81–87.
2. Miller ME, Dunn PM, Smith DW. Uterine malformation and fetal deformation. *J Pediatr*. 1979;94:387–390.
3. Takami M, Aoki S, Kurasawa K, et al. A classification of congenital uterine anomalies predicting pregnancy outcomes. *Acta Obstet Gynecol Scand*. 2014;93:691–697.
4. Bocca SM, Oehninger S, Stadtmauer L, et al. A study of the cost, accuracy, and benefits of 3-dimensional

sonography compared with hysterosalpingography in women with uterine abnormalities. *J Ultrasound Med.* 2012;31:81–85.

5. Bendarska-Czerwińska A, Zmarzły N, Morawiec E, et al. Endocrine disorders and fertility and pregnancy: an update. *Front Endocrinol (Lausanne)*. 2022;13:970439.
6. Saravelos SH, Cocksedge KA, Li TC. Prevalence and diagnosis of congenital uterine anomalies in women with reproductive failure: a critical appraisal. *Hum Reprod Update*. 2008;14:415–429.
7. Chan YY, Jayaprakasan K, Tan A, et al. Reproductive outcomes in women with congenital uterine anomalies: a systematic review. *Ultrasound Obstet Gynecol.* 2011;38:371–382.
8. Chifan M, Tîrnovanu M, Grigore M, et al. Cervical incompetence associated with congenital uterine malformations. *Rev Med Chir Soc Med Nat Iasi.* 2012;116:1063–1068.
9. Singh N, Singh U, Verma ML. Ruptured bicornuate uterus mimicking ectopic pregnancy: a case report. *J Obstet Gynaecol Res.* 2013;39:364–366.
10. Allen WL, Subba B, Yoong W, et al. Chronic abdominal pregnancy following rupture from a bicornuate uterus. *Arch Gynecol Obstet.* 2007;275:393–395.
11. Brady PC, Molina RL, Muto MG, Stapp B, Srouji SS. Diagnosis and management of a heterotopic pregnancy and ruptured rudimentary uterine horn. *Fertil Res Pract.* 2018;4:6.
12. Parveen R. Detection and management of pregnancy in rudimentary horn of uterus. *J Coll Physicians Surg Pak.* 2019;29(6):S70–s72.
13. Walker C, Collins L, Pham A, George J, Johnson S. Avoiding the fatal misdiagnosis of pregnancy in a noncommunicating rudimentary horn using 3D transvaginal ultrasound. *J Clin Ultrasound.* 2020;48(9):553–556.
14. Crabtree GS, Machin GA, Martin JME, et al. Fetal deformation caused by uterine malformation. *Pediatr Path.* 1984;2:305–312.
15. Zlotogora J, Arad I, Yarkoni S, et al. Newborn with multiple joint contractures due to maternal bicornuate uterus, Israel. *J Med Sci.* 1985;21:454–455.
16. Romero R, Chervenak FA, DeVore G, et al. Fetal head deformation and congenital torticollis associated with a uterine tumor. *Am J Obstet Gynecol.* 1981;141:839–840.
17. Graham Jr JM, Miller ME, Stephan MJ, et al. Limb reduction anomalies and early in utero limb compression. *J Pediatr.* 1980;96:1052–1056.
18. Fox NS, Roman AS, Saltzman DH, et al. Twin pregnancy in patients with a uterine anomaly. *J Matern Fetal Neonatal Med.* 2014;27:360–364.
19. Almusalam MM, Badawi A, Bushaqer N. Are deliveries by inverted T-incision on the rise due to fibroids?: A case report. *Cureus.* 2022;14(5):e24781.
20. Brady PC, Stanic AK, Styer AK. Uterine fibroids and subfertility: an update on the role of myomectomy. *Curr Opin Obstet Gynecol.* 2013;25:255–259.
21. Mahalingaiah S, Hart JE, Wise LA, et al. Prenatal diethylstilbestrol exposure and risk of uterine leiomyomata in the Nurses' Health Study II. *Am J Epidemiol.* 2013;179:186–191.
22. Matsunaga E, Shiota K. Ectopic pregnancy and myoma uteri: teratogenic effects and maternal characteristics. *Teratology.* 1980;21:61–69.
23. Lam SJ, Best S, Kumar S. The impact of fibroid characteristics on pregnancy outcome. *Am J Obstet Gynecol.* 2014;211:395. https://doi.org/10.1016/j.ajog.2014.03.066.
24. Ciavattini A, Clemente N, Delli Carpini G, et al. Number and size of uterine fibroids and obstetric outcomes. *J Matern Fetal Neonatal Med.* 2014;5:1–5.
25. Vila-Vives JM, Hidalgo-Mora JJ, Soler I, et al. Fetal arthrogryposis secondary to a giant maternal uterine leiomyoma. *Case Rep Obstet Gynecol.* 2012;2012:726–732. https://doi.org/10.1155/2012/726732.
26. Aminu MB, Sania I, Khairunnaesa M. Post-dated breech pregnancy in a non-obviously communicating rudimentary horn of a bicornuate uterus requiring hemi-hysterectomy. *J West Afr Coll Surg.* 2023;13(1):111–113.
27. Polishuk WZ, Ron MA. Familial bicornuate and double uterus. *Am J Obstet Gynecol.* 1974;119:982–987.
28. Miyazaki Y, Ebisuno S, Uekado Y, et al. Uterus didelphys with unilateral imperforate vagina and ipsilateral renal agenesis. *J Urology.* 1986;135:107–109.
29. Satey T, O'Reilly PH. Bicornuate and unicornuate uterus associated with unilateral renal aplasia and abnormal solitary kidneys: report of 3 cases. *J Urology.* 1986;135:110–111.
30. Marshall FF, Beisel DS. The association of uterine and renal anomalies. *Obstet Gynecol.* 1978;51:550–562.
31. Woodward PJ, Sobaey R, Wagner BJ. Congenital uterine malformations. *Curr Probl Diagn Radiol.* 1995;24: 178–197.
32. Herlin M, Højland AT, Petersen MB. Familial occurrence of Mayer-Rokitansky-Küster-Hauser syndrome: a case report and review of the literature. *Am J Med Genet A.* 2014;164A:2276–2286.
33. Acién P, Acién M. Unilateral renal agenesis and female genital tract pathologies. *Acta Obstet Gynecol Scand.* 2010;89:1424–1431.
34. Hua M, Odibo AO, Longman RE, et al. Congenital uterine anomalies and adverse pregnancy outcomes. *Am J Obstet Gynecol.* 2011;205:558 e1–e5.
35. Zhang Y, Zhao YY, Qiao J. Obstetric outcome of women with uterine anomalies in China. *Chin Med J.* 2010;123:418–422.
36. Saravelos SH, Cocksedge KA, Li TC. The pattern of pregnancy loss in women with congenital uterine anomalies and recurrent miscarriage. *Reprod Biomed Online.* 2010;20:416–422.
37. Martinez-Frias ML, Bermejo E, Rodriquez-Pinilla E, et al. Congenital anomalies in the offspring of mothers with a bicornuate uterus. *Pediatrics.* 1998;101:693–694.
38. Ben-Rafael Z, Seidman DS, Recabi K, et al. Uterine anomalies: a retrospective matched-control study. *J Reprod Med.* 1991;36:723–727.

39. Grimbizis GF, Camus M, Tarlatzis BC, et al. Clinical implications of uterine malformations and hysteroscopic treatment results. *Hum Reprod Update*. 2001;7:161–174.
40. Acién P, Acién M, Mazaira N, et al. Reproductive outcome in uterine malformations with or without an associated unilateral renal agenesis. *J Reprod Med*. 2014;59:69–75.
41. Heinonen PK. Pregnancies in women with uterine malformation, treated obstruction of hemivagina and ipsilateral renal agenesis. *Arch Gynecol Obstet*. 2013;287:975–978.
42. Sugiura-Ogasawara M, Lin BL, Aoki K, et al. Does surgery improve live birth rates in patients with recurrent miscarriage caused by uterine anomalies? *J Obstet Gynaecol*. 2015;35(2):155–158.
43. Saravelos SH, Yan J, Rehmani H, et al. The prevalence and impact of fibroids and their treatment on the outcome of pregnancy in women with recurrent miscarriage. *Hum Reprod*. 2011;26:3274–3279.
44. Fagherazzi S, Borgato S, Bertin M, et al. Pregnancy outcome after laparoscopic myomectomy. *Clin Exp Obstet Gynecol*. 2014;41:375–379.
45. Metwally M, Cheong YC, Horne AW. Surgical treatment of fibroids for subfertility. *Cochrane Database Syst Rev*. 2012 Nov 14;11:CD003857. https://doi.org/10.1002/14651858.CD003857.pub3.
46. Radosa MP, Owsianowski Z, Mothes A, et al. Long-term risk of fibroid recurrence after laparoscopic myomectomy. *Eur J Obstet Gynecol Reprod Biol*. 2014;180C:35–39.
47. Gupta JK, Sinha A, Lumsden MA, et al. Uterine artery embolization for symptomatic uterine fibroids. *Cochrane Database Syst Rev*. 2012 May 16;5:CD005073. https://doi.org/10.1002/14651858.CD005073.pub3.
48. Mara M, Kubinova K. Embolization of uterine fibroids from the point of view of the gynecologist: pros and cons. *Int J Womens Health*. 2014;6:623–629.
49. Islam MS, Protic O, Giannubilo SR, et al. Uterine leiomyoma: available medical treatments and new possible therapeutic options. *J Clin Endocrinol Metab*. 2013;98:921–934.
50. Pérez-López FR, Ornat L, Ceausu I, et al. EMAS position statement: management of uterine fibroids. *Maturitas*. 2014;79:106–116.
51. Bernardi TS, Radosa MP, Weisheit A, et al. Laparoscopic myomectomy: a 6-year follow-up single-center cohort analysis of fertility and obstetric outcome measures. *Arch Gynecol Obstet*. 2014;290:87–91.

CHAPTER 46

Oligohydramnios Sequence

KEY POINTS

- Amniotic fluid tends to decrease during the last trimester of pregnancy, and a serious deficiency can result in fetal constraint.
- Oligohydramnios may be caused by renal/urinary tract malformations or amniotic rupture, accompanied by constrictive amnion strands, which can lead to various birth defects.
- Renal oligohydramnios is predominantly caused by congenital abnormalities of the kidney and urogenital tract.
- Oligohydramnios is associated with poor placental function, intrauterine growth retardation, intrapartum asphyxia, and fetal demise.
- Oligohydramnios can lead to oligohydramnios sequence characterized by facial compression, limb deformities, fetal growth deficiency, and pulmonary hypoplasia.
- Severe oligohydramnios lasting longer than 14 days with rupture of membranes before 25 weeks has a high mortality rate.
- Amnioinfusion significantly improves perinatal outcome and prolongs the pregnancy in severe second-trimester oligohydramnios in both idiopathic cases and those involving premature rupture of the amniotic membranes.
- The recurrence risk for oligohydramnios sequence relates to the basic problem that gave rise to the oligohydramnios.

GENESIS

The relative and absolute amount of amniotic fluid tends to decrease during the last trimester as the fetus fills out the uterine cavity, as shown in Fig. 46.1. A serious deficiency of amniotic fluid will result in significant fetal constraint.[1] Oligohydramnios may be secondary to amniotic rupture and may be accompanied by constrictive, disruptive strands of amnion (Fig. 46.2).[2] The consequences of what has been called very early amnion rupture can include the compressive consequences of early constraint, such as scoliosis and clubfeet, as well as facial clefts, limb-body wall defects, and amniotic bands (see Chapter 49).[3,4] Such early defects can be lethal, resulting in spontaneous abortion.[5] Later rupture of the amnion may or may not be accompanied by amniotic bands, and if bands are present, they are usually limited to constrictive bands around various parts of one or more limbs.

A systematic review and metaanalysis of 15 studies comprising 8067 singleton pregnancies diagnosed with oligohydramnios compared with 27,526 pregnancies with normal amniotic fluid index (AFI) indicated that pregnancies with oligohydramnios had significantly higher rates of an infant with meconium aspiration syndrome, cesarean delivery for fetal distress, admission to the neonatal intensive care unit, and low birth weight.[6] A retrospective study from 2017 to 2019 characterized the degree of oligohydramnios in all low-risk pregnancies at a single institution by AFI (mild = 41–50 mm, moderate = 21–40 mm, and severe = 0–20 mm). Of 610 women, 202 were mild (33.1%), 287 were moderate (47.0%), and 121 were severe (19.8%). Low-risk pregnancies with isolated severe oligohydramnios at term have a higher tendency toward nonreassuring fetal monitoring requiring prompt delivery and adverse neonatal outcomes, thus suggesting a need for close intrapartum surveillance.[7]

Chronic leakage of amniotic fluid for several weeks prior to delivery is one cause of oligohydramnios sequence (Fig. 46.3).[1] In a cohort of 85 women with premature rupture of membranes (PROM; at 14–23.6 weeks' gestation) the survival rate was 49%. A genetic amniocentesis-related cause of PROM, gestational age at PROM, C-reactive protein >1 mg/dL, and oligohydramnios were significantly associated with fetal survival.[8] Among 49 patients with PROM at 16 to 23

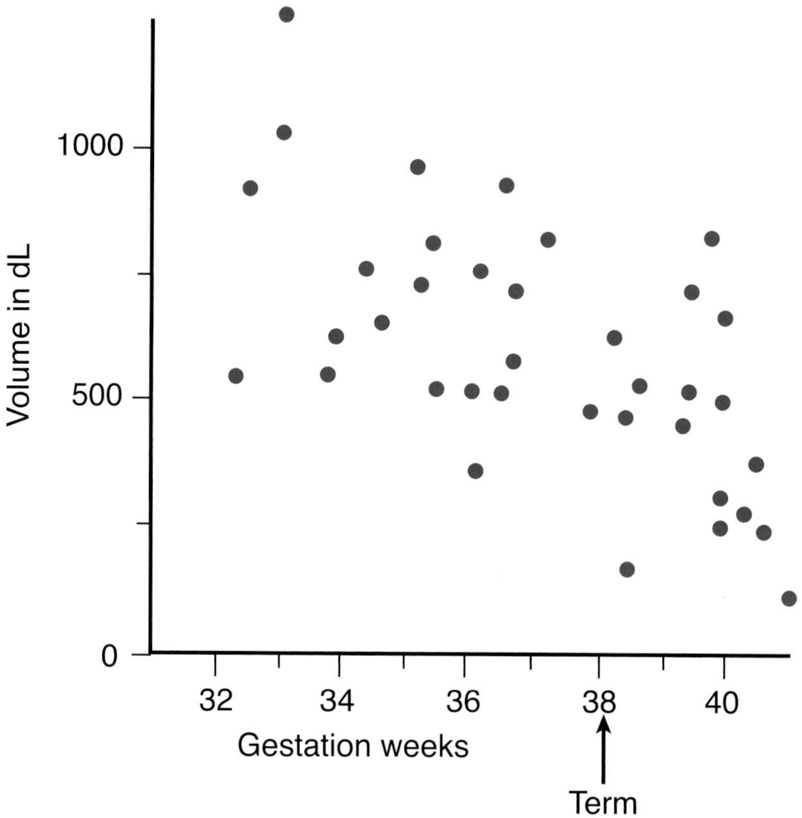

FIGURE 46.1 Progressive decrease in volume of amniotic fluid during the last trimester.

weeks' gestation from 1998 to 2003, 20 couples out of 49 chose medical termination of pregnancy. Among the remaining 29 continuing pregnancies, the mean delay to delivery after PROM was 2.1 weeks, and the mean gestational age at delivery was 23.2 weeks, with 19 patients delivering after 22 weeks.[9] The main factors predicting fetal survival were the initial AFI (2.9 cm vs. 0.8 cm) and gestational age at delivery (26.7 weeks vs. 22.6 weeks). About 2% of continuing pregnancies were complicated by maternal infection and 83% of the survivors had neonatal respiratory distress syndrome, with 41.2% developing sepsis. There was a uniformly poor prognosis with absent amniotic fluid and PROM before 21 weeks, whereas 63% of infants born after 24 weeks were still alive at 1 week.[9] To evaluate the respiratory and neurologic outcome data at 2 years of age, 15 infants born following PROM prior to 25 weeks with a prolonged latency (14 days) to delivery were compared with an age-matched group of 30 infants.[10] Survivors in this high-risk group (73%) had low morbidity at the time of discharge. Although there was no significant difference in the incidence of bronchopulmonary dysplasia between the groups, the length of hospitalization and respiratory morbidity during the first 2 years of life were significantly higher for infants born following a prolonged period of oligohydramnios, but developmental assessment at 20 to 24 months corrected for gestational age showed no difference between the two groups. A metaanalysis of 43 studies (244,493 fetuses) regarding prediction of amniotic fluid measurements for adverse pregnancy outcome demonstrated a strong association between oligohydramnios and birth weight <10th centile as well as mortality, but despite these strong associations with poor outcome, they did not accurately predict the outcome risk for individuals.[11]

Chronic abruption-oligohydramnios sequence is a clinical condition with prolonged vaginal bleeding and oligohydramnios owing to chronic placental abruption, which results in preterm labor, fetal growth restriction, and neonatal chronic lung disease. The duration of bleeding is a significant predictive factor for poor perinatal/neonatal outcomes, particularly

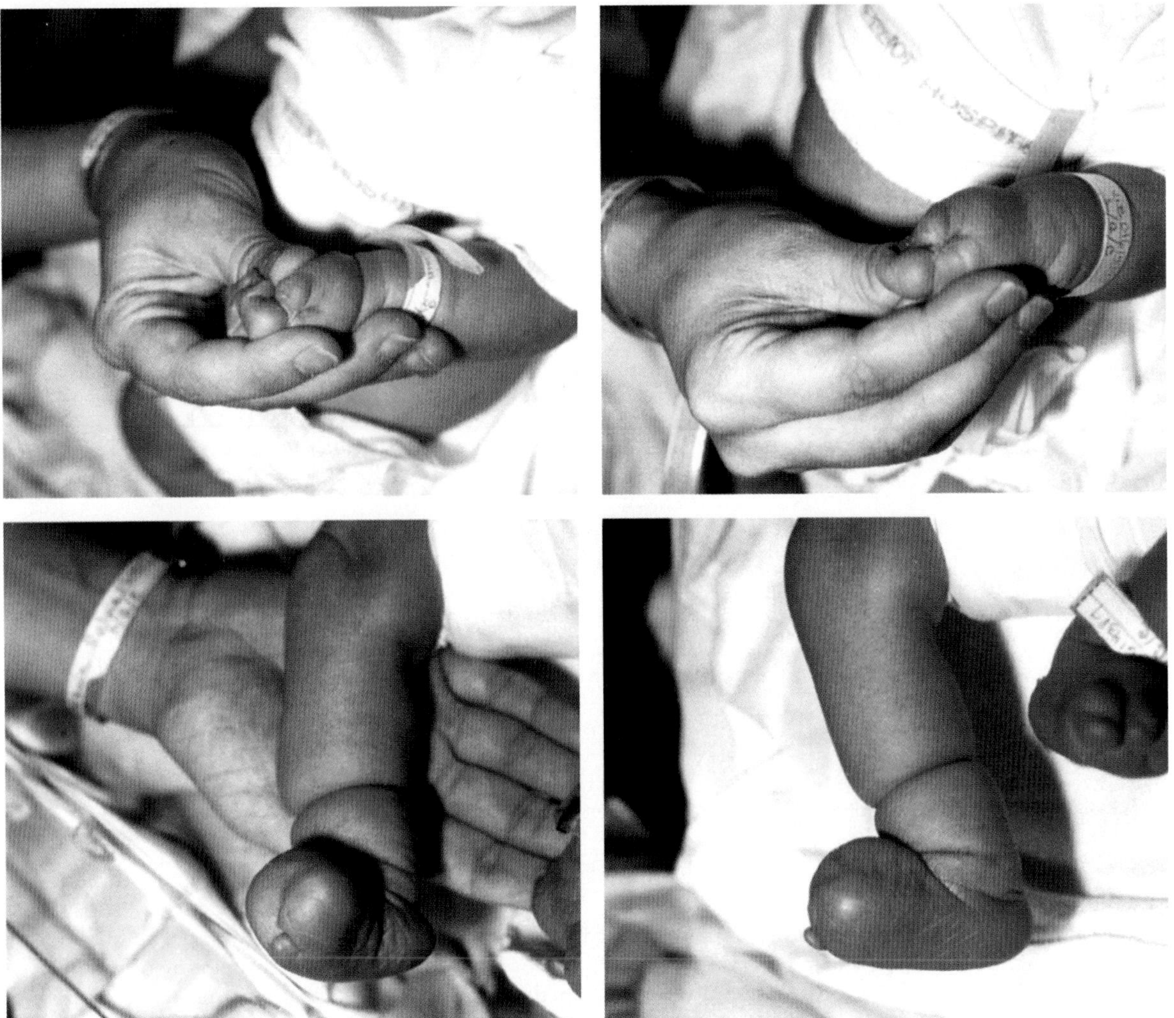

FIGURE 46.2 Examples of constrictive amniotic band disruption caused by early amniotic rupture.

when it begins during the first trimester.[12] Pulmonary hypoplasia in preterm infants in this condition is associated with oligohydramnios and diffuse chorioamniotic hemosiderosis caused by continuing intrauterine hemorrhage owing to chronic placental abuption.[13]

Fetal urination is the major source of amniotic fluid production, and the fetal kidneys begin to function at around 10 to 12 weeks. It is estimated that approximately 1000 to 1200 mL of fetal urine enters the amniotic space each day from the fetal kidneys, with additional fluid entering from the fetal lungs (half of which is swallowed). There is usually a complete turnover of amniotic fluid volume (about 800 mL at term) in less than 24 hours. Roughly 500 mL is swallowed each day (not including swallowed fetal lung fluid), with additional fluid moving into the maternal and fetal circulation through vessels in the amniotic membranes and placenta.[14] By 20 to 25 weeks of gestation fetal urine becomes the major constituent of amniotic fluid; hence oligohydramnios is predominantly a feature of renal or urinary tract malformations during the last half of gestation.

Among 34 cases of prenatal severe bilateral renal hypoplasia, 38% were liveborn and 62% underwent pregnancy termination. Oligohydramnios or anhydramnios was observed in 30 of 34 (88.2%) cases, with normal renal function in 4 of 13 liveborn cases. Overall, 30 of 34 (88.2%) cases had a poor outcome, and serum β_2-microglobulin accurately predicted

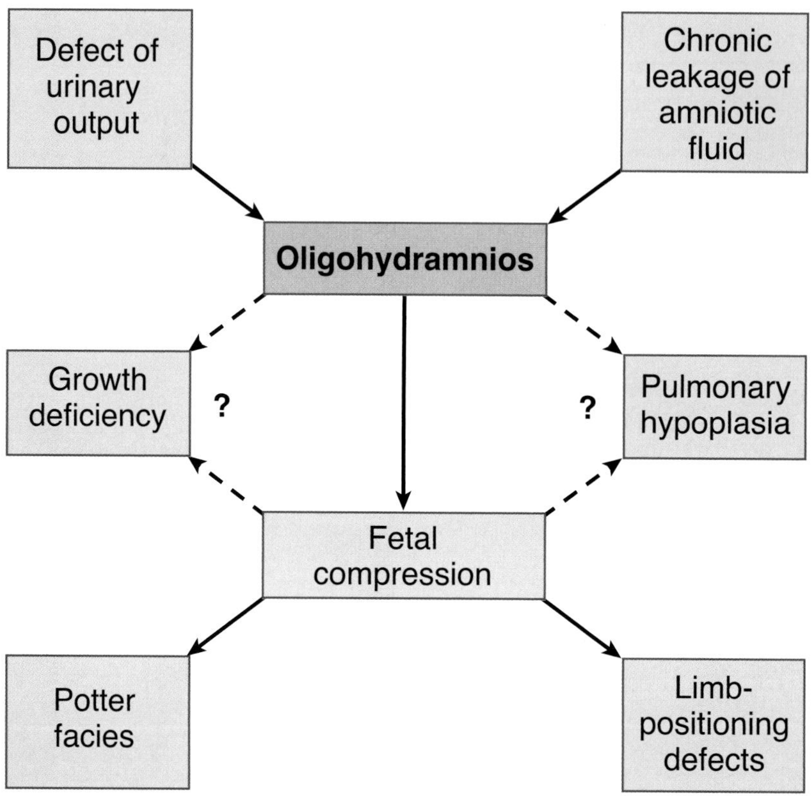

FIGURE 46.3 Origins and impact of oligohydramnios on the fetus.

poor renal outcome.[15] Renal oligohydramnios is predominantly caused by congenital abnormalities of the kidney and urogenital tract. Among 36 neonates with renal oligohydramnios treated between 1996 and 2007, the causes included obstructive uropathy (19), polycystic kidney disease (6), renal agenesis/dysplasia (10), and bilateral renal vein thrombosis (1). Overall survival was 58% (21 of 36), and seven patients died within 2 days of birth from respiratory failure, with a low oxygenation index and a diagnosis of renal oligohydramnios before 28 weeks' gestation predicting poor survival.[16] Among 71 pregnancies with renal oligohydramnios between 2000 and 2008, causes included cystic dysplasia (36), polycystic kidney disease (15), and hydronephrosis (20), with 23 (32%) demonstrating associated anomalies. In 49 fetuses (69%), the diagnosis was made before 24 weeks of gestational age, and 41 of those pregnancies were terminated. Among 25 liveborn neonates, 10 survived and 15 died. Prognostic factors for survival included gestational age at diagnosis (32.2 weeks for survivors vs. 28.1 weeks for nonsurvivors), diagnosis of hydronephrosis (seven in the survivors vs. four in the nonsurvivors), and isolated anomaly (nine in the survivors vs. seven in the nonsurvivors).[17]

Renal pathology is particularly important for genetic counseling. Among 14 cases of fetal or neonatal renal malformations, the results of postmortem examination disclosed renal malformations that were not diagnosed prenatally (86%), provided extensive additional information (50%), or confirmed the diagnosis hypothesis (14%).[18] Renal tubular dysgenesis (RTD) is a severe fetal disorder characterized by the absence or poor development of proximal tubules, early-onset and persistent anuria (leading to oligohydramnios sequence), and ossification defects of the skull. In most cases early death occurs from pulmonary hypoplasia, anuria, and refractory arterial hypotension.[19] RTD may be acquired during fetal development or inherited as an autosomal recessive condition. Inherited RTD is genetically heterogeneous and linked to mutations in the genes encoding the major components of the renin-angiotensin system: angiotensinogen, renin, angiotensin-converting enzyme, or angiotensin II receptor type 1.[20] Mutations result in either the absence of production or lack of efficacy of angiotensin II. Secondary RTD has been observed in various situations, particularly in the donor twin of severe twin-to-twin transfusion syndrome, in fetuses affected with congenital hemochromatosis, or in fetuses exposed to renin-angiotensin system blockers.[21] All causes result in renal hypoperfusion. These examples illustrate the importance of a functional renin-angiotensin system in the maintenance of blood pressure and renal blood flow during fetal life. The pathologic diagnosis of RTD in an anuric fetus with normal renal sonography can be very important for the management of the fetus or neonate.[19-21] A retrospective study of chromosomal microarray and exome sequencing in 126 fetuses with oligohydramnios revealed pathogenic or likely pathogenic copy number variants in 2 of 124 fetuses. Exome sequencing revealed pathogenic or likely pathogenic in 7 of 32 (21.8%), with 6 of 7 (85.7%) fetuses showing an autosomal recessive inheritance pattern and 3 of 7 (42.9%) variants related to the renin-angiotensin-aldosterone system, which are the known genetic causes of autosomal recessive RTD.[22]

Twin-twin transfusion syndrome is a serious condition that complicates 8% to 10% of twin pregnancies with monochorionic diamniotic placentation.[23] Diagnosis requires monochorionic diamniotic placentation and the presence of oligohydramnios in one sac and of polyhydramnios in the other sac. Serial sonographic evaluation should begin around 16 weeks and continue until delivery. More than 75% of cases remain stable or regress without invasive intervention, with perinatal survival of about 86%, but with advanced twin-twin transfusion syndrome there is a perinatal loss rate of 70% to 100%, particularly when it presents before 26 weeks.[24] Oligohydramnios may be a sign of danger in one member of a monozygotic twin pair because of placental vascular shunting. If one twin is transfusing the other, the donor tends to be hypovolemic with reduced renal blood flow, resulting in oligohydramnios.

Fetal immobilization during late gestation owing to oligohydramnios associated with renal agenesis or obstructive uropathy is associated with positional limb abnormalities but is not associated with reduced bone mass, whereas fetal immobilization owing to fetal akinesia sequence results in thin long bones with decreased bone mass, which suggests that muscular stress is a major factor in fetal periosteal bone growth.[24] Oligohydramnios may be a sign of poor placental function and is frequently associated with intrauterine growth retardation, intrapartum asphyxia, and fetal demise, because poor placental function (such as might occur with severe preeclampsia or pregnancy-induced maternal hypertension) leads to decreased fetal hydration, growth retardation, and decreased fetal urinary flow.

FEATURES

Amniotic fluid volume can be determined by ultrasound and may be predictive of some types of fetal and maternal problems, as described previously. Amniotic fluid volume rises progressively from 10 to 20 mL at 10 weeks to 800 mL at 24 weeks and then remains relatively constant at 700 to 800 mL until term (see Fig. 46.1). After 40 weeks amniotic fluid volume declines by about 8% per week, reaching 400 mL at 42 weeks.[25,26] Oligohydramnios (less than fifth percentile for gestational age) is approximately 300 mL. Amniotic fluid volume assessment is usually determined by ultrasound after 16 weeks to monitor patients with preterm PROMs. Mechanisms for recirculation of amniotic fluid include fetal breathing lung movements, swallowing, absorption through the fetal gastrointestinal tract, and excretion through fetal urine production. Oligohydramnios requires evaluation for fetal growth restriction and genitourinary issues, such as renal agenesis, multicystic dysplastic kidneys, RTD, ureteropelvic junction obstruction, and bladder outlet obstruction. Premature preterm rupture of membranes should also be considered as a cause of oligohydramnios.[27]

Persistent oligohydramnios may be an indication for prompt delivery, and antepartum testing with nonstress tests and fetal biophysical profiles can facilitate this decision. Perinatal mortality is increased when sonographic determination of amniotic fluid volume is marginal, and it is increased even more with severe oligohydramnios. A prospective study of 180 pregnant women at 37 to 40 weeks of gestation compared women with a mean AFI of 4.14 cm (AFI ≤fifth percentile) with a control group (mean AFI = 10.14 cm).[28] In the control group 53% of patients were induced for reasons other than oligohydramnios, whereas in the study group 86% of patients were induced for oligohydramnios, with 65% of patients in the study group and 24% in the control group demonstrating a nonreactive nonstress test. Among the control group, 33% had a cesarean section, whereas 67% delivered vaginally. In the study group, 34% delivered vaginally and 66% had a cesarean section. The 5-minute Apgar score was <7 in 34% of the study group and 11% of the control group, and 33% neonates in the control group and 64% in the study group had birth weights <2.5 kg.[28] A metaanalysis of 43 studies (244,493 fetuses) demonstrated a strong association between oligohydramnios, low birth weight, and perinatal mortality.[11] A second systematic review and metaanalysis used 12 studies and compared 2414 pregnancies with isolated oligohydramnios with 35,585 pregnancies with normal AFI and found oligohydramnios at term was associated with significantly higher rates of labor induction, cesarean sections, and short-term neonatal morbidity.[29]

The features of oligohydramnios sequence often include those of breech deformation sequence, because about 50% of infants experiencing oligohydramnios are in breech presentation at birth due to their inability to undergo normal version in late gestation. The term *oligohydramnios tetrad* describes the primary features in nonrenal cases: facial compression (flattened nose with enlarged, flattened ears), aberrant hand and foot positioning, fetal growth deficiency, and pulmonary hypoplasia (Fig. 46.4).[1]

Craniofacial

The head usually looks as though a silk stocking has been pulled down over it, causing a flattened nose and the appearance of low-set, flattened, enlarged external auricles (Fig. 46.5).

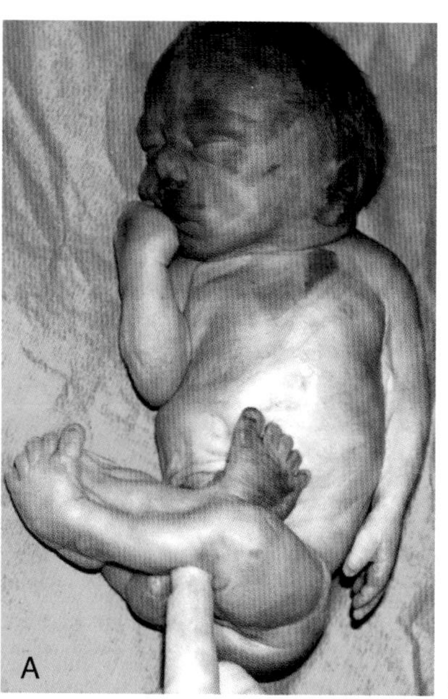

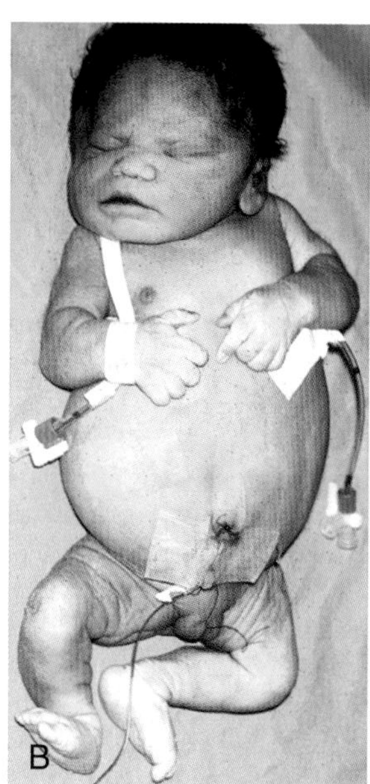

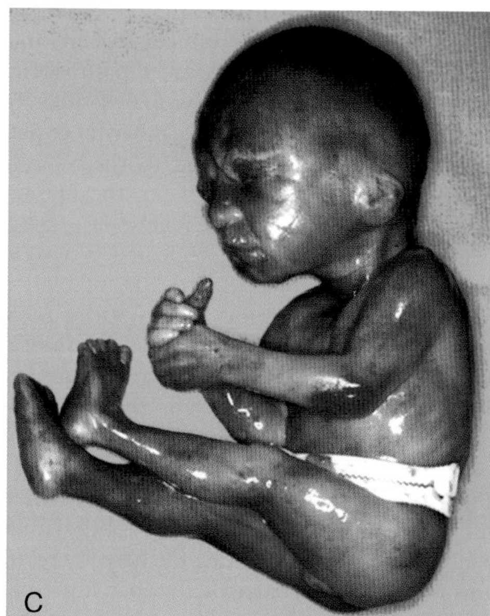

FIGURE 46.4 Oligohydramnios tetrad resulting from chronic leakage of amniotic fluid for 6 weeks before delivery, resulting in lethal pulmonary hypoplasia (A), cystic renal dysplasia (B), and bilateral renal agenesis (C).

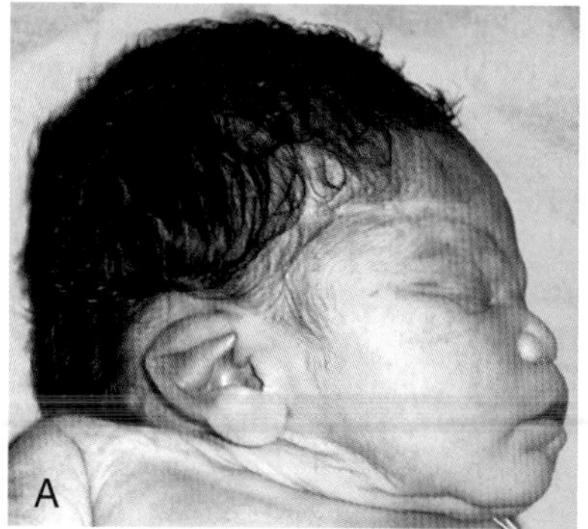

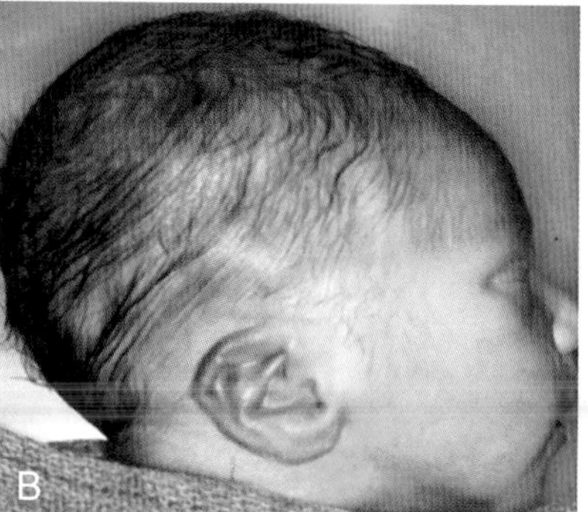

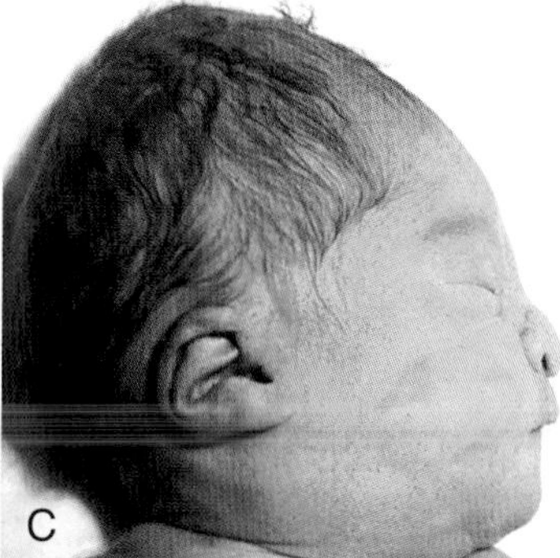

FIGURE 46.5 Oligohydramnios sequence facial features include flattened nose, auricle, and loose skin. Causes of oligohydramnios may include cystic renal dysplasia (A), renal agenesis in a 24-week terminated fetus (B), or renal agenesis in a term fetus (C). Note the compressed face, redundant skin, and accordion ear of a newborn infant with severe oligohydramnios secondary to renal agenesis (C).

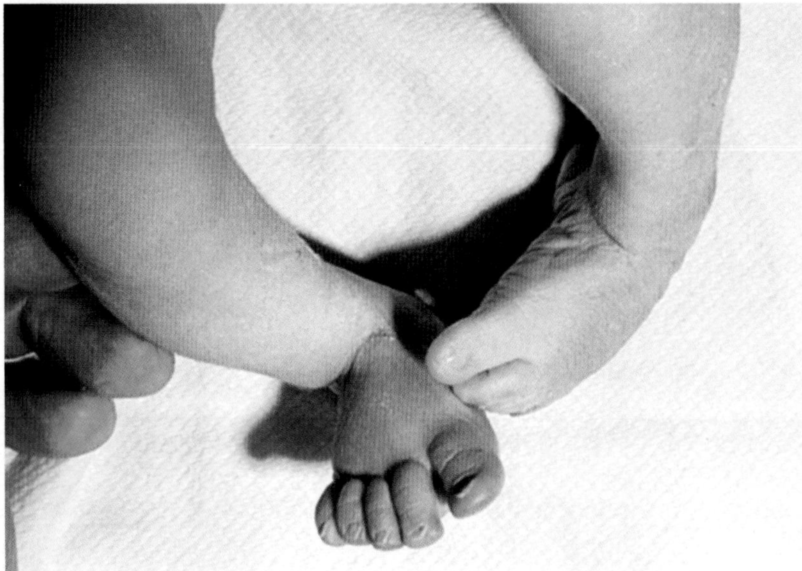

FIGURE 46.6 Renal agenesis with severe oligohydramnios and foot deformations at term delivery.

Limbs

The hands and feet may be edematous with positional deformation, and there is often stiffness of the joints, with flexion contractures of the elbows, knees, and feet (Fig. 46.6).[30] In surviving infants, these limb defects respond readily to physical therapy. A systematic review indicated congenital knee dislocation was associated with oligohydramnios in 20% of cases, and invasive genetic studies were performed in 55% of these 20 reviewed cases. In isolated cases, these studies were normal, but in 10 of 13 (77%) nonisolated cases, genetic syndromes were diagnosed.[31] In isolated cases, early postnatal treatment achieves success in most cases without surgical intervention (see Chapter 12). Hip dislocation may occur with oligohydramnios, especially with breech presentation. In a prospective study investigating of 27,731 live births over a 5-year period, breech position, family history, oligohydramnios, and foot deformations demonstrated significant association with developmental dysplasia of the hip ($P < .0001$).[32]

Thorax and Lungs

The chest circumference is decreased, and radiographs reveal a bell-shaped chest with small lung fields, an elevated diaphragm, and pneumothoraxes from high-pressure ventilation. Thoracic growth is restrained; this was initially hypothesized to cause the lungs to remain small and underdeveloped,[1] but it is inhibition of breathing movements (essential for lung growth) and/or abnormal fluid dynamics within the lungs themselves that result in decreased intraluminal fluid pressures and cause poor lung growth. Lung growth often does not progress beyond the 4- to 5-month level of development, leading to hypoplasia (Fig. 46.7), and because the lungs lack surfactant, they remain incapable of aerobic expansion and/or oxygen exchange. This respiratory insufficiency is the most common cause of demise in the immediate postnatal period, and peak inspiratory pressures of greater than 30 cm H_2O are required, often resulting in pneumothoraxes and interstitial emphysema (Fig. 46.8). Many infants die from hypoxemia, but some survive with pulmonary hypertension and pulmonary interstitial emphysema. Neonatal outcomes in 319 very-low-birth-weight infants with preterm PROM ($n = 141$) and/or oligohydramnios ($n = 54$) were compared with no PROM ($n = 178$) or no oligohydramnios ($n = 265$) during the study period of January 2013 to September 2018.[33] Oligohydramnios was significantly associated with neonatal death, air leak syndrome, and persistent pulmonary hypertension, while PROM per se was not associated with any adverse neonatal outcome. Thus oligohydramnios is a significant risk factor for adverse neonatal outcomes, which is presumably related to pulmonary hypoplasia.

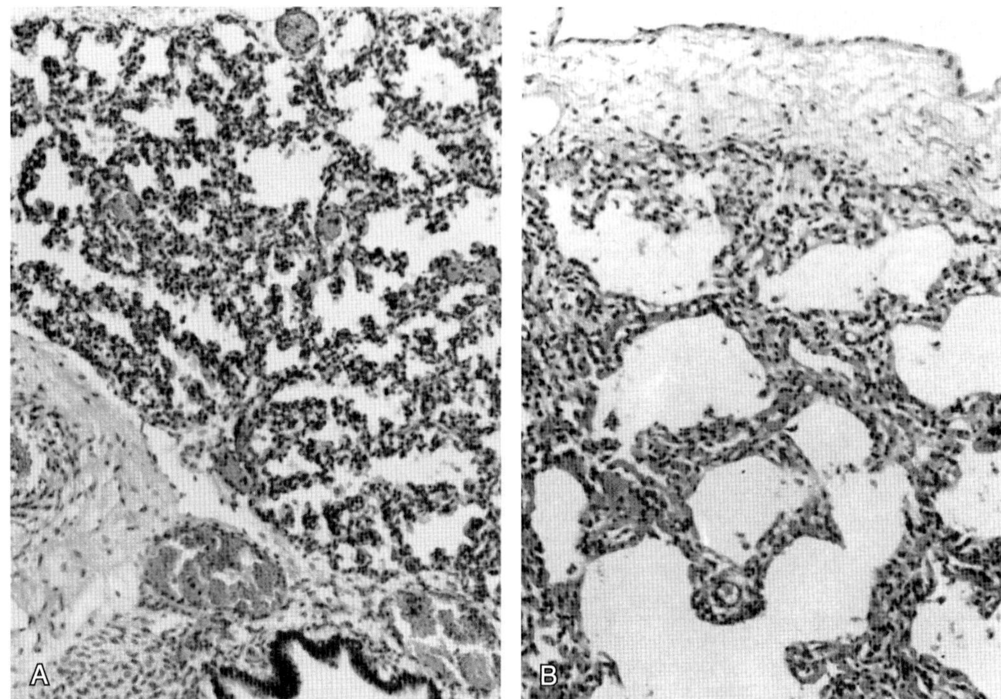

FIGURE 46.7 Lung hypoplasia secondary to severe oligohydramnios, yielding nonexpansile lung with limited aerobic exchange (**A**) in contrast to a normal lung (**B**). *(From Thomas IT, Smith DW. Oligohydramnios, cause of the non-renal features of Potter's syndrome. J Pediatr. 1974;84:811.)*

Skin

The skin tends to be redundant, which is presumably the result of overgrowth related to external constraint.[34] This gives rise to accentuated inner canthal and infraorbital skin folds, which contribute to the "Potter" facies and sometimes yield the false impression of a webbed neck (see Fig. 46.5).

Other

Concretions of amnion cells may build up on the relatively dry surface of the amnion, a feature termed *amnion nodosum*, and the umbilical cord is usually short. Amnion nodosum is the placental hallmark of severe and prolonged oligohydramnios. It consists of nodules of amorphous granular material present on the surface of the amnion. Among cases of amnion nodosum, amniotic bands, oligohydramnios, multiple pregnancy, perinatal mortality, macerated stillbirths, and chronic twin-twin transfusion were common associated clinical disorders.[35,36]

MANAGEMENT, PROGNOSIS, AND COUNSEL

If the oligohydramnios is caused by renal agenesis or another type of severe renal problem, attempts to artificially oxygenate the neonate are of little or no value. However, if the deficit of amniotic fluid is caused by chronic leakage of amniotic fluid, then survival hinges on the severity of oligohydramnios, the gestational age at which rupture occurs, and the duration of oligohydramnios, all of which determine the extent of pulmonary hypoplasia. The importance of gestational age at PROM is related to the histologic development of the lungs, which can be divided into three stages: (1) the pseudoglandular stage (5–17 weeks; all major lung elements are formed with the exception of those related to gas exchange); (2) canalicular stage (16–25 weeks; terminal bronchioles give rise to respiratory bronchioles and then to thin-walled terminal sacs); and (3) terminal sac stage (24 weeks to birth; an increase in the number of terminal sacs rapidly increases the gas

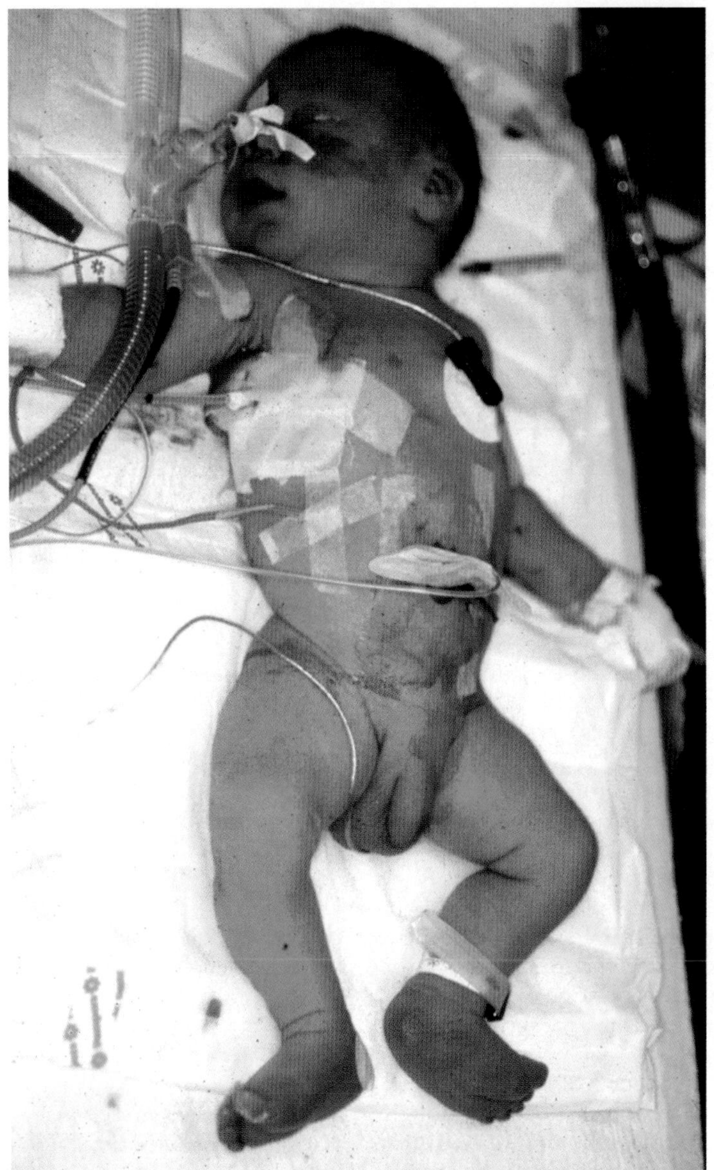

FIGURE 46.8 Renal agenesis in a newborn with lethal pulmonary hypoplasia and pneumothoraxes because of attempted ventilation and resuscitation.

exchange area). If oligohydramnios is limited to the terminal sac stage it does not affect lung growth, but when oligohydramnios occurs during the canalicular stage the result is a cumulative reduction in lung size.[37] Thus the risk for pulmonary hypoplasia diminishes when oligohydramnios occurs after 24 weeks of gestation.[38-41] The duration of severe oligohydramnios and the gestational age at which oligohydramnios had its onset are independent risk factors. Severe oligohydramnios lasting longer than 14 days with rupture of membranes before 25 weeks has a high mortality rate. Rupture at an early gestational age with severe oligohydramnios predisposes to joint contractures, and the risk for deformation relates to the duration of oligohydramnios.[30] If such an infant survives, there is usually catch-up growth within a few months after birth, with a restitution toward normal form with physical therapy.

For the obstetrician, management efforts are balanced between expectant management versus risks from prematurity if delivery is expedited, with attempts to prevent acute complications such as infection, cord prolapse, and placental abruption. When rupture occurs before 24 weeks, there is greater risk for pulmonary hypoplasia, and prompt delivery is generally untenable. With rupture after 24 weeks, it is unlikely that prolongation of the pregnancy beyond this time will further increase the risk of pulmonary hypoplasia, but it can affect the development of skeletal deformation; therefore delivery within 2 weeks of rupture seems feasible once the risk of complications from prematurity becomes low. Case series reveal that amnioinfusion significantly improves the perinatal outcome and prolongs pregnancy in severe second-trimester oligohydramnios in both idiopathic cases and those involving premature rupture of the amniotic membranes.[39–41] A prospective study of 80 cases of severe oligohydramnios treated with transabdominal amnioinfusion beginning at a mean age of 24 weeks gestation between 2011 and 2016 revealed perinatal and neonatal mortalities were 45% and 35%, respectively, with high perinatal mortality related to major fetal malformations diagnosed after the time of amnioinfusion.[42] Severe malformations of the kidney and urinary tract present early in pregnancy with renal oligohydramnios, and they are considered lethal due to pulmonary hypoplasia. Owing to the high rate of additional structural anomalies, genetic abnormalities, and associated syndromes, a detailed anatomic survey with genetic testing is necessary to determine which pregnancies are appropriate for fetal intervention.[43]

There is a lower frequency of perinatal complications and successfully prolonged gestation in iatrogenic preterm PROM after the amniopatch technique relative to population controls. In one series, the amniopatch resulted in a mean gestational age at delivery of 27.5 weeks, with an overall live birth rate of 68% and 55% survival to discharge.[44] Chronic abruption-oligohydramnios sequence, which is characterized by chronic vaginal bleeding and oligohydramnios, is associated with preterm delivery and lung problems in the infant. Fetal lung damage may be induced by not only oligohydramnios but also iron-induced oxidative stress through chronic aspiration of bloody substances in amniotic fluid. Management with repeated amnioinfusions resulted in a significant reduction of high concentrations of iron and lack of chronic lung disease.[45] A hypotonic aqueous composition with reduced chloride content like human amniotic fluid has been safely used for amnioinfusion.[46]

The recurrence risk for oligohydramnios sequence relates to the basic problem that gave rise to the oligohydramnios. Thus with chronic leakage of fluid, the recurrence risk would be very low unless the early rupture of amniotic membranes is caused by inherited Ehlers-Danlos syndrome. Classic Ehlers-Danlos syndrome is associated with early amnion rupture and is inherited in an autosomal dominant fashion. With defects such as obstructive uropathy or renal agenesis, the recurrence risk may be higher. Renal agenesis may recur and be associated with an increased risk of renal anomalies in first-degree relatives.[47] With infantile polycystic kidney disease and inherited renal tubule dysgenesis, the risk may be as high as 25% owing to autosomal recessive inheritance, and fetal autopsy studies are essential to make this diagnosis.[48] Prenatal diagnosis should be offered for subsequent pregnancies when oligohydramnios is caused by a fetal malformation problem. Oligohydramnios is a contraindication for external cephalic version of breech position at term.[49] Previous oligohydramnios is associated with a significantly higher incidence of oligohydramnios in second delivery, small for gestational age neonates, and overall placental related disorders of pregnancy. Thus pregnancies complicated by isolated oligohydramnios are associated with an increased risk of placental related disorders in subsequent pregnancy.[50]

DIFFERENTIAL DIAGNOSIS

Oligohydramnios sequence may be caused by failure to produce amniotic fluid due to renal or urinary tract malformations, which may be isolated defects or part of a syndrome. Some of these problems have a genetic or chromosomal basis, which may become evident from autopsy studies and is important information from a genetic counseling perspective with respect to natural history and recurrence risk. The recurrence risk for PROM depends on whether it is associated with an underlying connective tissue disorder such as Ehlers-Danlos syndrome. Most of the time, PROM is a sporadic occurrence, but this should not be assumed without further evaluation.

References

1. Thomas IT, Smith DW. Oligohydramnios, cause of the non-renal features of Potter's syndrome, including pulmonary hypoplasia. *J Pediatr.* 1974;84:811–814.
2. Czeizel A, Vitez M, Kodaj I, et al. Study of isolated apparent amniogenic limb deficiency in Hungary, 1975–1984. *Am J Med Genet.* 1983;46:372–378.
3. Higgenbottom MC, Jones KL, Hall BD, et al. The amniotic band disruption complex: timing of amniotic rupture and variable spectrum of consequent defects. *J Pediatr.* 1979;95:544–549.
4. Hunter AG, Seaver LH, Stevenson RE. Limb-body wall defect: is there a defensible hypothesis and can it explain all the associated anomalies? *Am J Med Genet A.* 2011;155A:2045–2059.
5. Kalousek DK, Bamforth S. Amnion rupture sequence in previable fetuses. *Am J Med Genet.* 1988;31:63–73.
6. Rabie N, Magann E, Steelman S, Ounpraseuth S. Oligohydramnios in complicated and uncomplicated pregnancy: a systematic review and meta-analysis. *Ultrasound Obstet Gynecol.* 2017;49(4):442–449.
7. Zilberman Sharon N, Pekar-Zlotin M, Kugler N, et al. Oligohydramnios: how severe is severe? *J Matern Fetal Neonatal Med.* 2022;35(25):5754–5760.
8. Acaia B, Crovetto F, Ossola MW, et al. Predictive factors for neonatal survival in women with periviable preterm rupture of the membranes. *J Matern Fetal Neonatal Med.* 2013;26:1628–1634.
9. Muris C, Girard B, Creveuil C, et al. Management of premature rupture of membranes before 25 weeks. *Eur J Obstet Gynecol Reprod Biol.* 2007;131:163–168.
10. Williams O, Michel B, Hutchings G, et al. Two-year neonatal outcome following PPROM prior to 25 weeks with a prolonged period of oligohydramnios. *Early Hum Dev.* 2012;88:657–661.
11. Morris RK, Meller CH, Tamblyn J, et al. Association and prediction of amniotic fluid measurements for adverse pregnancy outcome: systematic review and meta-analysis. *BJOG.* 2014;121:686–699.
12. Kobayashi A, Minami S, Tanizaki Y, et al. Adverse perinatal and neonatal outcomes in patients with chronic abruption-oligohydramnios sequence. *J Obstet Gynaecol Res.* 2014;40:1618–1624.
13. Yamada S, Marutani T, Hisaoka M, et al. Pulmonary hypoplasia on preterm infant associated with diffuse chorioamniotic hemosiderosis caused by intrauterine hemorrhage due to massive subchorial hematoma: report of a neonatal autopsy case. *Pathol Int.* 2012;62:543–548.
14. Moore TR. Clinical assessment of amniotic fluid. *Clin Obstet Gynecol.* 1997;40:303–313.
15. Spaggiari E, Stirnemann JJ, Heidet L, et al. Outcome following prenatal diagnosis of severe bilateral renal hypoplasia. *Prenat Diagn.* 2013;33:1167–1172.
16. Mehler K, Beck BB, Kaul I, et al. Respiratory and general outcome in neonates with renal oligohydramnios: a single-centre experience. *Nephrol Dial Transplant.* 2011;26:3514–3522.
17. Grijseels EW, van-Hornstra PT, Govaerts LC, et al. Outcome of pregnancies complicated by oligohydramnios or anhydramnios of renal origin. *Prenat Diagn.* 2011;31:1039–1045.
18. Giordano G, Fellegara G, Brigati F, et al. Value of autopsy in renal malformations: comparison of clinical diagnosis and post-mortem examination. *Acta Biomed.* 2011;82:230–243.
19. Gubler MC. Renal tubular dysgenesis. *Pediatr Nephrol.* 2014;29:51–59.
20. Gribouval O, Morinière V, Pawtowski A. Spectrum of mutations in the renin-angiotensin system genes in autosomal recessive renal tubular dysgenesis. *Hum Mutat.* 2012;33:316–326.
21. Plazanet C, Arrondel C, Chavant F, et al. Fetal renin-angiotensin-system blockade syndrome: renal lesions. *Pediatr Nephrol.* 2014;29:1221–1230.
22. Shi X, Ding H, Li C, et al. Clinical utility of chromosomal microarray analysis and whole exome sequencing in foetuses with oligohydramnios. *Ann Med.* 2023;55(1):2215539.
23. Simpson LL. Twin-twin transfusion syndrome. *Am J Obstet Gynecol.* 2013;208:3–18.
24. Palacios J, Rodriguea JI. Extrinsic fetal akinesia and skeletal development: a study in oligohydramnios sequence. *Teratology.* 1990;42:1–5.
25. Brace RA, Wolf EJ. Normal amniotic fluid volume changes throughout pregnancy. *Am J Obstet Gynecol.* 1989;161:382–388.
26. Brace RA. Physiology of amniotic fluid volume regulation. *Clin Obstet Gynecol.* 1997;40:280–289.
27. Jha P, Raghu P, Kennedy AM, et al. Assessment of amniotic fluid volume in pregnancy. *Radiographics.* 2023;43(6):e220146.
28. Bachhav AA, Waikar M. Low amniotic fluid index at term as a predictor of adverse perinatal outcome. *J Obstet Gynaecol India.* 2014;64:120–123.
29. Shrem G, Nagawkar SS, Hallak M, Walfisch A. Isolated oligohydramnios at term as an indication for labor induction: a systematic review and meta-analysis. *Fetal Diagn Ther.* 2016;40(3):161–173.
30. Christianson C, Huff D, McPherson E. Limb deformations in oligohydramnios sequence: effects of gestational age and duration of oligohydramnios. *Am J Med Genet.* 1999;86:430–433.
31. Cavoretto PI, Castoldi M, Corbella G, et al. Prenatal diagnosis and postnatal outcome of fetal congenital knee dislocation: systematic review of literature. *Ultrasound Obstet Gynecol.* 2023 Jun 8. https://doi.org/10.1002/uog.26283. Epub ahead of print. PMID: 37289939.
32. Poacher AT, Froud JLJ, Caterson J, et al. The cost effectiveness of potential risk factors for developmental dysplasia of the hip within a national screening programme. *Bone Jt Open.* 2023;4(4):234–240.
33. Kim MS, Kim S, Seo Y, Oh MY, Yum SK. Impact of preterm premature rupture of membranes and

oligohydramnios on in-hospital outcomes of very-low-birthweight infants. *J Matern Fetal Neonatal Med.* 2023;36(1):2195523.
34. Smith DW. Commentary: redundant skin folds in the infant: their origin and relevance. *J Pediatr.* 1979;94:1021–1022.
35. Stanek J, Adeniran A. Chorion nodosum: a placental feature of the severe early amnion rupture sequence. *Pediatr Dev Pathol.* 2006;9:353–360.
36. Adeniran AJ, Stanek J. Amnion nodosum revisited: clinicopathologic and placental correlations. *Arch Pathol Lab Med.* 2007;131:1829–1833.
37. Moessinger AC, Collins MH, Blanc WA, et al. Oligohydramnios-induced lung hypoplasia: the influence of timing and duration in gestation. *Pediatr Res.* 1986;20:951–954.
38. Kilbride HW, Yeast J, Thiebault DW. Defining limits of survival: lethal pulmonary hypoplasia after midtrimester premature rupture of membranes. *Am J Obstet Gynecol.* 1996;175:675–681.
39. Kozinszky Z, Sikovanyecz J, Pásztor N. Severe midtrimester oligohydramnios: treatment strategies. *Curr Opin Obstet Gynecol.* 2014;26:67–76.
40. Takahashi Y, Iwagaki S, Chiaki R, et al. Amnioinfusion before 26 weeks' gestation for severe fetal growth restriction with oligohydramnios: preliminary pilot study. *J Obstet Gynaecol Res.* 2014;40:677–685.
41. Porat S, Amsalem H, Shah PS, et al. Transabdominal amnioinfusion for preterm premature rupture of membranes: a systematic review and meta-analysis of randomized and observational studies. *Am J Obstet Gynecol.* 2012;207:393 e1–e11.
42. Ahmed B. Amnioinfusion in severe oligohydramnios with intact membrane: an observational study. *J Matern Fetal Neonatal Med.* 2022;35(25):6518–6521.
43. Miller JL, Baschat AA, Atkinson MA. Fetal therapy for renal anhydramnios. *Clin Perinatol.* 2022;49(4):849–862.
44. Richter J, Henry A, Ryan G, et al. Amniopatch procedure after previable iatrogenic rupture of the membranes: a two-center review. *Prenat Diagn.* 2013;33:391–396.
45. Morita A, Kondoh E, Kawasaki K, et al. Therapeutic amnioinfusion for chronic abruption-oligohydramnios sequence: a possible prevention of the infant respiratory disease. *J Obstet Gynaecol Res.* 2014;40:1118–1123.
46. Tchirikov M, Bapayeva G, Zhumadilov Z, et al. Treatment of PPROM with anhydramnion in humans: first experience with different amniotic fluid substitutes for continuous amnioinfusion through a subcutaneously implanted port system. *J Perinat Med.* 2013;41:657–663.
47. Morse RP, Rawnsley BE, Crow HC, et al. Bilateral renal agenesis in three consecutive siblings. *Prenat Diagn.* 1987;7:573–579.
48. Hartung EA, Guay-Woodford LM. Autosomal recessive polycystic kidney disease: a hepatorenal fibrocystic disorder with pleiotropic effects. *Pediatrics.* 2014;134:e833–e845.
49. Rosman AN, Guijt A, Vlemmix F, et al. Contraindications for external cephalic version in breech position at term: a systematic review. *Acta Obstet Gynecol Scand.* 2013;92:137–142.
50. Leytes S, Kovo M, Weiner E, Ganer Herman H. Isolated oligohydramnios in previous pregnancy is a risk factor for a placental related disorder in subsequent delivery. *BMC Pregnancy Childbirth.* 2022;22(1):912.

CHAPTER 47

Fetal Akinesia Deformation Sequence

KEY POINTS

- Fetal movement is crucial for normal joint development, and lack of movement can lead to joint contractures.
- Prenatal diagnosis of fetal akinesia may reveal additional structural abnormalities such as cystic hygroma, increased nuchal translucency, and hydrops fetalis.
- Fetal akinesia deformation sequence (FADS) is a term used to describe the causally heterogeneous conditions characterized by fetal akinesia and associated malformations.
- Experimental studies in animals have shown that fetal akinesia can lead to abnormalities similar to FADS.
- Myotonic dystrophy and myasthenia gravis are examples of conditions that can cause the fetal akinesia phenotype.
- FADS can be caused by intrinsic factors (neuromuscular abnormalities) or extrinsic factors (such as oligohydramnios or fetal crowding), and distinguishing between them is important for diagnosis and management.
- Prenatal diagnosis is challenging, and fetal pathology combined with genomic sequencing allows for proper counseling.

GENESIS

Fetal movement is essential to normal joint morphogenesis. Joints develop secondarily within the condensed mesenchyme of the developing bones, and chronic lack of movement leads to joint contractures.[1–4] Fetal akinesia is associated with a specific combination of clinical findings that was previously called the *Pena-Shokeir phenotype* because these signs were first described as part of Pena-Shokeir syndrome.[2] These findings include fetal growth retardation, congenital contractures with underdeveloped limbs, polyhydramnios, pulmonary hypoplasia, short umbilical cord, and craniofacial alterations such as micrognathia, occasional cleft palate, hypertelorism, and short neck (Fig. 47.1), and they are usually autosomal recessive and detectable through prenatal diagnosis.[3–5] Prenatal diagnosis of fetal akinesia may reveal cystic hygroma, increased nuchal translucency, nuchal edema, hydrops fetalis, arthrogryposis, pterygia, and other structural abnormalities. Genetic evaluation should include a differential diagnosis of neuromuscular junction disorders with genetic analysis for mutations in neuromuscular junction genes such as *CHRNA1*, *CHRND*, *CHRNG*, *CNTN1*, *DOK7*, *RAPSN*, and *SYNE1*. Genomic evaluation may unveil the pathogenetic cause of fetal akinesia deformation sequence (FADS) and multiple pterygium syndrome, which is helpful for genetic counseling and clinical management.[4]

Hall emphasized the causal heterogeneity of this condition,[6] and Moessinger[7] demonstrated that rat fetuses paralyzed by daily transuterine injections of curare from day 18 of gestation until term on day 21 demonstrated a consistent pattern of abnormalities that he termed the *fetal akinesia deformation sequence*. In a dramatic human example, the mother of an infant born with multiple joint contractures (arthrogryposis) had received tubocurarine for 19 days in early pregnancy for the treatment of tetanus.[8] This phenotype represents an etiologically heterogeneous deformation sequence that can result from neuropathy, myopathy, restrictive dermopathy, teratogens, or intrauterine constraint caused by prolonged oligohydramnios, which results in congenital contractures owing to extrinsic fetal immobilization. Among 30 cases of arthrogryposis associated with long-standing oligohydramnios (representing 1.2% of 2500 cases of arthrogryposis), none had renal agenesis or renal disease, 73% had a history of known rupture of membranes, and 50% had pulmonary hypoplasia, but only 2 died (7%), whereas 60% had multiple congenital contractures owing to the long-standing oligohydramnios and they responded well to physical therapy.[9]

Pena-Shokeir syndrome was first described in 1974 as an autosomal recessive type of fetal akinesia (see

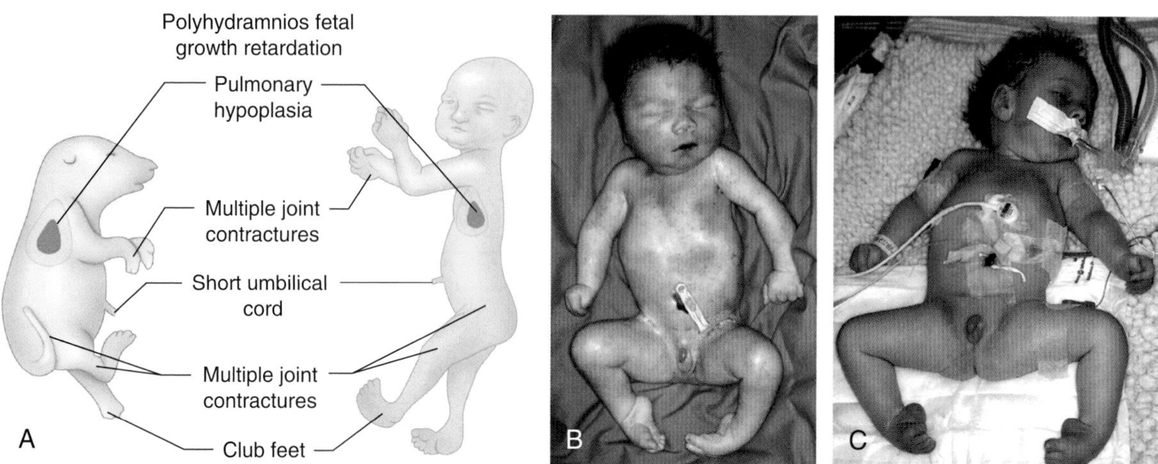

FIGURE 47.1 **A,** The fetal akinesia deformation sequence is a causally heterogeneous phenotype that can occur with a variety of congenital neuropathies and myopathies. **B** and **C,** These two newborn siblings with type I Pena-Shokeir syndrome were born with polyhydramnios, lethal pulmonary hypoplasia, and joint contractures. Attempts to diagnose recurrences during the second trimester were unsuccessful because the affected fetuses were still moving at this time, but polyhydramnios and limited fetal movement were evident during the third trimester. (**A,** From Moessinger AC. Fetal akinesia deformation sequence. An animal model. *Pediatrics*. 1983;72:857.)

the affected brothers in Fig. 47.1), and since that time multiple cases have been reported with a wide variety of associated findings, which suggest causal heterogeneity and warrant use of the more general term FADS.[2,6] It is very important to distinguish extrinsic factors that limit fetal movement (e.g., oligohydramnios or fetal crowding) from intrinsic factors owing to neuromuscular abnormalities (Fig. 47.2). Both types of problems can lead to abnormal fetal presentation, hence the association between breech presentation and fetal abnormalities.[10] Fetal immobilization during late gestation can also give rise to transient joint limitation in normal newborns. Both FADS and oligohydramnios sequence share phenotypic manifestations such as arthrogryposis, short umbilical cord, and lung hypoplasia, caused by decreased intrauterine fetal motility. Other characteristic manifestations found in oligohydramnios sequence, such as Potter facies and redundant skin, are produced by fetal compression. On the other hand, growth retardation, craniofacial anomalies, micrognathia, long bone hypoplasia, and polyhydramnios are found in FADS and related to intrauterine muscular weakness.[11]

There is ample evidence in both experimental animals and humans that fetal akinesia owing to a variety of causes can lead to multiple joint contractures and other manifestations of FADS.[12,13] The fetal akinesia phenotype occurs in Pena-Shokeir syndrome (see Fig. 47.1), an autosomal recessive disorder,[2,5,6] and also in a number of other genetic fetal malformation syndromes.[4] Myotonic dystrophy can produce this phenotype[14] (Fig. 47.2B), and similar effects have been noted in infants born to mothers with myasthenia gravis (Fig. 47.3). Among 176 births by 79 mothers with myasthenia gravis, 4 (2.2%) newborns (including one pair of twins) were born with severe lethal skeletal anomalies (3 with arthrogryposis multiplex congenita and 1 with FADS). The mother of the child with fetal akinesia had previously given birth to a child with neonatal myasthenia gravis, and the mother of the twins with arthrogryposis later gave birth to a child with neonatal myasthenia gravis, suggesting a genetic basis independent of the mother's clinical state.[15]

Congenital myasthenic syndromes are a heterogeneous group of disorders caused by genetic defects affecting neuromuscular transmission and leading to muscle weakness accentuated by exertion. Disease-causing genes coding for proteins that have a key role at the neuromuscular junction have been identified, such as *CHAT*, *CHRNA1*, *CHRNB1*, *CHRND*, *CHRNE*, *COLQ*, *RAPSN*, *SCN4A*, *MUSK*, *DOK7*, *LAMB2*, and *AGRN*; however, for half of congenital myasthenia patients, the genes underlying their disease have not yet been identified.[16]

The manifestations and severity of FADS depend on the timing, duration, and degree of fetal akinesia, with multiple pterygia and increased nuchal translucency resulting from early prolonged fetal akinesia (Fig. 47.4).

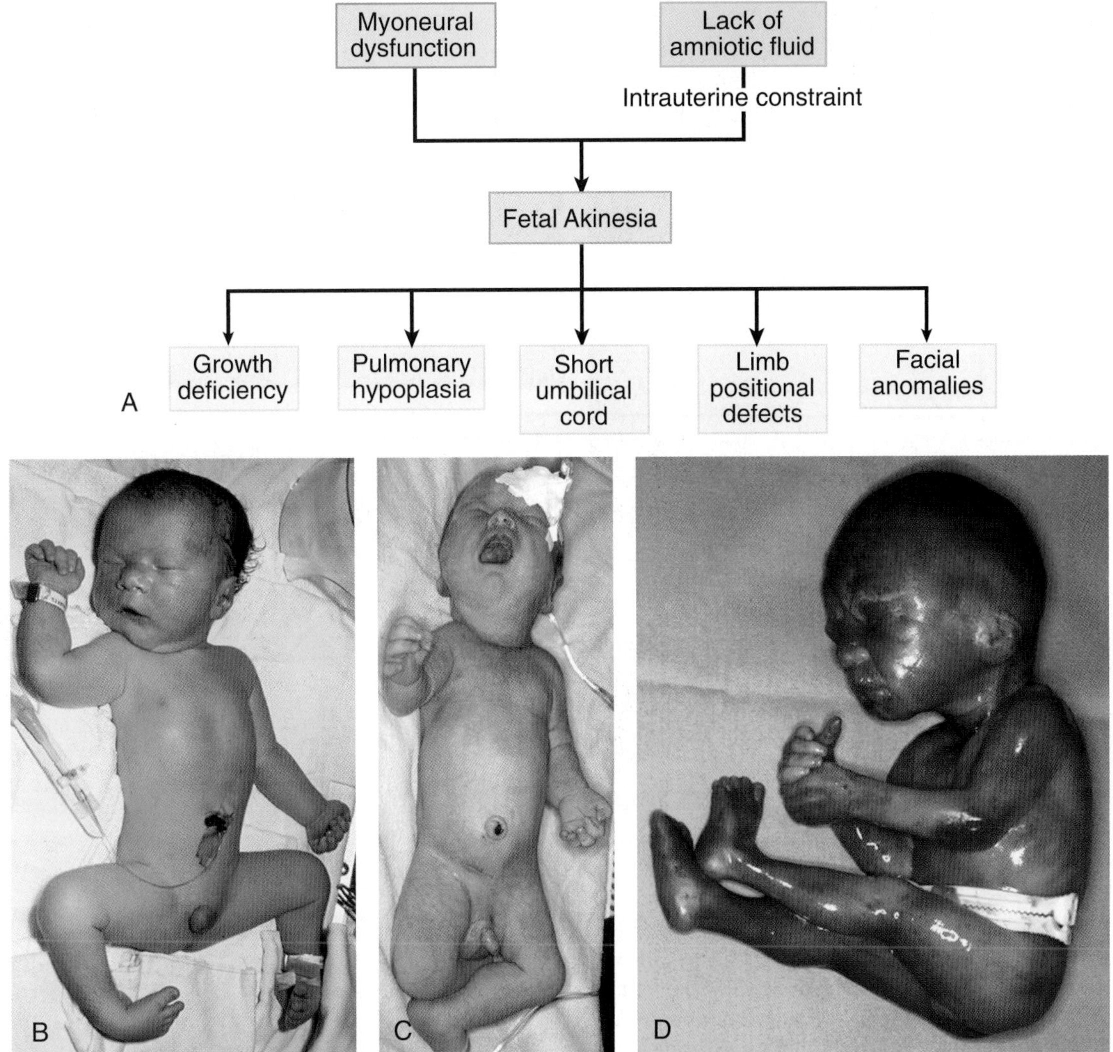

FIGURE 47.2 **A,** This diagram demonstrates the etiologically heterogeneous phenotype that results from fetal akinesia. **B,** This infant was born with myotonic dystrophy to a mother with the same condition. He had multiple joint contractures with thin bones and respiratory insufficiency. **C,** This infant was immobilized in a transverse lie after amnion rupture at 26 weeks. **D,** This fetus had bilateral renal agenesis resulting in oligohydramnios.

Prolonged neuromuscular akinesia limits bone growth, which affects subperiosteal growth in bone breadth much more severely than linear growth. This leads to the development of thin bones that are susceptible to fractures.[17] The size of a muscle relates to the magnitude and frequency of forces it brings to bear across a joint, and with diminished function, muscles tend to atrophy. Thus prolonged fetal akinesia results in low birth weight. Absence of flexion creases implies that the joint has never functioned, and, because most joints flex by the early second trimester, this implies an early cessation of fetal movement. Polyhydramnios is a relatively late manifestation of fetal akinesia sequence, which is usually associated with micrognathia caused by diminished fetal swallowing. Fetal lung movements are necessary for normal pulmonary growth and maturation, and deficient diaphragmatic function can lead to pulmonary hypoplasia. The importance of fetal respiratory movements in normal lung morphogenesis was highlighted by a case report that described an

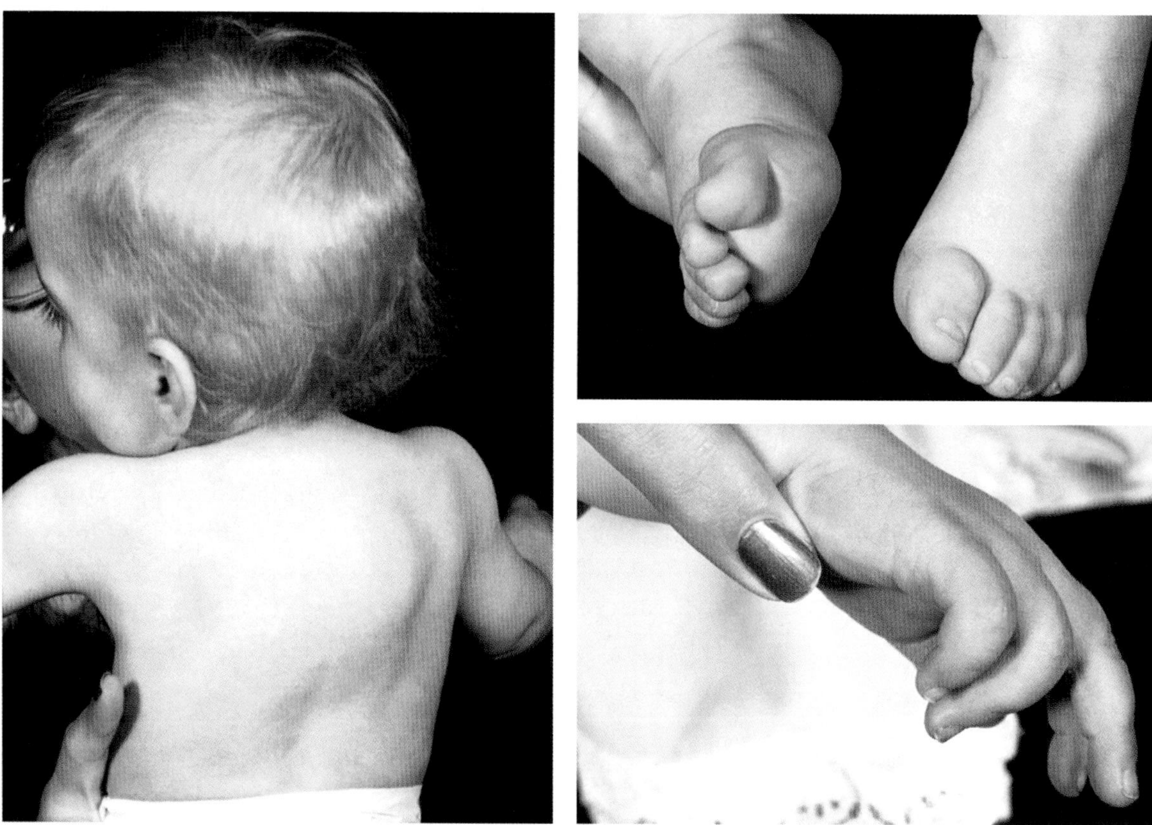

FIGURE 47.3 This female infant was born to a mother with myasthenia gravis. Both the infant and a subsequent sibling were born with hypotonia, multiple joint contractures, and severe scoliosis. (Courtesy Mark Stephan, Madigan Army Hospital, Tacoma, WA.)

infant with pulmonary hypoplasia caused by phrenic nerve agenesis and diaphragmatic amyoplasia.[18] In an experimental fetal rabbit model, destruction of the fetal cervical spinal cord in the C4 to C6 region caused complete atrophy of the diaphragm in addition to cutting off motor pathways from the respiratory center. Higher lesions at C1 to C3 preserved the phrenic nerve supply and hence allowed normal diaphragmatic growth but prevented any coordinated fetal respiratory activity. Each operation, when performed at 23 days of gestation during the late pseudoglandular phase of lung development, resulted in severe lung hypoplasia.[19] Consequently, with severe fetal akinesia that inhibits fetal swallowing and fetal lung movements, the fetus is usually born with micrognathia, polyhydramnios, and respiratory insufficiency from pulmonary hypoplasia.

The association of a shortened umbilical cord implies that fetal akinesia began during or prior to the second trimester. Umbilical cord growth is influenced by tensile forces and depends on both fetal motion and the amount of space available for fetal movement.[20] This has been demonstrated in both humans and rats.[20,21] Oligohydramnios can severely limit fetal movement during the last half of gestation, and there is overlap between oligohydramnios sequence and FADS, but oligohydramnios does not limit fetal long bone growth to the same extent seen with neuromuscular akinesia, which also results in thin, fragile bones.[17] Compression of skin in oligohydramnios sequence leads to skin redundancy,[9] whereas fetal akinesia is associated with thin, tight skin with few flexion creases.

Restrictive dermopathy is a rare, lethal, autosomal recessive disorder characterized by extreme tautness of the skin causing restricted intrauterine movement and FADS with characteristic facial features (e.g., large anterior fontanelle; hypertelorism; a short, narrow, upturned nose; blepharophimosis with swollen lids

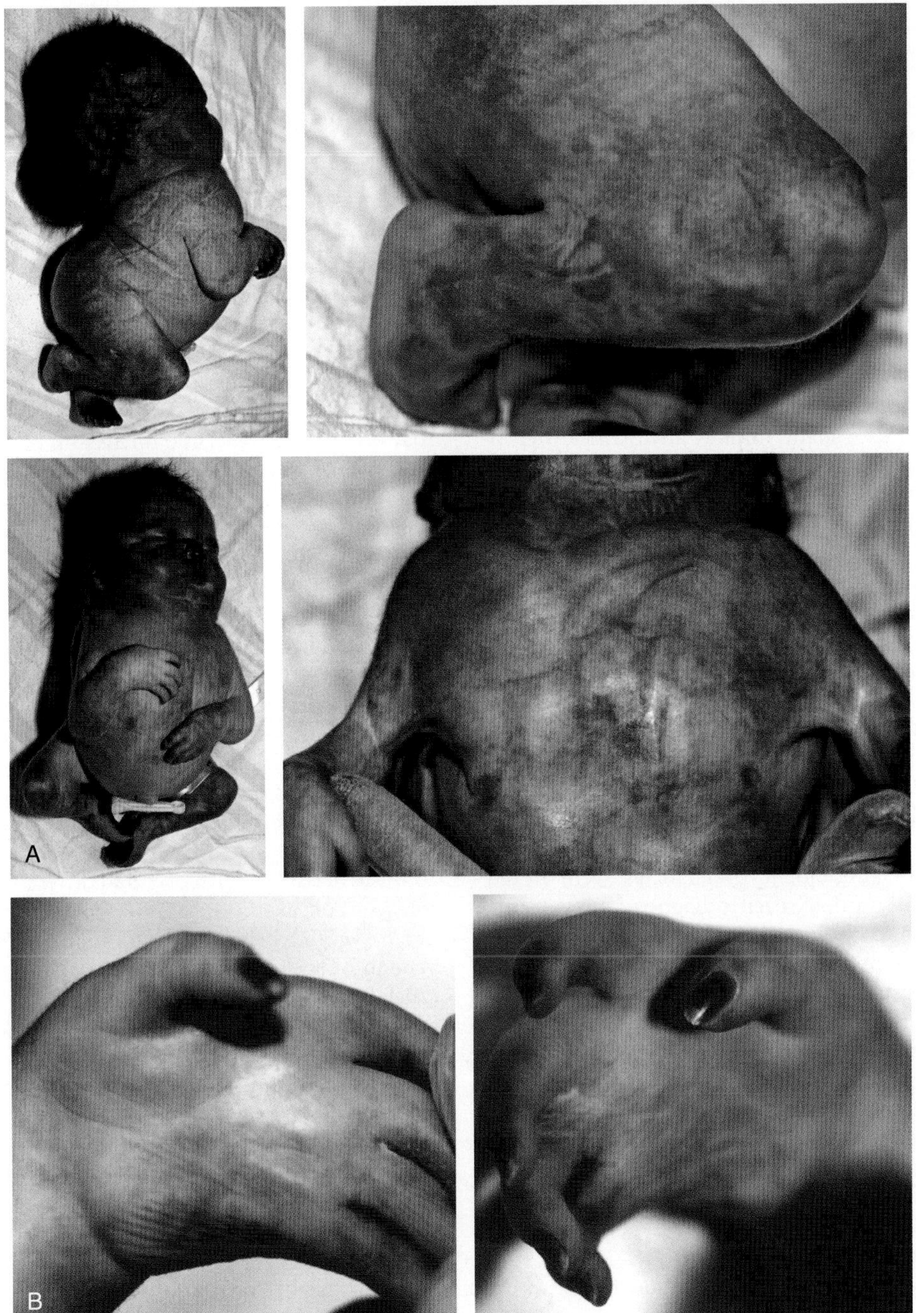

FIGURE 47.4 **A,** This fetus was recognized by prenatal ultrasound as having virtually no fetal movement and a large nuchal cystic hygroma. The hands were clenched, with no finger creases on examination. Amniocentesis revealed a normal karyotype, and multiple pterygia were noted postnatally. This illustrates the severe consequences of prolonged fetal akinesia in a fetus with lethal multiple pterygium syndrome and nuchal cystic hygroma. Muscle pathology demonstrated neurogenic atrophy. Some cases of lethal multiple pterygium syndromes have inactivating mutations in an embryonal acetylcholine receptor γ-subunit gene (*CHRNG*). **B,** Absent flexion creases in the fetus with lethal multiple pterygium syndrome and nuchal cystic hygroma.

and exophthalmos; a small, open mouth; and micrognathia).[22-24] Dermatopathology findings include thin dermis consisting of compactly arranged collagen fibers, scant elastic fibers, and poorly developed skin appendages.[22] The epidermal rete ridges are flattened and the dermal-hypodermal border is remarkably straight.[23] *LMNA* and *ZMPSTE24* have been identified as causative genes, offering an opportunity for prenatal genetic diagnosis.[24] Exome sequencing of two siblings with lethal multiple pterygium syndrome revealed *GBE1* mutations, which results in glycogen storage disease type IV, which was confirmed biochemically, and muscle pathology revealed storage material.[25]

When foot deformations are associated with polyhydramnios, this usually implies an intrinsic neuromuscular abnormality, whereas foot deformations associated with oligohydramnios suggest extrinsic constraint. In a study of 30 fetuses with FADS, detailed neuropathologic studies that included the brain, spinal cord, and muscles allowed a specific diagnosis to be made in 16 cases (53%).[26] Of these 16 cases, 9 had central nervous system abnormalities, 1 had spinal cord abnormality (spinal muscular atrophy I), 3 had a primary myopathy (nemaline myopathy and myotonic dystrophy), and 3 had a recognizable syndrome. In 10 other cases, neuromuscular pathology was evident but no specific diagnosis could be established. Only four patients had normal neuromuscular findings with no apparent etiology for FADS. Most importantly, recurrences in subsequent pregnancies were noted among all three groups (specific diagnosis, nonspecific neuromuscular pathology, and normal neuromuscular pathology).[26] Subsequently other autopsy studies have revealed different novel causes for FADS, such as loss/absence of Purkinje cells in the cerebellum in siblings.[27] A female fetus with hypoplasia of the cerebellum, corpus callosum, and optic nerves had nuclear cataracts and widespread axonal spheroids throughout the central and peripheral nervous systems with normal *PLA2G6* sequencing, ruling out infantile neuroaxonal dystrophy and related disorders.[28] Other postmortem case reports revealed evidence for a hypoxic-ischemic cause of FADS.[29,30]

Pathological examination of female fetuses with severe FADS, multiple pterygia, and muscular hypoplasia showed massive cystic dilatation of the cerebral ventricles (hydranencephaly) with calcification of the basal ganglion and brainstem, and a proliferative vasculopathy throughout the central nervous system. These findings in two female siblings suggested autosomal recessive inheritance of the Fowler type of hydranencephaly.[31] Mutations in *FLVCR2* were associated with this proliferative vasculopathy and hydranencephaly-hydrocephaly syndrome (Fowler syndrome) in other cases.[32]

FEATURES

As described above, the etiology of FADS is heterogeneous, and the severity of the phenotype varies from severe, generalized, early-onset disorders to milder defects that present later in pregnancy. The features of FADS often include breech head and features of Pena-Shokeir syndrome,[2] an autosomal recessive disorder that occurs in 1 in 12,000 births and has an extremely heterogeneous pathogenesis, hence the use of the term Pena-Shokeir phenotype as an alternative to FADS; however, the latter terminology is the preferred designation because Pena-Shokeir syndrome is thought to be one subtype of FADS. FADS is etiologically heterogeneous, with an estimated incidence of approximately 1 in 3000 live births and a much higher incidence when prenatally diagnosed cases are included owing to high intrauterine mortality. The condition can have an extrinsic etiology due to fetal crowding from uterine structural abnormalities, fibroids, or multiple gestation, or it can have an intrinsic etiology due to single-gene disorders affecting the brain, spinal cord, peripheral nerves, neuromuscular junction, muscle, or connective tissues, with over 320 different genes implicated.[33] For example, homozygotic and compound heterozygotic pathogenic variants in *TTN* (the largest gene in our genome) with autosomal recessive inheritance have been associated with FADS.[34,35] Ryanodine receptor type 1-related disorder is the most common subgroup of congenital myopathies with a wide phenotypic spectrum ranging from mild hypotonia to lethal fetal akinesia.[36]

Clinical findings of FADS include fetal growth retardation, congenital contractures with underdeveloped limbs, polyhydramnios, pulmonary hypoplasia, short umbilical cord, and craniofacial alterations such as micrognathia, occasional cleft palate, hypertelorism, and short neck. The findings of prenatal-onset growth deficiency with polyhydramnios may suggest a neuromuscular cause, and fetal pathology with genomic sequencing can help establish a more specific diagnosis in many cases. Polyhydramnios may result in premature delivery with severe respiratory distress due to pulmonary hypoplasia. As described above, a variety of congenital neuropathies and myopathies can limit fetal movement, and neuropathologic analysis with genomic sequencing of such lethally affected neonates is critically important to provide accurate genetic counseling. There are well-conceived clinical guidelines for the diagnosis of FADS so that families can receive appropriate diagnosis and counseling.[33,37–39] In a retrospective study of 41 prenatal cases with suspected fetal arthrogryposis congenita, this diagnosis was confirmed in 27 cases (66%), and hydrops was present in 53% of cases resulting in termination of pregnancy versus 0% of 8 surviving children. Absent stomach filling was found in 67% of the children with neonatal death. Scoliosis, nuchal edema, and absent stomach filling suggested a neurological etiology.[37] Specific suggestions for prenatal evaluation and counseling have been promulgated.[38,39]

Micrognathia may occur with a small mouth, depressed tip of the nose, and limited extension of the head. The eyes appear wide set and the ears appear low set. The hands and feet tend to be fixed in aberrant positions, leading to camptodactyly and equinovarus foot deformations. The long bones and ribs may be thin and brittle, with decreased muscular bulk. There is pulmonary hypoplasia with low lung weight or a low lung-body weight ratio at autopsy. Deficient alveolarization with decreased surfactant may lead to fetal respiratory insufficiency in the perinatal period. The skin appears thin and tight, with deficient or absent flexion creases. Webbing of skin across joints (pterygia) may occur with early limitations of movement. The umbilical cord is short, and there may be occasional cryptorchidism or hip dislocation. Hall has thoroughly delineated the full spectrum of deformations and prenatal clinical features associated with FADS and arthrogryposis.[40]

MANAGEMENT, PROGNOSIS, AND COUNSEL

If the akinesia is caused by either prolonged oligohydramnios or a congenital neuropathy or myopathy, attempts to oxygenate the neonate may be unsuccessful owing to underlying pulmonary hypoplasia. If late gestational constraint has immobilized the fetus, then vigorous orthopedic management and physical therapy are merited, and the prognosis is good. The recurrence risk relates to the basic problem that gave rise to the FADS. With congenital neuropathies and myopathies, the recurrence risk may be quite high.

DIFFERENTIAL DIAGNOSIS

Prolonged limitation of fetal movement leads to a generalized pattern of anomalies termed FADS, and it is critical to determine the cause for reduced fetal movement. Generally, the etiology can be classified into one of five categories: neuropathy, myopathy, restrictive dermopathy, teratogen exposure, or restricted movement caused by fetal constraint such as oligohydramnios deformation sequence. Prenatal hydrops, nuchal edema, scoliosis, and absent stomach filling are strongly associated with a neuromuscular etiology and unfavorable outcome.[37] Neurogenic causes include type 1 Pena-Shokeir syndrome (see Fig. 47.1), lethal multiple pterygium syndrome (see Fig. 47.4), Gaucher disease, neuronal dystrophy, Fowler syndrome, and Neu-Laxova syndrome, which are well-defined autosomal recessive disorders that can lead to FADS. Other, less common disorders with varying modes of inheritance have also been reported.[24–36] Full expansion of the pathogenic dominantly inherited trinucleotide repeat in myotonic dystrophy can result in FADS (see Fig. 47.2B). The amyoplasia subtype of arthrogryposis multiplex, in which early denervation leads to fibrous fatty muscle replacement, is a frequent cause of FADS. This is a sporadic disorder that can result from vascular disruption within the developing spinal cord, and it is occasionally associated with twinning and gastroschisis; it has a good prognosis for survival with normal cognitive function.[41] FADS in twins is also heterogeneous, and autopsy studies with genomic sequencing can help distinguish between autosomal recessive myogenic etiologies and sporadic anoxic-ischemic damage.[29,42]

Lethal multiple pterygium syndrome is a myopathic disorder that causes fetal akinesia in association with soft tissue webbing (antecubital and popliteal pterygia) around the contracted joints.[43] Lethal multiple pterygium syndrome is usually an autosomal recessive disorder associated with antecubital and popliteal skin webs, as well as variable nuchal cystic hygroma (see Fig. 47.4), but some cases may manifest X-linked inheritance.[43–45] When inherited as an autosomal recessive trait, it can result from acetylcholine receptor dysfunction caused by mutations in *CHRNG*. Germline mutations in the *CHRNG* gene that encodes the γ subunit of the embryonal acetylcholine receptor can also cause the nonlethal Escobar syndrome, or the lethal form of multiple pterygium syndrome. In addition, *CHRNG* mutations and mutations in other components of the embryonal acetylcholine receptor may present with FADS without pterygia.[43] Analysis of *CHRNG* mutations in 100 families with a clinical diagnosis of FADS identified mutations in 11 of 41 (27%) families with Escobar syndrome and 5 of 59 (8%) with lethal multiple pterygium syndrome. Most patients with a detectable *CHRNG* mutation (87.5%) had pterygia, and no *CHRNG* mutations were detected in the presence of central nervous system anomalies. There is a 95% chance that a subsequent affected sibling will have the same multiple pterygium syndrome phenotype. Other features include generalized edema with loose skin, nuchal cystic hygromas, ocular hypertelorism, and cleft palate; most cases demonstrate generalized amyoplasia (muscle replaced by fibrous fatty tissue) without degeneration of anterior horn cells. Prenatal diagnosis has been made as early as 14 weeks. An X-linked form of myotubular myopathy can cause FADS, which is usually fatal in early infancy because of bulbar muscle weakness, and this disorder is associated with characteristic centronucleated hypotrophic myofibers.[45]

The suggested workup for fetuses with FADS detected prenatally includes fetal pathology of the brain, spinal cord, and muscle. Storage material in a muscle biopsy should result in a workup for glycogen storage disease. Prenatal diagnosis of FADS is often possible, but variability in the cessation of fetal movement within a given family may make early diagnosis a challenge.[3-5,37-39,46-48] Increased nuchal translucency can be an early sign of FADS, and three-dimensional ultrasonography can be quite helpful in confirming this diagnosis. Restrictive dermopathy is an autosomal recessive cause of fetal akinesia associated with tight, rigid, shiny skin and mutations in *LMNA* or *ZMPSTE24*, and skin histopathology is diagnostic. Mutations in *FLVCR2* are associated with FADS, and autopsy reveals distinctive proliferative vasculopathy with ultrasound findings of hydranencephaly-hydrocephaly syndrome (Fowler syndrome). Parents should be checked for myotonic dystrophy and myasthenia gravis. First-trimester exposure to curare can cause FADS,[8] as can prolonged oligohydramnios.[9] Transplacental infection with coxsackievirus B3 infection was confirmed by molecular techniques after prenatal ultrasound detected a severe reduction of fetal movements during the 27th week. Late-onset FADS with mild arthrogryposis, necrotic meningoencephalitis with vascular calcifications, interstitial pneumonitis, mild myocardial hypertrophy, and chronic monocytic placental villitis were the cardinal findings at fetal autopsy.[49] The facial features in oligohydramnios deformation sequence usually lack the micrognathia seen in association with neurogenic causes, which typically result in polyhydramnios caused by diminished fetal swallowing. Because of the high recurrence risks for many of these disorders, it is critically important to establish a specific diagnosis through genomic sequencing to provide accurate genetic counseling.

References

1. Drachman DB, Coulombre AJ. Experimental clubfoot and arthrogryposis multiplex congenital. *Lancet.* 1962;2:523–526.
2. Pena SD, Shokeir MH. Syndrome of camptodactyly, multiple ankyloses, facial anomalies and pulmonary hypoplasia: a lethal condition. *J Pediatr.* 1974;85:373–375.
3. Hoellen F, Schröer A, Kelling K, et al. Arthrogryposis multiplex congenita and Pena-Shokeir phenotype: challenge of prenatal diagnosis: report of 21 cases, antenatal findings and review. *Fetal Diagn Ther.* 2011;30:289–298.
4. Chen CP. Prenatal diagnosis and genetic analysis of fetal akinesia deformation sequence and multiple pterygium syndrome associated with neuromuscular junction disorders: a review. *Taiwan J Obstet Gynecol.* 2012;5:12–17.
5. Santana EF, Oliveira Serni PN, Rolo LC, et al. Prenatal diagnosis of arthrogryposis as a phenotype of Pena-Shokeir Syndrome using two- and three-dimensional ultrasonography. *J Clin Imaging Sci.* 2014;4:20. https://doi.org/10.4103/2156-7514.131642. eCollection 2014.
6. Hall JG. Pena-Shokeir phenotype (fetal akinesia deformation sequence) revisited. *Birth Defects Res A Clin Mol Teratol.* 2009;85:677–694.
7. Moessinger AC. Fetal akinesia deformation sequence: an animal model. *Pediatrics.* 1983;72:857–863.
8. Jago RH. Arthrogryposis following treatment of maternal tetanus with muscle relaxants. *Arch Dis Child.* 1970;45:277–279.
9. Hall JG. (2014). Oligohydramnios sequence revisited in relationship to arthrogryposis, with distinctive skin changes. *Am J Med Genet A.* 2014;164A:2775–2792. https://doi.org/10.1002/ajmg.a.36731.
10. Braun FH, Jones KL, Smith DW. Breech presentation as an indication of fetal abnormality. *J Pediatr.* 1975;86:419–421.
11. Rodríguez JI, Palacios J. Pathogenetic mechanisms of fetal akinesia deformation sequence and oligohydramnios sequence. *Am J Med Genet.* 1991;40:284–289.
12. Hall JG, Reed SD. Teratogens associated with congenital contractures in humans and in animals. *Teratology.* 1982;25:173.
13. Swinyard CA. Concept of multiple congenital contractures (arthrogryposis) in man and animals. *Teratology.* 1982;25:247–258.
14. Hunter AG, Jacob P, Ottoy K, et al. Decrease in size of the myotonic dystrophy CTG repeat during transmission from parent to child: implications for genetic

counseling and genetic anticipation. *Am J Med Genet.* 1993;45:401–407.

15. Hoff JM, Daltveit AK, Gilhus NE. Arthrogryposis multiplex congenita: a rare fetal condition caused by maternal myasthenia gravis. *Acta Neurol Scand Suppl.* 2006;183:26–27.
16. Huze C, Bauche S, Richard P, et al. Identification of an Agrin mutation that causes congenital myasthenia and affects synapse function. *Amer J Hum Genet.* 2009;85:155–167.
17. Rodriquez JI, Garcia-Alix A, Pastor I, et al. Effects of immobilization on fetal bone development: a morphometric study in newborns with congenital neuromuscular diseases with intrauterine onset. *Calcif Tissue Int.* 1988;43:335–339.
18. Goldstein JD, Reid LM. Pulmonary hypoplasia resulting from phrenic nerve agenesis and diaphragmatic amyoplasia. *J Pediatr.* 1980;97:282–287.
19. Wigglesworth JS, Desai R. Effects on lung growth of cervical cord section in the rabbit fetus. *Early Hum Dev.* 1979;3:51–65.
20. Miller ME, Higginbottom MC, Smith DW. Short umbilical cords: its origin and relevance. *Pediatrics.* 1981;67:618–621.
21. Moessinger AC, Blanc WA, Marone PA, et al. Umbilical cord length as an index of fetal activity: experimental study and clinical implications. *Pediatr Res.* 1982;16:109–112.
22. Nijsten TE, De Moor A, Colpaert CG, et al. Restrictive dermopathy: a case report and a critical review of all hypotheses of its origin. *Pediatr Dermatol.* 2002;19:67–72.
23. Khanna P, Opitz JM, Gilbert-Barness E. Restrictive dermopathy: report and review. *Fetal Pediatr Pathol.* 2008;27:105–118.
24. Kim JY, Kim SH, Ji HY, et al. A case of restrictive dermopathy with novel *ZMPSTE24* gene mutation. *Pediatr Dev Pathol.* 2012;15:393–396.
25. Ravenscroft G, Thompson EM, Todd EJ, et al. Whole exome sequencing in foetal akinesia expands the genotype-phenotype spectrum of *GBE1* glycogen storage disease mutations. *Neuromuscul Disord.* 2013;23:165–169.
26. Witters I, Moerman P, Fryns J-P. Fetal akinesia deformation sequence: a study of 30 consecutive in utero diagnoses. *Am J Med Genet.* 2002;113:23–28.
27. Nayak SS, Kadavigere R, Mathew M, et al. Fetal akinesia deformation sequence: expanding the phenotypic spectrum. *Am J Med Genet A.* 2014;164:2643–2648.
28. Rakheja D, Uddin N, Mitui M, et al. Fetal akinesia deformation sequence and neuroaxonal dystrophy without *PLA2G6* mutation. *Pediatr Dev Pathol.* 2010;13:492–496.
29. Mayumi M, Obata-Yasuoka M, Ogura T, et al. Discordance in Pena-Shokeir phenotype/fetal akinesia deformation sequence in a monoamniotic twin. *J Obstet Gynaecol Res.* 2013;39:344–346.
30. Rudzinski ER, Kapur RP, Hevner RF. Fetal akinesia deformation sequence with delayed skeletal muscle maturation and polymicrogyria: evidence for a hypoxic/ischemic pathogenesis. *Pediatr Dev Pathol.* 2010;13:192–201.
31. Witters I, Moerman P, Devriendt K, et al. Two siblings with early onset fetal akinesia deformation sequence and hydranencephaly: further evidence for autosomal recessive inheritance of hydrocephaly, Fowler type. *Am J Med Genet.* 2002;108:41–44.
32. Meyer E, Ricketts C, Morgan NV, et al. Mutations in *FLVCR2* are associated with proliferative vasculopathy and hydranencephaly-hydrocephaly syndrome (Fowler syndrome). *Am J Hum Genet.* 2010;86:471–478.
33. Niles KM, Blaser S, Shannon P, Chitayat D. Fetal arthrogryposis multiplex congenita/fetal akinesia deformation sequence (FADS)-aetiology, diagnosis, and management. *Prenat Diagn.* 2019;39(9):720–731.
34. Alkhunaizi E, Martin N, Jelin AC, et al. Fetal akinesia deformation sequence syndrome associated with recessive TTN variants. *Am J Med Genet A.* 2023;191(3):760–769.
35. Di Feo MF, Lillback V, Jokela M, et al. The crucial role of titin in fetal development: recurrent miscarriages and bone, heart and muscle anomalies characterise the severe end of titinopathies spectrum. *J Med Genet. jmg.* 20232022-109018.
36. Baker EK, Al Gharaibeh FN, Bove K, et al. A novel *RYR1* variant in an infant with a unique fetal presentation of central core disease. *Am J Med Genet A.* 2023;191(6):1646–1651.
37. Busack B, Ott CE, Henrich W, Verlohren S. Prognostic significance of prenatal ultrasound in fetal arthrogryposis multiplex congenita. *Arch Gynecol Obstet.* 2021;303(4):943–953.
38. Tjon JK, Tan-Sindhunata MB, Bugiani M, et al. Care pathway for foetal joint contractures, foetal akinesia deformation sequence, and arthrogryposis multiplex congenita. *Fetal Diagn Ther.* 2021;48(11–12): 829–839.
39. Filges I, Jünemann S, Viehweger E, Tercanli S. Fetal arthrogryposis: what do we tell the prospective parents? *Prenat Diagn.* 2023;43(6):798–805.
40. Hall JG. Deformations associated with arthrogryposis. *Am J Med Genet A.* 2021;185A:2676–2682.
41. Hall JG, Aldinger KA, Tanaka KI. Amyoplasia revisited. *Am J Med Genet A.* 2014;164A:700–730.
42. Ho NC. Monozygotic twins with fetal akinesia: the importance of clinicopathological work-up in predicting risks of recurrence. *Neuropediatrics.* 2000;31:252–256.
43. Vogt J, Morgan NV, Rehal P, et al. *CHRNG* genotype-phenotype correlations in the multiple pterygium syndromes. *J Med Genet.* 2012;49:21–26.
44. Vogt J, Morgan NV, Marton T, et al. Germline mutation in *DOK7* associated with fetal akinesia deformation sequence. *J Med Genet.* 2009;46:338–430.
45. Meyer-Cohen J, Pai GS, Conradi S. Lethal multiple pterygium syndrome in four male fetuses in a family: evidence for an X-linked recessive subtype? *Am J Med Genet.* 1999;82:97–99.

46. Chen M, Chan GS, Lee CP, et al. Sonographic features of lethal multiple pterygium syndrome at 14 weeks. *Prenat Diagn*. 2005;25:475–478.
47. Donker ME, Eijckelhof BH, Tan GM, et al. Serial postural and motor assessment of fetal akinesia deformation sequence (FADS). *Early Hum Dev*. 2009;85:785–790.
48. Makrydimas G, Sotiriadis A, Papapanagiotou G, et al. Fetal akinesia deformation sequence presenting with increased nuchal translucency in the first trimester of pregnancy. *Fetal Diagn Ther*. 2004;19:332–335.
49. Konstantinidou A, Anninos H, Spanakis N, et al. Transplacental infection of coxsackievirus B3 pathological findings in the fetus. *J Med Virol*. 2007;79:754–757.

CHAPTER 48

Abdominal Pregnancy (Extrauterine Pregnancy)

KEY POINTS

- Ectopic pregnancy occurs when a fertilized ovum implants outside the uterus, most commonly in the fallopian tube.
- Risk factors for ectopic pregnancy include tubal damage, prior ectopic pregnancy, use of intrauterine devices, tubal sterilization, infertility, pelvic inflammatory disease, genital infections, multiple sexual partners, endometriosis, and cigarette smoking.
- Abdominal pregnancies have a higher maternal mortality rate compared with tubal pregnancies and intrauterine pregnancies due to massive maternal hemorrhage.
- Clinical presentation of abdominal pregnancy varies, and maternal morbidity includes hemorrhage, infection, toxemia, disseminated intravascular coagulation, pulmonary embolism, and fistula formation.
- Advanced extrauterine pregnancies have a low chance of live birth and high rates of fetal anomalies and maternal complications, with significant fetal deformational problems.
- The management of abdominal pregnancy involves prompt recognition, surgical skill, access to blood products, postoperative care, and assessment of the newborn.

GENESIS

Ectopic pregnancy, defined as the implantation of a fertilized ovum outside the uterus, occurs most commonly in the fallopian tube (95.5% of all ectopic pregnancies), with 70% implanting in the ampulla, 12% in the isthmus, 11% in the fimbrial end, 2% in the interstitial region, and 3% ovarian (Fig. 48.1 A).[1] Only 1.3% of ectopic pregnancies are abdominal, occurring with direct implantation onto the peritoneal surface (see Fig. 48.1B).[1] Abdominal pregnancies are classified as either primary or secondary to tubal or ovarian pregnancies, which rupture into the peritoneal cavity and reimplant for a second time. Reported sites of implantation have included the posterior cul-de-sac, posterior uterine wall (most commonly), uterine serosa, uterine ligaments, omentum, almost all intraperitoneal organs, diaphragm, and retroperitoneal space.[2] Abdominal pain in different locations is the most common presenting symptom. The incidence of ectopic pregnancies increased from 4.5 per 1000 pregnancies in 1970 to 19.7 per 1000 pregnancies in 1992, with this increase attributed to the increasing use of assisted reproductive techniques. Risk factors for ectopic pregnancy include previous *Chlamydia trachomatis* infection (adjusted odds ratio [aOR]: 3.18), prior ectopic pregnancy (aOR: 2.72), previous adnexal surgery (aOR: 2.09), previous infertility (aOR: 2.18), use of an intrauterine device (aOR: 1.72), previous appendectomy (aOR: 1.64), use of in vitro fertilization, pelvic inflammatory disease, multiple sexual partners, endometriosis, and cigarette smoking.[3-7] The risk of ectopic pregnancy increased with a prior ectopic pregnancy, prior tubal ligation, use of intrauterine device (IUD), and prior pelvic/abdominal surgery in a sample of 150 Iranian women with ectopic pregnancy compared with 300 controls.[4] A case-control study in women with planned pregnancy included 900 women diagnosed with ectopic pregnancy (case group) and 889 women with intrauterine pregnancy as the control group. Ectopic pregnancy was associated with previous adnexal surgery, uncertainty of previous pelvic inflammatory disease, and positive serum *C. trachomatis* immunoglobulin G antibody. A history of infertility including tubal infertility, nontubal infertility, and in vitro fertilization treatment was correlated with the

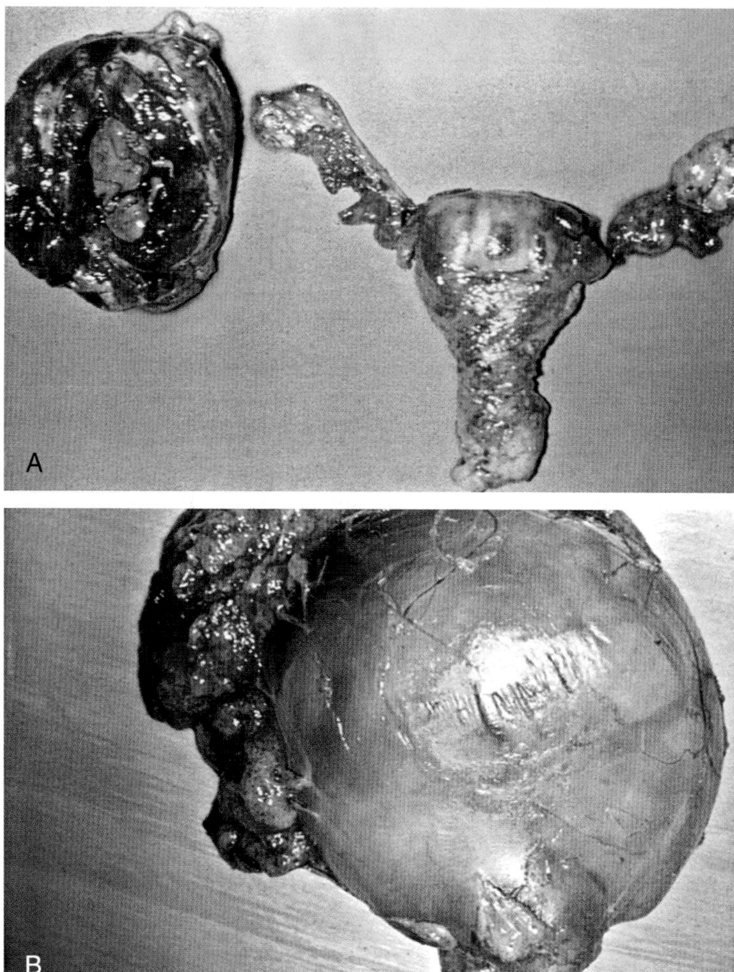

FIGURE 48.1 **A,** Ovarian pregnancy involving the right ovary. **B,** Abdominal pregnancy implanted on the omentum with an intact amniotic sac.

risk of ectopic pregnancy in an umbrella review of risk factors prior to conception.[5] Metaanalyses and systematic reviews carried out through June 25, 2021 graded two risk factors as suggestive evidence: *C. trachomatis* (odds ratio [OR]: 3.03) and smoking (OR: 1.77). Two other risk factors were graded as weak evidence: endometriosis (OR: 2.66) and tubal ligation (OR: 9.3).[7] Currently, the incidence of ectopic pregnancy is 1.3% to 2.4%, with suspicion starting after a positive serum pregnancy test and failure to visualize the intrauterine gestational sac by transvaginal ultrasonography,[8] which is superior to abdominal ultrasonography.[9]

There is usually less early compression and disruption with abdominal pregnancy compared with tubal ectopic pregnancy, and the fetus is more likely to survive. The maternal mortality rate of abdominal pregnancy is seven to eight times higher than that of tubal pregnancy and 90-fold higher than that of intrauterine pregnancy.[10] Most of this increased risk is caused by massive maternal hemorrhage from partial or total placental separation. Clinical presentation is extremely variable, and the maternal mortality rate is approximately 6%.[11] Maternal morbidity includes massive hemorrhage, infection, toxemia, disseminated intravascular coagulation, pulmonary embolism, and formation of a fistula between the amniotic sac and intestine. Some ruptured tubal ectopic pregnancies result in abdominal pregnancies; thus abdominal pregnancy affects about 1 in 6000 to 1 in 10,000 deliveries.[7] A history of pelvic pain along with an abnormal beta human chorionic gonadotropin level should trigger an evaluation for an ectopic pregnancy. The fallopian tube is the most common location for an ectopic pregnancy, and 88% of tubal ectopic pregnancies are diagnosed by absence of a gestational sac and presence of an adnexal mass that is separate from the uterus during transvaginal ultrasound.[8]

Other types of ectopic pregnancy include cornual (an ectopic pregnancy within a malformed uterus),[12] ovarian (Fig. 48.1A),[13] cesarean scar,[14] cervical, intraabdominal, and heterotopic pregnancy.[15] Interstitial pregnancy occurs when the gestational sac implants in the myometrial segment of the fallopian tube.[16] Cornual pregnancy refers to the implantation of a blastocyst within the cornua of a bicornuate or septate uterus.[12] An ovarian pregnancy occurs when an ovum is fertilized and retained within the ovary (see Fig. 48.1A).[13] Cervical pregnancy results from an implantation within the endocervical canal. In a scar pregnancy, implantation takes place within the scar of a prior cesarean section.[14] In an intraabdominal pregnancy, implantation occurs within the intraperitoneal cavity. Heterotopic pregnancy occurs when an intrauterine and an extrauterine pregnancy occurs simultaneously.[15] IUD is a contraceptive method that prevents 99.5% intrauterine implantations, and if implantation occurs with an IUD in place, it is a tubal implantation in 95% of cases and rarely in other places such as the ovary.[17] Cervical heterotopic pregnancy is a very rare event that almost universally results from infertility treatment.[18]

Because most diagnoses of advanced abdominal pregnancy are missed preoperatively, even with the use of sonography, the cornerstones of successful management seem to be quick intraoperative recognition, surgical skill, and ready access to blood products, with meticulous postoperative care and thorough assessment of the newborn. It is usually easier to appreciate an abdominal pregnancy at the end of the first trimester or early in the second trimester, when the pelvic organs are best visualized. The most specific findings to diagnose abdominal pregnancy are the absence of an intrauterine gestational sac combined with a clearly extrauterine gestational sac, fetus, and/or placenta. During the second or third trimester, sonographic findings include the absence of intervening myometrium between amniotic fluid and adjacent maternal pelvic or abdominal viscera, and the inability to establish continuity between the cervical canal and the amniotic cavity. Advanced extrauterine pregnancy is an extremely rare, life-threatening pregnancy complication. Management of such pregnancies presents significant challenges, especially when they have progressed to an advanced stage of fetal viability. With high rates of maternal and fetal mortality associated with this complication, delivery or pregnancy interruption should be expedited following diagnosis. Localization of the placenta and its blood supply is critical to preoperative planning.[19] Because the placentation in advanced abdominal pregnancy is presumed to be inadequate, advanced abdominal pregnancy can be complicated by preeclampsia, which is another condition with high maternal and perinatal morbidity and mortality.[20] After the baby is extracted, because the placenta is implanted in an abnormal site, its removal can result in massive intraoperative bleeding necessitating blood and blood product transfusion and the administration of factor VII to control the bleeding.[21]

Abdominal pregnancies usually arise when a fertilized ovum ruptures from within the fallopian tube and implants within the peritoneal cavity, and only rarely does fertilization of the ovum take place outside the fallopian tube. In other instances, rupture of one horn of a bicornuate uterus can lead to a secondary abdominal pregnancy, and presence of a congenital uterine malformation is a known risk factor for abdominal pregnancy.[22] Cocaine use has also been associated with a 20% increase in the incidence of abdominal pregnancy.[23,24] Ovarian pregnancies are included within the broader category of extrauterine pregnancies, comprising 0.5% to 1% of all ectopic gestations (see Fig. 48.1A), and the presence of an IUD is one risk factor.[17] These pregnancies present similarly to ruptured tubal ectopic pregnancy or ruptured hemorrhagic ovarian cyst, with severe hypogastric abdominal pain, irregular vaginal bleeding, and clinical shock in some cases.

FEATURES

Abdominal pregnancies are located within the peritoneal cavity and exclude tubal, ovarian, and intraligamentous pregnancies (see Fig. 48.1B). In ovarian pregnancy, the fallopian tube is intact and separated from the ovary (see Fig. 48.1A). The gestational sac occupies the position of the ovary and connects to the uterus via the utero-ovarian ligament, and ovarian tissue is evident in the walls of the gestational sac. If an ovarian pregnancy remains unruptured after the second trimester, it is likely to remain intact with

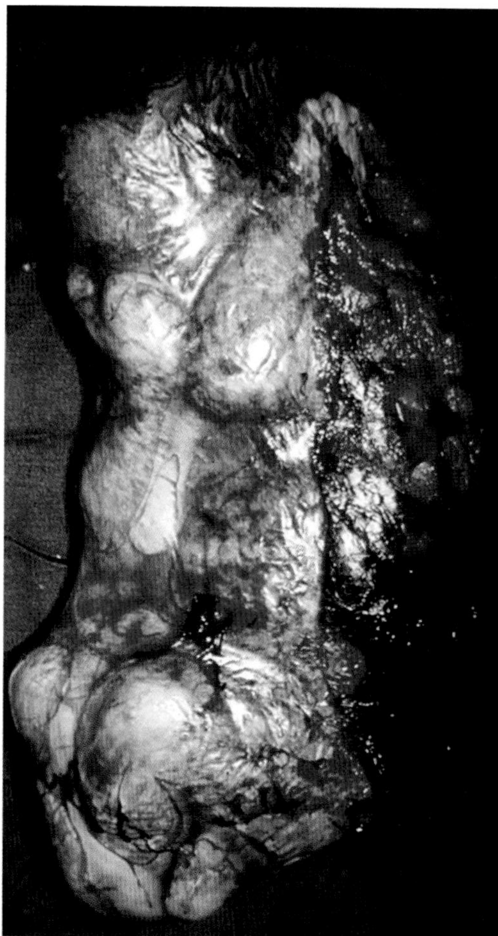

FIGURE 48.2 This extrauterine pregnancy shows an intact amniotic sac that contains no amniotic fluid and completely envelopes the compressed fetus. (Courtesy Dr. James Scott, Professor of Obstetrics and Gynecology, University of Leeds School of Medicine, Leeds, UK.)

resultant fetal problems owing to oligohydramnios, similar to those seen in abdominal pregnancy.[25,26] For advanced extrauterine pregnancies, there is a 10% to 25% chance of a live birth, the rate of fetal anomalies is high, and only 50% of neonates survive longer than 1 week.[26] Problems commonly seen in surviving neonates (Figs. 48.2–48.4) are primarily deformational and/or caused by oligohydramnios (torticollis, plagiocephaly, facial asymmetry, joint contractures, hip dislocation, scoliosis, talipes equinovarus, and pulmonary hypoplasia).[27-29] (See Chapter 46 concerning the oligohydramnios deformation sequence.) Less common malformations include neural tube defects, hydrocephalus, microcephaly, cleft lip and/or palate, omphalocele, imperforate anus, or limb deficiency; the combined rate for both malformations and deformations is 21.4%.[29] The type of limb deficiency seen with abdominal pregnancy appears to be caused by vascular disruption rather than a result of limb malformation, and, in some cases, it may be attributed to the severity of early fetal compression.[29]

MANAGEMENT

When extrauterine pregnancy occurs, the embryo/fetus seldom survives, and oligohydramnios is frequent. If survival does occur, there is likely to be severe constraint of fetal development, and survival is greatly improved if the amniotic sac remains intact.[27] The overall mortality rate for the embryo/fetus is 75% to 95%,[30] with death usually resulting from pulmonary hypoplasia caused by oligohydramnios and possibly fetal thoracic compression.[31] In a 1993 literature review concerning abdominal pregnancies, the maternal mortality rate dropped from 18.2% to 4.5% during the preceding 20 years, and the survival rate for infants at 30 weeks' gestation or older was 63%.[29] During surgery for an abdominal pregnancy, the fetus should be removed and the cord clamped close to the placenta with minimal manipulation. Placental manipulation can lead to significant blood loss because there is no normal cleavage plane and no intrinsic mechanism similar to uterine contractility to control bleeding.[32] There is a 53.8% risk of peritonitis, intraabdominal abscess, sepsis, or other febrile morbidity with advanced abdominal pregnancies, and a reported colonization of the gestational cavity with group B *Streptococcus* has been attributed to a ruptured tubal ectopic pregnancy that seeded the abdominal cavity with vaginal flora. Thus preoperative prophylactic antibiotics and intraoperative cultures of the abdominal cavity and gestational sac have been suggested.[32] Most ovarian pregnancies (92%) fail to survive beyond the first trimester, and they present earlier than abdominal pregnancies because of the vascularity of the ovary and associated maternal hemorrhage.[24] Whereas the traditional treatment of advanced abdominal pregnancy was with laparotomy, the use of improved diagnostic techniques, such as transvaginal ultrasonography, have enabled new, minimally invasive laparoscopic techniques, selective embolization of vessels that supply the placenta, and medical management of the placenta with methotrexate.[33-38]

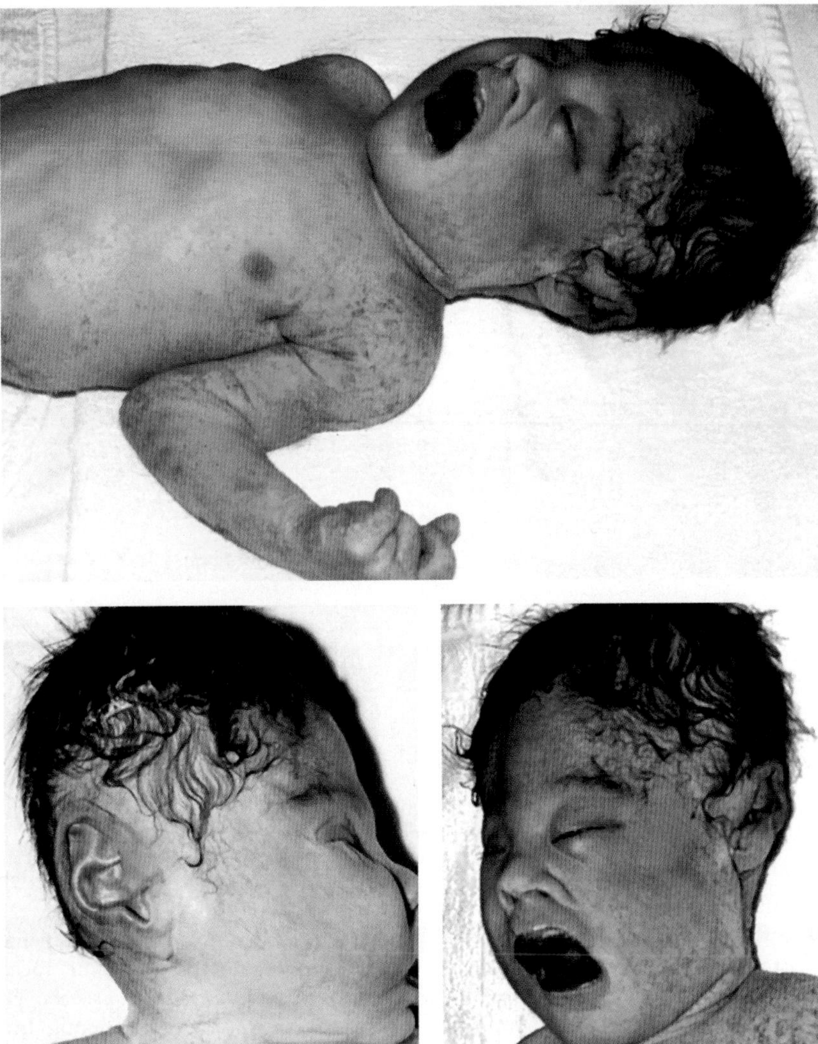

FIGURE 48.3 This infant was delivered abdominally from an extrauterine location behind the uterus. Note the marked distortion of the face and compressive overgrowth of the right ear. Respiratory insufficiency associated with oligohydramnios led to death shortly after birth. (Courtesy Dr. Will Cochran, Beth Israel Hospital and Harvard Medical School, Boston, MA.)

Given high fetal and maternal mortality, use of a single dose of methotrexate for ectopic tubal pregnancy has a similar success rate to surgical treatment, but the presence of fetal heart sounds, β-human chorionic gonadotropin levels >5000 mIU/mL, and size >4 cm are relative contraindications to using methotrexate for an ectopic pregnancy.[8] Methotrexate has advantages over surgery, particularly salpingectomy, in improved subsequent natural pregnancy outcomes. A decrease of 10% in β-human chorionic gonadotropin between days 0 and 7 and 19% between days 0 and 4 are good predictors of treatment success.[39]

DIFFERENTIAL DIAGNOSIS

Differential diagnosis includes pelvic sepsis, food poisoning, and ruptured ectopic pregnancy.[11] Ovarian pregnancies are rare events (about 10 times less common than abdominal pregnancies), and they must be

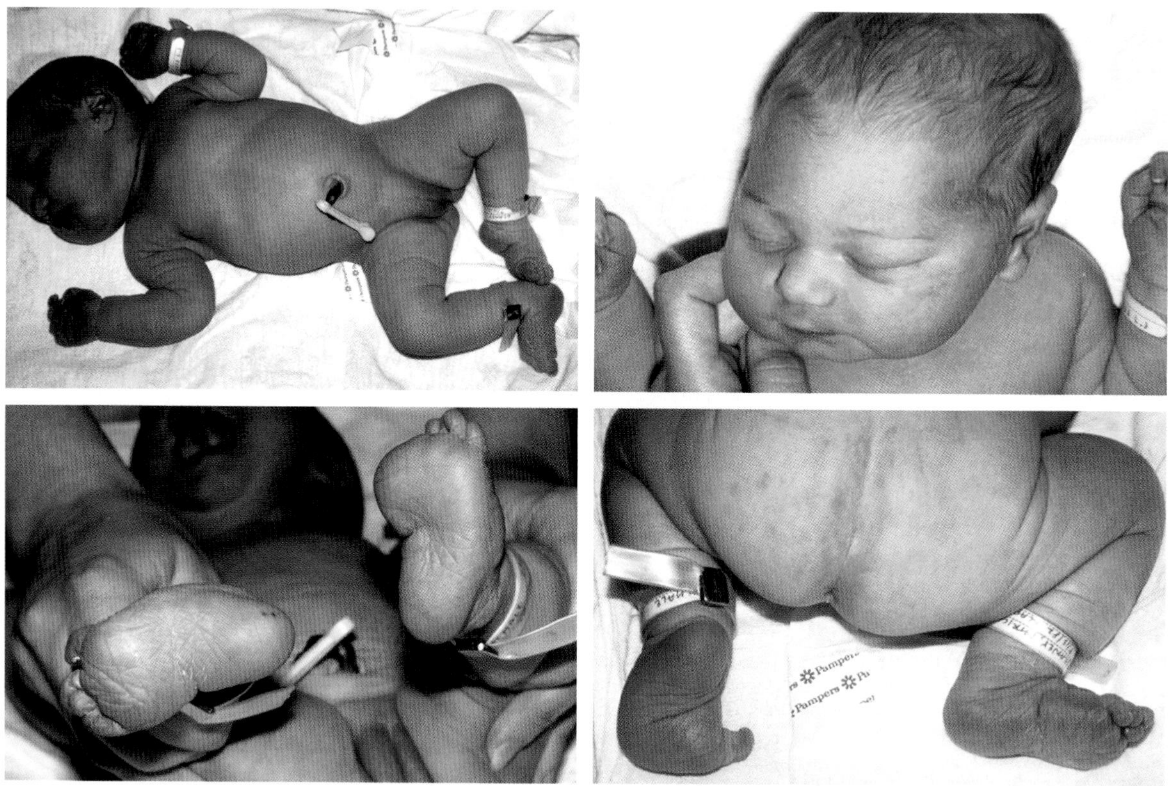

FIGURE 48.4 This infant was an abdominal pregnancy, with her head under the stomach and feet under the gallbladder. (Courtesy Dr. Will Cochran, Beth Israel Hospital and Harvard Medical School, Boston, MA.)

distinguished from tubal ectopic pregnancy, hemorrhagic ovarian cyst, and primary ovarian choriocarcinoma.[24,40] Careful ultrasound assessment is indicated for every hemodynamically stable patient with a suspected ectopic pregnancy, and failure to respond to induction is a classic clue that the pregnancy might be extrauterine. If the pregnancy is not visualized in the uterus or tubes, then unusual locations such as the cervix, cornua, ovaries, and pouch of Douglas should be checked, because the rare forms of ectopic pregnancy are generally more dangerous than tubal ectopic pregnancies. Unexplained abdominal ascites in a patient with a positive pregnancy test and no intrauterine gestational sac may be associated with abdominal pregnancy.[41] An ectopic pregnancy that implanted on the diaphragm and resulted in spontaneous hemothorax owing to trophoblastic invasion of the pleura has also been reported.[42] Nontubal ectopic pregnancies account for less than 5% of all ectopic pregnancies but result in approximately 20% of the fatalities; therefore additional measures such as laparoscopy and other imaging modalities (e.g., magnetic resonance imaging) may aid in diagnosis and management.[24,42] The most commonly reported anatomic locations of primary peritoneal implantations are the pouch of Douglas and the posterior uterine wall, but other reported locations have included the liver, spleen, intestines, retroperitoneum, diaphragm, broad ligament, omentum, ovary, and within a cesarean scar.[34,41–44] The key to early and successful diagnosis and management appears to be strong clinical suspicion and, simply put, "knowing where to look."

References

1. Bouyer J, Coste J, Fernandez H, et al. Sites of ectopic pregnancy: a 10-year population-based study of 1800 cases. *Hum Reprod.* 2002;17:3224–3230.
2. Eisner SM, Ebert AD, David M. Rare ectopic pregnancies: a literature review for the period 2007-2019 on locations outside the uterus and fallopian tubes. *Geburtshilfe Frauenheilkd.* 2020;80(7):686–701.
3. Pisarska MD, Carson S. Incidence and risk factors for ectopic pregnancy. *Clin Obstet Gynecol.* 1999;42:2–8.

4. Parashi S, Moukhah S, Ashrafi M. Main risk factors for ectopic pregnancy: a case-control study in a sample of Iranian women. *Int J Fertil Steril.* 2014;8:147–154.
5. Li C, Meng CX, Zhao WH, et al. Risk factors for ectopic pregnancy in women with planned pregnancy: a case-control study. *Eur J Obstet Gynecol Reprod Biol.* 2014;181:176–182.
6. Li C, Zhao WH, Zhu Q, et al. Risk factors for ectopic pregnancy: a multi-center case-control study. *BMC Pregnancy Childbirth.* 2015 Aug 22;15:187, 2015.
7. Jenabi E, Ayubi E, Khazaei S, Soltanian AR, Salehi AM. The environmental risk factors associated with ectopic pregnancy: an umbrella review. *J Gynecol Obstet Hum Reprod.* 2023;52(2):102532.
8. Obaid M, Abu-Faza M, Abdelazim IA, Al-Khatlan HS, Al-Tuhoo AM. Undisturbed tubal pregnancies with positive fetal heart treated medically: case study. *J Mother Child.* 2023;26(1):124–126. 22.
9. Hu HJ, Sun J, Feng R, Yu L. Comparison of the application value of transvaginal ultrasound and transabdominal ultrasound in the diagnosis of ectopic pregnancy. *World J Clin Cases.* 2023;11(13):2945–2955.
10. Atrash HK, Friede A, Hogue CJ. Abdominal pregnancy in the United States: frequency and maternal mortality. *Obstet Gynecol.* 1987;69:333–337.
11. Ombelet W, Vandermerwe JV, Assche FA. Advanced extrauterine pregnancy: description of 38 cases with literature survey. *Obstet Gynecol.* 1988;59:386–397.
12. Dhanju G, Goubran A, Zimolag L, Chartrand R, Matthew F, Breddam A. Distinguishing between cornual, angular and interstitial ectopic pregnancy: a case report and a brief literature review. *Radiol Case Rep.* 2023;18(7):2531–2544.
13. Shao M, Wang X, Zhou X. Case Report: Ovarian pregnancy, a rare but lethal condition: an analysis of 112 cases. *Front Surg.* 2023;10:1062228.
14. Thakur B, Shrimali T. Rare concomitant cesarean scar ectopic pregnancy with tubal ectopic pregnancy: a case report. *Cureus..* 2023;15(4):e37434.
15. Elsayed S, Farah N, Anglim M. Heterotopic pregnancy: case series and review of diagnosis and management. *Case Rep Obstet Gynecol.* 20232124191, 2023.
16. Dunphy L, Haresnape C, Furara S. Interstitial ectopic pregnancy successfully treated with methotrexate. *BMJ Case Rep.* 2023;16(4):e252588.
17. Ghasemi Tehrani H, Hamoush Z, Ghasemi M, et al. Ovarian ectopic pregnancy: a rare case. *Iran J Reprod Med.* 2014;12:281–284.
18. Moragianni VA, Hamar BD, McArdle C, et al. Management of a cervical heterotopic pregnancy presenting with first-trimester bleeding: case report and review of the literature. *Fertil Steril.* 2012;98:89–94.
19. Smrtka MP, Gunatilake R, Miller MJ, et al. Improving the management of an advanced extrauterine pregnancy using pelvic arteriography in a hybrid operating suite. *AJP Rep.* 2012;2:63–66.
20. Masukume G, Sengurayi E, Muchara A, et al. Full-term abdominal extrauterine pregnancy complicated by post-operative ascites with successful outcome: a case report. *J Med Case Rep.* 2013;7:10. https://doi.org/10.1186/1752-1947-7-10. 2013.
21. Dahab AA, Aburass R, Shawkat W, et al. Full-term extra-uterine abdominal pregnancy: a case report. *J Med Case Rep.* 2011;5:531.
22. Jayaprakash S, Muralidhar L, Sampathkumar G, et al. Rupture of bicornuate uterus. *BMJ Case Rep.* Oct 28;2011. https://doi.org/10.1136/bcr.08.2011.4633. pii: bcr0820114633.
23. Audain L, Brown WE, Smith DM, et al. Cocaine use as a risk factor for abdominal pregnancy. *J Natl Med Assoc.* 1998;90:277–283.
24. Nisenblat V, Leibovitz Z, Tal J, et al. Primary ovarian ectopic pregnancy misdiagnosed as first-trimester missed abortion. *J Ultrasound Med.* 2005;24:539–543.
25. Lee W, Voet RL, Poliak J. Combined intrauterine and ovarian pregnancy: a case report. *J Reprod Med.* 1985;30:563.
26. Hallet JG. Abdominal pregnancy: a study of twenty-one consecutive cases. *Am J Obstet Gynecol.* 1985;152:444–449.
27. Tan KL, Goon SM, Wee JH. The pediatric aspects of advanced abdominal pregnancy. *J Obstet Gynaec Br Commonw.* 1969;76:1021–1028.
28. Uglow MG, Clarke NM. Congenital dislocation of the hip in extrauterine pregnancy. *J Bone Joint Surg Br.* 1996;78:751–753.
29. Stevens CA. Malformations and deformations in abdominal pregnancy. *Am J Med Genet.* 1993;47:1189–1195.
30. Delke I, Veridanio NP, Tancer ML. Abdominal pregnancy: review of current management and addition of 10 cases. *Obstet Gynecol.* 1982;60:200–204.
31. Bell JB, Gerdes JS, Bhutani VK, et al. Chronic lung disorder following abdominal pregnancy. *Am J Dis Child.* 1987;141:1111–1113.
32. Bergstrom R, Mueller G, Yankowitz J. A case illustrating the continued dilemmas in treating abdominal pregnancy and a potential explanation for the high rate of postsurgical febrile morbidity. *Gynecol Obstet Invest.* 1998;46:268–270.
33. Rahamon J, Berkowitz R, Mitty H, et al. Minimally invasive management of an advanced abdominal pregnancy. *Obstet Gynecol.* 2004;103:1064–1068.
34. Graesslin O, Dedecker F, Quereux C, et al. Conservative treatment of ectopic pregnancy in a cesarean scar. *Obstet Gynecol.* 2005;105:869–871.
35. Krissi H, Hiersch L, Stolovitch N, et al. Outcome, complications and future fertility in women treated with uterine artery embolization and methotrexate for non-tubal ectopic pregnancy. *Eur J Obstet Gynecol Reprod Biol.* 2014;182C:172–176.
36. Yu Y, Xu W, Xie Z, et al. Management and outcome of 25 heterotopic pregnancies in Zhejiang, China. *Eur J Obstet Gynecol Reprod Biol.* 2014;180:157–161.

37. OuYang Z, Yin Q, Xu Y, et al. Heterotopic cesarean scar pregnancy: diagnosis, treatment, and prognosis. *J Ultrasound Med.* 2014;33:1533–1537.
38. Headley A. Management of cervical ectopic pregnancy with uterine artery embolization: a case report. *J Reprod Med.* 2014;59:425–428.
39. Aiob A, Shqara RA, Mikhail SM, Sharon A, Odeh M, Lowenstein L. Alternative beta-hCG follow-up protocols after single-dose methotrexate therapy for ectopic pregnancy: a retrospective cohort study. *Eur J Obstet Gynecol Reprod Biol.* 2023;284:120–124.
40. Heo EJ, Choi CH, Park JM, et al. Primary ovarian choriocarcinoma mimicking ectopic pregnancy. *Obstet Gynecol Sci.* 2014;57:330–333.
41. Ross JA, Hacket E, Lawton F, et al. Massive ascites due to abdominal pregnancy. *Hum Reprod.* 1997;12:390–391.
42. Fishman DA, Padilla LA, Joob A, et al. Ectopic pregnancy causing hemothorax managed by thorascopy and actinomycin D. *Obstet Gynecol.* 1998;91:837–838.
43. Deshpande N, Mathers A, Acharya U. Broad ligament twin pregnancy following in-vitro fertilization. *Hum Reprod.* 1999;14:852–854.
44. Valley MT, Pierce JG, Daniel TB, et al. Cesarean scar pregnancy: imaging and treatment with conservative surgery. *Obstet Gynecol.* 1998;91:838–840.

CHAPTER 49

Early Embryonic Compression or Disruption

Tubal Ectopic Pregnancy, Early Amnion Rupture, Limb-Body Wall Complex, and Body Stalk Anomaly

KEY POINTS

- Compression during early morphogenesis (the first trimester) can result in three types of defects: molded deformations, incomplete morphogenesis, and disruptions of morphogenesis.
- Experimental animal studies showed that early amniotic sac puncture caused defects similar to Pierre Robin sequence, cleft palate, syndactyly, and limb-reduction defects.
- Limb-body wall complex is a rare defect characterized by extensive extremity and body wall defects, often associated with low birth weight and younger maternal age.
- Amniotic band sequence can lead to craniofacial defects, extremity defects, abdominal wall defects, and spinal column abnormalities.
- Recurrent malformation associations affecting the development of the embryo, such as LBWC, MURCS, OEIS, and VACTERL, are now termed recurrent constellations of embryonic malformations (RCEM).
- Pathogenic variants in *CSX2*, *TBXT* (sacral agenesis), and *CSX1* (anorectal malformations) have been discovered in a number of early caudal malformations such as sirenomelia, persistent cloaca, and imperforate anus with renal, urogenital, vertebral, and limb defects.

GENESIS

Constraint that occurs during the latter period of gestation can cause molded deformations with good prospects for spontaneous or assisted return to normal form; however, when constraint occurs during early morphogenesis, it can have more severe and lasting impacts on form. The types of defects that can be produced by such compression during this early period of organogenesis (i.e., within the first trimester) fall into three categories: molded deformations, incomplete morphogenesis, and disruptions of morphogenesis (Table 49.1). All three types of defects were produced experimentally by Poswillo after early amniotic sac puncture in rat embryos at 15.5 days' gestation.[1] At this stage of gestation, the rat embryo is at a period of development equivalent to that of the 6- to 7-week human embryo, and mesenchymal condensations have formed bones within the developing limbs but the fingers are not fully separated (Fig. 49.1). The lip has fused, but the palatal shelves have not yet closed (Table 49.2). Amniotic bands were only present in 19% of the rat fetuses in Poswillo's study, and there were no defects in control animals.[1] Treated animals showed a small jaw that was caused by compression of the mandible against the sternum. In all but one rat fetus, this caused the tongue to be thrust between the posterior palatal shelves, thereby preventing closure of the palatal shelves (similar to what is seen in Pierre Robin sequence). Poswillo found that 29% of these rat fetuses with Robin sequence defects induced by oligohydramnios and compression also had limb defects.[1] Defects such as cleft palate and syndactyly were also interpreted as incomplete morphogenesis secondary to compression. Limb-reduction defects involving the radius, femur, and other long bones were interpreted as resulting from vascular disruption due to focal hemorrhage and necrosis.

Vascular disruption is the most common cause of limb deficiency. In a hospital-based surveillance program of 161,252 infants born in the years 1972 to 1974 and 1979 to 1994, the overall prevalence of limb-reduction defects was 0.69 per 1000 live births, with 34% of these defects attributed to vascular disruption (a prevalence of 0.22 per 1000 live births).[2] Kennedy and Persaud demonstrated that early amnion puncture, particularly on day 15 in the rat, leads to edema and hemorrhage, thereby causing tissue damage and resorption within the distal limbs, and these researchers showed that lower limbs are more affected than upper limbs (Figs. 49.2 and 49.3).[3] Webster et al. demonstrated that a broad variety of uterine manipulations in pregnant mice during a similar early stage of gestation can result in hemorrhagic disruption of various fetal structures,[4] and this may be mediated through fetal hypoxia.[5] Animal studies indicate that hypoxic episodes in the first trimester of human pregnancy could occur by temporary constriction of the uterine arteries, and this could be a consequence of exposure to cocaine, misoprostol, or severe shock. There is evidence that these exposures have resulted in hypoxia-related malformations in humans, and the

Table 49.1 TYPES OF DEFECTS PRODUCED BY CONSTRAINT IN EARLY GESTATION

Defect	Description
Molded deformations	Similar to those produced in late fetal life but often more severe; more difficult to return to normal form because of early onset
Incomplete morphogenesis	Constraint may limit or prevent full completion of a normal stage in morphogenesis
Disruption of morphogenesis	Constraint may cause edema, hemorrhage, and focal necrosis with loss of previously formed tissue

Table 49.2 DEFECTS IN RAT FETUSES AFTER AMNION PUNCTURE AT 15.5 DAYS[a]

Defect	Prevalence
Molded deformations	100%
Micrognathia	100%
Talipes	5%
Incomplete morphogenesis	97%
Failure of palatal closure	97%
Syndactyly	9%
Disruption of morphogenesis	12%
Absent radius, femur	6%
Phocomelia	6%

[a]15.5 days in the rat fetus is similar to 42 to 45 days in the human fetus.
From Poswillo D. Observations of fetal posture and causal mechanisms of congenital deformity of the palate, mandible and limbs. *J Dent Res*. 1966;45:583.

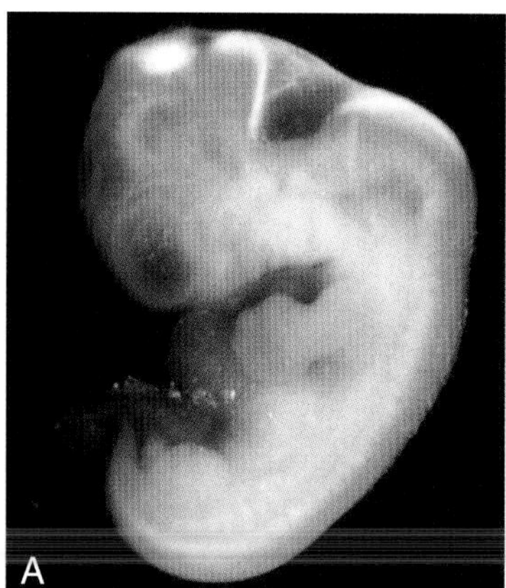

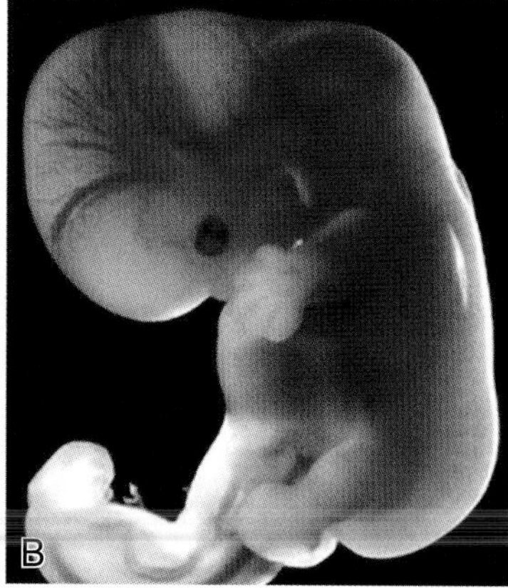

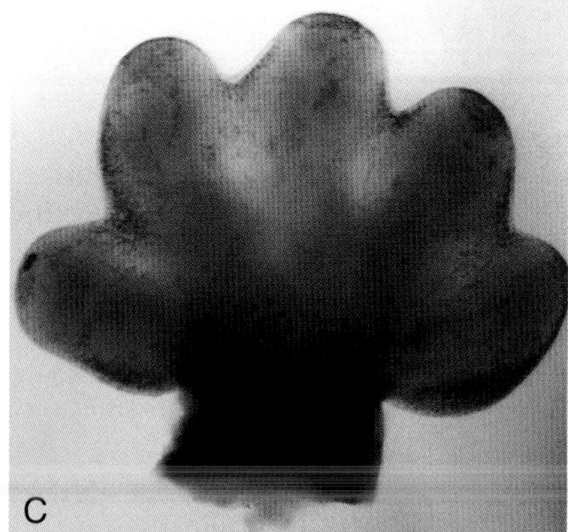

FIGURE 49.1 Human embryo at 32–36 days of development (**A**), with the hand plate formed but no separation of the finger rays. By day 44 (**B**), the process of apoptosis removes soft tissue between the digits (**C**). Around this time constraint of the developing limb has been found in animal studies to cause edema, hemorrhage, and resorptive necrosis with loss of previous limb tissues. The process of separation of the digits may also be impaired, yielding syndactyly.

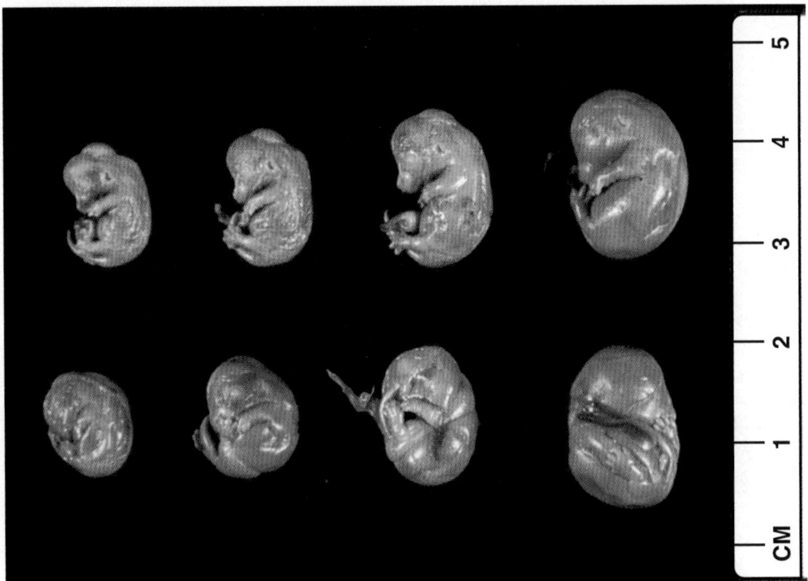

FIGURE 49.2 After early amnion puncture on day 15, rat fetuses are compressed in a cephalocaudal fashion with the developing mandible thrust against the sternum. From left to right, rat embryos are shown at 12, 24, 36, and 48 hours after amniotic puncture *(bottom row)*; a control fetus of the same gestational age is shown in the top row. (Courtesy TVN Persauds, Department of Anatomy, University of Manitoba, Winnipeg, Manitoba, Canada.)

strongest evidence of hypoxia causing birth defects in humans comes from studies of fetuses lacking hemoglobin F. Such fetuses are hypoxic from the middle of the first trimester and show a range of birth defects, particularly transverse limb-reduction defects.[5] Hypoxia in the developing human fetus can lead not only to the more commonly accepted disruptive-type defects but also to patterns of anomalies that suggest a more classic teratogenic effect, such as abnormal embryonic neuronal migration and organization resulting in polymicrogyria, cortical dysplasia, or dysgenesis, and some types of focal cortical dysplasia.[6]

The combination of early embryonic compression with vascular disruption that results in extensive extremity and body wall defects in humans has been termed *limb-body wall complex* (LBWC) (Fig. 49.4).[7-12] This defect occurs with a birth prevalence of 0.26 per 10,000 births, with half of the cases being stillborn, and there is a strong association with very low birth weight, short gestational age, and younger maternal age.[12] The spectrum of defects can include variable combinations of body wall defects with evisceration of thoracic and/or abdominal organs, limb deficiency, neural tube defects, and facial clefts, with or without amniotic bands and renal agenesis. Lower limbs are more severely and consistently affected than upper limbs, with distal structures more involved than proximal structures, similar to what is seen in rats subjected to early amnion puncture on day 15, which suggests a vascular pathogenesis.[12] Several theories have been suggested to explain this complex: early amnion rupture (operating through uterine pressure and/or disruption by amniotic bands), vascular compromise (primarily hypoperfusion), and an early intrinsic defect of the developing embryo. These associations of malformations originate as early as the embryonic disc stage, since some of the observed associated anomalies are secondary complications of a primary disturbance in embryogenesis.[13]

There are patterns of malformation whose pathogenesis has not been firmly established, such as sirenomelia, vertebral anal cardiac tracheo-esophageal fistula renal limb defects (VACTERL) association, omphalocele exstrophy imperforate anus spinal defects (OEIS) complex, limb-body wall complex (LBWC), urorectal septum malformation (URSM) sequence, and Müllerian duct aplasia renal anomalies cervico-thoracic somite dysplasia (MURCS) association, all of which predominantly affect caudal structures. Based on the overlap of component malformations, Stevenson proposed a common pathogenesis for these early patterns of malformation.[14] A single umbilical

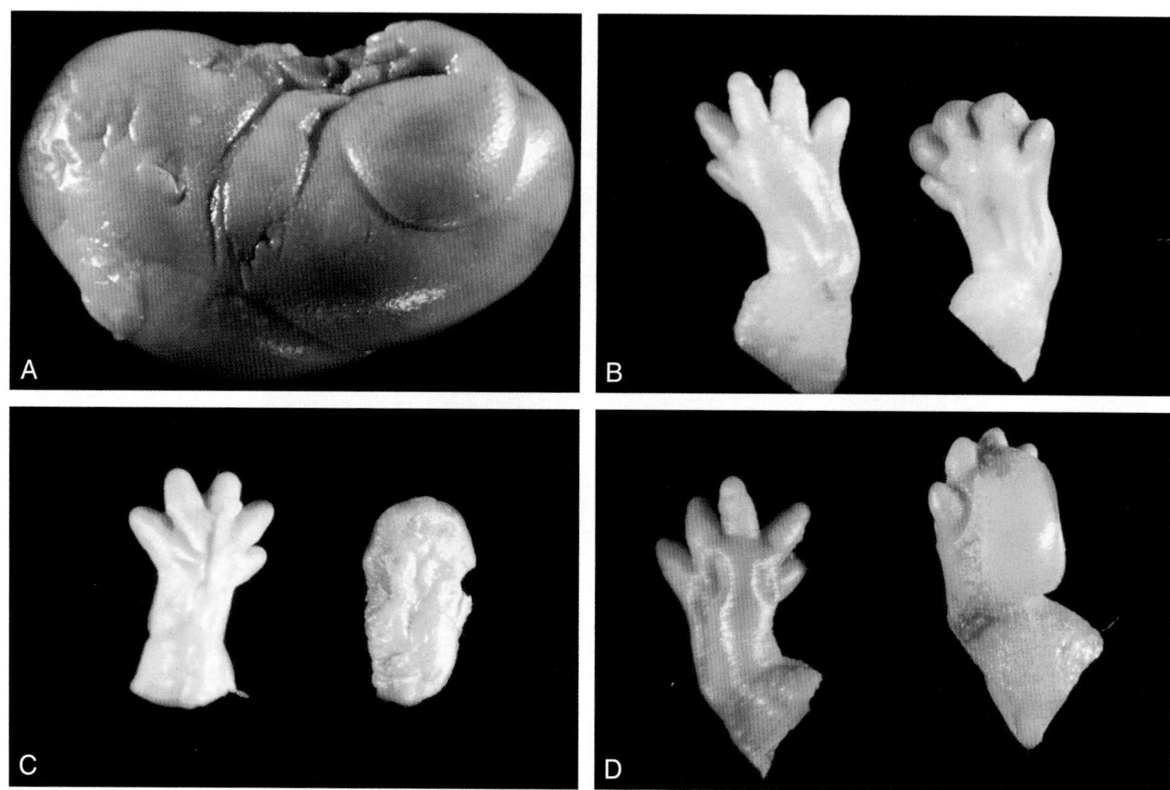

FIGURE 49.3 Limb compression leads to edema and hemorrhage, thereby causing tissue damage and resorption within the distal limbs, with lower limbs more affected than upper limbs. A, The rat fetus is shown 48 hours after amnion puncture on day 15 with edema, compression, and banding around a digit on the right foot. Individual paws are shown 36 hours after puncture with adactyly (B) and 48 hours after puncture with blebs (C, D). Control paws of the same gestational age are shown on the left in B to D. (Courtesy TVN Persauds, Department of Anatomy, University of Manitoba, Winnipeg, Manitoba, Canada.)

artery is present in all cases of sirenomelia and 30% to 50% of cases of VACTERL association, OEIS complex, URSM sequence, and LBWC. This single artery arises from the descending aorta high and redirects blood flow from the developing caudal structures of the embryo to the placenta, a phenomenon termed vitelline vascular steal.[14] As more genomic sequencing has been done in patients with caudal malformations such as sirenomelia, persistent cloaca, and imperforate anus with renal, urogenital, vertebral, and limb defects, pathogenic variants in *CSX2*, *TBXT* (sacral agenesis), and *CSX1* (anorectal malformations) have been discovered.[15] Recurrent malformation associations affecting the development of the embryo such as LBWC, MURCS, oculo-auricul-vertebral spectrum (OAVS), OEIS, pentalogy of Cantrell (POC), and VACTERL are now termed recurrent constellations of embryonic malformations (RCEM), which are characterized by an excess of reported monozygotic discordant twins and lack of familial recurrence.[16]

There have been several attempts to subcategorize infants with amniotic rupture sequence. Among 1,706,639 births reported to the Polish Registry of Congenital Malformations between 1998 and 2006, there were 47 infants with a diagnosis of amniotic rupture sequence (presenting with fibrous bands, possibly as a result of amniotic tear in the first trimester of gestation), 38 infants with only limb involvement, and 9 infants with associated body wall defects.[17] The cases with body wall defects were more frequently affected by other congenital defects, particularly urogenital malformations, suggesting this combination arose at an earlier stage of development. In both groups, limb-reduction defects occurred in approximately 80% of cases; however, minor distal limb defects (phalangeal or digital amputation, pseudosyndactyly,

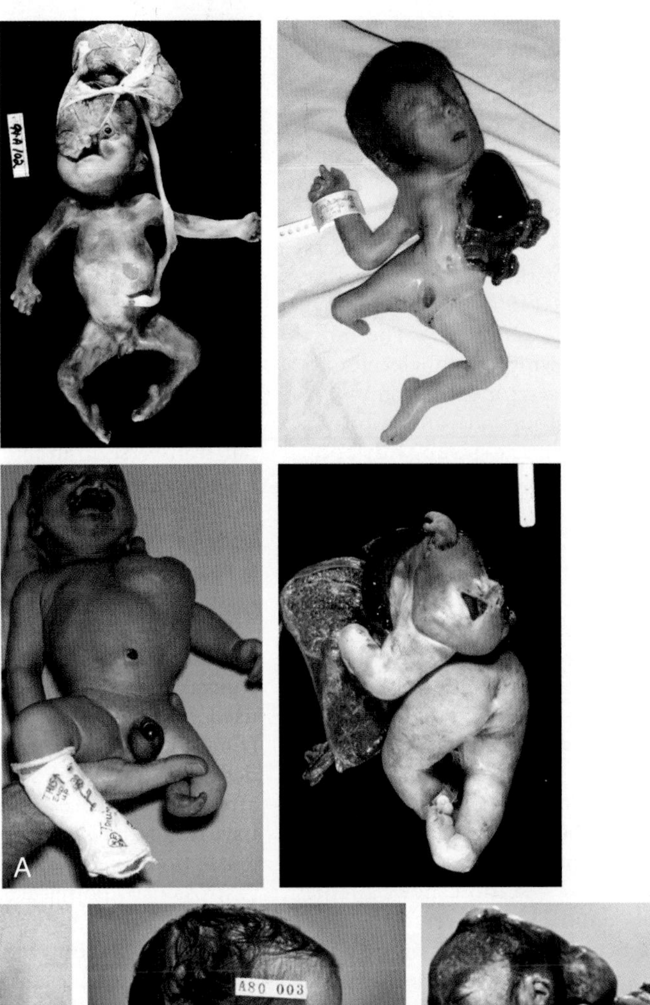

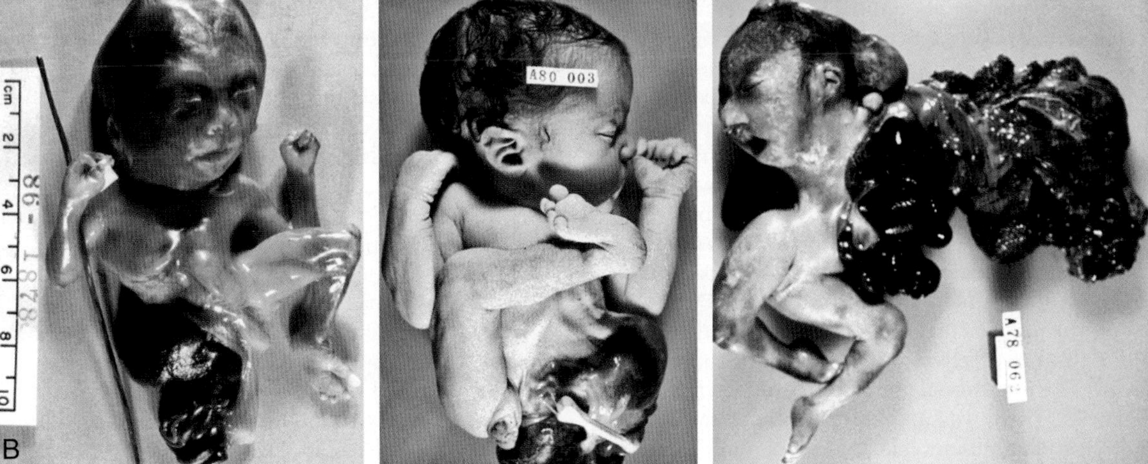

FIGURE 49.4 Examples of very early amnion rupture in lethally affected fetuses with facial clefts, amniotic disruption of limbs and facial structures, and limb-body wall defects. (From Graham JM Jr, Miller ME, Stephan MJ, et al. Limb reduction anomalies and early in-utero limb compression. *J Pediatr.* 1980;96:1052.)

constriction rings) predominated in the group with only limb involvement, which also had a higher frequency of hand and upper limb involvement.[17] Among 50 cases with prenatal diagnosis of amniotic band sequence from 1993 to 2010, the mean maternal age was 25.7 ± 6.9 years, and 54% (27 of 50) were primiparous, compared with 22% (11 of 50) who had three or more previous pregnancies.[18] Craniofacial defects were seen in 78% (39 of 50) of the cases, followed by defects of the extremities 70% (35 of 50), abdominal wall, spine, and/or thorax 52% (26 of 50). The most frequent defects were the following: encephalocele and facial clefts in the craniofacial group; shortening at any level in the limb defects group; and alterations of the spinal column curvature in the group with body wall defects.[18] Among eight fetuses encountered over a 3-year period with limb-body wall defect, 50% of mothers were younger than 25 years and in their first pregnancy (62.5%). Craniofacial defects were verified in three patients (37.5%), thoracic/abdominal abnormalities in six (75%), and limb defects in all eight (100%). Congenital heart defects were observed in five patients (62.5%).[19] Complementary examinations, such as fetal magnetic resonance imaging (MRI) and echocardiography, have been used to better define the observed defects.[19,20]

Body stalk anomaly is a rare lethal malformation of unknown cause that has been reported with discordant occurrence in four monoamniotic pregnancies.[21] Ultrasound at 10 to 14 weeks' gestation shows a fetus with a large anterior abdominal wall defect, with most of the abdominal contents and almost half of the body in the celomic cavity, in association with severe kyphoscoliosis and a very short umbilical cord. Exteriorized abdominal contents and lower limbs within the extraembryonic celom, with an intact amniotic membrane, have been visualized by fetal MRI at 14 weeks' gestation.[22] Among 16 Danish infants with body stalk anomaly, representing 3.4% of 469 infants ascertained in a nationwide dataset of live- and stillborn infants born with abdominal wall defects during 1970 to 1989, the prevalence was 0.12 per 10,000 live- and stillborn infants, and all affected infants died at or shortly after birth.[23] The gestational age at birth varied from 33 to 40 weeks. There was an excess of males (M/F ratio: 2.2:1.0), and all infants had associated malformations: severe limb-reduction defects (56%), absence of one kidney associated with malformations of genitalia and/or urinary bladder (62%), scoliosis (82%), and anal atresia (57%). There were two sets of twins; one discordant and one concordant.[23]

Infants with limb-reduction defects resulting from early exposure to misoprostol or chorion villus sampling (CVS) have asymmetric digit loss, constriction rings, and syndactyly owing to vascular disruption in limb structures that had formed normally (Fig. 49.5). These defects can resemble amniotic band disruption.[2] The underlying mechanism of such vascular disruption is embryonic hypotension and hypoxia followed by endothelial cell damage, hemorrhage, and necrosis with tissue loss.[4] Such defects are more likely to involve distal structures in the upper body (hands and tongue) than proximal structures or the lower body, with middle digital rays more affected than medial or lateral rays (see Fig. 49.5).[2,24–27] The frequency of terminal transverse limb-reduction defects is significantly higher after CVS than in nonexposed pregnancies, with earlier procedures resulting in more severe types of defects.[26,27] Absence of the distal portion of the third finger, with tapering and stiff joints, appears to be a distinctive feature of exposure to CVS.[27]

Misoprostol, a synthetic analog of prostaglandin E_1, increases the amplitude and frequency of uterine contractions and stimulates uterine bleeding. When used illegally to induce abortions during the first trimester, it has been associated with limb-reduction defects and Möbius sequence.[28–31] Other unsuccessful attempts to induce abortion during the first trimester have resulted in similar defects as well as other vascular disruption defects such as arthrogryposis, amyoplasia, gastroschisis, bowel atresia, and scalp defects. Other types of defects may occur because of incomplete morphogenesis or compression, such as scoliosis, facial clefts, heart defects, cortical gyral abnormalities, camptodactyly, and syndactyly.[32–35] Similar defects have resulted after severe abdominal trauma in early pregnancy,[36–40] and also after high maternal fever in early pregnancy.[41] These defects have also been reproduced experimentally through early amnion puncture, uterine manipulations, or hyperthermia in pregnant rats and mice.[1,3–5]

Matsunaga and Shiota recognized early spatial limitation as a significant factor in constraint-induced malformations, noting that 11.6% of 43 embryos and fetuses recovered from ectopic tubal pregnancies had structural defects, as did 6.2% of 97 fetuses from myomatous pregnancies, in contrast to a 3.3% incidence of structural defects among 3474 normally implanted therapeutic abortuses from nonmyomatous uteri.[42] Amelia was present in two of the five fetuses with structural defects who implanted in a fallopian tube (Fig. 49.6), which is consistent with the notion that

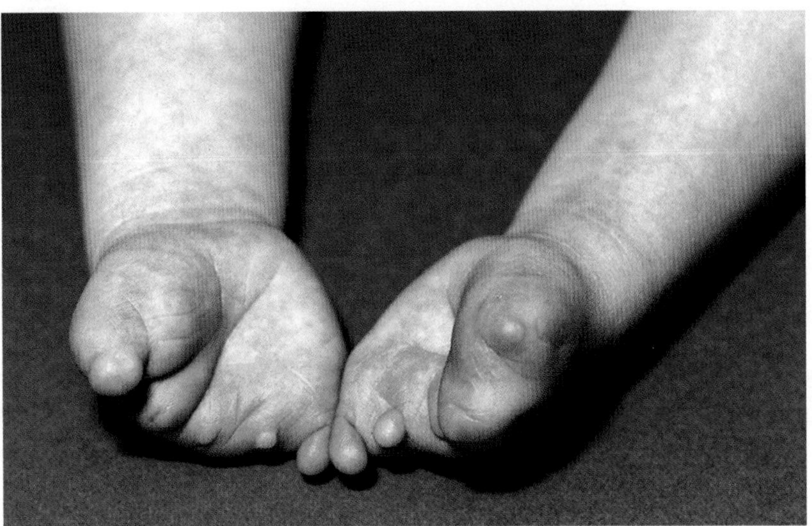

FIGURE 49.5 Disruptive loss of fingers in the hand (affecting central digits more severely) as a consequence of chorion villus sampling performed at 7 to 8 weeks of gestation.

early fetal disruption leads to more severe limb-reduction defects.[42] *Ectopic pregnancy*, defined as the implantation of a fertilized ovum outside the uterus, occurs most commonly in the fallopian tube (see Fig. 49.6), with 70% implanting in the ampulla, 12% in the isthmus, 11% in the fimbrial end, 2% in the interstitial region, and 3% ovarian.[43] The incidence of ectopic pregnancies increased from 4.5 per 1000 pregnancies in 1970 to 19.7 per 1000 pregnancies in 1992, with risk factors including tubal damage or sterilization, use of an intrauterine device, infertility, previous genital infections, multiple sexual partners, and cigarette smoking.[44] Ectopic pregnancy is also associated with previous adnexal surgery, pelvic inflammatory disease, positive serum *Chlamydia trachomatis* immunoglobulin G antibody, a history of infertility including tubal infertility, and nontubal infertility. In vitro fertilization has also been correlated with the recent increased risk of ectopic pregnancy.[45]

FEATURES

Among patients with body wall complex, with or without amniotic bands, observed defects have included scoliosis, joint contractures, Robin sequence, syndactyly, body wall defects with evisceration of thoracic and/or abdominal organs, limb deficiency, neural tube defects, and facial clefts, with or without amniotic bands. These defects are of a type that cannot be readily explained by amniotic band constriction alone, and lower limbs are more severely and consistently affected than upper limbs, with distal structures more involved than proximal structures, which suggests a vascular pathogenesis with internal anomalies that might be secondary complications of a primary disturbance in embryogenesis.[13-16] This must be distinguished from body stalk anomaly, which consists of a large anterior abdominal wall defect, with most of the abdominal contents and almost half of the body in the celomic cavity, in association with severe kyphoscoliosis and a very short umbilical cord. Fetal MRI can distinguish body stalk anomaly from limb-body wall defect, confirming a large anterior wall defect with herniation of the liver and bowel and a short or absent umbilical cord.[22]

Defects associated with CVS include terminal transverse limb-reduction defects (with or without nubbins), amniotic bandlike anomalies of the hands (e.g., digital fusion, syndactyly, constriction rings, loss of distal digits, tapered fingers with stiff joints, with digits two to four especially affected), hypoglossia, cranial nerve dysfunction, hemangiomas, intestinal atresia, clubfoot, and gastroschisis.[46-48] Defects associated with unsuccessful attempts at pregnancy termination or early abdominal trauma include arthrogryposis, amyoplasia, gastroschisis, bowel atresia, scalp defects, limb defects, Möbius sequence, scoliosis, facial clefts, heart defects, cortical gyral abnormalities, hydrocephaly, porencephaly, camptodactyly, and syndactyly.

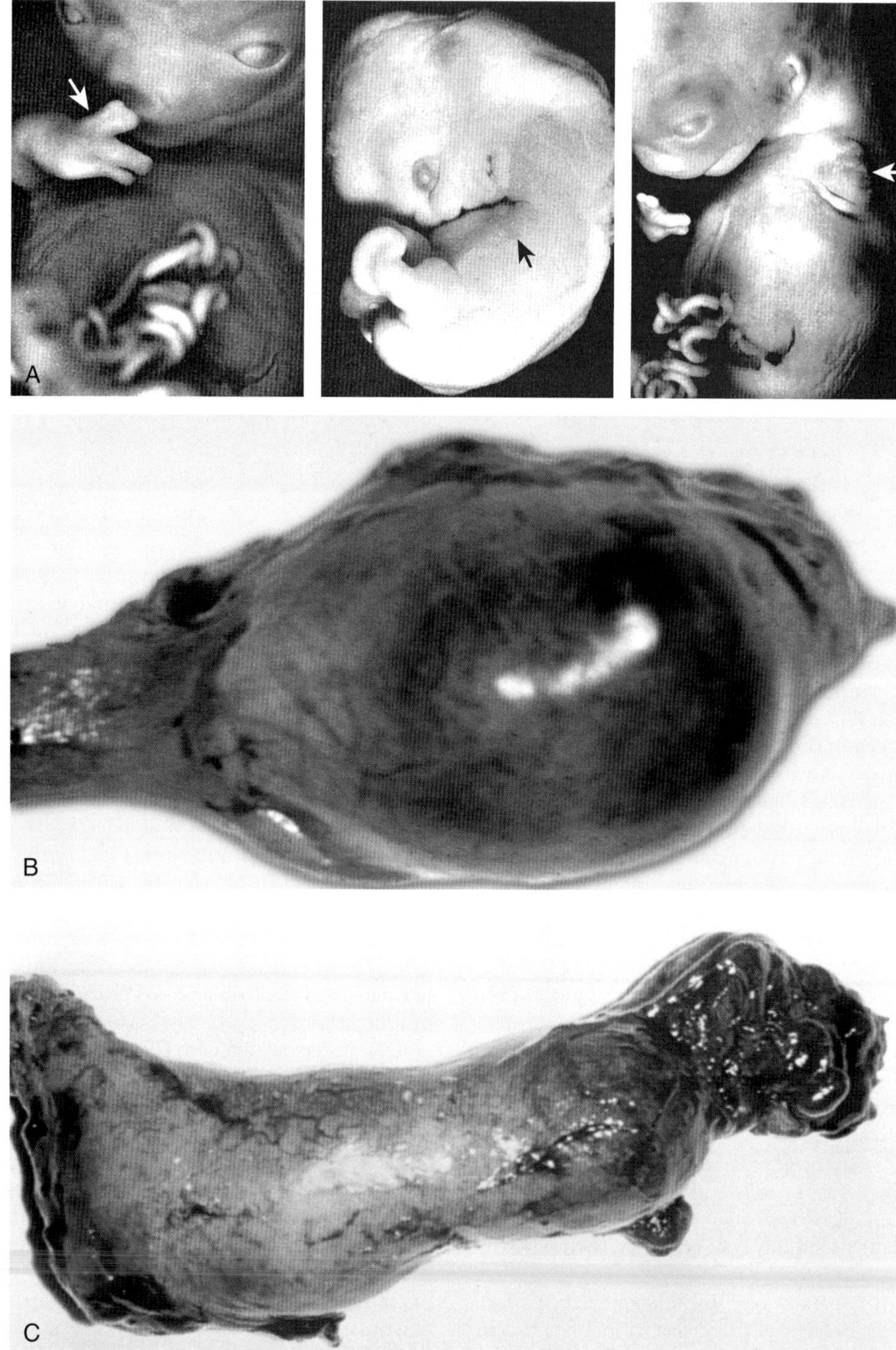

FIGURE 49.6 Embryos recovered from resected fallopian tubes showing amelia and syndactyly (A). Ectopic pregnancies occur most commonly in the fallopian tube (95.5% of all ectopic pregnancies). These examples of tubal pregnancies demonstrate fimbrial implantation (B) (11% of all ectopic pregnancies) and isthmus implantation (C) (12% of all ectopic pregnancies).

A metaanalysis of four studies of misoprostol involving 4899 cases of congenital anomalies and 5742 controls revealed increased risks for Möbius sequence (odds ratio: 25.31; 95% confidence interval: 11.11–57.66) and terminal transverse limb defects (odds ratio: 11.86; 95% confidence interval: 4.86–28.90).[49] Limb defects of all three types described in Table 49.2 have been noted in individuals who have been reared in constrictive environments, such as a fallopian tube, bicornuate uterus, or a uterus with large fibroids (see Chapter 45). Unilateral limb defects of the type shown in Fig. 49.7 are typical of those seen with early limb compression.

MANAGEMENT, PROGNOSIS, AND COUNSEL

Corrective surgery to improve limb function may be indicated, and in some cases of terminal transverse limb-reduction defects, the use of prostheses can be beneficial. In most cases, infants learn to use the limbs they are born with much more readily than those who experience traumatic amputations after birth. Prenatal diagnosis of lethal malformations such as limb-body wall defect and body stalk anomaly can be very helpful.

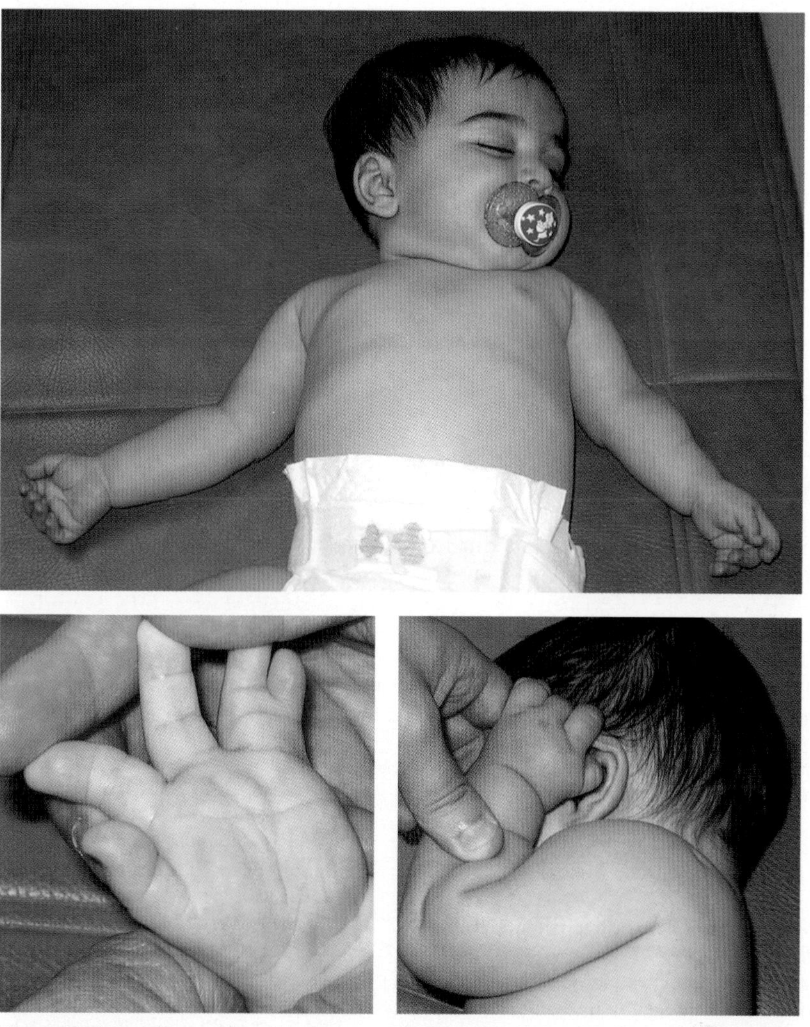

FIGURE 49.7 This infant with hypoplasia and compression-related dimpling of his left arm has hypoplasia with syndactyly of digits four and five of the left hand, which suggests early compression of the left arm and shoulder.

DIFFERENTIAL DIAGNOSIS

Occasionally, distal limb-reduction defects occur with scalp vertex aplasia because of the genetic disorder Adams-Oliver syndrome (see Fig. 39.7). Adams-Oliver syndrome is a genetically heterogeneous condition that typically includes a combination of congenital scalp defects and terminal transverse limb defects. Gain-of-function mutations in *ARHGAP31* and *RBPJ* cause autosomal dominant Adams-Oliver syndrome, which can vary from severe terminal transverse limb-reduction defects to mild or clinically unaffected carriers.[50,51] Other features can include acrania, constriction rings, encephaloceles, large scalp defects, aplasia cutis congenita, and bilateral cleft lip and palate. Adams-Oliver syndrome is genetically heterogeneous. Variants in *ARHGAP31* (<5%), *DLL4* (10%), *NOTCH1* (23%), and *RBPJ* (<10%) are inherited in an autosomal dominant manner, while variants in *DOCK6* (17%) and *EOGT* (<10%) are inherited in an autosomal recessive manner, with 40% to 50% of cases of unknown genetic etiology.[52] Death of one monozygotic co-twin can result in vascular disruption defect in the surviving co-twin.[53] It should be kept in mind that arthrogryposis has many other causes that are much more common than failed obstetric termination procedures. Such procedures are usually recorded in the medical records (unless they are performed illegally); thus with a careful history and pathologic examination of the products of conception, there should be little confusion as to the pathogenesis of such defects. Terminal transverse hemimelia has been associated with familial defects in anticoagulation,[54] and this can be investigated in the affected child and the mother by performing a thrombophilia evaluation. If defects are found, further treatment during subsequent pregnancies may be merited.

References

1. Poswillo D. Observations of fetal posture and causal mechanisms of congenital deformity of the palate, mandible and limbs. *J Dent Res*. 1966;45:584–596.
2. McGuirk CK, Westgate MN, Holmes LB. Limb deficiencies in newborn infants. *Pediatrics*. 2001;108:e64.
3. Kennedy LA, Persaud TVN. Pathogenesis of developmental defects induced in the rat by amniotic sac puncture. *Acta Anat*. 1977;97:23–35.
4. Webster WS, Lipson AH, Brown-Woodman PDC. Uterine trauma and limb defects. *Teratology*. 1987;35:253–260.
5. Webster WS, Abela D. The effect of hypoxia in development. *Birth Defects Res C Embryo Today*. 2007;81:215–228.
6. Adam AP, Payton KSE, Sanchez-Lara PA, Adam MP, Mirzaa GM. Hypoxia: a teratogen underlying a range of congenital disruptions, dysplasias, and malformations. *Am J Med Genet A*. 2021;185(9):2801–2808.
7. Pagon RA, Stephens TD, McGillivray BC, et al. Body wall defects with reduction limb anomalies: report of fifteen cases. *BDOAS*. 1979;15(5A):171–185.
8. Graham Jr JM, Miller ME, Stephan MJ, et al. Limb reduction anomalies and early in-utero limb compression. *J Pediatr*. 1980;96:1052–1056.
9. Graham JM. Jr: Causes of limb reduction defects: the contribution of fetal constraint and/or vascular disruption. *Clin Perinatol*. 1986;13:575–591.
10. Van Allen MI, Curry C, Gallagher L. Limb body wall complex: I. Pathogenesis. *Am J Med Genet*. 1987;28:529–548.
11. Van Allen MI, Curry C, Walden CE, et al. Limb body wall complex: II. Limb and spine defects. *Am J Med Genet*. 1987;28:549–565.
12. Martinez-Frias ML. Clinical and epidemiological characteristics of infants with body wall complex with and without limb deficiency. *Am J Med Genet*. 1997;73:170–175.
13. Hunter AG, Seaver LH, Stevenson RE. Limb-body wall defect: is there a defensible hypothesis and can it explain all the associated anomalies? *Am J Med Genet A*. 2011;155A:2045–2059.
14. Stevenson RE. Common pathogenesis for sirenomelia, OEIS complex, limb-body wall defect, and other malformations of caudal structures. *Am J Med Genet A*. 2021;185(5):1379–1387.
15. Stevens SJC, Stumpel CTRM, Diderich KEM, et al. The broader phenotypic spectrum of congenital caudal abnormalities associated with mutations in the caudal type homeobox 2 gene. *Clin Genet*. 2022;101(2):183–189.
16. Adam AP, Curry CJ, Hall JG, Keppler-Noreuil KM, Adam MP, Dobyns WB. Recurrent constellations of embryonic malformations re-conceptualized as an overlapping group of disorders with shared pathogenesis. *Am J Med Genet A*. 2020;182(11):2646–2661.
17. Jamsheer A, Materna-Kiryluk A, Badura-Stronka M, et al. Comparative study of clinical characteristics of amniotic rupture sequence with and without body wall defect: further evidence for separation. *Birth Defects Res A Clin Mol Teratol*. 2009;85:211–215.
18. Guzmán-Huerta ME, Muro-Barragán SA, Acevedo-Gallegos S, et al. Amniotic band sequence: prenatal diagnosis, phenotype descriptions, and a proposal of a new classification based on morphologic findings. *Rev Invest Clin*. 2013;65:300–306.
19. Gazolla AC, da Cunha AC, Telles JA, et al. Limb-body wall defect: experience of a reference service of fetal medicine from Southern Brazil. *Birth Defects Res A Clin Mol Teratol*. 2014;100(10):739–749.
20. Aguirre-Pascual E, Epelman M, Johnson AM, et al. Prenatal MRI evaluation of limb-body wall complex. *Pediatr Radiol*. 2014;44(11):1412–1420.
21. Tavares MV, Domingues AP, Tavares M, et al. Monoamniotic twins discordant for body stalk anomaly. *J Matern Fetal Neonatal Med*. 2015;28(1):113–115.
22. Higuchi T, Sato H, Iida M, et al. Early second-trimester diagnosis of body stalk anomaly by fetal magnetic resonance imaging. *Jpn J Radiol*. 2013;31:289–292.

23. Bugge M. Body stalk anomaly in Denmark during 20 years (1970–1989). *Am J Med Genet A*. 2012;158A:1702–1708.
24. Burton BK, Schulz CJ, Burd LI. Limb anomalies associated with chorionic villus sampling. *Lancet*. 1992;79:726–730.
25. Los FJ, Brandenburg H, Niermeijer MF. Vascular disruptive syndromes after exposure to misoprostol or chorionic villus sampling. *Lancet*. 1999;353:843–844.
26. Brumback BA, Holmes LB, Ryan LM. Adverse effects of chorionic villus sampling: a meta-analysis. *Stat Med*. 1999;18:2163–2175.
27. Golden CM, Ryan LM, Holmes LB. Chorionic villus sampling: a distinctive teratogenic effect on fingers? *Birth Defects Res (Part A)*. 2003;67:557–562.
28. Gonzalez CH, Vargas FR, Perez ABA, et al. Limb deficiency with or without Mobius sequence in seven Brazilian children associated with misoprostol use in the first trimester of pregnancy. *Am J Med Genet*. 1993;47:59–64.
29. Pastuszak AL, Schuler L, Speck-Martins CE, et al. Use of misoprostol during pregnancy and Mobius syndrome in infants. *N Engl J Med*. 1998;338:1881–1885.
30. Oriolli IM, Castilla EE. Epidemiological assessment of misoprostol teratogenicity. *Br J Obstet Gynaecol*. 2000;107:519–523.
31. Vargus FR, Schuler-Faccini L, Brunoni D, et al. Prenatal exposure to misoprostol and vascular disruption defects: a case-control study. *Am J Med Genet*. 2000;95:302–306.
32. Reid CO, Hall JG, Anderson C, et al. Association of amyoplasia with gastroschisis, bowel atresia and defects of the muscular layer of the trunk. *Am J Med Genet*. 1986;78:451–457.
33. Lipson AH, Webster WS, Brown-Woodman PD, et al. Moebius syndrome: animal model, human correlations, and evidence for a brainstem vascular etiology. *Teratology*. 1989;40:339–350.
34. Holmes LB. Possible fetal effects of cervical dilatation and uterine curettage during the first trimester of pregnancy. *J Pediatr*. 1995;126:131–134.
35. Hall JG, Arthrogryposis AMC. associated with unsuccessful attempts at termination of pregnancy. *Am J Med Genet*. 1996;63:293–300.
36. Meyer H, Cummins H. Severe maternal trauma in early pregnancy: congenital amputations in infant at term. *Am J Obstet Gynecol*. 1941;40:150–160.
37. Steigner M, Stewart RE, Setoguchi Y. Combined limb deficiencies and cranial nerve dysfunction: report of 6 cases. *BDOAS*. 1975;11:133–141.
38. Ossipoff V, Hall BD. Etiologic factors in the amniotic band syndrome in a study of 24 patients. *BDOAS*. 1977;13:117–132.
39. Traboulsi EI, Maumene IH. Extraocular muscle aplasia in Moebius syndrome. *J Pediatr Ophthalmol*. 1986;23:120–122.
40. Viljoen DL. Porencephaly and terminal transverse limb defects following severe maternal trauma in early pregnancy. *Clin Dysmorphol*. 1995;4:75–78.
41. Martinez-Frias ML, Garcia-Mazario MJ, Feito-Caldas C, et al. High maternal fever during gestation and severe limb disruptions. *Am J Med Genet*. 2001;98:201–203.
42. Matsunaga E, Shiota K. Ectopic pregnancy and myoma uteri: teratogenic effects and maternal characteristics. *Teratology*. 1980;21:61–69.
43. Bouyer J, Coste J, Fernandez H, et al. Sites of ectopic pregnancy: a 10-year population-based study of 1800 cases. *Hum Reprod*. 2002;17:3224–3230.
44. Pisarska MD, Carson S. Incidence and risk factors for ectopic pregnancy. *Clin Obstet Gynecol*. 1999;42:2–8.
45. Li C, Meng CX, Zhao WH, et al. Risk factors for ectopic pregnancy in women with planned pregnancy: a case-control study. *Eur J Obstet Gynecol Reprod Biol*. 2014;181:176–182.
46. Firth HV, Boyd PA, Chamberlain P, et al. Severe limb abnormalities after chorionic villus sampling at 56-66 days' gestation. *Lancet*. 1991;337:762–763.
47. Mahoney MJ. Limb abnormalities and chorionic villus sampling. *Lancet*. 1991;337:1422–1423.
48. Stoler JM, McGuirk CK, Lieberman E, et al. Malformations reported in chorionic villus sampling exposed children: a review and analytic synthesis of the literature. *Genet Med*. 1999;1:315–322.
49. da Silva DAL, Pizzol T, Knop FP, et al. Prenatal exposure to misoprostol and congenital anomalies: systematic review and meta-analysis. *Reprod Toxicol*. 2006;22:666–671.
50. Isrie M, Wuyts W, Van Esch H, et al. Isolated terminal limb reduction defects: extending the clinical spectrum of Adams-Oliver syndrome and *ARHGAP31* mutations. *Am J Med Genet A*. 2014;164A:1576–1579.
51. Southgate L, Machado RD, Snape KM, et al. Gain-of-function mutations of *ARHGAP31*, a Cdc42/Rac1 GTPase regulator, cause syndromic cutis aplasia and limb anomalies. *Am J Hum Genet*. 2011;88:574–585.
52. Lehman A., Wuyts W., Patel M.S. 2016 Adams-Oliver Syndrome. In: Adam MP, Mirzaa GM, Pagon RA, et al., eds. GeneReviews [Internet]. Seattle (WA): University of Washington, Seattle; 1993–2023.
53. Zankl A, Brooks D, Boltshauser E, et al. Natural history of twin disruption sequence. *Am J Med Genet*. 2004;127:133–138.
54. Hunter AG. A pilot study of the possible role of familial defects in anticoagulation as a cause for terminal limb reduction malformations. *Clin Genet*. 2000;57:197–204.

CHAPTER 50

First-Trimester Vascular Disruption

KEY POINTS

- The underlying mechanism for most defects related to problems associated with failed first-trimester obstetric procedures is vascular disruption.
- With chorionic villus sampling, removal of villi may result in embryonic hypotension, hypoxia, endothelial damage, hemorrhage, and necrosis with tissue loss involving distal structures in the upper body (hands and tongue), with middle digital rays more affected than medial or lateral rays.
- Failed dilatation and uterine curettage in early pregnancy has also been associated with fetal oromandibular limb hypogenesis syndrome, which is consistent with the role of hypoxic trauma in inducing fetal structural defects in early pregnancy.
- Maternal hyperthermia during the late first trimester, resulting in fever greater than 39°C for more than 2 days, can cause severe congenital limb disruption with hypoglossia, hypodactylia, terminal transverse hemimelia, and Möbius sequence.
- Infants who survive attempted termination of pregnancy (both surgical and medical) are at increased risk to be born with arthrogryposis and intellectual disability as well as terminal transverse hemimelia and Möbius sequence.

GENESIS

The underlying mechanism for most defects related to problems associated with failed obstetric procedures is vascular disruption. With chorionic villus sampling (CVS), removal of villi may result in embryonic hypotension, hypoxia, endothelial damage, hemorrhage, and necrosis with tissue loss.[1] Defects are more likely to involve distal structures in the upper body (hands and tongue) than proximal structures or the lower body, with middle digital rays more affected than medial or lateral rays (Fig. 50.1).[1-4] Absence of the distal portion of the third finger, with tapering and stiff joints, appears to be a distinctive effect of exposure to CVS.[2]

Following blunt trauma to the placenta, Quintaro et al.[5] noted numerous ecchymoses that might be related to the increased frequency of hemangiomas in CVS-exposed infants.

Limb defects caused by vascular disruption have a birth prevalence of 0.22 per 1000, accounting for 34% of all limb-reduction defects (which occur with a prevalence rate of 0.69 per 1000).[6] The frequency of terminal transverse limb-reduction defects is significantly higher after CVS than in nonexposed pregnancies, with earlier procedures resulting in more severe types of defects and a higher frequency of procedure-related defects.[7] The estimated risk for terminal transverse defects after early CVS is estimated to be between 1:1000 and 1:3000.[8] Therefore it is recommended that CVS only be performed after 10 weeks of gestation. Most experienced operators try to insert the CVS catheter into the chorion frondosum because if the catheter enters the decidua, it can cause hemorrhages. Loss rates after CVS increase with the number of insertions, and inexperienced operators usually require more insertions to obtain adequate samples.

The embryo is normally in a state of partial hypoxia, and because of this state of partial hypoxia, disturbances in the embryo's oxygen supply can more easily lead to a damaging degree of hypoxia. In an experimental setting, mammalian embryos show a surprising degree of resilience to hypoxia, with many organogenic-stage embryos able to survive 30 to 60 minutes of anoxia, but in some embryos this degree of hypoxia causes abnormal development, particularly transverse limb reduction defects.[9] These abnormalities are preceded by hemorrhage, edema, and tissue necrosis. Other parts of the embryo are also susceptible to such

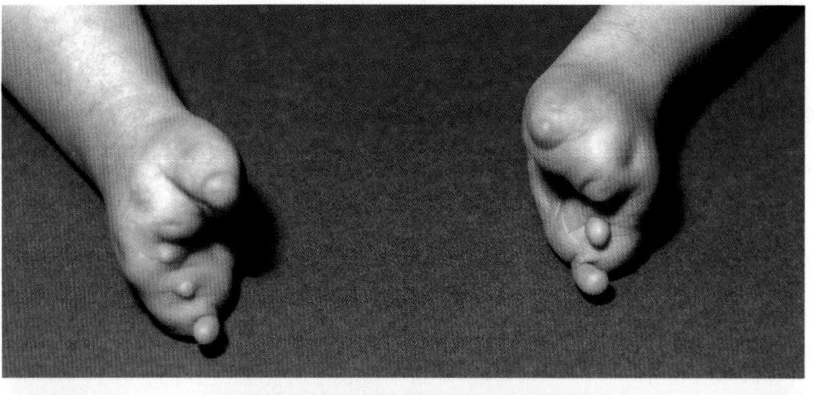

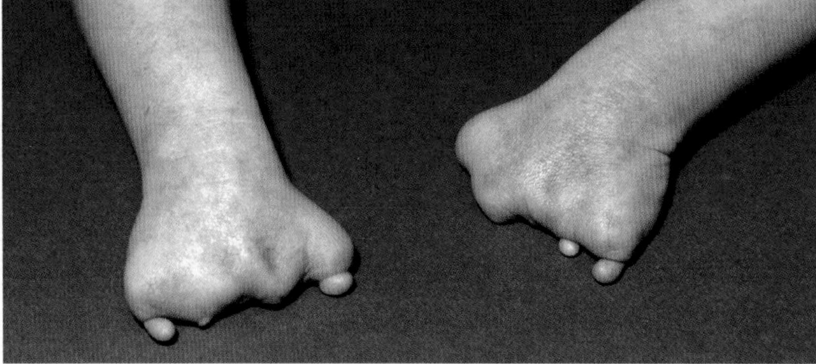

FIGURE 50.1 Disruptive loss of fingers in the hand (affecting central digits more severely). The mother of this fetus underwent chorionic villus sampling at 7–8 weeks and, in addition to these digital-reduction defects, there was a flank hemangioma.

hypoxia-induced damage, and these include the genital tubercle, the developing nose, the tail, and the central nervous system. Animal models of hypoxia during early stages of organ development result in patterns of limb defects with more severe destruction of the feet compared with the hands and hypoplasia of digits two through four, particularly the third digit. In human fetuses with hypoxia due to homozygous alpha thalassemia, this same pattern of distal limb deficiency has been identified.[10] Animal studies indicate that hypoxic episodes in the first trimester of human pregnancy could occur by temporary constriction of the uterine arteries.[9] This also could be a consequence of exposure to cocaine, misoprostol, or severe shock resulting from failed attempts at pregnancy termination.

Similar exposures have resulted in hypoxia-related malformations in the human, and fetal limb-reduction defects have been reported after early hypoxic injury, such as CVS before 66 days' gestation. Failed dilatation and uterine curettage in early pregnancy has been associated with fetal oromandibular limb hypogenesis syndrome,[11] which is consistent with this hypothesis concerning the role of hypoxic trauma in inducing fetal structural defects in early pregnancy.

Case reports of infants born after failed attempts at dilatation and curettage describe vascular disruption defects such as limb-reduction defects and amniotic band–related defects affecting the limbs, facial clefts, and cranium.[12,13] Failed termination of pregnancy is a relatively rare occurrence, with estimates ranging from 0.02% to 0.07% when termination is undertaken by dilation and curettage or dilation and extraction.[14] Among 2500 unselected patients with arthrogryposis, there were 11 cases of failed termination of pregnancy in which the individuals were subsequently born with arthrogryposis.[14] Infants who survive attempted termination of pregnancy (both surgical and medical) are at increased risk to be born with multiple congenital contractures. Among infants who survived attempted termination of pregnancy and had arthrogryposis, more than half also had intellectual disability. Maternal cocaine use during pregnancy has been associated with congenital contractures, suggesting that vascular compromise may play a role in this type of limb anomaly, and maternal trauma also leads to vascular compromise of the fetus and arthrogryposis.[14] A woman who conceived with an intrauterine device in place had the device removed at 7 weeks' gestation, and her sonogram at 25 weeks' gestation revealed transverse limb reduction of the right forearm.[15] A dichorionic-diamniotic twin was born with hydrocephalus, clubfeet, and hypoplastic toes following myomectomy at 12 weeks' gestation for a 10-cm posterior retroplacental subserous uterine myoma.[16] Severe abdominal trauma at 52 days postconception, caused by blunt trauma to the abdomen, resulted in terminal transverse limb-reduction defects and porencephaly.[17]

Maternal hyperthermia during the late first trimester, resulting in fever greater than 39 °C (102.2 °F) for more than 2 days, can cause severe congenital limb disruption with hypoglossia, terminal transverse hemimelia, and Möbius sequence (Fig. 50.2).[18–23] In a meta-analysis of 22 studies, maternal influenza exposure was defined as any reported influenza, influenza-like illness, or fever with influenza, with or without serologic or clinical confirmation during the first trimester of pregnancy. First-trimester maternal influenza exposure was associated with an increased risk for neural tube defects (odds ratio [OR]: 3.33; 95% confidence interval [CI]: 2.05–5.40), hydrocephaly (OR: 5.74; 95% CI: 1.10–30.00), congenital heart defects (OR: 1.56; 95% CI: 1.13–2.14), aortic valve atresia or stenosis (OR: 2.59; 95% CI: 1.21–5.54), ventricular septal defect (OR: 1.59; 95% CI: 1.24–2.14), cleft lip (OR: 3.12; 95% CI: 2.20–4.42), digestive system abnormalities (OR: 1.72; 95% CI: 1.09–2.68), and limb-reduction

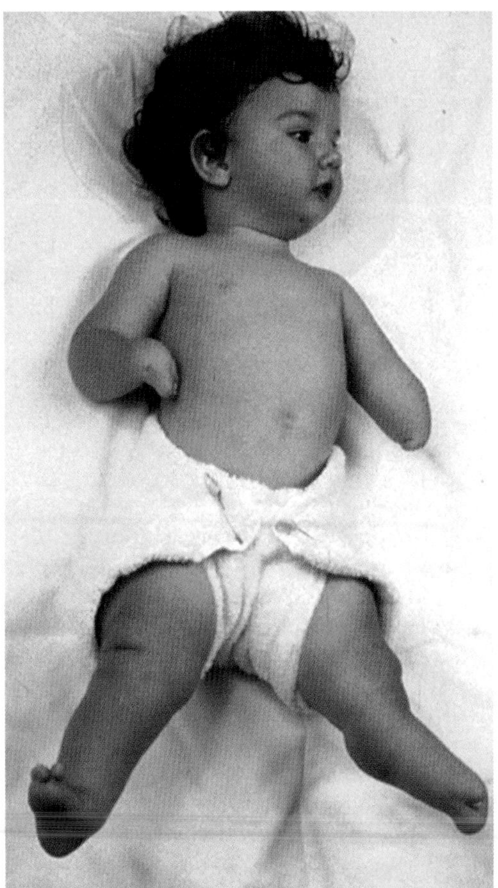

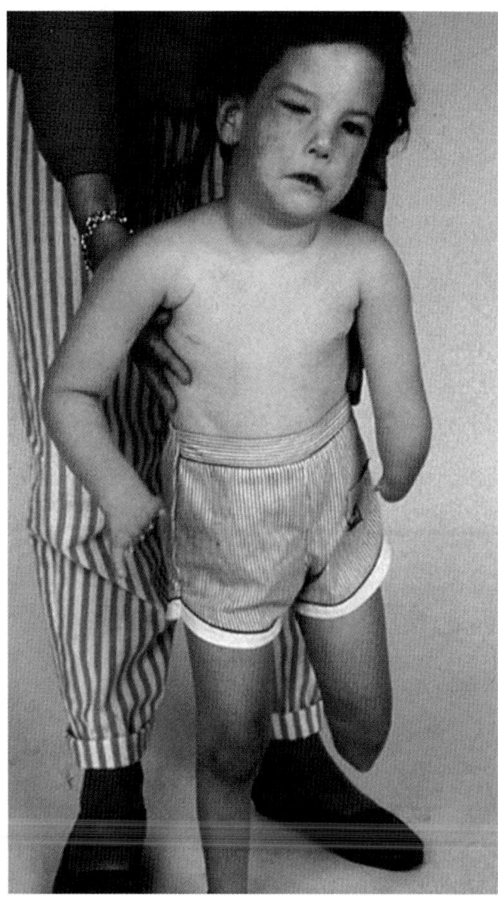

FIGURE 50.2 These children were born following prolonged high fever at 7 weeks' gestation with terminal transverse limb-reduction defects, ankyloglossia, missing teeth, and bilateral sixth and seventh cranial nerve palsies. This same pattern of defects has been induced experimentally in animals following exposure to heat at an equivalent stage of gestation. (Courtesy Tony Lipson, Camperdown Children's Hospital, Sydney, Australia.)

defects (OR: 2.03; 95% CI: 1.27–3.27).[22] Associations between maternal reports of periconceptional fever and transverse limb deficiency and intercalary limb deficiency were confirmed in a subsequent large study, which found no association with longitudinal limb deficiency, which is more likely to have a genetic basis.[23] This study also noted associations between maternal fever and intestinal atresia, as well as spina bifida. When there is a history of significant first-trimester hyperthermia in an infant with a transverse limb-reduction defect with or without other defects, the possibility of a febrile illness causing these defects should be considered.

When administered inappropriately, first-trimester misoprostol and/or methotrexate for induction of abortion can result in damage to a continuing pregnancy. In 1998, it became apparent that misoprostol, a synthetic prostaglandin E1 analog used in the prophylaxis and treatment of peptic ulcers, was being used to induce abortion in South and Central America where abortions are illegal. A study of 42 infants from São Paulo, Brazil, who were exposed to misoprostol during the first trimester revealed distinctive patterns of birth defects due to vascular disruption: 17 infants had equinovarus with cranial nerve defects and 10 had equinovarus as part of more extensive arthrogryposis. The most distinctive phenotypes were arthrogryposis confined to the legs (five cases) and terminal transverse limb defects (nine cases) with or without Möbius syndrome.[24] In a study of 265 women exposed to misoprostol during the first trimester and followed through delivery, the main indication for misoprostol was voluntary abortion (60.9%). Ten major malformations (5.5%; 95% CI: 2.65–9.82%) were reported, and five of them were consistent with the pattern of malformations attributed to misoprostol: Möbius sequence, hydrocephalus, terminal transverse limb reduction associated with a clubfoot, syndactyly, and posterior encephalocele.[25] A prospective study of first-trimester misoprostol exposure after medical prescriptions found the malformation rate was higher among 236 exposed pregnancies (4%) than in 255 controls (1.8%). Three malformations in the exposed group were consistent with the misoprostol-specific spectrum (2%).[26] In a systematic review and metaanalysis of 4899 cases of congenital anomalies and 5742 controls, prenatal exposure to misoprostol was associated with an increased risk of Möbius sequence and terminal transverse limb defects.[27]

Methotrexate is a folate antagonist that is used to treat malignancies and rheumatoid or inflammatory autoimmune diseases. It is also used for the nonsurgical treatment of ectopic pregnancies and the elective termination of pregnancy, and it is teratogenic when used in high doses for cancer or termination of tubal pregnancy. A prospective study of women exposed to low-dose methotrexate for rheumatologic conditions revealed one case of typical methotrexate embryopathy (Fig. 50.3) among the eight exposed pregnancies.[28] Among 188 postconception methotrexate-exposed pregnancies at dosages typically used in the treatment of rheumatic diseases, there was an increased risk of spontaneous abortion (42.5%) and major birth defects (6.6%) when compared to a cohort of disease-matched controls and to women without autoimmune disease.[29] Occasionally, methotrexate and misoprostol are used together to terminate a pregnancy. Data from eight patients who were exposed to both medications in the first trimester indicated a significant teratogenic risk. Reported anomalies included growth deficiency, absence or hypoplasia of the frontal bones, craniosynostosis, large fontanelle, ocular hypertelorism, short palpebral fissures, wide nasal bridge, malformed and low-set ears, micrognathia, syndactyly, short forearms, missing ribs, dislocated hips, and talipes equinovarus.[30]

FEATURES

Defects in CVS-exposed pregnancies include terminal transverse limb-reduction defects (with or without nubbins), amniotic band-like anomalies of the hands (digital fusion, syndactyly, constriction rings, loss of distal digits, and tapered fingers with stiff joints; digits two to four are especially affected; see Fig. 50.1), hypoglossia, cranial nerve dysfunction, hemangiomas, intestinal atresia, clubfoot, and gastroschisis.[31–34]

Maternal fever resulting in significant hyperthermia during the first trimester can cause malformations such as spina bifida and heart defects, as well vascular disruptions such as transverse limb-reduction defects and intestinal atresia. Hypoglossia with transverse limb-reduction defects (see Fig. 50.2) is not genetic and should lead to consideration of various causes for vascular disruption. The use of misoprostol and/or methotrexate during the first trimester can result in vascular disruptive defects such as terminal transverse limb-reduction defects, arthrogryposis, equinovarus, and Möbius sequence, which results from vascular disruption involving the territory of the subclavian artery occurring in a critical period of embryonic life between 6 and 8 weeks postconception.[35]

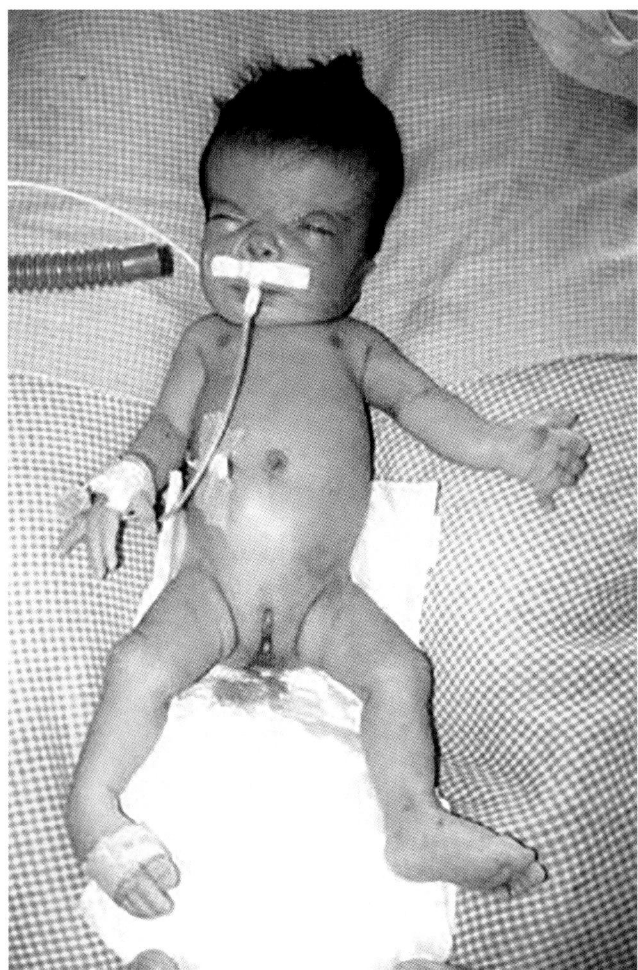

FIGURE 50.3 This newborn was born with methotrexate embryopathy after exposure to low-dose weekly methotrexate (7.5 mg) during the first trimester of pregnancy. They were born with intrauterine growth restriction at 31 weeks with microcephaly, wide anterior fontanel, high forehead, low nasal bridge, ocular proptosis, dysplastic low-set ears, high arched palate, short neck, narrow chest, abnormal fifth fingers, and right clubfoot. Brain ultrasound showed moderate dilatation of the lateral ventricles. Radiographs of the hands showed absence of the fifth metacarpal bone and phalanges bilaterally. (From Martín MC, Barbero P, Groisman B, Aguirre MÁ, Koren G. Methotrexate embryopathy after exposure to low weekly doses in early pregnancy. *Reprod Toxicol.* 2014;43:26–29.)

MANAGEMENT, PROGNOSIS, AND COUNSEL

Surgery to improve limb function may be indicated for some terminal transverse limb-reduction defects, and sometimes the use of prostheses can be beneficial. In most cases, infants learn to use their deficient limbs more readily than those who experience traumatic amputations after birth. Such sporadic limb-reduction defects caused by obstetric procedures have no significant recurrence risk, and in many instances they can be prevented or minimized by performing procedures at the proper time and under real-time ultrasound guidance.

DIFFERENTIAL DIAGNOSIS

Occasionally terminal transverse limb-reduction defects occur with aplasia cutis congenita of the scalp due to a genetic disorder, Adams-Oliver syndrome (Fig. 39.7), which is genetically heterogeneous. Variants in *ARHGAP31* (<5%), *DLL4* (10%), *NOTCH1* (23%), and *RBPJ* (<10%) are inherited in an autosomal dominant manner, while variants in *DOCK6* (17%) and *EOGT* (<10%) are inherited in an autosomal recessive manner, with 40% to 50% of cases of unknown genetic etiology.[36] A large four-generation family with isolated terminal limb defects segregating in an autosomal dominant fashion was found to have a truncating mutation in *ARHGAP31*. This finding underscores the relevance of sequencing *ARHGAP31* in similar recurrences of isolated terminal transverse limb defects, even if there are no other features of Adams-Oliver syndrome.[37,38] There is extensive variability in clinical features among mutation carriers, which can vary from severe terminal transverse limb-reduction defects to mild or clinically unaffected carriers. In other families with Adams-Oliver syndrome, other features can include acrania, constriction rings, encephaloceles, large scalp defects, aplasia cutis congenita, heart defects, and bilateral cleft lip and palate. Autosomal recessive mutations in *DOCK6* can also result in abnormal actin cytoskeleton organization and cause Adams-Oliver syndrome.[39]

References

1. Holmes LB. Teratogen-induced limb defects. *Am J Med Genet.* 2002;112:297–303.
2. Golden CM, Ryan LM, Holmes LB. Chorionic villus sampling: a distinctive teratogenic effect on fingers? *Birth Defects Res (Part A).* 2003;67:557–562.
3. Los FJ, Brandenburg H, Niermeijer MF. Vascular disruptive syndromes after exposure to misoprostol or chorionic villus sampling. *Lancet.* 1999;353:843–844.
4. Light TR, Ogden JA. Congenital constriction band syndrome: pathophysiology and treatment. *Yale J Biol Med.* 1993;66:143–155.
5. Quintaro RA, Romero R, Mahoney MJ, et al. Fetal hemorrhagic lesions after chorionic villus sampling. *Lancet.* 1992;339:193.
6. McGuirk CK, Westgate M-N, Holmes LB. Limb deficiencies in newborn infants. *Pediatrics.* 2001;108:e64–e76.
7. Brumback BA, Holmes LB, Ryan LM. Adverse effects of chorionic villus sampling: a meta-analysis. *Stat Med.* 1999;18:2163–2175.
8. Olney RS, Khoury MG, Alo CJ, et al. Increased risk for terminal transverse digital deficiency after chorionic villus sampling: results of the United States Multistate Case-Control Study, 1988–1992. *Teratology.* 1995;51:20–29.
9. Webster WS, Abela D. The effect of hypoxia in development. *Birth Defects Res C Embryo Today.* 2007;81: 215–228.
10. Adam AP, Payton KSE, Sanchez-Lara PA, Adam MP, Mirzaa GM. Hypoxia: a teratogen underlying a range of congenital disruptions, dysplasias, and malformations. *Am J Med Genet A.* 2021;185(9):2801–2808.
11. Allanson E, Dickinson JE, Charles AK, et al. Fetal oromandibular limb hypogenesis syndrome following uterine curettage in early pregnancy. *Birth Defects Res A Clin Mol Teratol.* 2011;91:226–229.
12. Holmes LB. Possible fetal effects of cervical dilatation and uterine curettage during the first trimester of pregnancy. *J Pediatr.* 1995;126:131–134.
13. Hall JG. Arthrogryposis (AMC) associated with unsuccessful attempts at termination of pregnancy. *Am J Med Genet.* 1996;63:293–300.
14. Hall JG. Arthrogryposis (multiple congenital contractures) associated with failed termination of pregnancy. *Am J Med Genet Part A.* 2012;158A:2214–2220.
15. Weissmann-Brenner A, Lerner A, Peleg D. Transverse limb reduction and intrauterine device: case report and review of the literature. *Eur J Contracept Reprod Health Care.* 2007;12:294–297.
16. Danzer E, Hotzgreve W, Batukan P, et al. Myomectomy during the first trimester associated with fetal limb anomalies and hydrocephalus in a twin pregnancy. *Prenat Diagn.* 2001;21:848–851.
17. Viljoen DL. Porencephaly and terminal transverse limb defects following severe maternal trauma in early pregnancy. *Clin Dysmorphol.* 1995;4:75–78.
18. Lipson AH, Webster WS, Woodman-Brown PDC, et al. Moebius syndrome animal model: human correlations and evidence for brainstem vascular etiology. *Teratology.* 1989;40:339–350.
19. Superneau DW, Wertelecki W. Brief clinical report: similarity of effects—experimental hyperthermia as a teratogen and maternal febrile illness associated with oromandibular and limb defects. *Am J Med Genet.* 1985;21:575–580.
20. Martinez-Frias ML, Garcia Mazario MJ, Feito Caldas C, et al. High maternal fever during gestation and severe congenital limb disruptions. *Am J Med Genet.* 2001;98: 201–203.
21. Graham JM Jr, Edwards MJ, Edwards MJ. Teratogen update: gestational effects of maternal hyperthermia due to febrile illnesses and resultant patterns of defects in humans. *Teratology.* 1998;58:209–221.
22. Luteijn JM, Brown MJ, Dolk H. Influenza and congenital anomalies: a systematic review and meta-analysis. *Hum Reprod.* 2014;29:809–823.
23. Mohan Dass NL, Botto LD, Tinker SC, et al. National Birth Defects Prevention Study. Associations between maternal reports of periconceptional fever from miscellaneous causes and structural birth defects. *Birth Defects Res.* 2022;114(15):885–894.
24. Gonzalez CH, Marques-Dias MJ, Kim CA, et al. Congenital abnormalities in Brazilian children associated with misoprostol misuse in first trimester of pregnancy. *Lancet.* 1998;351(9116):1624–1627.

25. Auffret M, Bernard-Phalippon N, Dekemp J, et al. Misoprostol exposure during the first trimester of pregnancy: is the malformation risk varying depending on the indication? *Eur J Obstet Gynecol Reprod Biol.* 2016;207:188–192.
26. Vauzelle C, Beghin D, Cournot MP, Elefant E. Birth defects after exposure to misoprostol in the first trimester of pregnancy: prospective follow-up study. *Reprod Toxicol.* 2013;36:98–103.
27. da Silva Dal Pizzol T, Knop FP, Mengue SS. Prenatal exposure to misoprostol and congenital anomalies: systematic review and meta-analysis. *Reprod Toxicol.* 2006;22(4):666–671.
28. Martín MC, Barbero P, Groisman B, Aguirre MÁ, Koren G. Methotrexate embryopathy after exposure to low weekly doses in early pregnancy. *Reprod Toxicol.* 2014;43:26–29.
29. Weber-Schoendorfer C, Chambers C, Wacker E, et al. Pregnancy outcome after methotrexate treatment for rheumatic disease prior to or during early pregnancy: a prospective multicenter cohort study. *Arthritis Rheumatol.* 2014;66(5):1101–1110.
30. Kozma C, Ramasethu J. Methotrexate and misoprostol teratogenicity: further expansion of the clinical manifestations. *Am J Med Genet Part A.* 2011;155:1723–1728.
31. Firth HV, Boyd PA, Chamberlain P, et al. Severe limb abnormalities after chorionic villus sampling at 56–66 days' gestation. *Lancet.* 1991;337:762–763.
32. Mahoney MJ. Limb abnormalities and chorionic villus sampling. *Lancet.* 1991;337:1422–1423.
33. Stoler JM, McGuirk CK, Lieberman E, et al. Malformations reported in chorionic villus sampling exposed children: a review and analytic synthesis of the literature. *Genet Med.* 1999;1:315–322.
34. Gruber B, Burton BK. Oromandibular-limb hypogenesis syndrome following chorionic villus sampling. *Int J Pediatr Otorhinolaryngol.* 1994;29:59–63.
35. Marques-Dias MJ, Gonzalez CH, Rosemberg S. Möbius sequence in children exposed in utero to misoprostol: neuropathological study of three cases. *Birth Defects Res A Clin Mol Teratol.* 2003;67(12):1002–1007.
36. Lehman A., Wuyts W., Patel M.S. 2016 Adams-Oliver Syndrome. In: Adam MP, Mirzaa GM, Pagon RA, Wallace SE, Bean LJH, Gripp KW, Amemiya A, editors. GeneReviews®[Internet]. Seattle (WA): University of Washington, Seattle; 1993–2023.
37. Isrie M, Wuyts W, Van Esch H, et al. Isolated terminal limb reduction defects: extending the clinical spectrum of Adams-Oliver syndrome and *ARHGAP31* mutations. *Am J Med Genet A.* 2014;164A:1576–1579.
38. Southgate L, Machado RD, Snape KM, et al. Gain-of-function mutations of *ARHGAP31*, a Cdc42/Rac1 GTPase regulator, cause syndromic cutis aplasia and limb anomalies. *Am J Hum Genet.* 2011;88:574–585.
39. Shaheen R, Faqeih E, Sunker A, et al. Recessive mutations in *DOCK6*, encoding the guanidine nucleotide exchange factor DOCK6, lead to abnormal actin cytoskeleton organization and Adams-Oliver syndrome. *Am J Hum Genet.* 2011;89:328–333.

CHAPTER 51

Fetal Disruption

KEY POINTS

- Fetal vascular disruption defects refer to structural defects that occur after a structure has formed normally, and they are usually limited to tissues within a defined area that are supplied by the affected blood vessels.
- Decreased blood flow to the affected area leads to hypoxia, endothelial cell damage, hemorrhage, tissue loss, and repair.
- Defects attributed to vascular defects included amniotic band defects, terminal transverse limb-reduction defects (most of which had associated digit-like nubbins), Poland anomaly, hydranencephaly, defects attributed to twin-twin transfusion, and jejunal atresia.
- Because of the normal vascular interchange between monozygous twins, vascular disruptions from a deceased co-twin with disseminated intravascular coagulation can cause embolization defects in the surviving twin, such as hydranencephaly.
- Selective reduction of one abnormal monozygotic twin can result in loss or disruption in the surviving twin.
- Fetal brainstem disconnection syndrome is a vascular disruption defect with characteristic postnatal brain imaging findings (disconnection between the upper pons and the medulla oblongata with cerebellar hypoplasia).
- Early amniocentesis (at 11 to 12 weeks instead of 15 to 16 weeks) has been implicated as one cause of clubfoot.
- Amniocentesis is the presumed cause of many types of penetrating fetal injuries, including skin puncture marks; ocular perforation; limb, chest, and abdominal trauma; cranial nerve injuries; porencephaly; and arteriovenous fistulae, with most of these injuries occurring in the era before ultrasound-guided amniocentesis.
- Congenital Zika virus infection can result in severe microcephaly with fetal brain disruption sequence, as well as joint contractures resembling amyoplasia arthrogryposis.

GENESIS

Fetal vascular disruption defects refer to structural defects that occur after a structure has formed normally, and they are usually limited to tissues within a defined area that are supplied by the affected blood vessels. Decreased blood flow to the affected area leads to hypoxia, endothelial cell damage, hemorrhage, tissue loss, and repair. In a Boston hospital-based study of 7020 infants born with structural defects among 289,365 consecutive births surveyed over 41 years (1972 to 2012), 105 infants had defects attributed to vascular defects. These included 40 infants with amniotic band defects, 31 infants with terminal transverse limb-reduction defects (most of which had associated digit-like nubbins), 15 infants with Poland anomaly, 7 infants with hydranencephaly, 7 infants with defects attributed to twin-twin transfusion, 2 infants with limb deficiencies associated with homozygous alpha-thalassemia (with altered hemoglobin leading to hypoperfusion), 2 infants exposed to chorionic villus sampling, and 1 infant with jejunal atresia.[1] Another study of the prevalence of defects attributed to vascular defects in Europe and the United Kingdom found similar prevalence in the United Kingdom and Europe for both transverse limb-reduction defects (2.16 vs. 2.14 per 10,000) and small intestinal atresia (0.85 vs. 0.86 per 10,000), as well as Poland anomaly and hydranencephaly (0.07–0.08 per 10,000).[2]

Hydranencephaly is a rare congenital condition that occurs in which cerebral structures are often limited to only the brainstem and thalamus, with cerebral spinal fluid filling a membranous sac that is normally inhabited by the cerebral cortex. Because of the normal vascular interchange between monozygous twins, vascular disruptions from a deceased co-twin with disseminated intravascular coagulation can cause embolization defects in the surviving twin. In one of six such twin pairs, all the surviving monozygous twins had central nervous system infarcts and three had multiple-organ infarcts, and fetal death in utero occurred 1 to 11 weeks before the live birth of the monozygous survivor.[3] In a larger study of brain imaging, zygosity, sex, and fetal demise in 56 proband twins and 7 less affected co-twins, brain disruptions were seen in 11 individuals with hydranencephaly, porencephaly, or white matter loss without cysts.[4] Recurrent associations with twin-twin transfusion syndrome, intrauterine growth retardation, and other prenatal factors support disruption of vascular perfusion as the most likely unifying cause. Hydranencephaly can also result from autosomal recessive mutations in *FLVCR2*, and rarely *LAMB1* or *CEP55*.[5–7]

In 2016, a marked increase in the number of cases with severe congenital microcephaly and other defects in Brazil led to the discovery of Zika virus encephalopathy.[8,9] Zika is an RNA virus that is related to other arborviruses such as dengue, yellow fever, Japanese encephalitis, and Nile viruses, and it is spread by the bite of *Aedes* species mosquitoes. Effects on infants born to prenatally infected mothers include structural birth defects and developmental problems. The risk of a structural birth defect among infants born to mothers with Zika virus infection during pregnancy range from 5% to 10%, with first-trimester risks higher than later exposures.[9] Among 6799 live-born infants in the US Zika Pregnancy and Infant Registry born during December 1, 2015 to March 31, 2018, 4.6% had any Zika-associated birth defect; in a subgroup of pregnancies with a positive nucleic acid amplification test for Zika virus infection, the percentage was 6.1% among live-born infants. The brain and eye defects most frequently reported included microcephaly, corpus callosum abnormalities, intracranial calcification, abnormal cortical gyral patterns, ventriculomegaly, cerebral or cortical atrophy, chorioretinal abnormalities, and optic nerve abnormalities.[10] A distinctive phenotype (the congenital Zika syndrome) was characterized with five features that were rarely seen with other congenital infections: (1) severe microcephaly with a partially collapsed skull; (2) thin cerebral cortices with subcortical calcifications; (3) macular scarring and focal pigmentary retinal mottling; (4) congenital contractures; and (5) marked early hypertonia with symptoms of extrapyramidal involvement.[11] Anomalies of shape of skull and redundancy of the scalp (fetal brain disruption sequence) were present in 70% of 83 infants with congenital Zika syndrome who were born in Brazil with congenital Zika syndrome from July 2015 to March 2016 (Figs. 51.1 and 51.2).[12] In addition, these infants with congenital Zika syndrome manifested features consistent with fetal immobility, ranging from dimples (30.1%), distal hand/finger contractures (20.5%), and feet malpositions (15.7%) to generalized arthrogryposis (9.6%). These defects all appear to be secondary to vascular disruption, and in addition to arthrogryposis, terminal transverse limb defects have been reported.[13]

Fetal brainstem disconnection syndrome is a severe, rare brain disorder resulting from a midbrain-hindbrain segmentation defect resulting in neurological defects (hypotonia, absent eye contact, clinical signs of thermoregulatory dysfunction, and paralysis of some cranial nerves), respiratory distress, early death, and characteristic postnatal brain imaging findings (disconnection between the upper pons and the medulla oblongata with cerebellar hypoplasia). In 70% of cases, the basilar artery was noted to be quite hypoplastic (Fig. 51.3).[14–17] A review of 14 cases suggested a vascular disruption defect in 9 cases based on imaging findings, with confirmation by autopsy in at least 2 cases.[14] In previously reported cases, nine patients died early during the first days or months of life, while three patients reached 1 year of life and two patients were still alive after that age with severe disability.[14]

Early amniocentesis (at 11 to 12 weeks instead of 15 to 16 weeks) has been associated with a 1% to 2% risk for talipes equinovarus.[18,19] Amniotic fluid leakage before 22 weeks was the only significant factor associated with clubfoot, there being a 15% risk with leakage but only a 1.1% risk without leakage (Fig. 51.4). None of the cases had persistent leakage at 18 to 20 weeks. In some circumstances early amniocentesis might result in a developmental arrest of the foot as it transitions from a normal equinus position at 9 weeks to a neutral position at 12 to 13 weeks. The lateral side of the distal tibia grows faster than the medial side, which may result in pressure necrosis of the lateral distal tibia at 11 to 12 weeks.[20]

Needle injuries from amniocentesis have been reported, primarily in the era before ultrasound-guided procedures (Figs. 51.5 and 51.6).[21–31] Most of these injuries result from direct trauma, vascular disruption, or amniotic band disruption. Midtrimester amniocentesis with concurrent ultrasound guidance appears to be associated with a procedure-related rate of excess pregnancy loss of 0.6% and reductions in the incidence of needle punctures and bloody amniotic fluid.[32]

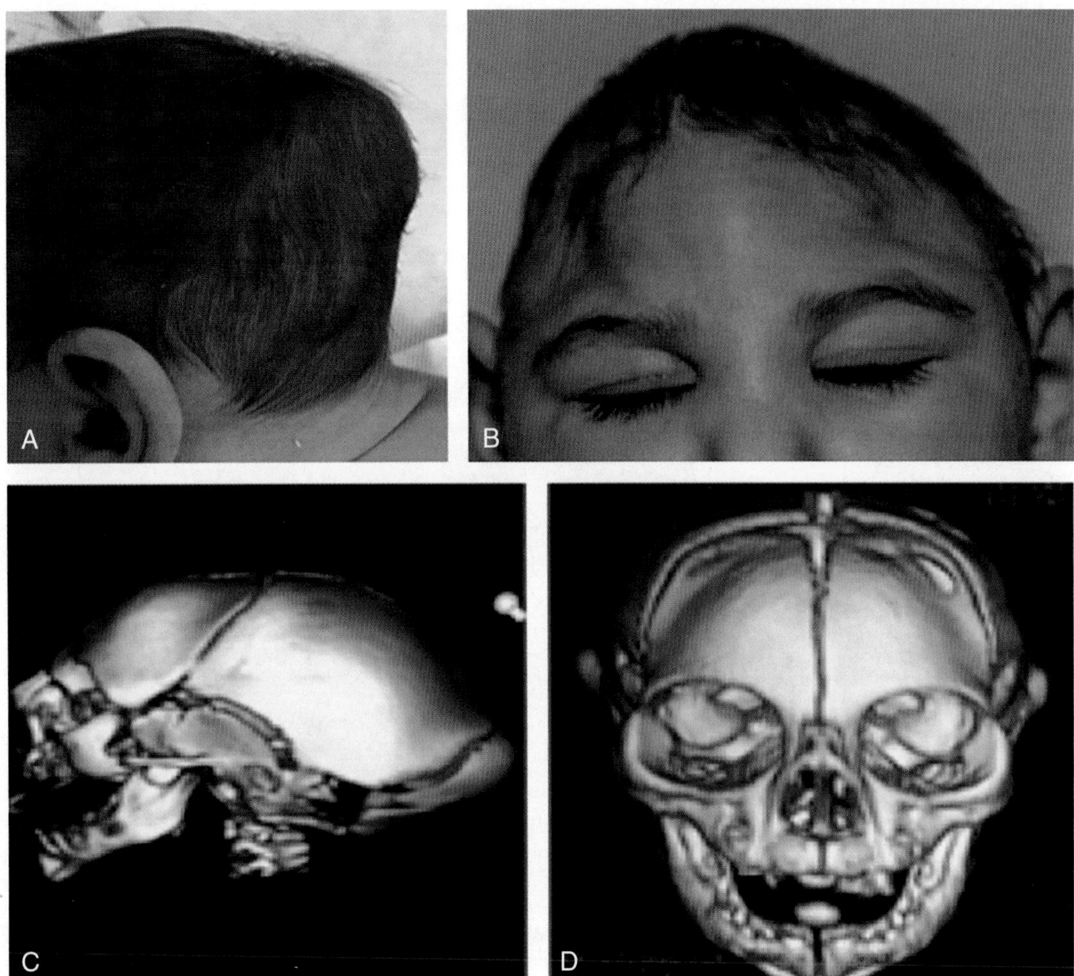

FIGURE 51.1 The occipital prominence is pronounced (**A**) with a very hypoplastic occipital bone on reconstructed computed tomography (CT) image (**C**). A frontal midline bulge is apparent due to significant depression of the lateral aspects on the frontal bone (**B**), which appear more depressed than the parietal bones along with obvious supratemporal depression on CT (**C** and **D**). The vertical dimension of the cranium is reduced and the parietal vault is narrow (**B** and **D**). (From Del Campo M, Feitosa IM, Ribeiro EM, et al.; Zika Embryopathy Task Force-Brazilian Society of Medical Genetics ZETF-SBGM. The phenotypic spectrum of congenital Zika syndrome. *Am J Med Genet A*. 2017;173(4):841–857.)

FEATURES

Early amniocentesis at 11 to 12 weeks has been associated with a 1% to 2% risk for talipes equinovarus (see Fig. 51.4)[18-20] Amniocentesis is the presumed cause of many types of penetrating fetal injuries, including skin puncture marks (see Fig. 51.5), ocular perforation, limb, chest, and abdominal trauma, cranial nerve injuries, porencephaly (see Fig. 51.6), and arteriovenous fistulae, with most of these injuries occurring in the era before ultrasound-guided amniocentesis.[32]

When attempted pregnancy termination fails, terminal transverse hemimelia suggests possible vascular disruption (Fig. 51.7). A terminal transverse limb defect with absence of the forearm and hand or just the hand is an uncommon limb defect in an otherwise healthy newborn. Among 194 newborns and fetuses with limb deficiency, 24 out of 28 affected infants also had tiny digit-like nubbins on the stump of the

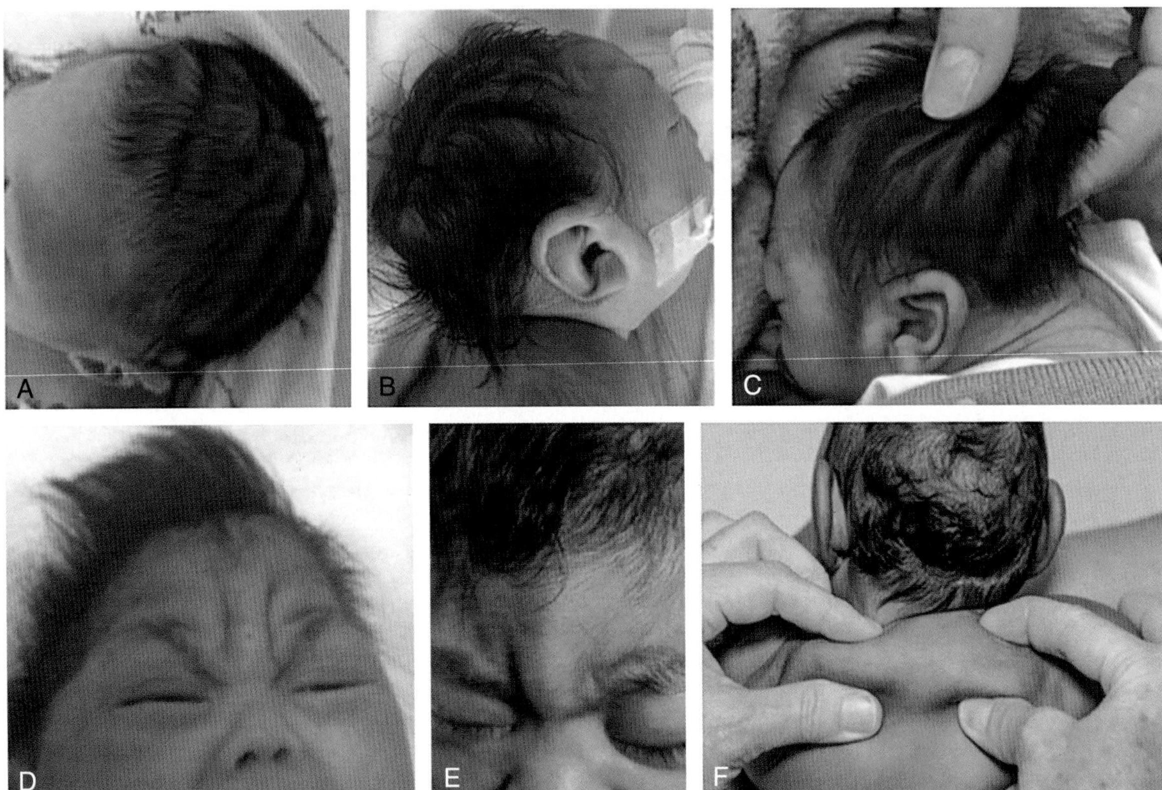

FIGURE 51.2 Redundant skin of the scalp creating transverse folds, that is, "cutis rugata" (**A**), or more cerebriform patterns, that is, "cutis gyrata" (**B**). In other cases, redundant skin is obvious only over the occipital region (**C**) or the glabellar region, where it can create several furrows (**D**) or a bulging single fold, with a crease above the nose, epicanthal folds and full periorbital tissues (**E**). **F** The excess skin can also be observed in the back, possibly secondary to prolonged fetal immobility and compression. (From Del Campo M, Feitosa IM, Ribeiro EM, et al.; Zika Embryopathy Task Force-Brazilian Society of Medical Genetics ZETF-SBGM. The phenotypic spectrum of congenital Zika syndrome. *Am J Med Genet A.* 2017;173(4):841–857.)

affected limb.[33] Another 17 infants had central digit hypoplasia consisting of hypoplasia of the thumb and fifth finger with nubbins of soft tissue in place of fingers 2, 3, and 4 at the level of the metacarpal–phalangeal joint, which should be distinguished from the terminal transverse limb defect that ends at the wrist and amniotic band defects. Another 14 infants had symbrachydactyly, with hypoplastic middle and distal phalanges of the fingers and toes.[34]

MANAGEMENT, PROGNOSIS, AND COUNSEL

Surgery to improve limb function may be indicated for some terminal transverse limb-reduction defects, and sometimes the use of prostheses can be beneficial. In most cases, infants learn to use their deficient limbs more readily than those who experience traumatic amputations after birth. Such sporadic limb-reduction defects caused by obstetric procedures have no significant recurrence risk, and in many instances they can be prevented or minimized by performing procedures at the proper time and under real-time ultrasound guidance.[32] A careful examination of the placenta is indicated to search for placental infarcts and clots, which might suggest that placental thrombosis contributed to terminal transverse limb-reduction defects (Fig. 51.8). In addition, underlying inherited thrombophilias may predispose toward vascular disruption in some terminal transverse limb-reduction defects. Because the risk of vascular disruption may be increased when certain common mutations within the coagulation pathway are present in the fetus and/or mother,

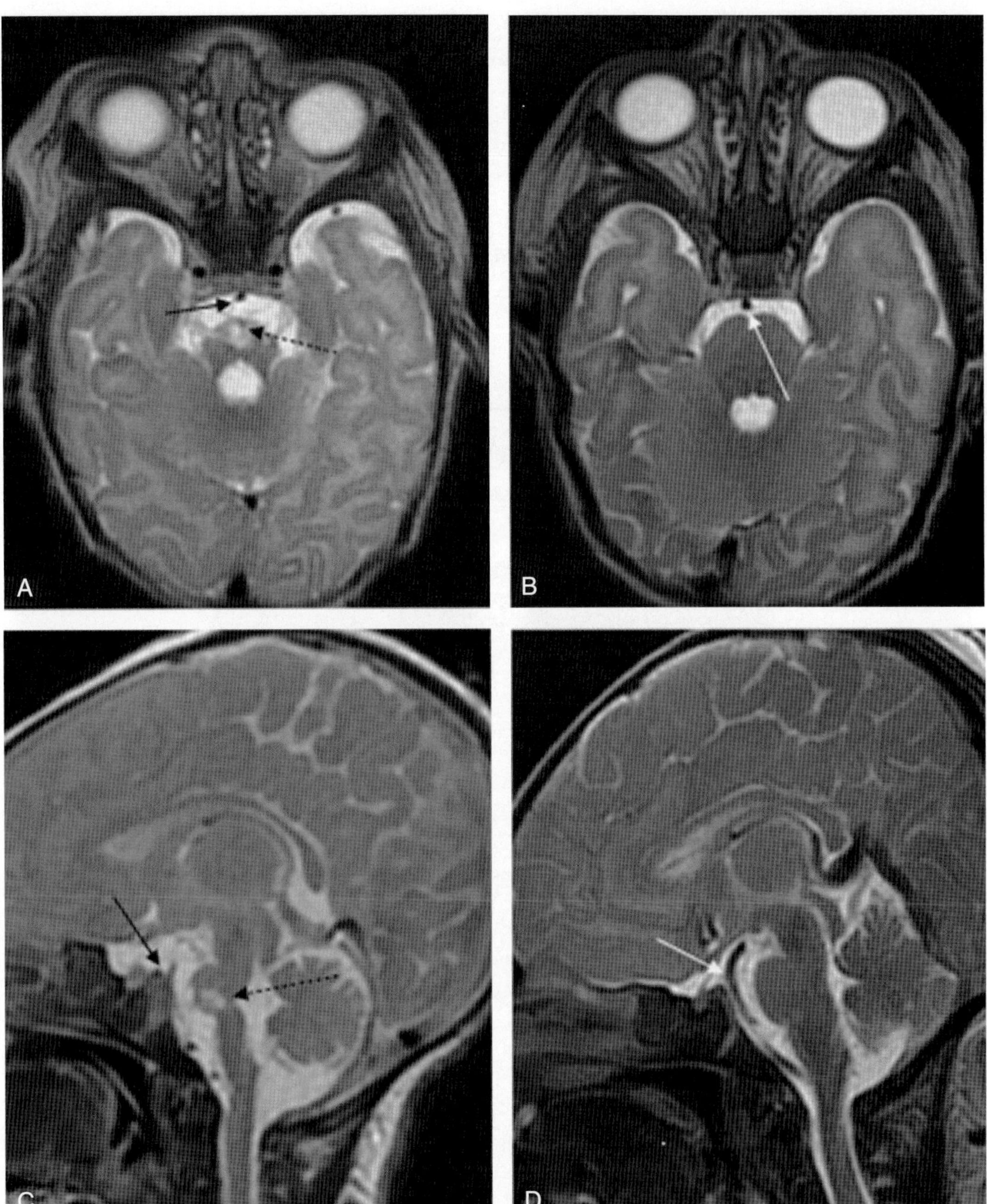

FIGURE. 51.3 Postnatal magnetic resonance image on day 1 of life. T2-weighted sequences (axial (**A**) and midsagittal (**C**)) reveal cerebellar and vermian hypoplasia associated with severe brainstem anomalies. A focal hyperintense signal in the pons *(dotted arrow)* is consistent with the presence of an ischemic/hemorrhagic lesion. On axial (**A**) and sagittal (**C**) T2-weighted sequences, the diameter of the basilar artery appears thin *(black arrow)* compared with age-matched controls (**B**) and (**D**; *white arrow*). (From Vekemans MA, Maurice P, Lachtar M, et al. Additional evidence for the vascular disruption defect hypothesis in a novel case of brainstem disconnection syndrome. *Birth Defects Res.* 2022;114(19):1298–1306.)

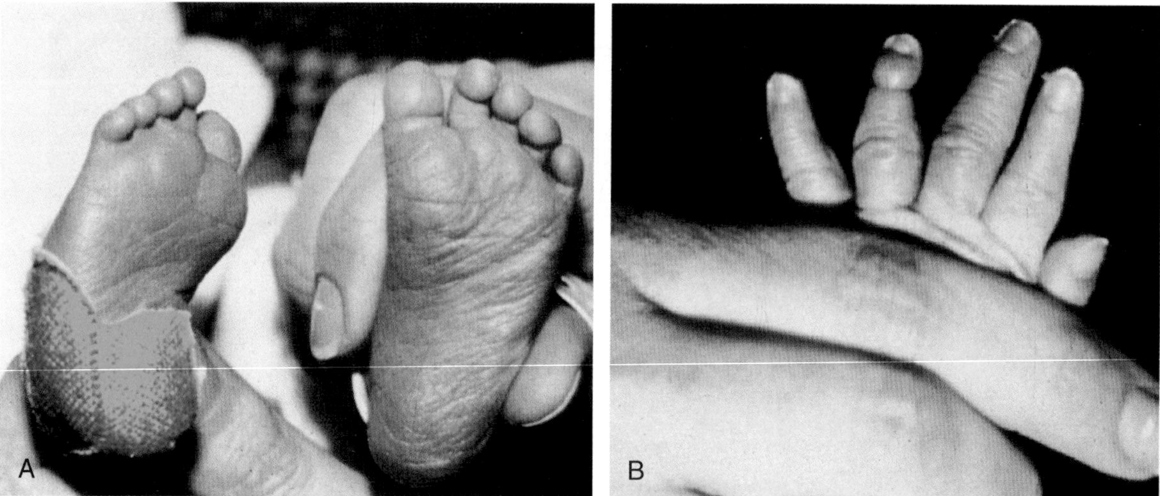

FIGURE 51.4 This rigid equinovarus foot deformity (**A**) was associated with an amniotic band around a finger (**B**) and a history of amniotic fluid leakage at 11 to 12 weeks.

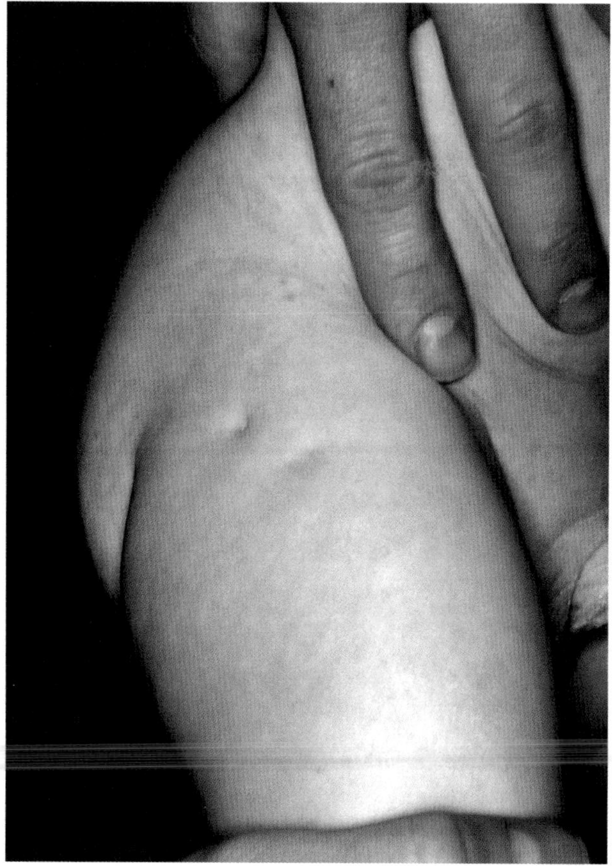

FIGURE 51.5 Amniocentesis puncture needle marks on an infant's thigh. The parent previously reported that the amniocentesis was carried out without ultrasound guidance and that the needle had to be repositioned several times before eventually drawing bloody amniotic fluid, which yielded a normal male karyotype.

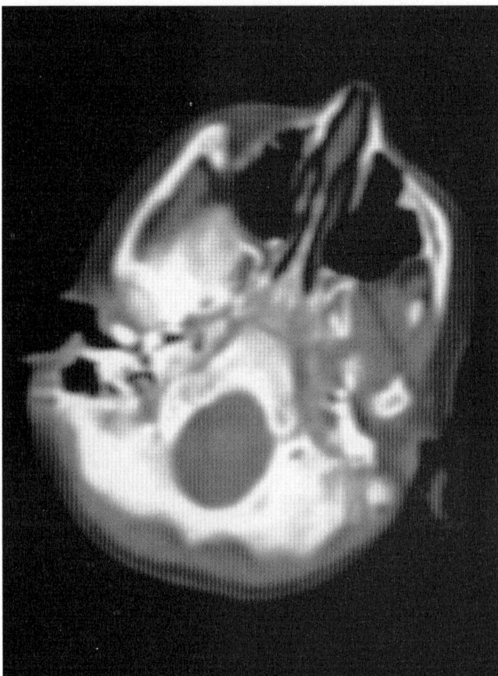

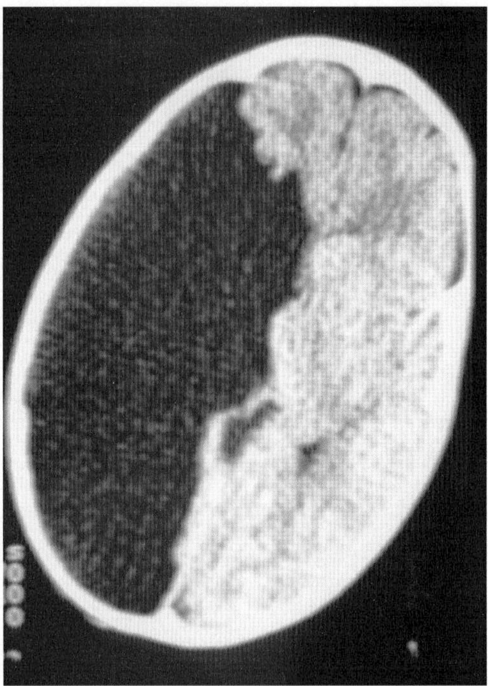

FIGURE 51.6 Amniocentesis-induced porencephaly following amniocentesis done on monozygotic twins during the 16th week without ultrasound guidance. This twin was the first to be tapped after ultrasound was used to identify a fluid pocket and then removed to prep the abdomen. Because the first two needle insertions went through apparent obstructions without yielding fluid, a third insertion was made, and chromosomally normal bloody fluid was obtained. The other twin had a separate amniotic sac and was tapped without incident. The first twin was born with porencephaly resulting from loss of flow in the right carotid artery, causing loss of tissue in the distribution of the right middle and posterior cerebral arteries. An external puncture site was evident just above the right ear, and she had severe intellectual disability with seizures and a left hemiparesis. Magnetic resonance imaging confirmed the porencephaly and demonstrated normal carotid cranial foramina.

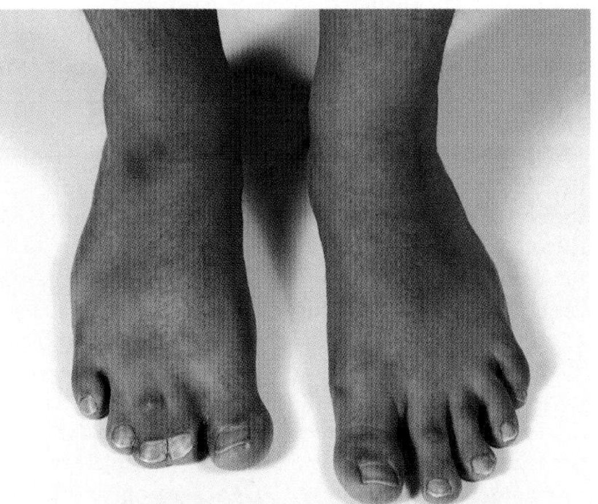

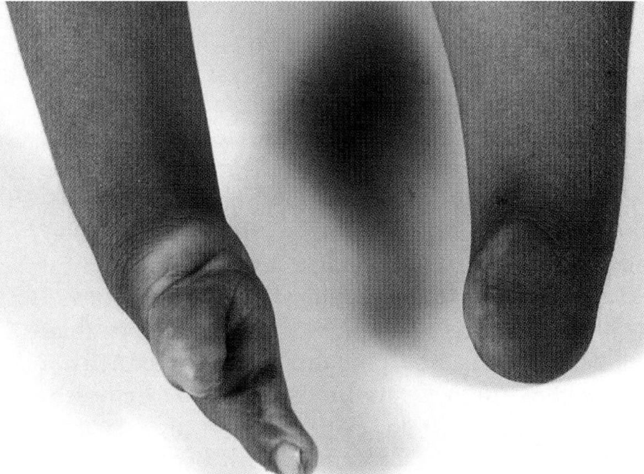

FIGURE 51.7 This child was born with asymmetric terminal transverse limb-reduction defects of the hand and wrist, short left lower leg and foot, syndactyly of the middle digits of the right foot, hypoglossia, and missing teeth. At 12 weeks' gestation, the mother went to an emergency department for vaginal bleeding and a ring forceps was passed into the uterine cavity, resulting in passage of blood-tinged amniotic fluid and uterine cramping. The boy was diagnosed as having hypoglossia-hypodactyly resulting from vascular disruption.

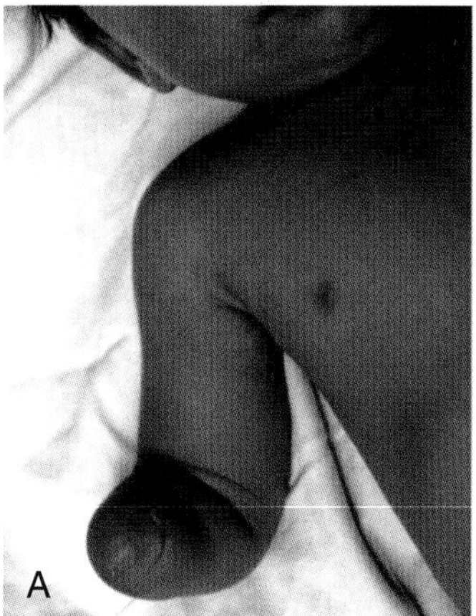

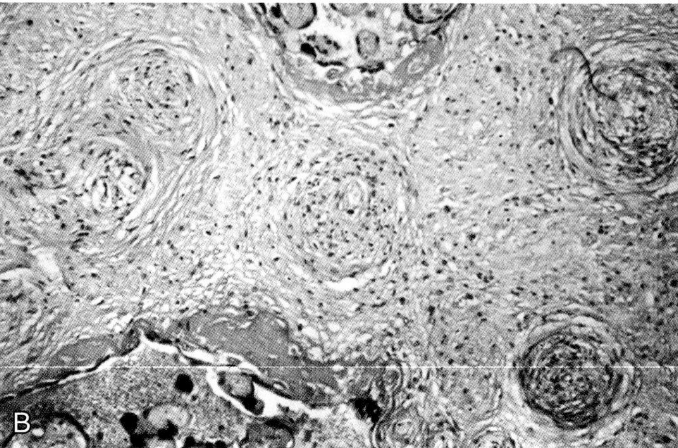

FIGURE 51.8 A, This infant was born at term with a right terminal transverse limb-reduction defect. **B,** Examination of the placenta revealed multiple areas of occlusion and thrombosis of large fetal vessels with normal blood supply to the intervillous spaces. (Courtesy H. Eugene Hoyme, Stanford University Medical Center, Palo Alto, CA.)

and because such mutations can be inherited from an asymptomatic parent, a thrombophilia evaluation of the child and parents should be considered in any birth with an unexplained vascular limb-reduction defect.[35] Arthrogryposis has many different causes that are much more common than failed obstetric termination procedures.[36] Such obstetric procedures are usually recorded in the medical records along with pathologic examination of the products of conception, so there should be little confusion as to the pathogenesis of such defects.

Approximately 1% to 2% of twin pregnancies manifest a defect in one of the twins, causing prenatal care providers to consider selective feticide. In dichorionic pregnancy, the passage of substances and thromboembolic debris from one twin into the circulation of the co-twin is unlikely because of the lack of placental anastomoses; hence potassium chloride can be injected safely into the circulation of the affected twin to produce fetal asystole. In monochorionic twin pregnancies, selective termination can only be performed after complete and permanent occlusion of both the arterial and venous flows in the umbilical cord of the affected twin. Bipolar cord coagulation or radiofrequency ablation under ultrasound guidance is associated with a 56% to 84% survival rate in the unaffected co-twin, depending on the indication.[37-40] Survival rates vary by indication for the procedure, with better survival in fetal growth restriction (83%), twin-reversed arterial perfusion sequence (80%), and lower survival with twin-twin transfusion syndrome (73%) and major fetal anomalies (61%).[39-41] This procedure is not without risk for the surviving co-twin.[42,43]

References

1. Holmes LB, Westgate MN, Nasri H, Toufaily MH. Malformations attributed to the process of vascular disruption. *Birth Defects Res*. 2018;110(2):98–107.
2. Morris JK, Wellesley D, Limb E, et al. Prevalence of vascular disruption anomalies and association with young maternal age: a EUROCAT study to compare the United Kingdom with other European countries. *Birth Defects Res*. 2022;114(20):1417–1426.
3. Szymonowicz W, Preston H, Yu VY. The surviving monozygotic twin. *Arch Dis Child*. 1986;61(5):454–458.
4. Park KB, Chapman T, Aldinger KA, et al. The spectrum of brain malformations and disruptions in twins. *Am J Med Genet A*. 2021;185(9):2690–2718.
5. Radio FC, Di Meglio L, Agolini E, et al. Proliferative vasculopathy and hydranencephaly-hydrocephaly syndrome or Fowler syndrome: report of a family and insight into the disease's mechanism. *Mol Genet Genomic Med*. 2018;6(3):446–451.
6. Sen K, Kaur S, Stockton DW, Nyhuis M, Roberson J. Biallelic variants in *LAMB1* causing hydranencephaly: a severe phenotype of a rare malformative encephalopathy. *AJP Rep*. 2021;11(1):e26–e28.
7. Rawlins LE, Jones H, Wenger O, et al. An Amish founder variant consolidates disruption of *CEP55* as a cause of hydranencephaly and renal dysplasia. *Eur J Hum Genet*. 2019;27(4):657–662.
8. Rasmussen SA, Jamieson DJ, Honein MA, Petersen LR. Zika virus and birth defects: reviewing the evidence for causality. *N Engl J Med*. 2016 May 19;374(20):1981–1987.
9. Rasmussen SA, Jamieson DJ. Teratogen update: Zika virus and pregnancy. *Birth Defects Res*. 2020 Sep; 112(15):1139–1149.
10. Roth NM, Reynolds MR, Lewis EL, et al. Zika-associated birth defects reported in pregnancies with laboratory evidence of confirmed or possible Zika virus infection:

U.S. Zika Pregnancy and Infant Registry, December 1, 2015-March 31, 2018. *MMWR Morb Mortal Wkly Rep.* 2022 Jan 21;71(3):73–79.
11. Moore CA, Staples JE, Dobyns WB, et al. Characterizing the pattern of anomalies in congenital Zika syndrome for pediatric clinicians. *JAMA Pediatr.* 2017 Mar 1;171(3):288–295.
12. Seeds JW. Diagnostic midtrimester amniocentesis: how safe? *Am J Obstet Gynecol.* 2004;191:608–616.
13. [No authors listed]. Randomized trial to assess safety and fetal outcome of early and midtrimester amniocentesis: the Canadian Early and Mid-trimester Amniocentesis Trial (CEMAT) Group. *Lancet.* 1998;351:242–247.
14. Del Campo M, Feitosa IM, Ribeiro EM, et al. Zika Embryopathy Task Force-Brazilian Society of Medical Genetics ZETF-SBGM: the phenotypic spectrum of congenital Zika syndrome. *Am J Med Genet A.* 2017 Apr;173(4):841–857.
15. Contreras-Capetillo SN, Palma-Baquedano JR, Valadéz-González N, et al. Case report: congenital arthrogryposis and unilateral absences of distal arm in congenital Zika syndrome. *Front Med (Lausanne).* 2021 Apr 13;8499016.
16. Vekemans MA, Maurice P, Lachtar M, et al. Additional evidence for the vascular disruption defect hypothesis in a novel case of brainstem disconnection syndrome. *Birth Defects Res.* 2022;114(19):1298–1306.
17. Duffield C, Jocson J, Wootton-Gorges SL. Brainstem disconnection. *Pediatr Radiol.* 2009;39(12):1357–1360.
18. Barth PG, de Vries LS, Nikkels PG, Troost D. Congenital brainstem disconnection associated with a syrinx of the brainstem. *Neuropediatrics.* 2008;39(1):1–7.
19. Jurkiewicz E, Dobrzańska A, Nowak K, Pleskaczyńska A. MRI findings in the young infant with brainstem disconnection and extracerebral features: report of one case and review of the literature. *Brain Dev.* 2010;32(6):495–498.
20. Farrell SA, Summers AM, Dallaire L, et al. Club foot, an adverse outcome of early amniocentesis: disruption or deformation? CEMAT. Canadian Early and Mid-Trimester Amniocentesis Trial. *J Med Genet.* 1999;36:843–846.
21. Broome DP, Wilson MG, Weiss B, et al. Needle puncture of fetus: a complication of second trimester amniocentesis. *Am J Obstet Gynecol.* 1976;126:247–252.
22. Naylor G, Roper JP, Willshaw HE. Ophthalmic complications of amniocentesis. *Eye.* 1990;4:845–849.
23. Rummelt V, Rummelt C, Naumann GOH. Congenital nonpigmented epithelial iris cyst after amniocentesis: clinicopathologic report on two children. *Ophthalmology.* 1993;100:776–781.
24. Creasman WT, Lawrence RA, Thiede HA. Fetal complications of amniocentesis. *JAMA.* 1968;204:949–952.
25. Epley SL, Hanson JW, Cruikshank DP. Fetal injury with midtrimester amniocentesis. *Obstet Gynecol.* 1979;53:77–80.
26. Egley CC. Laceration of fetal spleen during amniocentesis. *Am J Obstet Gynecol.* 1973;116:582–583.
27. Patel CK, Taylor DSI, Russell-Eggitt IM, et al. Congenital third nerve palsy associated with mid-trimester amniocentesis. *Br J Ophthal.* 1993;77:530–533.
28. Chong SKF, Levitt GA, Lawson J, et al. Subarachnoid cyst with hydrocephalus: a complication of mid-trimester amniocentesis. *Prenat Diagn.* 1989;9:677–679.
29. Youroukos S, Papdelis F, Matsanoitis N. Porencephalic cyst after amniocentesis. *Arch Dis Child.* 1980;55:814–815.
30. Cromie WJ, Bates RB, Duckett JW. Penetrating renal trauma in the neonate. *J Urol.* 1978;119:259–260.
31. Ledbetter DJ, Hall DG. Traumatic arteriovenous fistula; a complication of amniocentesis. *J Ped Surg.* 1992;27:720–721.
32. Williamson RA, Varner MW, Grant SS. Reduction in amniocentesis risks using a real-time needle guide procedure. *Obstet Gynecol.* 1985;65:751–755.
33. Holmes LB, Nasri HZ. Terminal transverse limb defects with "nubbins". *Birth Defects Res.* 2021;113(13):1007–1014.
34. Holmes LB, Nasri HZ. Hypothesis: central digit hypoplasia. *Am J Med Genet A.* 2022;188(6):1746–1751.
35. Hunter AGW. A pilot study of the possible role of familial defects in anticoagulation as a cause for terminal limb reduction malformations. *Clin Genet.* 2000;57:197–204.
36. Hall JG. Arthrogryposis (multiple congenital contractures) associated with failed termination of pregnancy. *Am J Med Genet Part A.* 2012;158A:2214–2220.
37. Peng R, Xie HN, Lin MF, et al. Clinical outcomes after selective fetal reduction of complicated monochorionic twins with radiofrequency ablation and bipolar cord coagulation. *Gynecol Obstet Invest.* 2016;81(6):552–558.
38. Li N, Sun J, Wang J, et al. Selective termination of the fetus in multiple pregnancies using ultrasound-guided radiofrequency ablation. *BMC Pregnancy Childbirth.* 2021 Dec 10;21(1):821.
39. Rahimi-Sharbaf F, Ghaemi M, Nassr AA, Shamshirsaz AA, Shirazi M. Radiofrequency ablation for selective fetal reduction in complicated Monochorionic twins: comparing the outcomes according to the indications. *BMC Pregnancy Childbirth.* 2021;21(1):189.
40. Wang H, Zhou Q, Wang X, et al. Influence of indications on perinatal outcomes after radio frequency ablation in complicated monochorionic pregnancies: a retrospective cohort study. *BMC Pregnancy Childbirth.* 2021(1):41.
41. Tang HR, Dai CY, Li J, et al. Fetoscopy-guided bipolar cord coagulation in selective fetal reduction with complicated monochorionic diamniotic twins: a prospective cohort study. *J Matern Fetal Neonatal Med.* 2022;35(25):7744–7747.
42. Rana A, Dadhwal V, Shainy P, Sharma KA. Pseudoamniotic band syndrome after bipolar cord coagulation in monochorionic twins complicated by twin-to-twin transfusion syndrome. *BMJ Case Rep.* 2021;14(7):e244471.
43. Gupta R, Sharma A. Amyoplasia in monochorionic monozygotic pregnancy following interstitial laser. *Am J Med Genet A.* 2022;188(7):2178–2183.

Section XII
Mechanics in Morphogenesis

CHAPTER 52

Principles of Human Biomechanics

KEY POINTS

- The direction and magnitude of forces affect the form of the developing fetus.
- Abnormal mechanical forces give rise to deformation in humans in much the same fashion as abnormal forces may deform a tree.
- The tissues of a human fetus are especially pliable and easily molded, especially as a fetus fills out the uterus in late gestation.
- Many factors can lead to an aberrant fetal position in late gestation, and shortly after birth the position of comfort for an infant can provide insight into their position during late gestation.
- The actual alignment of the fibrils in the extracellular space appears to be determined predominantly by mechanical forces.
- The stress of muscle-tendon tension on a bone affects the growth and form of the bone.
- Current medical practice uses custom-designed orthotic molding helmets to reshape infant heads that have become deformed by their resting positions.

Rather simple principles apply for the role of mechanical factors in morphogenesis. These are that the direction and magnitude of forces affect the form of the developing individual, as illustrated in Fig. 52.1. Some of the factors that affect the magnitude and direction of forces are summarized in Box 52.1. One major influence on the nature and alignment of forces is growth. Thus the rate and shape of growth in a particular basic tissue will determine the magnitude and direction of the forces it exerts on adjacent tissues. The plasticity of a tissue is another factor that affects its liability to be altered by mechanical forces. The tissues of a human fetus are especially pliable and easily molded, especially as a fetus fills out the uterus in late gestation (Fig. 52.2). Many factors can lead to an aberrant fetal position in late gestation, and shortly after birth the position of comfort for an infant can provide insight into their position during late gestation.

Another major influence is tension or compression related to muscle pull, gravity, or local constraint. The orientation of fibers within a structure made from connective tissue, such as bone, cartilage, tendon, ligament, or suture, is determined by such forces. For example, collagen fibrils, the basic threads of tensile strength within connective tissues, align in the direction of stress (Fig. 52.3). These fibrils are synthesized by fibroblasts under genetic direction, but the actual alignment of the fibrils in the extracellular space appears to be determined predominantly by

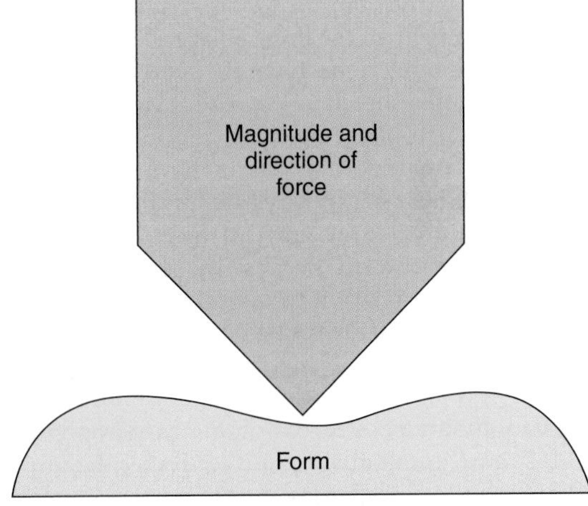

FIGURE 52.1 The basic principles relative to deformation are simple: the magnitude and direction of forces have their impact on form. The response of a given tissue is dependent on its pliability and stage of development.

BOX 52.1 FACTORS THAT AFFECT THE MAGNITUDE AND DIRECTION OF MECHANICAL FORCES

External resistance to growth and/or movement
Growth rate and shape of basic tissue
Forces of fluid flow (or pressure)
Plasticity of the fetus
Forces of muscle pull
Forces of gravity

mechanical forces. If there is no consistent direction for the mechanical forces, the collagen strands may be haphazardly arranged. Given a sustained direction of forces, they become organized and woven in relation to those forces.

The general precepts of mechanical engineering are relevant to human biology, as is the nomenclature (Table 52.1). In many tissues there is an integral interaction between growth and the forces of tension and compression.[1] This is readily evident in the relationship between muscle usage and the size of muscle mass. The greater the forces, the larger the muscle mass tends to become. In turn, the stress of muscle-tendon tension on a bone affects the growth and form of the bone. With greater pull by a muscle on a bone, the size of the bony promontory at the site of the muscle attachment to the bone enlarges. For example, the prominent bony ridge down the center of the skull in the male gorilla shown in Fig. 52.4 relates to the size of the attachment of the powerful temporalis chewing muscles. The female gorilla does not have such a prominent ridge because her muscles are less powerful.

Humans are ruled by gravity, which has a major impact on human form. Because their surface area is relatively small in relation to overall volume, humans are more heavily influenced by gravitational forces than smaller mammals. In contrast, the impact of gravity is less significant to very small animals that have a high surface area to-volume ratio, and their world is more dominated by surface forces. Examples of the impact of mechanical forces on morphogenesis abound in nature. The magnitude and direction of growth on form are dramatically reflected in the chambered nautilus, whose shell represents the successively larger living quarters occupied by this mollusk as it outgrows and creates one new chamber after another, resulting in an equiangular, logarithmic spiral shell, as shown in Fig. 52.5. This exemplifies the basic orderliness of growth and its biomechanical consequences on the development of the form of an organism.

Another beautiful example from nature of the impact of the size and direction of forces on form is the alignment of cellulose fibers in a tree. The reason the tree grows straight up relates to the alignment of cellulose fibers in the direction of the stress force of gravity. Extrinsic forces, such as compression by snow during the winter, may deform the young tree. However, once released from such temporary constraint, the sapling will again tend to grow in the direction of the force of gravity. The forces of prevailing winds may be sufficient to deform a tree (Fig. 52.6), and controlled external forces may be used to deform a young tree into a form that will be maintained after the tree is fully grown.

The collagen fibrils within developing bone may be compared with the cellulose fibers of a tree. They are the basic structural elements and they also align in the direction of stress in such a manner as to resist shear forces, as previously indicated. This is dramatically evidenced in the longitudinal section of the human femur shown in Fig. 52.7. The bony spicules are aligned in the direction of the stress of gravitational weight bearing and in relation to muscle pull. The form of the upper femur relates to the combined forces of weight bearing plus the pull of major muscle groups. This results in a sloping "neck" of the femur and the two large promontories of bone in this region of the femur, the greater and lesser trochanters.

The force lines that are evident in the form of such a bone may be of value to the engineer in their design of somewhat similar structures. D'Arcy Thompson relates the story of a Zürich engineer, Professor Culmann, who became famous for his design of a mechanical crane. In the design of his crane he used stress forces that he observed in a longitudinal section of the human femur in 1871.[2] When he was shown the section of the femur by his friend, Professor Hermann von Meyer of the Anatomy Institute of the University of Zürich, Professor Culmann exclaimed, "There is my crane!" Possibly, there should be a closer interchange between biology and engineering, as the biomechanically determined "lines of stress" are naturally evident in many living creatures. The differences in these lines of stress will vary with the function of a bone. In the wings of a soaring bird, such as a vulture, the lines of stress relate to forces above and beneath the wing. The bony form in the pneumatized bone of a vulture is aligned accordingly, and it appears remarkably like the form that engineers learned to use in the wing girders of early airplanes, as well as in bridge trusses.

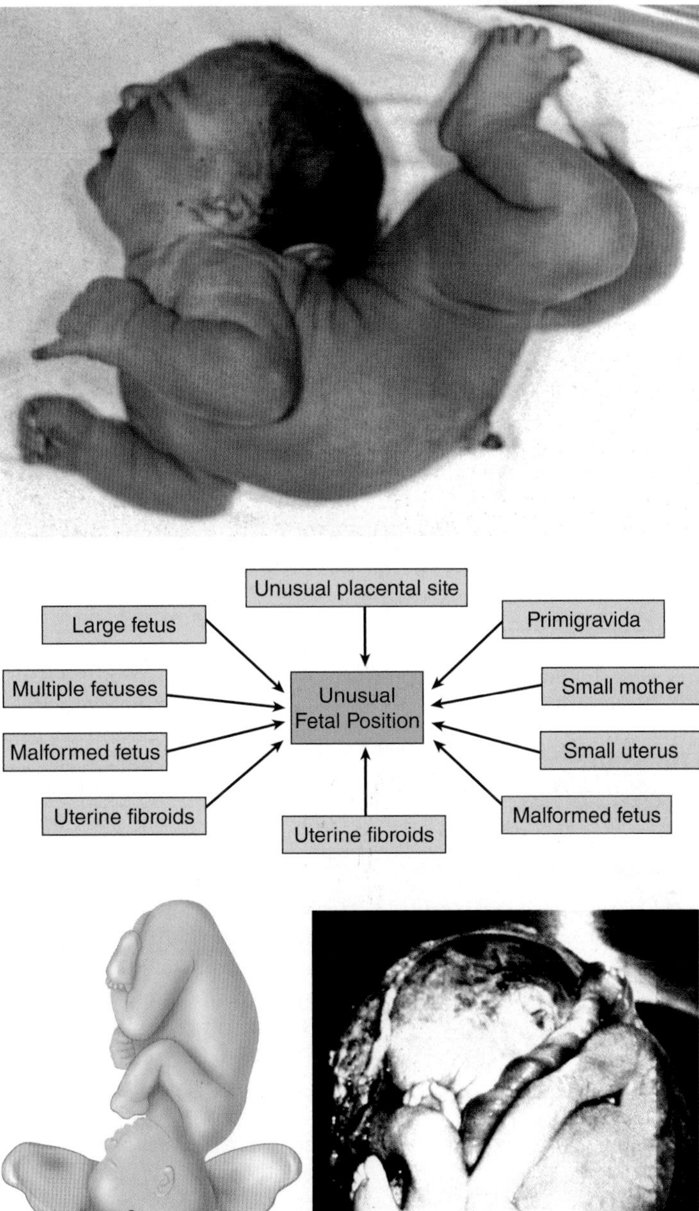

FIGURE 52.2 Many constraining factors may lead to a nonvertex fetal presentation, as depicted by this diagram. The resting position of the infant after birth often reflects the prenatal position of the fetus. This is shown dramatically by the top fetus, which was in breech presentation with a hyperextended head. Within the first few weeks, this infant developed a more normal position of comfort. The term fetus on the bottom right was in breech position when its mother died in an automobile accident, which illustrates the constraining impact of breech presentation on late gestation on pliable fetal tissues. (*Top*, Courtesy Dr. Will Cochran, Beth Israel Hospital and Harvard Medical School, Boston, MA.)

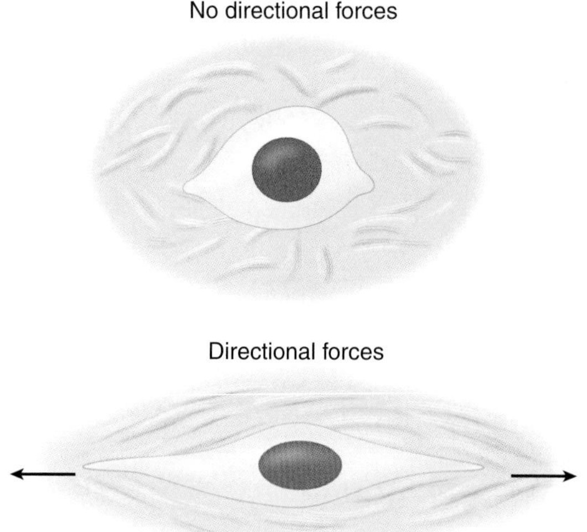

FIGURE 52.3 Schematic depiction of fibroblasts producing collagen fibrils. When there are no directional forces, the extruded fibrils tend to be haphazardly oriented *(top)*. When there are directional forces, the collagen fibrils align in the direction of the forces, thus affecting the form of the tissue. (Based on discussions with Gian Töndury, Anatomisches Institute, University of Zürich, Zürich, Switzerland.)

Table 52.1 MECHANICAL ENGINEERING TERMS APPLICABLE TO HUMAN BIOLOGY

Term	Definition
Deformation	Altered form caused by unusual forces
Stress	Intensity of force (force per unit area)
Strain	Sufficient force to cause deformation
Tension	Stretching forces
Compression	Compressive forces
Torsion	Twisting forces
Shear forces	Forces contrary to the main orientation of a tissue
Axial forces	Forces parallel to the main orientation of a tissue

Mechanical forces play a major role in the form of an individual and relate to the function of that individual; for example the pneumatized lightweight but strong bones of the larger soaring birds. The largest soaring mammal was the extinct Pteranodon, with a wingspan of 21 feet (7 meters). It apparently had pneumatized wing bones. The form and dimension of the reconstructed Pteranodon are considered aerodynamically ideal for the soaring function of this animal. Because its femora were delicately built and could not withstand compressive stress, it was necessary for this mammal to hang upside down from cliffs as compensation for reduction in bone weight for flight. This adaptation is also true of the bat. The evolutionary impact of forces on form is also beautifully evidenced in the form of three different classes of sea creatures (Fig. 52.8).

Abnormal mechanical forces give rise to deformation in humans in much the same fashion as abnormal forces may deform a tree. In addition to those extrinsic deformations that relate to uterine constraint, abnormal forces can be seen in the deformations wrought by past societies in the name of beauty or custom by application of external forces after the time of birth (Figs. 52.9–52.14). Constraint forces were used to mold infant heads by a number of groups, including the so-called "Flathead Indians," whose name was derived from this practice.[3] Current medical practice uses custom-designed orthotic molding helmets to reshape infant heads, which have become deformed by their resting positions (see Fig. 52.10).[4,5] Deformational plagiocephaly is the leading cause of head shape abnormalities in children, with mild cases affecting 40% of infants under 12 months of age. Deformational plagiocephaly can cause facial asymmetry, eventual malocclusion requiring orthodontic treatment, and social stigmatization later in life. Most often, it is detected by the child's parents or pediatrician through simple visual assessment, and subsequent monitoring of the abnormal head shape is crucial because the progression of deformity can indicate the need for additional intervention (such as treatment of persistent torticollis) or an undiagnosed sutural fusion (craniosynostosis) requiring surgical treatment.[6]

In the past, the Chinese custom of binding the feet of infant girls resulted in small, misshapen feet (see Fig. 52.11).[7] The practice was initiated at around 3 years of age, when all toes but the first toes were broken and bound with tight cloth over the next 2 years so as to keep the feet less than 10 cm in length, with a marked concavity of the sole.[8] Through contact with Western culture, this practice decreased at the beginning of the 20th century after its first ban in 1912, although some continued this practice in secret. In 1997, a study on foot binding recruited 193 Beijing women and found that the majority were between the ages of 70 and 79 years, while 93 were above the age of 80 years.[8]

In other societies in the Americas and Africa, various techniques were designed to cause deformations. The insertion of stretching devices into the earlobes

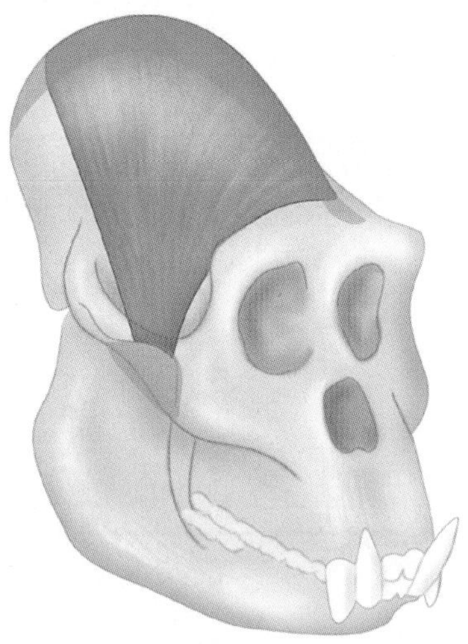

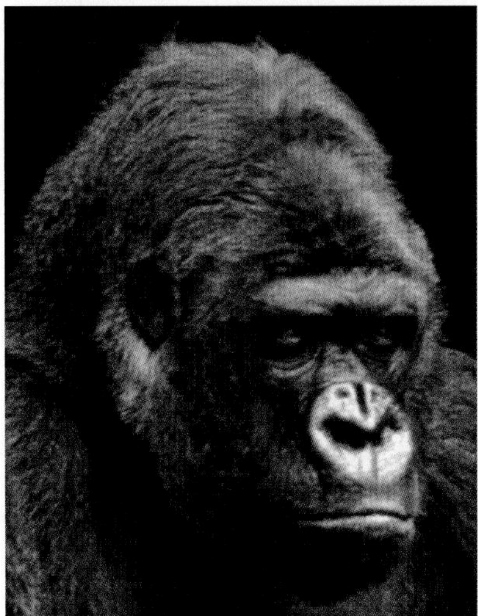

FIGURE 52.4 Male gorilla skull with prominent bony ridge down the center of the calvarium, which is the consequence of the pull of the powerful temporalis muscles that insert at this location.

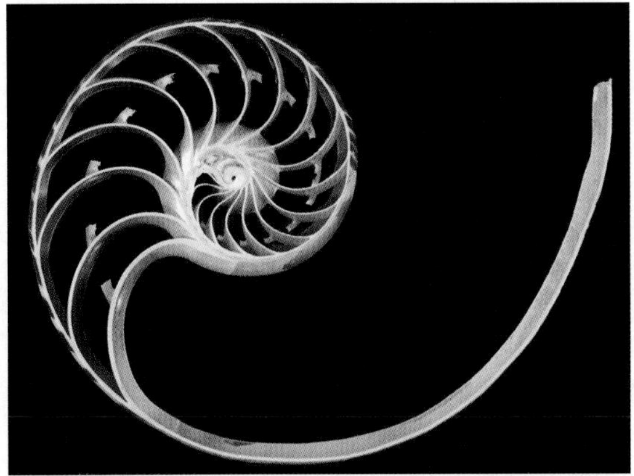

FIGURE 52.5 The growing nautilus mollusk outgrows one chamber after another, thus creating an equiangular, logarithmic spiral shell.

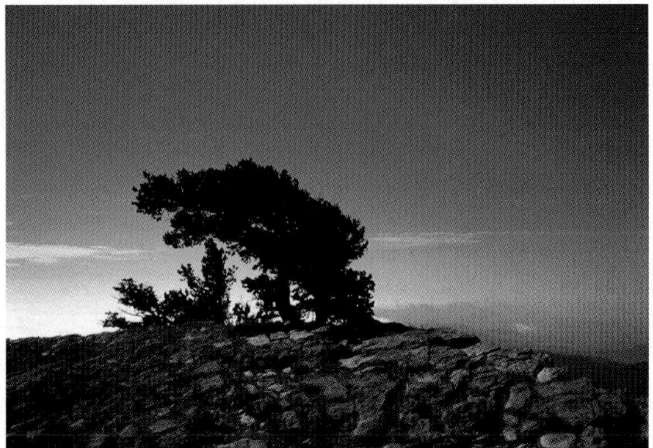

FIGURE 52.6 Ridgetop tree showing deformation by the prevailing winds that blow from right to left.

resulted in excessive skin in this region, as did similar practices with the lips. Successive heavy metal rings were placed around the necks of young girls to elongate their necks. Other practices, such as the swaddling or papoose board immobilization of infants, may have inadvertently increased the likelihood of such deformations as hip dislocation.

Many types of cranial deformation were practiced in pre-Columbian Peru.[3,9] Highland Peruvians applied circumferential bandages to elongate the calvarium (see Figs. 52.12 and 52.13). In coastal areas of Peru, banding was combined with the application of occipital boards to mold the skull into a bilobed shape or a "tower skull" configuration. Anthropologic observations suggest that the practice of artificial cranial deformation was quite widespread, occurring throughout the world, as shown by similar head-binding practices among the Mangbetu people (see Fig. 52.14).[3] Such anular deformation results in a head shape like that seen with persistent vertex molding.[10]

Just as some past societies were knowledgeable about mechanical means for producing deformations after birth, other societies successfully used biomechanical means to treat some congenital deformations. In India, some women specialized in reshaping cranial deformations by daily massage and manipulation. Among Polynesian societies, where talipes equinovarus was a common deformity, some older women

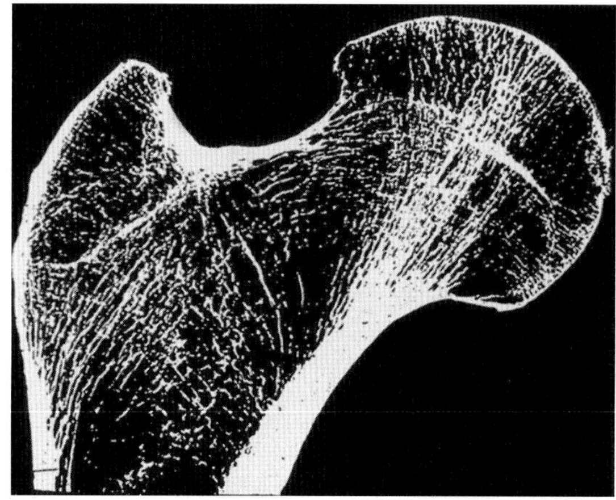

FIGURE 52.7 This section of the proximal human femur beautifully illustrates the relationship between function and form in the alignment of the bone spicules, which relate to the orientation of collagen fibrils. (From Thompson D. *On Growth and Form. A New Edition*. Cambridge, UK: Cambridge University Press; 1942.)

specialized in manipulating and binding such feet. The deformation was deliberately corrected only partially because such feet were ideal for climbing coconut trees, and no shoes were needed in their environment.

SPECIFIC MECHANICAL IMPACTS ON MORPHOGENESIS

Mechanical forces play an important role in the normal morphogenesis of most tissues, and different tissues have their own limited repertoire of responses to forces. The abnormalities mentioned in this section are used predominantly to illustrate specifically how mechanical factors are relevant to the normal morphogenesis of specific tissues. Many of these examples relate to the impact of forces during early morphogenesis, when extrinsic constraint deformation would be unlikely to occur; however, they do provide the reader with some clinically relevant illustrations of the impact of mechanical forces on form in morphogenesis.

Overall Growth

Constraint may limit the intrauterine growth of an infant.[11,12] When the onset of constraint-related growth deficiency occurs during late fetal life, there will usually be catch-up growth into the normal range once the constraint is relieved after birth.[12] This appears to be the reason why the first born infant, who must distend the mother's uterus and abdominal wall for the first time, averages about 200–300 g smaller than subsequent offspring. With more constraint, there is greater deceleration of growth. This is dramatically evident in most multiple births. Twins grow at a normal rate for the first 30–34 weeks of gestation. After they have achieved a combined weight of 4.0 kg, they become constrained and their growth rate tends to slow, as also noted in animal studies. If only one animal is reared in a uterine horn, the newborn is appreciably larger at birth than when many are reared in the same uterine horn.[13] Situations other than multiple births may limit the available intrauterine space and cause it to yield a smaller baby, such as oligohydramnios, uterine malformation, and uterine fibroids (Fig. 52.15).

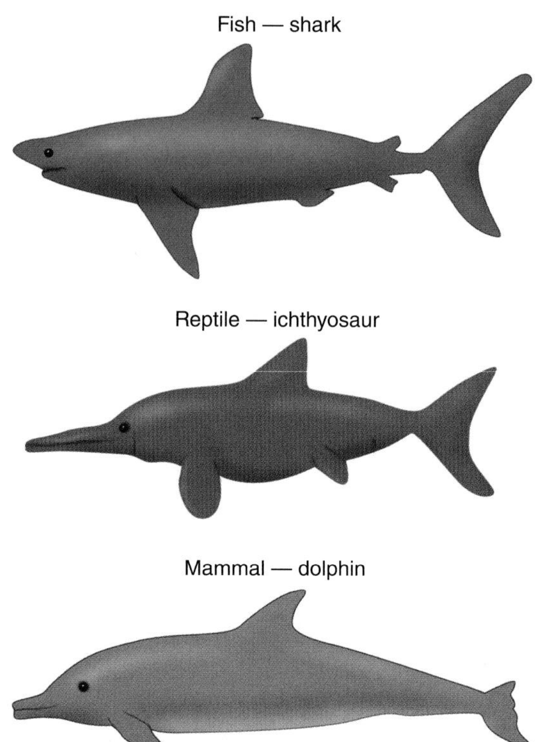

FIGURE 52.8 The adaptation of the form toward reducing turbulence and toward ease of free movement in water is beautifully exemplified by the similarities of form in a larger free-swimming fish, a reptile, and a mammal. In this environment, gravity is of less importance than is the buoyancy of the sea in shaping form. (Adapted from Bunnell S, McIntyre J. *Mind in the Water*. New York: Charles Scribner & Sons; 1974.)

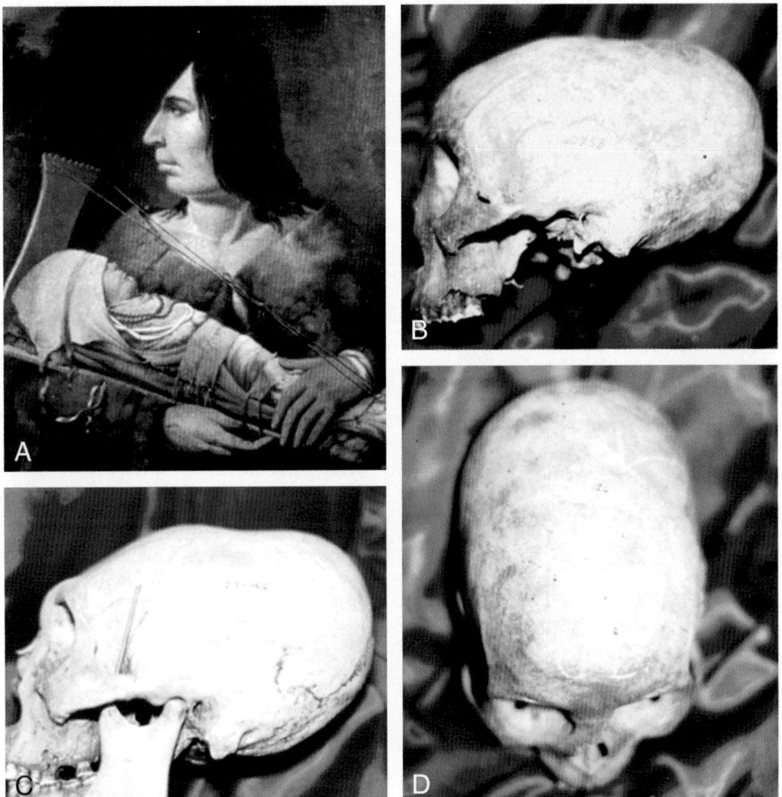

FIGURE 52.9 The Kwakiutl Native Americans of the Pacific Northwest used cedar boards and leather thongs to mold infants' heads. Boys were molded for 5 months, and girls were generally molded for 7 months. (**A,** Courtesy Bill Holm, Burke Museum of Natural History and Culture, Seattle, CA; **B–D,** courtesy Dr. Kate Donahue, Department of Anthropology, Plymouth State College, Plymouth, NH.)

Effects on Specific Tissues

Bone

The early cartilage models of different long bones appear to be genetically specified, but the alignment of collagen fibrils and bone trabeculae relate to mechanical forces, as do the bony promontories. Collagen fibrils align in the same direction as stress forces, thereby helping to resist shear forces, and sites of muscle attachment relate to muscle tension. For example, the size and shape of the greater trochanter relate to the relatively massive pull of five muscles at that site, including the very strong gluteus maximus muscle. The lesser trochanter only has one major muscle attaching at that site, the psoas minor. The combined forces of weight bearing plus muscle pull affect the form of the upper femur, including the normal configuration of the "neck" of the femur. Prolonged muscle weakness in the growing child may give rise to smaller trochanters and a straighter neck of the femur, termed *coxa valga deformity* (Fig. 52.16). It is important that these bony findings be interpreted as secondary deformations caused by a more primary neuromuscular problem, rather than as additional malformations involving the skeletal system.

The impact of increasing weight is also evident in the breadth of bone, whereas linear growth is only mildly affected by muscle weakness. Thus paralysis or immobility of a limb results in only a 5% to 10% reduction in its rate of linear growth; however subperiosteal growth in bone breadth is much more dramatically affected. Hence with muscle weakness or lack of use, the growing bone tends to become slender (Fig. 52.17).

The adaptive capacity of bone is beautifully exemplified by the realization that the amount of bone and its alignment are influenced by the very forces that the bone is required to withstand. Bone appears to have a critical strain or stress threshold, above which there

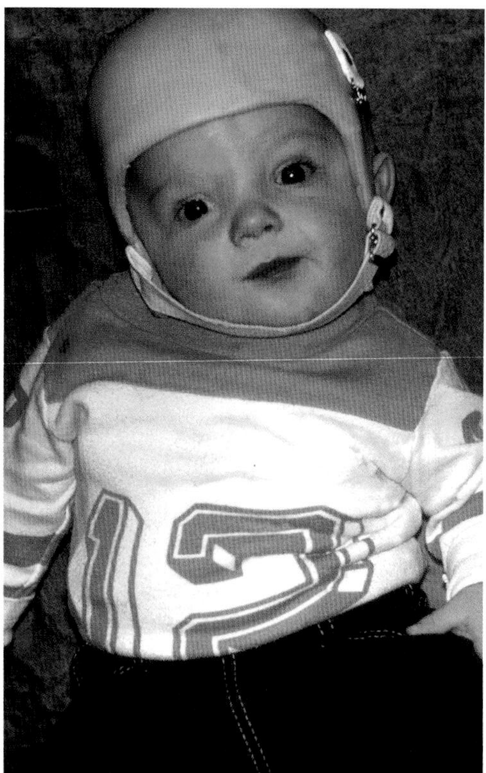

FIGURE 52.10 Cranial orthotic devices are used today to reshape the heads of infants with deformational posterior plagiocephaly not associated with craniosynostosis.

tends to be bone deposition and below which there tends to be bone resorption. Intermittent stress on a bone tends to foster local growth of bone, as exemplified in bony promontories at sites of muscle attachment. One example is the bony spurs that are liable to develop in the arch of the foot because of the strain of long-distance running. The medial longitudinal arch of the foot is a critical shock absorber during standing and movement. Studies have indicated that childhood obesity can damage and flatten the arch structure as early as age 8 years, with increases in BMI correlated with decreases in arch height, leading to medial longitudinal arch deformation at BMIs above 20 kg/m^2 that diminishes the functional structure of the foot arch architecture.[14]

Persistent stress on cranial bone, such as that caused by continuous external compression, can lead to a decrease in bone. This is dramatically exemplified by constraint-induced vertex craniotabes. This abnormality commonly results from prolonged pressure on the fetal vertex as a consequence of the head being "engaged" for a prolonged period of time before birth.[15] A similar effect of persistent pressure on the calvarium was deduced by G. E. Smith from his evaluation of ancient Egyptian skulls.[16] He recognized that the upper-class Egyptians, who lived during the fourth to nineteenth dynasties and wore heavy headdresses, had notable thinning of the calvarium. Smith deduced that this was the consequence of the *continuous pressure* exerted by these heavy headdresses.

Joints

Joints develop secondarily within the condensed mesenchyme of the developing bones. Movement is an important factor in joint morphogenesis. The embryo starts moving by 7.5 weeks' gestation, and 2 to 3 weeks later general movements, isolated limb and head movements, hiccups, and breathing movements appear.[17] Chronic lack of movement tends to give rise to multiple joint contractures and a pattern of problems called the *fetal akinesia deformation sequence* (Fig. 52.18).[18,19] This can be of extrinsic etiology resulting from intrauterine crowding secondary to congenital structural uterine abnormalities (e.g., bicornuate or septate uterus), uterine tumors (e.g., fibroid), or multifetal pregnancy, or of intrinsic fetal etiology due to functional abnormalities in the brain, spinal cord, peripheral nerves, neuromuscular junction, muscles, bones, or restrictive dermopathies, tendons, and joints. Unlike many intrinsic primary fetal cases, which are difficult to treat, secondary fetal akinesia deformation sequence can be treated with physical therapy. Primary cases may present prenatally with fetal akinesia associated with joint contractures and occasionally brain abnormalities, decreased muscle bulk, polyhydramnios, and nonvertex presentation, while the secondary cases usually present with isolated contractures.[19] One dramatic example was an infant with multiple joint contractures (termed *arthrogryposis*) whose mother had received tubocurarine for 19 days in early pregnancy for the treatment of tetanus.[20] Such medically induced early immobilization was considered to be the cause of the joint contractures in her fetus. Similar defects have been induced experimentally by the injection of curare into pregnant rats (Fig. 52.19).[21] Physical constraint caused by prolonged oligohydramnios can also cause joint contractures. Hall summarized 30 cases with multiple congenital contractures due to long-standing oligohydramnios among a total of 2500 cases of arthrogryposis. All 30 cases had "Potter" facies (flattened face and nose, short columella, puffy eyelids, micrognathia, and enlarged flattened ears) with remarkable skin changes (soft

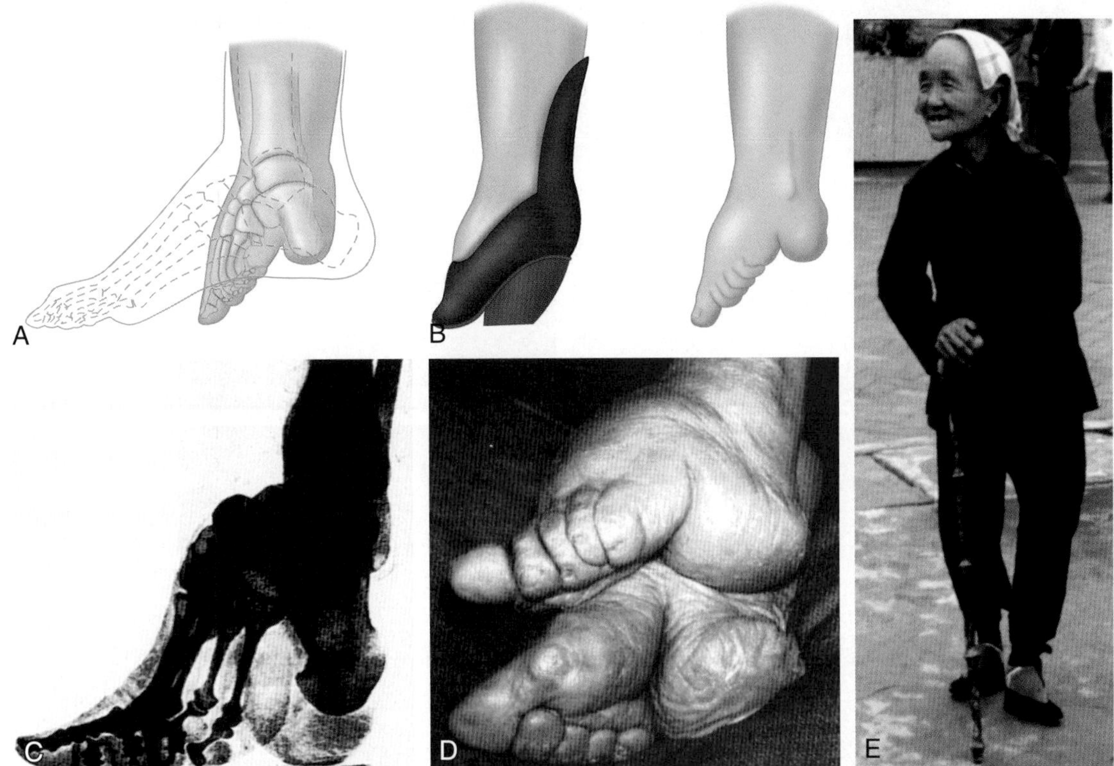

FIGURE 52.11 For almost 1500 years, certain young Chinese girls were subjected to the harrowing experience of molding their feet for several years in order to produce the desired small feet. These feet were deemed sexually attractive. The form into which the deformed feet were molded is demonstrated by a diagram (**A**), along with a drawing of the special shoe and foot position (**B**), a radiograph (**C**), and images of actual deformed feet (**D** and **E**). (**A** and **B** From Levy HS. *Chinese Footbinding*. New York: Walton Rawl; 1966.)

hyperextensible skin with excessive creases on the forehead, face, and neck), 50% had pulmonary hypoplasia at birth, and 60% had multiple congenital contractures that responded well to therapy.[22] Fig. 52.20 demonstrates the multiple consequences on bones and joint development in constrained twins carried to term by a small primigravida woman.

Muscles

Muscle cells align in the direction of muscle pull, which has obvious importance for muscle function. The size of a muscle relates to the magnitude and frequency of the forces it exerts, and the larger the forces, the greater the muscle bulk. Conversely, with diminished function a muscle becomes smaller in size, and lack of muscle function will result in a diminished, hypoplastic muscle. Based on a study of muscle-tendon insertions in genetic limb-reduction defects and sites of juncture in conjoined twins (in whom genetic instructions for such altered anatomy could not be predetermined), there appears to be a hierarchy for the determination of muscle-tendon attachment sites. Tendons attach preferentially to bone, and in the absence of the bone to which a tendon would normally attach, the tendon attaches to the next closest bone. If no such bone is available, tendons may attach to other tendons or to the fascia of another muscle. If there is no connective tissue attachment site, then there is no muscle, which implies a need for muscle to function in the development and maintenance of muscle.[23] The biomechanical impact of muscle strength on bone form and growth has already been emphasized.

Organ Capsules

Organ capsules may be viewed as exoskeletons that provide connective tissue support for specific tissues.

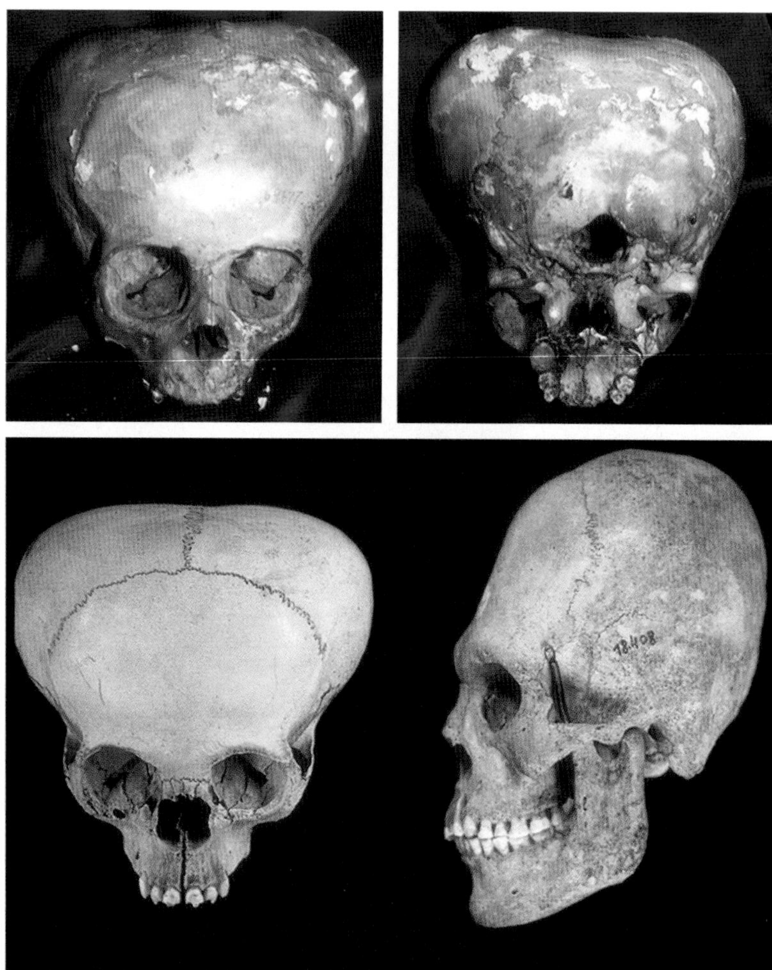

FIGURE 52.12 These bilobed, brachycephalic skulls from coastal Peru resulted from the application of boards to the occiput with pads to the frontal region and circumferential banding. Molding devices were applied until around 8 months of age and then discarded because the desired deformation would persist. (Courtesy Dr. Kate Donahue, Department of Anthropology, Plymouth State College, NH.)

Included within this category are the dura mater of the brain, the sclera and outer covering of the eye, the pericardium of the heart, the pleura of the lung, the peritoneum of the intestine, the capsule of the kidney, and the tunica albuginea of the testes. The skin may also be interpreted as an organ capsule, as it is the capsule for the entire organism. The only organ capsule that becomes ossified is that of the brain. The dura mater is responsible for the development and ossification of the calvarium. (This is considered in more depth in the craniofacial section of this book.) None of these organ capsules appear to have any basic impetus for growth. Rather, they grow in accordance with the mechanical forces imposed by the expansion of the underlying organ or tissue that they envelope. All organ capsules are composed of connective tissues within which the collagen fibrils align, in accord with the growth stretch imposed by the internal expansile growth of the respective organ. The direction of such forces is curvilinear, as is readily evident in the alignment of the collagen fibrils within these organ capsules.

Skin and Its Derivatives

Skin does not appear to have any basic impetus for growth but instead grows in accordance with

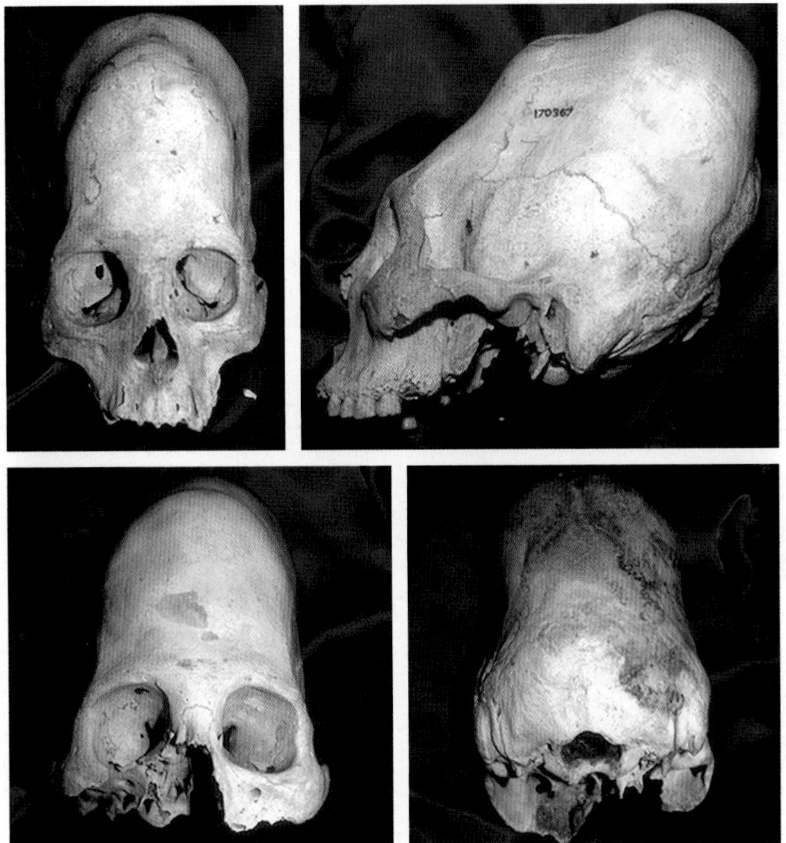

FIGURE 52.13 Highland Peruvians applied circumferential bandages to the calvarium to achieve a conic head shape. Coastal Peruvians applied boards to the occiput and pads to the frontal region along with circumferential banding. (Courtesy Dr. Kate Donahue, Department of Anthropology, Plymouth State College, NH.)

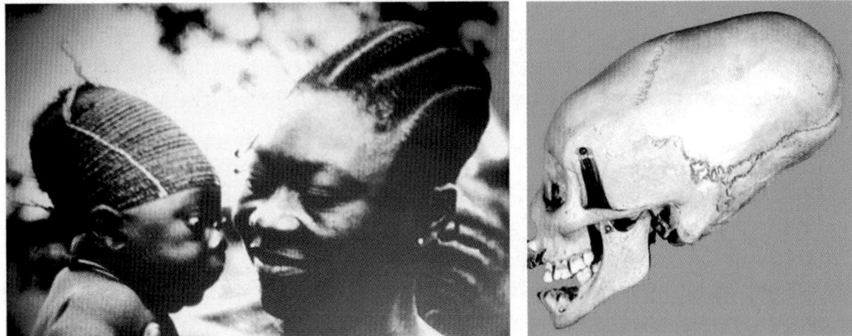

FIGURE 52.14 Among the Mangbetu people, circumferential binding was used to achieve a conic head shape that persisted throughout adulthood, as shown by this adult female as well as the skull. (Courtesy Dr. Tim Littlefield, Cranial Technologies, Tempe, AZ.)

mechanical forces.[24] Under normal circumstances, such forces are exerted by the growth of underlying tissues. If there is unusual growth of underlying tissues, the skin will respond accordingly. Thus if hydrocephalus is present, the skin will grow in accordance with the enlarged head. The excessive skin of the pterygium colli that may occur in Turner syndrome and certain other disorders is secondary to a more primary

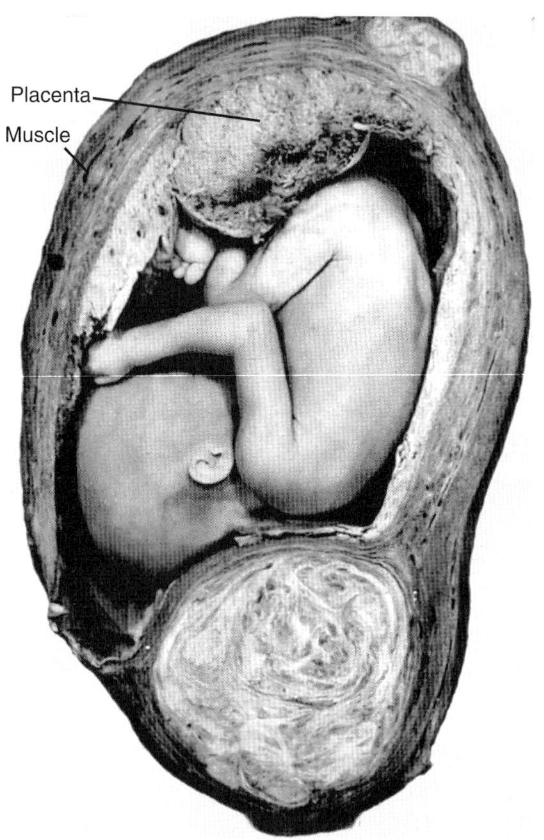

FIGURE 52.15 Diminished uterine cavity because of a large uterine fibroid.

problem in the development of the lymphatic system, as shown in Figs. 52.21 and 52.22. A lag in the development of a channel between the juguloaxillary lymph sac and the internal jugular vein results in grossly distended jugular lymph sacs, which distend the overlying skin in the posterolateral regions of the neck.[25] This lymphaticovenous communication channel usually develops by the 40th day after conception, thus draining the distended lymphatic sacs. The excess skin remains as redundant folds of skin from the mastoid region toward the shoulder, a deformational clue to the nature of the problem that engendered the webbed neck. Another condition that may leave a residuum of redundant skin is the urethral obstruction malformation sequence. When the prostatic urethra fails to hollow out, obstructed urine flow can massively distend the bladder in early fetal life.[26] This will usually be lethal unless the bladder decompresses, which then yields a wrinkled "prune belly" abdomen with redundant folds of abdominal skin evident at birth.

The skin appears to respond to external pressure by overgrowth in a fashion like its response to internal expansile stretch. For example, when there has been external pressure on the skin, such as occurs with oligohydramnios, there may be loose, redundant folds of skin at birth. Such accentuated folds in the face may account for the "Potter facies" noted with external constraint resulting from oligohydramnios.[22] Redundant loose folds have also been noted on the back of the neck in infants who have been in prolonged breech presentation with the head hyperextended, yielding the breech head deformation sequence (see Chapter 42). This is presumed to be the consequence of excessive pressure of the basiocciput on the posterior neck, resulting in localized overgrowth of the skin in this region. Similarly, skin overgrowth in the anterior neck and chin region may be noted with prolonged face presentation (see Chapter 44). Thus the finding of redundant excessive skin at birth may implicate either previous internal expansile growth stretch or previous external compression of a considerable duration.

An occasional finding in an otherwise normal baby is a small, raw, punched-out lesion in the skin of the scalp (Fig. 52.23). Such lesions are also a frequent feature in babies with trisomy 13 syndrome, as shown in Fig. 52.23B, but they can also occur in otherwise normal individuals as an autosomal dominant trait (Fig. 52.23A). These areas of aplasia cutis congenita tend to occur near the parietal hair whorl (see Chapter 39). The parietal hair whorl may represent the apical point from which growth stretch is exerted by the domelike outgrowth of the brain. This point in the developing skin of the scalp would therefore be the most liable to break down during the period of rapid brain growth, which stretches the skin away from this point. With this hypothesis, the ulceration would be the result of the interaction of mechanical forces plus increased liability of the skin to break down at this point of maximal stretch.[27] The development of dermal appendages and dermal ridges also follows mechanical principles, as follows:

1. *Hair directional patterning*: As the hair follicles grow downward from the germinative layer of the skin at 10 to 18 weeks of development, they take on a sloping angulation (Fig. 52.24).[28,29] This angulation is considered to be the consequence of the direction and magnitude of growth stretch exerted on the surface skin during the period of down growth of the hair follicles, which have a sloping angulation as a result of differential lag. When the keratinized rods of hair are extruded at 16 to 18 weeks of

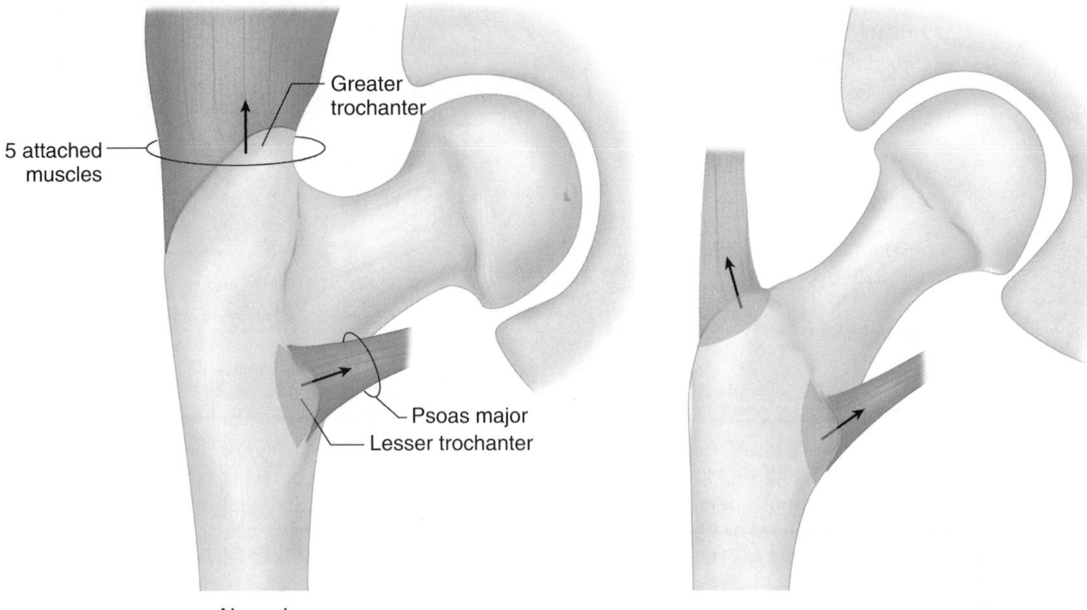

FIGURE 52.16 Impact of muscle weakness on the form of the proximal femur. The coxa valga and slimmer bone is secondary to the diminished forces exerted on the bone.

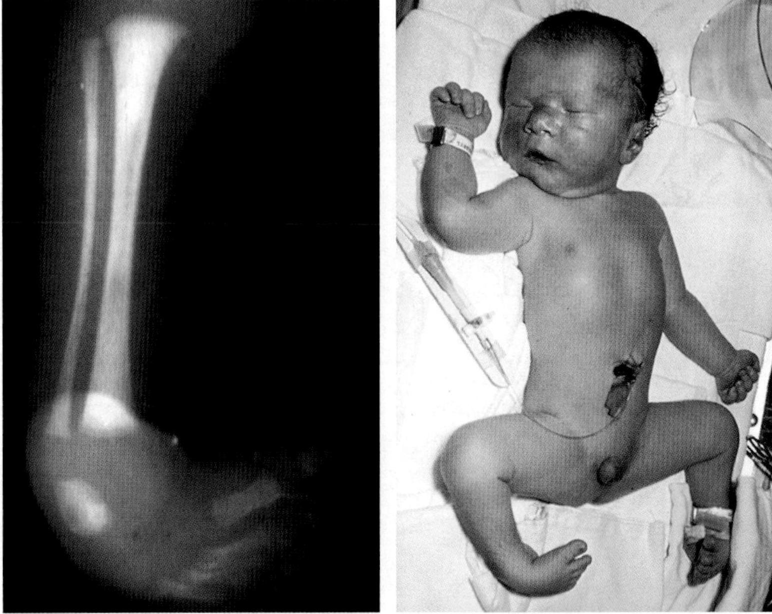

FIGURE 52.17 These slim lower leg bones are secondary to long-standing neuromuscular weakness in a newborn with myotonic dystrophy whose mother had this dominantly inheritable disorder.

development, the direction of the hair appears to be set for life and reflects the magnitude and direction of growth stretch exerted on the skin during the 11- to 16-week period (Figs. 52.25 and 52.26). On any expanding sphere or hemisphere there is one immobile point, away from which all other points

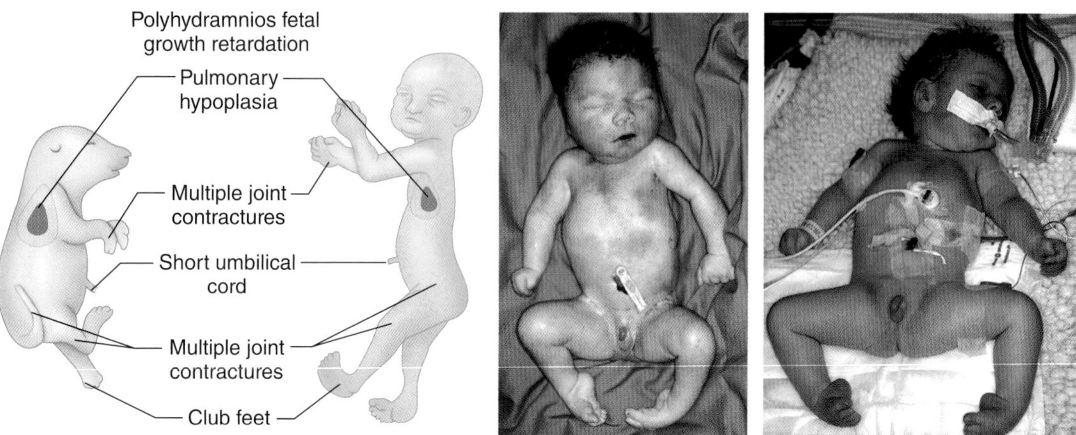

FIGURE 52.18 Fetal akinesia sequence results from decreased movement in utero. The consequent anomalies consisted of intrauterine growth curtailment, micrognathia, multiple joint contractures, pulmonary hypoplasia, short umbilical cords, and polyhydramnios. These defects result from intrinsic deformation resulting from myoneural dysfunction, as shown in these brothers with fetal akinesia deformation sequence caused by type I Pena-Shokeir syndrome, a lethal autosomal recessive disorder resulting from pulmonary hypoplasia. (From Moessinger AC. Fetal akinesia deformation sequence: an animal model. *Pediatrics*. 1983;72:857.)

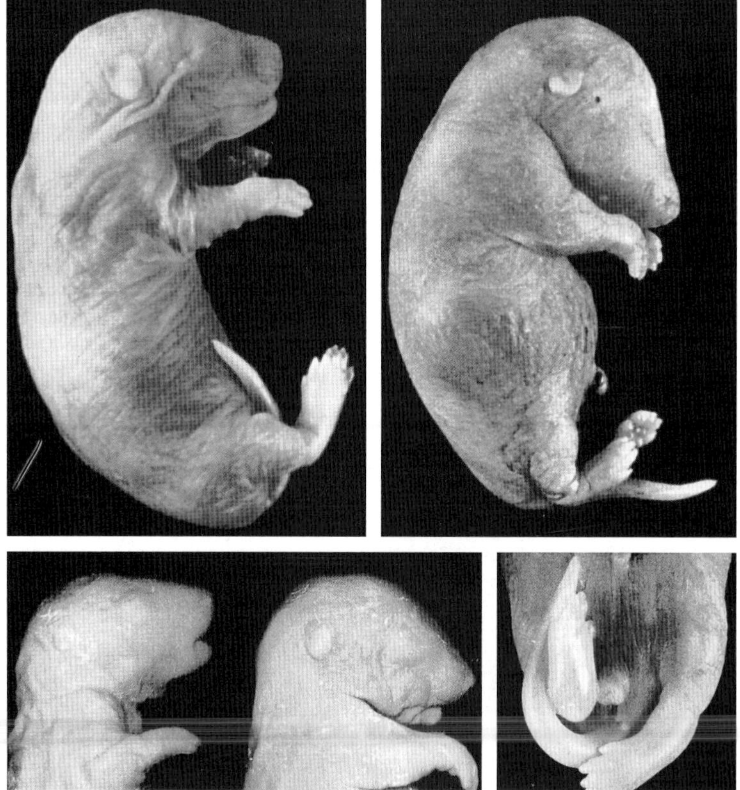

FIGURE 52.19 Moessinger modeled fetal akinesia sequence experimentally in rat fetuses, which were paralyzed by daily transuterine injections of curare from day 18 of gestation until term (day 21). Compared with the control fetuses *(left)*, the experimental fetuses demonstrated tight skin, micrognathia, and joint contractures. (From Moessinger AC. Fetal akinesia deformation sequence: an animal model. *Pediatrics*. 1983;72:857.)

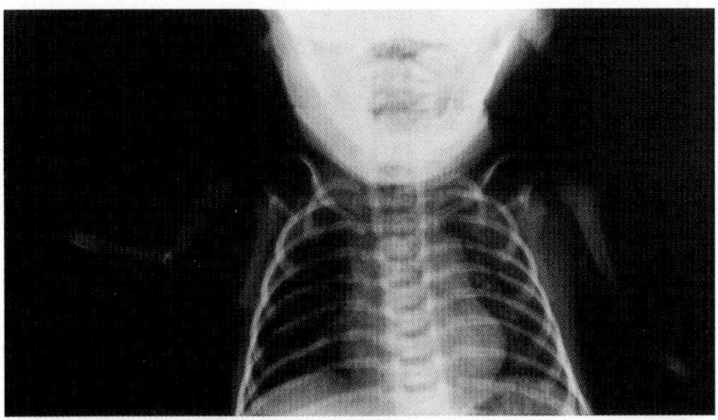

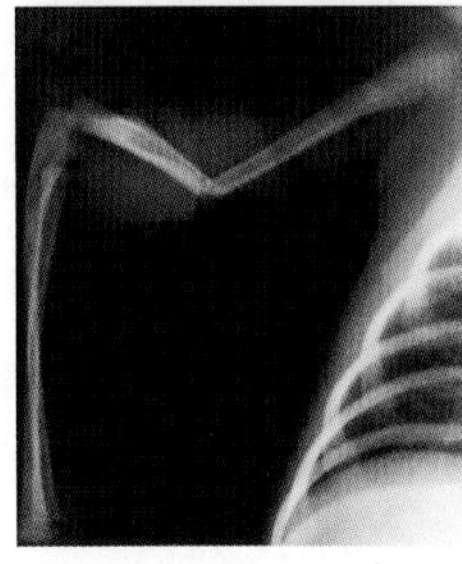

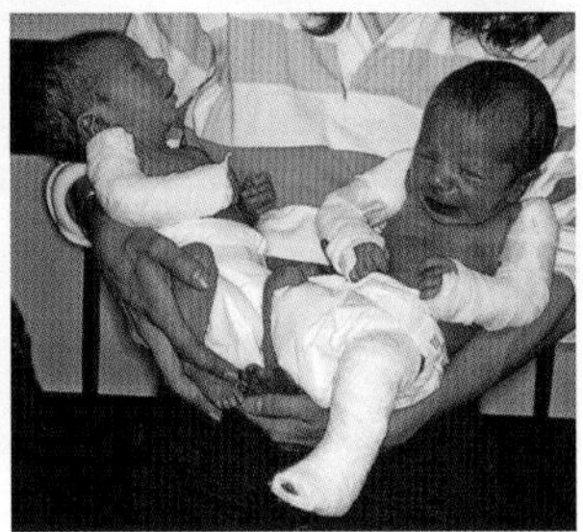

FIGURE 52.20 This 62-inch, 98-lb primiparous mother delivered these twins at term with a combined weight of 10 lb, 11 oz. There was marked fetal crowding during the last half of gestation to the extent that this small mother had such difficulty eating that she experienced a 2-lb weight loss during the course of her pregnancy. She noted very little fetal movement during the third trimester, and both twins were born with severe joint contractures, which resulted in 60- to 90-degree limitation of extension at the elbows and 30-degree limitation of extension at the knees. Twin A was born from a vertex presentation with thin bones, resulting in a fracture postnatally during routine handling. Twin B was delivered vaginally from a breech presentation with thin bones and fractured both humeri during delivery; he also had a right equinovarus foot deformity. Both twins had markedly redundant skin and large ears from prolonged compression. By the time photographs were taken at 12 days of age, the joint contractures had shown marked improvement and the twins were beginning to fill out their loose skin. The prognosis for continued improvement was excellent.

are moving. Over the scalp, this point is usually in the parietal region and this is considered to result in the parietal hair whorl, or crown. This is a beautiful example of the impact of mechanical forces on form. Thus differences in brain growth and form are the primary reason for most differences in scalp hair directional patterning, including those that exist between humans and other primates (Fig. 52.27). Of special clinical relevance are the aberrant hair directional patterns that may be secondary to early problems of brain morphogenesis, examples of which are shown in Figs. 52.28–52.30. Such findings not only tend to implicate a problem in brain morphogenesis, but also suggest that the disorder had its advent before 16 weeks of fetal life.

2. *Nails*: Each nail is a keratinized plate derived from the germinative layer of skin, like what is seen with hair follicles. The nail tends to conform to the shape of the underlying distal phalanx (Fig. 52.31). Thus if the distal phalanx is short and broad, then the nail is short and broad, as seen in brachydactyly D (Fig. 52.32). If the distal phalanx is hypoplastic, the nail is hypoplastic, as seen in fetal alcohol syndrome and fetal hydantoin syndrome (Fig. 52.33). If the distal phalanx is bifid, the nail is bifid. The impact of forces on the early form of the nails caused by peripheral lymphedema in Turner syndrome is illustrated in Fig. 52.34.
3. *Dermal ridge patterning*: As with other primates, humans have dermal ridges on the thickened skin of the volar surfaces of the hands and feet. This parallel ridging provides an important frictional surface for the palms and soles. These ridges develop at 13 to 19 weeks of fetal life and appear to form at right angles to the plane of growth stretch in the skin.[30,31] Dermal ridges resemble the ridges of sand that develop on the beach at right angles to the direction of the flow of water or wind. The surface characteristics over underlying pads give rise to curvilinear dermal ridge patterns that reflect the shape of the pads at the time of dermal ridge development (Figs. 52.35 and 52.36). If the fingertip pad is low, the pattern forms an arch; however, if the pads are very prominent, a whorl develops, with the center of the whorl representing the apex of the pad. A high proportion of loops, the most common fingertip pattern, has little clinical relevance. The finding of six or more arches on the 10 fingertips is unusual (found in only 3% of normal individuals), and the finding of eight or more whorls on the fingertips is also unusual. Altered dermal ridge patterning is generally a nonspecific deformation, providing evidence of the nature of the topographic growth dynamics in the volar surfaces of the hands and feet at 13 to 19 fetal weeks.
4. *Dermal creases*: The dermal creases (Fig. 52.37) are simply deep wrinkles that reflect the flexional planes of functional folding in the thickened skin of the palms and soles. Creases occur in relation to joints and provide evidence of the functional movement at such joints. Over the palm, the thenar flexion crease relates to the flexional plane of oppositional flexion of the thumb and first metacarpal. The upper palmar crease reflects the sloping plane

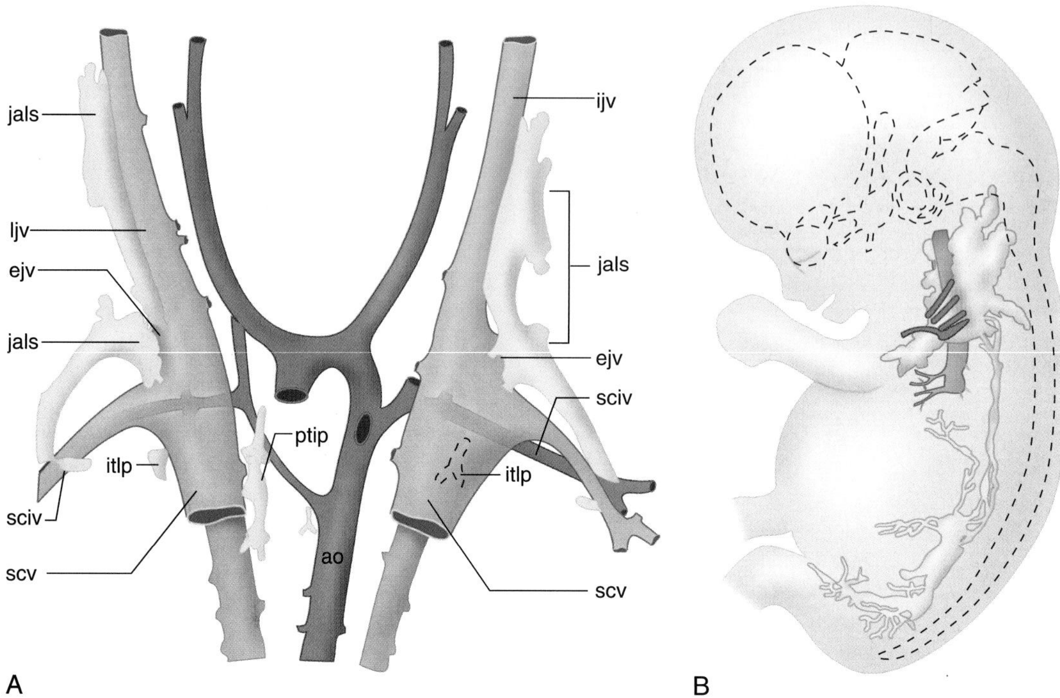

FIGURE 52.21 A, The early developing lymph channels drain into the venous system. In the cervical region the jugular lymph sac *(jals)* drains into the jugular vein *(ejv* and *ijv).* **B,** This occurs at 40 days of development, by which time the jugular and axillary lymph sacs (in yellow) empty into the jugular vein (in blue). (**A,** From van de Putte SC. The development of the lymphatic system in man. *Adv Anat Embryol.* 1975;51:1. **B,** From Töndury G, Kubik S. *Zur Ontogenese des Lymphatischen Systems. Handbuch der Allgemeinen Pathologie*. Berlin: Springer-Verlag; 1975.)

of flexional folding of the third, fourth, and fifth metacarpophalangeal joints, and the midpalmar crease simply reflects the folding plane in the skin between the other two palmar creases.[32] Small differences in the shape or form of the hand can result in a single upper palmar crease, sometimes termed a *simian crease* (Fig. 52.38A). This highly nonspecific finding is found unilaterally in 4% and bilaterally in 1% of normal individuals, and it is also observed in more than 50% of individuals with Down syndrome (trisomy 21). In 2010, Park et al. examined the palmar creases of 3216 normal Koreans and found that 12.6% had a single palmar crease, with right being more frequent then left.[33] Absent creases often reflect absent or deficient function of a flexional plane across the surface of a joint (see Fig. 52.38).[34]

Craniofacial Region

The normal formation of the brain is genetically determined. The growth of the brain in size (magnitude) and shape (direction) exerts a major mechanical impact on the form of the tissues that surround and relate to the brain in the craniofacial region.[35,36] Early neural structures have a major impact. Thus the brain affects the development of the calvarium and its sutures,[37,38] the outgrowth of the optic cup has a major impact on the development of the orbit,[39,40] the invaginating olfactory placodes are primarily responsible for the subsequent formation of the nose, and the invaginating auditory placodes form the inner ear structures and determine the orientation of the temporal wing of the sphenoid bone. The role of pressure on the regulation of craniofacial bone growth was beautifully demonstrated by comparing the orbital growth in 8-week-old kittens, which were evenly divided into three surgical groups for unilateral operations: (1) orbital evisceration alone; (2) orbital evisceration followed by a silastic implant; and (3) orbital evisceration followed by a tissue expander. Only group 3 experienced normal orbital growth, whereas group 1 showed a 23.4% reduction in size and group 2 showed a 9% reduction in size.[41] Therefore the

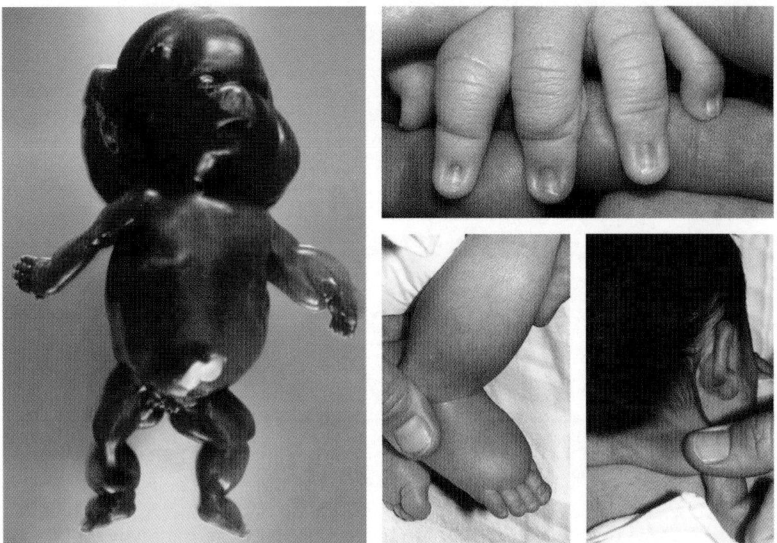

FIGURE 52.22 If there is a delay or failure in the development of the communication between the lymphatic system and the venous system, the lymphatic system distends to cause lymphedema, as is evident in this fetus with 45,X Turner syndrome. Such lymphedema is the major reason why most fetuses with Turner syndrome fail to survive. In newborn infants with Turner syndrome, the distended jugular lymph sacs result in excess skin in the lateral neck (pterygia coli). Distended lymphatic sacs can also interfere with the developing aorta, thus infants with Turner syndrome and a web neck should be closely examined for aortic coarctation. Lymph accumulation may also cause peripheral lymphedema that results in puffy hands and feet, and prior lymph accumulation may yield such residual features as loose skin in the face and a lax abdomen.

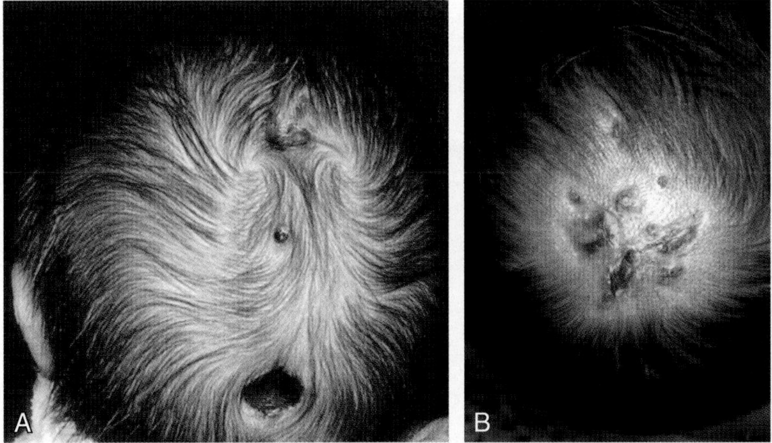

FIGURE 52.23 Small areas of vertex cutis aplasia resembling ulcerations can occur in otherwise normal newborns as an autosomal dominant trait (**A**) and in newborns with trisomy 13 syndrome (**B**). Note that these lesions tend to occur at or near the site of the parietal hair whorl, the location of maximal stretch exerted on the developing skin of the scalp by the domelike outgrowth of the brain.

statement that the "face reflects the brain" has much evidence to support it. Individual features in the craniofacial region are summarized in this section. Fig. 52.39 emphasizes the integral relationship that exists between the face and the brain. Beyond the mechanical impacts of brain development on facial form, there are indirect effects of neuromuscular function on facial form. Such effects are depicted in Figs. 52.40 and 52.41.

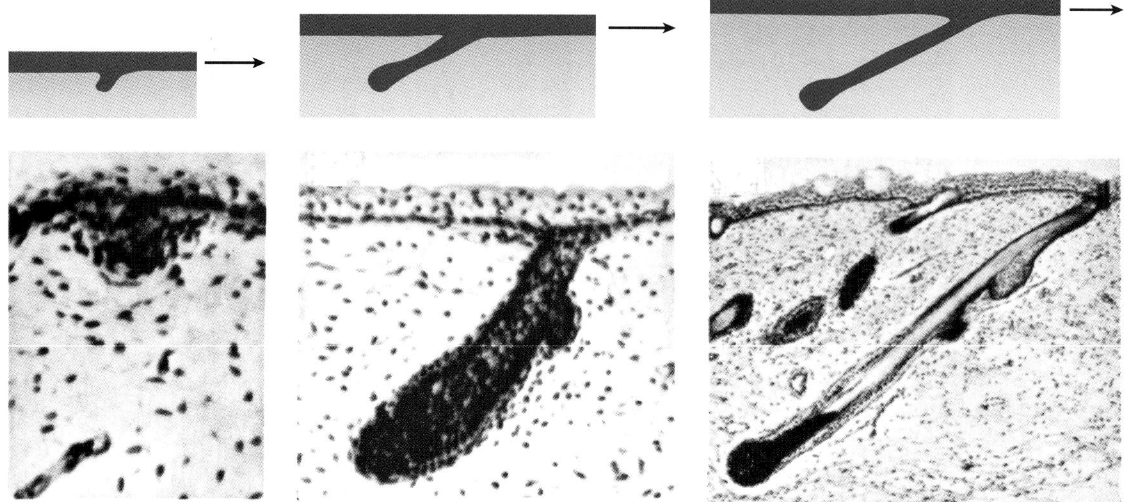

FIGURE 52.24 As a hair follicle grows downward, its direction of angulation is determined by the forces exerted via the underlying growth of the brain. These stretch forces, which are greater at the surface than in deeper tissues, affect the hair directional patterning, which is usually set by about 16 weeks. (From Smith DW, Gong BT. Scalp-hair patterning: its origin and significance relative to early brain and upper facial development. *Teratology*. 1974;9:17.)

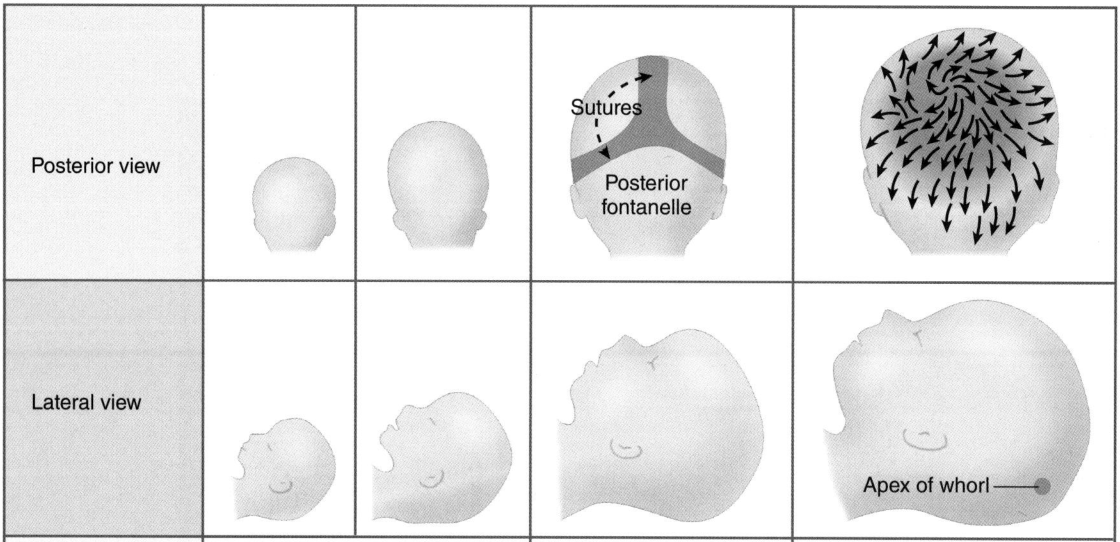 Posterior view			Sutures Posterior fontanelle	
Lateral view				Apex of whorl
Hair	Early hair follicles with sloping downgrowth		Hair being produced	Surface hair patterning evident
Gestational age	11 weeks	12 1/2 weeks	16 1/2 weeks	18 weeks
C-R length	71 mm	83 mm	122 mm	145 mm

FIGURE 52.25 The rapid domelike projection of the brain during the period of hair follicle downgrowth is evident in these proportionate drawings of the early fetal head at this time. (From Smith DW, Gong BT. Scalp-hair patterning: its origin and significance relative to early brain and upper facial development. *Teratology*. 1974;9:17.)

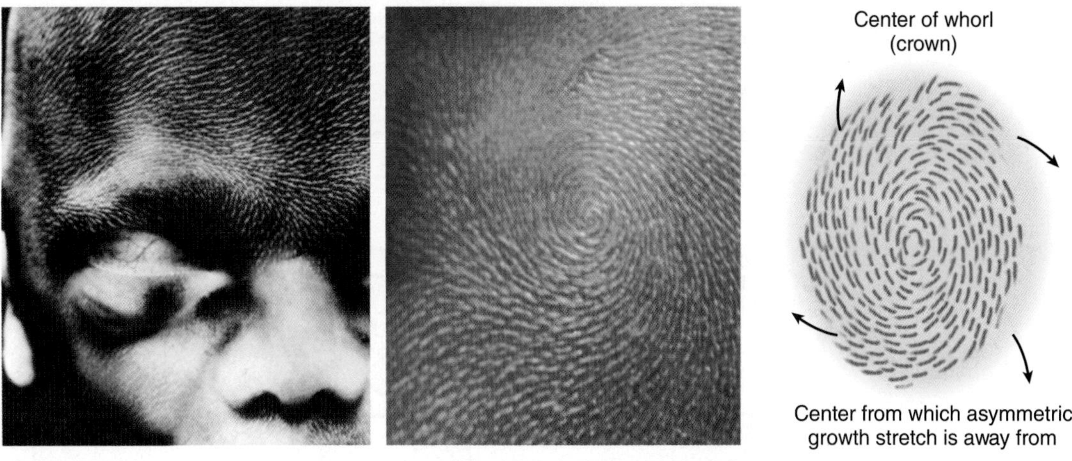

FIGURE 52.26 As the fetal hairs emerge at about 18 weeks, the hair directional patterns are beautifully evident. Over the forehead the "frontal hair stream" emanating from the fixed skin points of the ocular puncta meets with the down-sweeping parietal hair stream, which emanates from the parietal hair whorl (crown). On any expanding sphere or hemisphere there must be at least one fixed point from which all other points are moving. Presumably, it is the mild asymmetry of forces that conveys the whorl pattern. (From Smith DW, Gong BT. Scalp-hair patterning: its origin and significance relative to early brain and upper facial development. *Teratology*. 1974;9:17.)

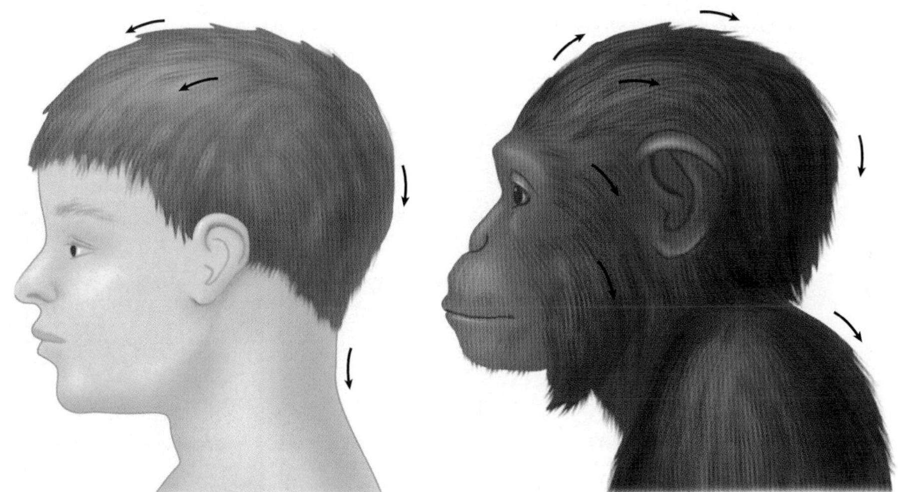

FIGURE 52.27 Head hair patterning in a boy compared with that in a young chimpanzee. In the human, the large domelike brain has generated a parietal whorl and the hair "streams" from that spot, with the parietal hair stream sweeping forward to meet with the frontal hair stream on the forehead. Because the chimpanzee has a much smaller brain, the frontal hair stream simply sweeps directly back over the head with no parietal whorl or parietal hair stream. (From Kidd W. *The Direction of Hair in Animals and Man*. London: Adam and Charles Black; 1903.)

Calvarium

The growth and shape of the brain normally determines the shape of the calvarium. Thus in the absence of problems in calvarial development, such as constraint molding or craniosynostosis, it is the brain that determines the shape of the calvarium.[38] For example, a narrow forehead means a narrow forebrain, and a brachycephalic skull (that is not excessively widened because of deformation) means a brain of short length. The organ capsule of the brain, the dura mater, is literally the mother tissue in the development of the bony calvarium and its sutures (Figs. 52.42–52.44). The

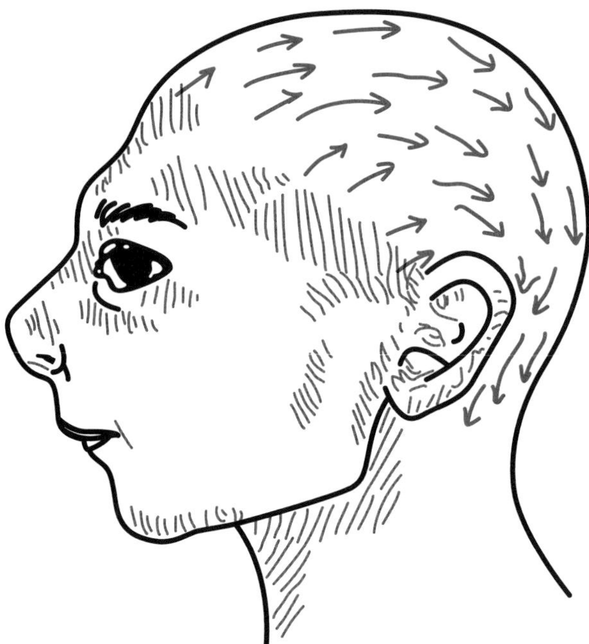

FIGURE 52.28 Child with severe microcephaly and midfacial defect. There is no parietal hair whorl, and the frontal hair stream sweeps back over the scalp in a fashion similar to that found in the chimpanzee. (Modified from Smith DW, Gong BT. Scalp-hair patterning: its origin and significance relative to early brain and upper facial development. *Teratology*. 1974;9:17. Illustration by Zen Sanchez.)

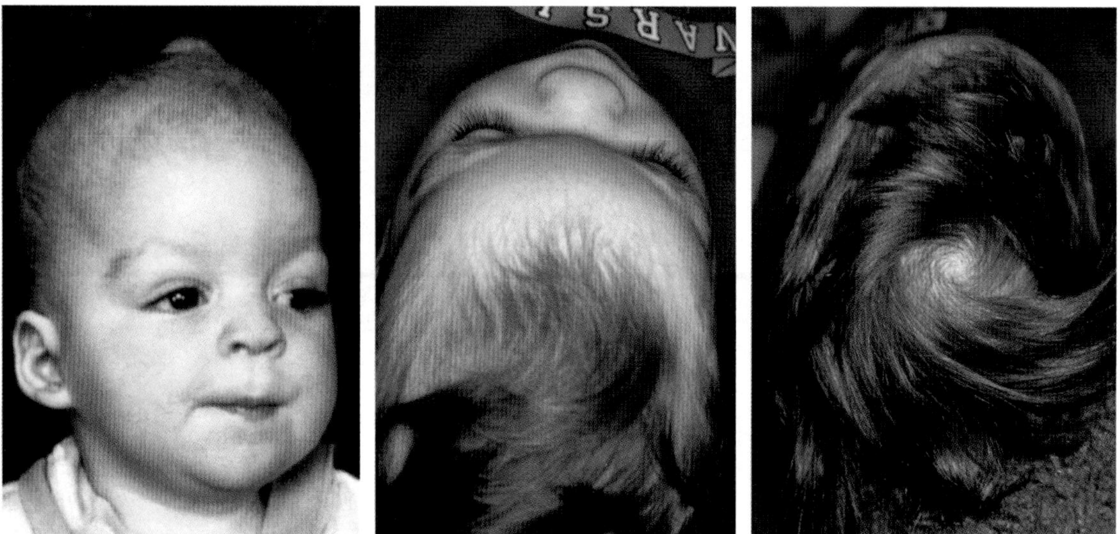

FIGURE 52.29 This profoundly intellectually disabled child was exposed to 40- to 60-mg Accutane per day from the 2nd through the 20th week of gestation and had microcephaly, a brain hamartoma protruding from the scalp, and a markedly altered scalp hair pattern.

calvarium consists of bony plates joined by strips of unmineralized dura, the sutures. These sutures relate directly to the form of the early brain and reflect dural folds into the surface of the brain. As the brain grows, it stretches the overlying dura mater. The brain is not a smooth hemisphere, and dural reflections occur into

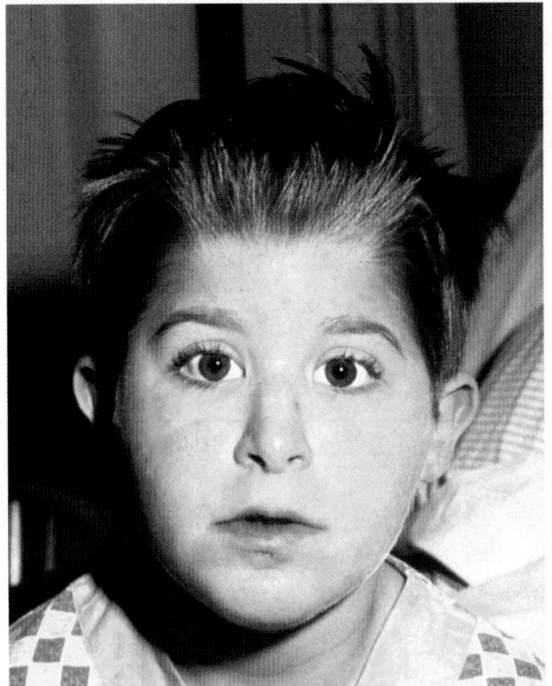

FIGURE 52.30 Frontal brain deficiency may result in the frontal hair stream sweeping upward into the scalp region and giving rise to a frontal upsweep, more commonly referred to as a "cowlick." This occurs in mild degrees in about 3% of normal individuals. This figure represents an unusual degree in a child with Rubinstein-Taybi syndrome. (From Smith DW, Gong BT. Scalp-hair patterning: its origin and significance relative to early brain and upper facial development. *Teratology*. 1974;9:17.)

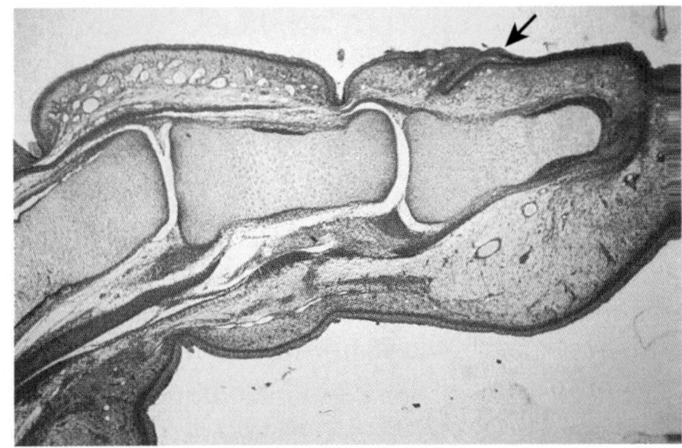

FIGURE 52.31 Longitudinal section of the finger in an 11-week fetus showing the orientation of the early nail plate *(arrow)* to the distal phalanx. The growing cells of the nail plate become a keratinized nail that generally reflects the form of the underlying distal bony phalanx. (Courtesy of Gian Töndury, University of Zürich, Zürich, Switzerland.)

the recesses of the brain. These dural reflections are shown in Figs. 52.42 and 52.43. Normally, no ossification overlies these dural reflections if brain growth stretch continues (see Fig. 52.44), and these are the usual sites of the sutures.[37] The metopic and sagittal sutures relate to the sites of the dural reflections into the interhemispheric fissure and the falx cerebri. The lambdoid sutures relate to the sites of the dural reflection between the cerebrum and cerebellum, the falx cerebelli. The coronal sutures relate to the insular sulci of the brain, with its dural reflections off the sphenoid wings, which faithfully fills in this sulcus in the brain.[37] Between the sites of dural reflection, ossification begins within the membranous dura as niduses of ossification spread outward toward the sites of the sutures. The radial orientation of the spreading ossification appears to relate to tensile forces within the dura. At the sites of initial ossification in the calvarium, there may be small external promontories, which are most evident in infancy and childhood. These promontories may be noted toward the center of each frontal bone, each parietal bone, and each lateral portion of the occipital bone. They appear to be normal features. The major era for the early development of the calvarium is from 12 to 16 weeks. In areas of the developing calvarium where the stretch forces may be diminished, such as in the region of the parietal bone near the posterior fontanel and along the lambdoid sutures, multiple small centers of ossification may develop and then coalesce. These are referred to as *Wormian bones*.[42] When posterior occipital pressure occurs because of molding or when the skull is demineralized, the dura may become relaxed, and Wormian bones will form in increased numbers, especially within the posterior sutures.

The implication of these principles is that early brain form determines the sites of dural reflections and thereby the location of sutures. This thesis is supported by aberrations of early brain morphogenesis that give rise to altered dural reflections and thereby affect the location of sutures, as shown in Figs. 52.45 and 52.46. The sutures of the calvarium may be altered by several means, including primary defects of brain morphogenesis, problems in suture development, genetic syndromes, metabolic problems, and external constraint (primarily nulliparity, plurality, macrosomia).[43] A serious deficit of brain growth with a lack of growth stretch at suture sites, whether owing to primary microcephaly or overshunted hydrocephalus, may allow for mineralization of one or more sutures.[44,45] This secondary craniosynostosis may then

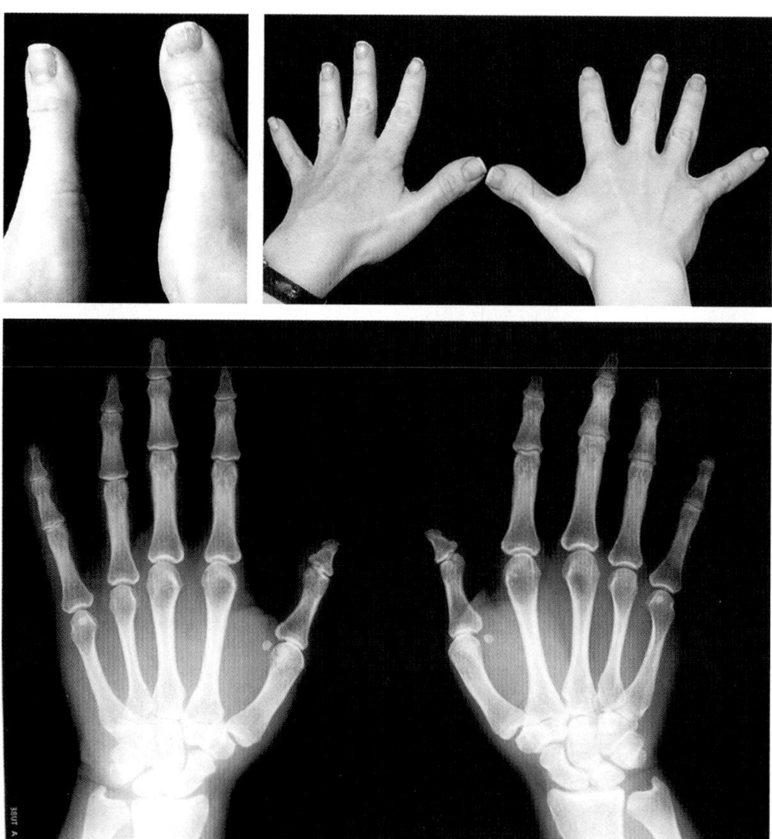

FIGURE 52.32 This figure compares the short, wide distal nail and phalanx in the thumb of a woman with brachydactyly D (an autosomal dominant trait) with that of a normal woman *(left)*.

lead to further problems. A primary defect of brain formation may affect the presence or site of dural reflections and thus the presence and site of the sutures. One example is holoprosencephaly, in which a primary failure of diverticulation of the two cerebral vesicles may result in a single cerebral ventricle and no interhemispheral fissure. This is usually, but not always, accompanied by the lack of a metopic suture (see Fig. 52.46).[46]

External constraint of the developing fetal head may result in a lack of growth stretch at a given suture, thereby causing craniosynostosis (see Chapters 29–34). This appears to be a common cause for this problem.[43,47] The impact of craniosynostosis on craniofacial form depends on the age of onset of sutural closure and the suture(s) involved. Sagittal craniosynostosis limits lateral growth of the calvarium, resulting in a narrow, elongated, scaphocephalic head shape. Coronal synostosis limits anteroposterior growth, resulting in a short and wide (brachycephalic) head shape. Early coronal synostosis also prevents the forward growth of the brain and hence the anterior growth of the cranial base. Because the cranial base is the roof of the face, the midface tends to be retrusive, the orbits become shallow, the eyes become more widely spaced, and the forehead becomes high and wide.

Craniosynostosis of both the sagittal and coronal sutures will limit the capacity for brain growth and will usually result in increased intracranial pressure. Radiographs of the skull may show a "beaten-copper" appearance, partially because of a more vertical orientation of the bone fibrils within the calvarium, which tend to align in relation to the altered stress forces. The head tends to become tower shaped, which leads to oxycephaly, acrocephaly, or turricephaly. The head is quite malleable, especially during fetal life. This is a normal and obviously necessary phenomenon during vaginal delivery. During delivery, the bony plates of

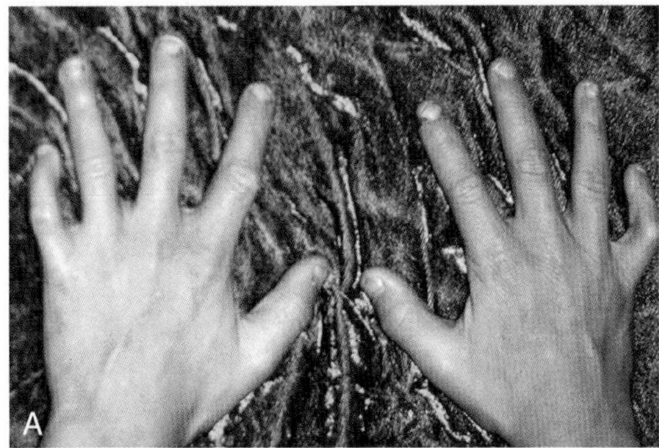

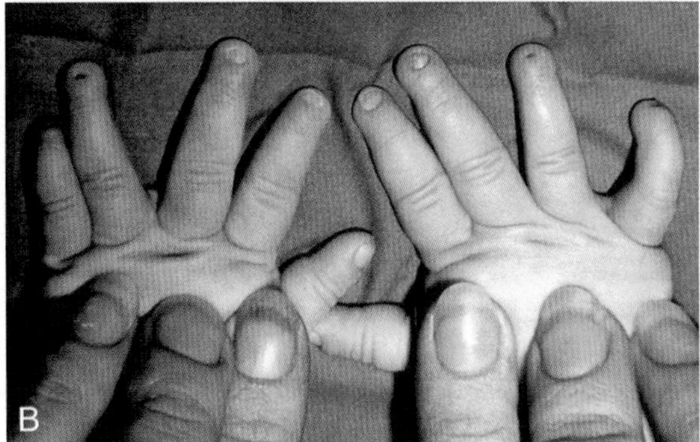

FIGURE 52.33 Distal phalangeal and nail hypoplasia in the hands of a person with fetal alcohol syndrome (**A**) and fetal hydantoin syndrome (**B**).

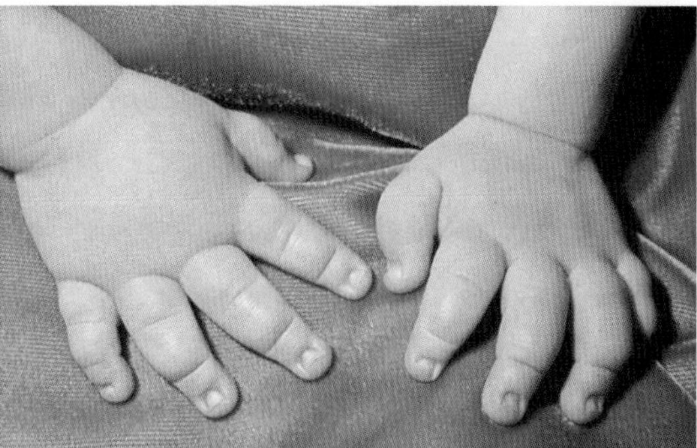

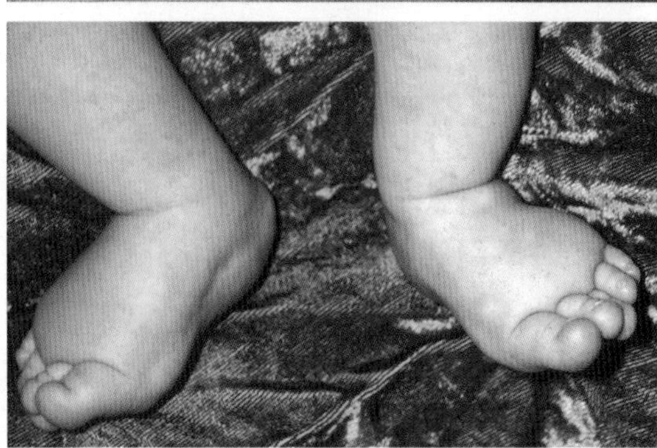

FIGURE 52.34 Fetal lymphedema may distort the form of the nails, as exemplified in a newborn with peripheral lymphedema caused by Turner syndrome. The narrow, hyperconvex nails with the appearance of a deep-set nail base are the residual consequences of prior lymphedema.

the calvarium overlap at the sutures, sometimes to a surprising degree. Such normal vertex molding is usually transient and limited in duration to a few days. Prolonged uterine constraint with compression of the fetal head during late fetal life may give rise to deformations of the head that usually slowly resolve over time; cases of extensive molding may require management to achieve a more normal resolution.[48]

Cranial Base

The anterior cranial base develops from cartilage that becomes ossified, with persisting growth centers posterior and anterior to the sella turcica. The region anterior to the sella turcica, which is designated as the anterior cranial base, tends to grow forward in accordance with frontal brain growth. Hence cranial base growth parallels normal brain growth. The modern human brain is only 25% of its adult size at birth and continues to grow at a rapid rate throughout the first year of life, when it reaches 50% of its adult size.[49] Human brains are 95% of adult size by 10 years of age. In comparison, a chimpanzee brain is already 40% of its adult size by birth and reaches 80% of the adult volume by the end of the first year. A 1-year-old *Homo erectus* brain was closer to apes in its growth pattern, measuring 72% to 84% of adult size at that age, which implies differences in the development of *Homo erectus'* cognitive abilities when compared with modern humans.[49] It is important to appreciate that the anterior cranial base is the roof of the face, from which the maxilloethmoid complex projects downward to form the anterior portion of the nasal bridge. A deficit of frontal brain growth may yield a shorter cranial base and a less prominent nasal bridge. A shorter cranial base will generally yield a flatter facial profile with a tendency toward a hypoplastic, retrusive midface.

Eyes

Early outpouchings from the diencephalon, the optic cups, induce the formation of the lenses in the overlying ectoderm; thus begins the formation of the eye.

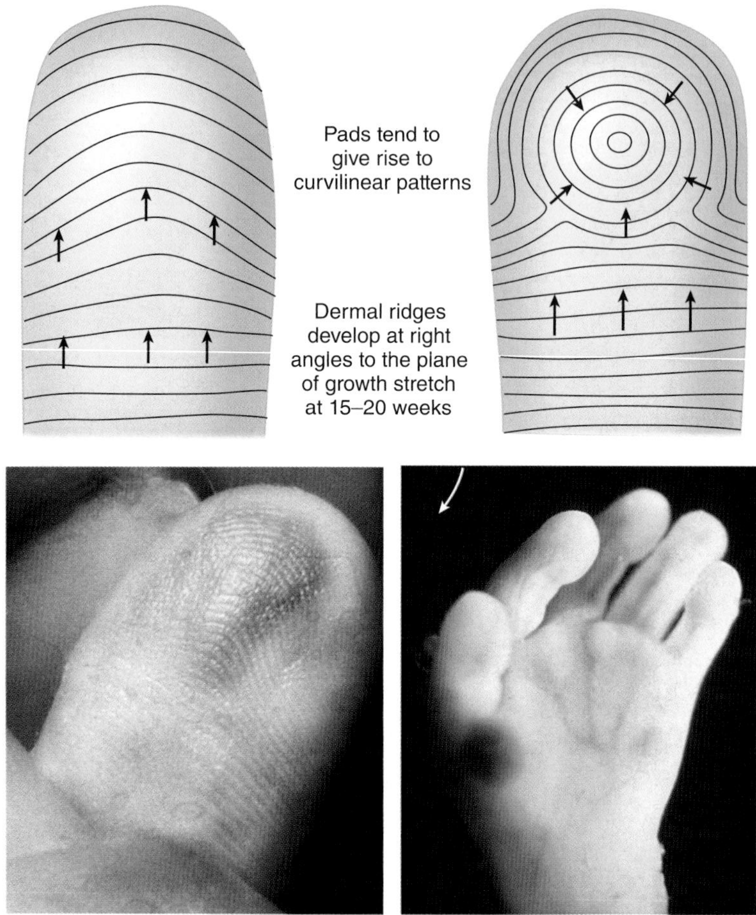

FIGURE 52.35 The dermal ridges tend to develop at right angles to the growth stretch exerted on the skin by the development of the underlying tissues. Where there are pads, such as those shown in the fingertips and interdigital areas of the palm of an 8.5-week fetus *(right)*, the result is the development of curvilinear ridge patterns.

Zones of periocular hair growth suppression determine the frontal hair pattern and are strongly influenced by the size and location of the eyes (Fig. 52.47). Surrounding mesenchymal cells condense to form the globular eye capsule within which the collagen fibrils align in relation to fluid pressure from within the eye. Around the eye, the mesenchymal tissues condense to form the bony orbit, which conforms to and is shaped in relation to the eye.[39] Excessive fluid pressure within the eye may result in increased glaucoma. This tends to distort the shape of the tense eye toward increased anterior globular prominence. It may also result in cloudiness of the cornea and destructive changes within the eye, which can lead to eventual blindness. A small eye (microphthalmia) yields a small orbit. A lack of any optic cup results in no orbit, and loss of an eye in early childhood arrests orbital growth unless a tissue expander is maintained in the eye socket.[39,40] The accessory tissues around the eye, which consist of muscles, lacrimal ducts, eyebrows, eyelids, and eyelashes, all relate to the development of the early optic cup.[39] For example, an altered position of the early orbit is accompanied by predictable secondary development of all these accessory structures in relation to the aberrant position of the optic vesicle (see Fig. 52.47).

Ears

The different parts of the ear are derived from different areas of the developing embryo, as follows:

1. *Inner ear*: The otic placode, which is neural tissue, invaginates from the surface ectoderm to become

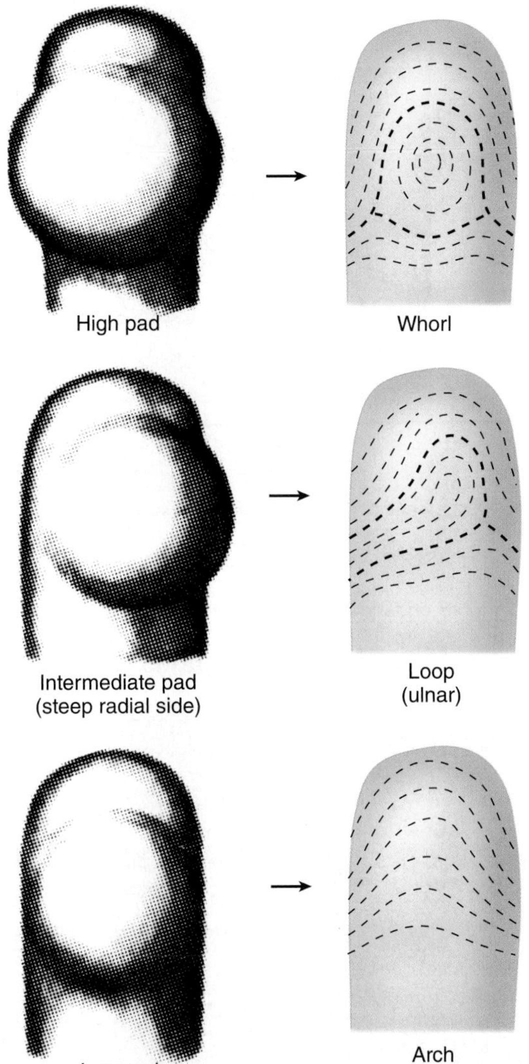

FIGURE 52.36 The fingertip dermal ridge patterning appears to relate to the form of the fingertip pads at the time of development of the dermal ridges. (From Mulvihill JJ, Smith DW. Genesis of dermatoglyphics. *J Pediatr*. 1969;75:579.)

the otocyst. The differential growth of the otocyst leads to the spiral form of the cochlea and the form of the vestibular apparatus. The mesenchyme around the otic placode is induced to form cartilage that faithfully conforms to its shape and exerts a major role in the development of the sphenoid wing.

2. *Middle ear*: The derivatives of the second and third branchial arches form the malleus, incus, and stapes as a connecting functional link between the tympanic membrane and the round window of the cochlea, thus transmitting auditory vibrations to the cochlea. Any ankylosis within the joints between these bones may result in conductive hearing loss.
3. *External ear*: The external auricle forms from the cartilaginous cores of the six auricular hillocks, which blend into a sheet of cartilage that grows throughout life. Mild to moderate deformations of the external auricle are common in the newborn because of constraint of the pliable auricle in late fetal life. Oligohydramnios accentuates such deformation and may result in an "accordion" ear and/or an ear that is enlarged and flattened against the skull. The shoulder may be pressed up under the auricle in such situations as breech presentation, resulting in uplifting of the lower auricle. These distortions tend to resolve toward normal form after birth and are benign deformations. Localized compression that affects one ear more than the other may result in overgrowth of the compressed ear.[50] Distended jugular lymph sacs, such as frequently occurs in the fetus with Turner syndrome, may distort the auricles, making them more prominent and slanted than usual (see Fig. 52.22).[25]

The position and form of the cartilaginous folds of the auricle relate largely to the sites of insertion and origin of the auricular muscles.[51] Therefore some defects in the form of the external auricle may be the consequence of aberrant development and/or function of particular ear muscles (Fig. 52.48). Absence of the posterior auricular ear muscle, which normally holds the ear against the calvarium, results in a protruding auricle. On the other hand, absence of the superior auricular ear muscle results in a folded-over "lop" ear that may appear low in placement. The inner conchal plical folds appear to relate to the intrinsic auricular ear muscles, and defects in their development may result in varying degrees of a simplified conchal form. Experimental studies in the rodent have shown that early denervation of the seventh nerve, which supplies the auricular ear muscles, will result in a simple auricle that lacks the usual conchal folds. Similar defects are seen with the ears in CHARGE syndrome (coloboma, heart disease, atresia choanae, curtailed growth and development, genital hypoplasia, and ear anomalies and/or hearing loss) resulting from seventh nerve weakness. With profound muscular hypotonia or lax connective tissues, the ears may protrude (Fig. 52.49).

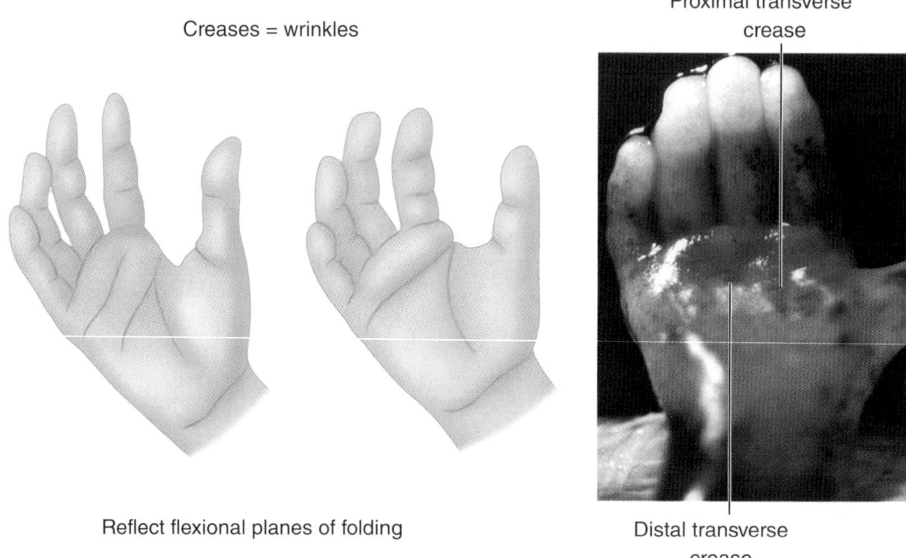

FIGURE 52.37 Creases relate to flexional planes of folding, always being secondary to mechanical forces. The upper palmar crease relates to the sloping plane of folding of the third, fourth, and fifth metacarpophalangeal joints, the thenar crease relates to the flexion of the thenar region, and the midpalmar crease represents the folding plane between these two.

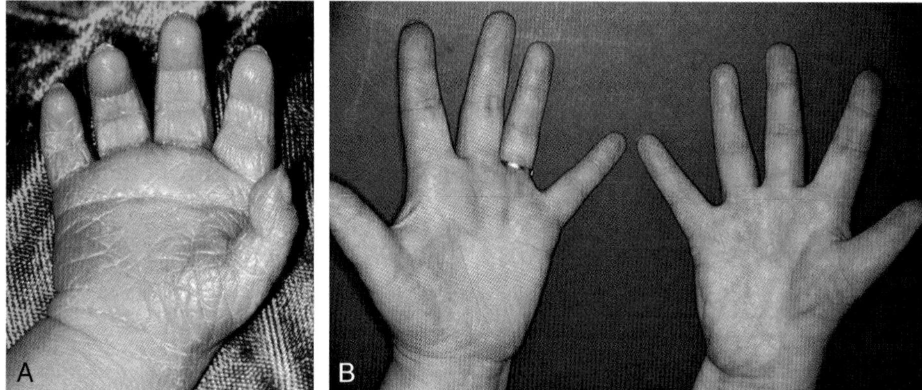

FIGURE 52.38 **A,** Minor differences in the form of the hand in Down syndrome can result in a single crease across the upper palm (simian crease). This hand also has a short fifth finger and a single crease as a consequence. **B,** These hands have absent or hypoplastic thenar creases with absent interphalangeal thumb creases, indicating a functional deficit in oppositional flexional folding of the thenar region (which was inherited as a variably expressed autosomal dominant trait).

Nose and Nasopharynx

The neural olfactory pits invaginate from the surface ectoderm and then send axons to synapse with those of the olfactory lobes. Later, when the base of the skull becomes cartilage and bone, these axons create the sites of "perforation" in the cribriform plate. Around the edges of the olfactory pit, the medial and lateral nasal swellings rapidly grow out and coalesce with the maxillary swelling to form much of the external nose and fuse inferiorly to form the upper lip. The invaginating olfactory pits meet posteriorly with the foregut, and the epithelium between them breaks down, thus providing a communication between the nasal and oral cavities. The cartilaginous nasal septum is in direct continuity with the anterior base of the skull, and hence alterations in growth of the base of the skull may secondarily affect nasal morphogenesis. The fusion of the maxillary

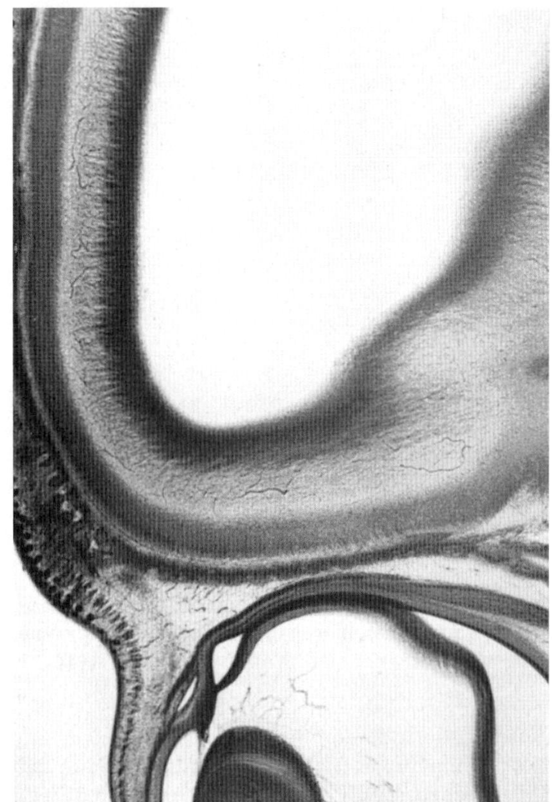

FIGURE 52.39 At 10 weeks, the cerebrum, which has only one cortical layer at this stage, is molding the forehead. The upper face is influenced by the early brain derivatives, the eyes. The mesenchymal tissues will soon condense and organize the supportive skeletal framework in accordance with these neural tissues. The growth of the cranial base anterior to the pituitary will occur in relationship to the frontal growth of the brain.

palatal shelves and the nasal septum separates the nasal cavity from the mouth proper. Cartilaginous plates develop in the ala nasi, which have muscle attachments that allow for constriction of the nares. Within the nose, the cartilaginous turbinates grow, and evaginations from the nasal cavity invade the surrounding bone. These evaginations become sinuses, which aerate the surrounding bones. This substantially reduces their weight while still providing excellent structural support. Sinus development is largely incomplete at birth. The first pharyngeal pouch persists as the eustachian tube and middle ear. Evaginations from the middle ear aerate the mastoid portion of the temporal bone, in a fashion like that of the sinuses.

Late uterine constraint may distort the nose. Most commonly it becomes compressed to one side during the neonate's transition through the birth canal. After birth, this usually resolves spontaneously, although some manual pulling and remolding may be merited. Persisting compression may limit the growth of the nose, as in a face presentation. However, postnatal catch-up growth will usually result in a restoration toward normal form. As previously mentioned, aberrations of the growth of the cranial base, such as occur with problems of frontal brain growth, may alter both the relative position of the nasal bridge and the size and form of the nose. Problems with the development and/or function of the musculature of the ala nasi may result in a narrow nose with small alar wings. The sinuses tend to extend well into the solid bone that surrounds them. If there is a loss of permanent teeth from the upper jaw, the maxillary sinus will extend farther than usual, coming into proximity with the alveolar ridge at the sites of the missing teeth.

Palate and Tongue

The palatal shelves, which initially project downward alongside the tongue, undergo a shift into their horizontal position and then fuse from front to back with each other and with the nasal septum. If the mandible is unusually small, there may be posterior displacement of the tongue, which will tend to occlude closure of the palatal shelves, giving rise to a U-shaped soft palatal defect (Fig. 52.50).[52] The posteriorly displaced tongue may obstruct the posterior pharynx, giving rise to partial upper airway obstruction at birth. The initiating problem in mandibular size may be a malformation, and thus the consequences are termed the *early micrognathia malformation sequence* or the *Robin malformation sequence*.[53] Among 175 children with Robin sequence, 45 of 45 (100%) children with Robin sequence without cleft palate were classified as syndromic, while 83 of 130 (64%) children with Robin sequence with cleft palate were classified as syndromic.[54] Therefore Robin sequence is etiologically heterogeneous, and a review of 39 articles revealed 56% of the cases were syndromic, 22% were associated with other malformations, and the remaining cases were nonsyndromic. Genetic mutations were found in 31% of the 300 cases, with *SOX9* the most common gene associated with both syndromic and nonsyndromic Robin sequence.[55] The small mandible could also be the result of early fetal constraint with limitation of mandibular growth (in such an instance the anomaly

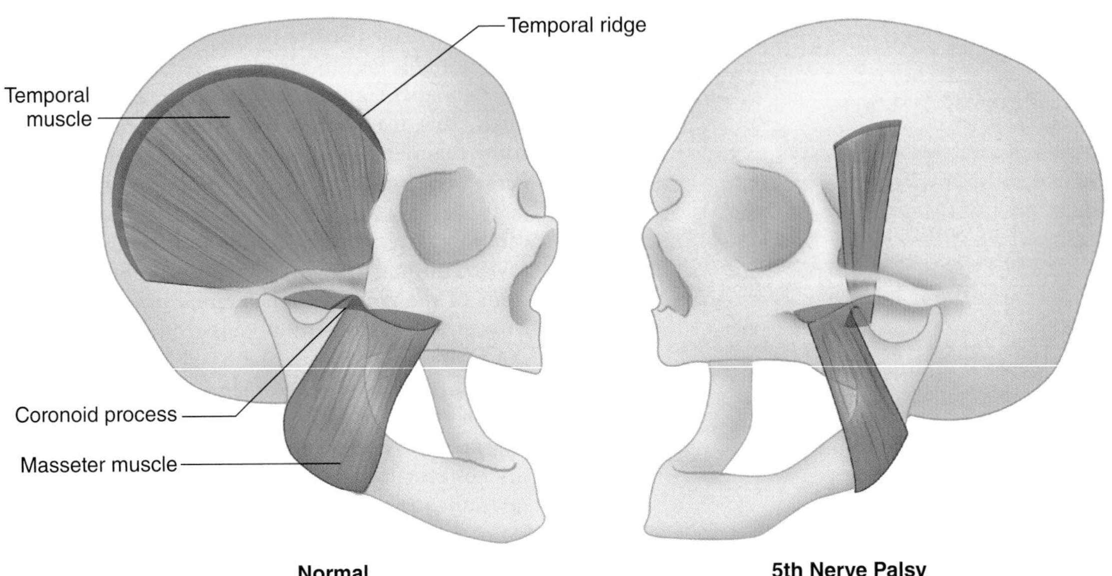

FIGURE 52.40 Mechanical force relationships between function and form as illustrated in a 60-year-old man who had unilateral fifth nerve palsy from early in life. On the affected side the facial muscles are quite small, and all the sites of muscle attachment were less prominent on the affected side.

could be termed the *early micrognathia deformation sequence*), which possibly explains why isolated Robin sequence is associated with twinning and discordantly expressed.[56] Not only does the tongue play a significant mechanical role in palatal closure, but it also exerts a major impact on palatal form. Normally lateral palatine ridges extend from the palate on the lingual side of the alveolar ridges (Fig. 52.51).[57] These ridges are prominent in fetal life and are composed of mucopolysaccharide-rich connective tissue and numerous small salivary glands. The force of tongue thrust tends to smooth out these ridges during fetal life. Any disorder that limits tongue thrust into the palate (e.g., hypotonia, other neurologic deficits, or microglossia) will result in prominent lateral palatine ridges (see Fig. 52.51), often giving the appearance of a narrow, high-arched palate. At the other extreme, an enlarged tongue may result in relative flattening and broadening of the hard palate. Thus the tongue, a very strong muscle, exerts a major impact on the palate.

Alveolar Ridge, Teeth, and Mandible

The tooth anlagen develop as ectodermal downgrowths that interact with the underlying mesenchyme to form the teeth, which then erupt, usually through the channel of their original downgrowth. If there is a failure of tooth development, then the alveolar ridge lacks prominence at that region. Thus the major mass of the alveolar ridges relates to the presence of teeth. The form of the enamel and the crown of a tooth, which is produced by the ectodermal component, are genetically determined, and they allow for interdigitation between the upper and lower teeth. The forces of biting and chewing tend to foster alignment of the teeth. The growth of the mandible tends to follow the lead of the upper jaw. This applies to lateral growth as well. Thus if the maxilla is narrow, the mandible also tends to be narrow. If there is a deficit of mandibular function, the mandible will slow its growth rate and remain hypoplastic. The muscles of the mandible are powerful, and their sites of attachment give rise to bony promontories. Fig. 52.40 shows the impact of a unilateral fifth nerve palsy on these muscles and therefore on the bony form of the face. The impact of the facial muscles on bony promontories is dramatically exemplified by experimental studies in rodents. For example, early resection of the masseter muscle results in a complete lack of the coronoid process, its site of insertion on the mandible (Fig. 52.52). If the teeth are crowded, one or more may erupt in an aberrant alignment. Usually the easiest management is removal of the "crowded-out" tooth. Malalignment of the teeth is common, and orthodontic methods of constraint

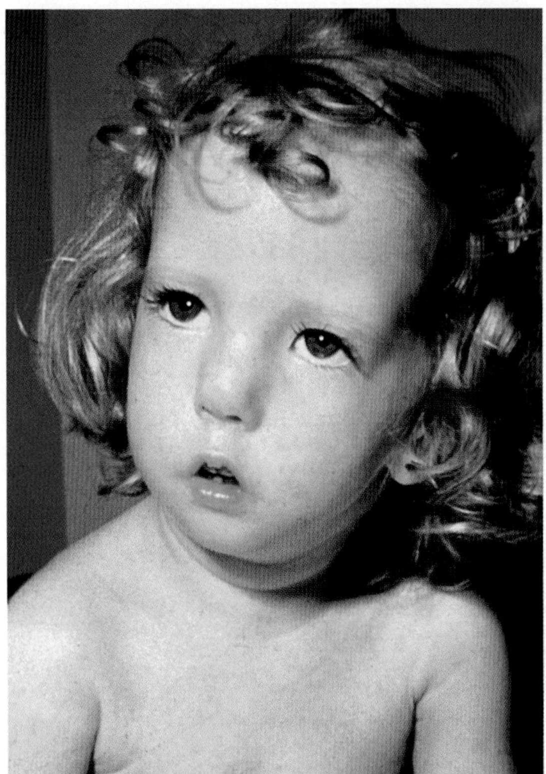

FIGURE 52.41 This girl is lacking sixth and seventh nerve function (Möbius malformation sequence). The facial impact is secondary to the long-standing deficit of forces in the developing face. The almond-shaped eye is interpreted as being secondary to a deficiency of orbicularis oculi function, the small alae nasae to a deficit in the muscles that attach to this cartilage, and the small mouth to a lack of orbicularis oris muscle function. The shallow temporal region is ascribed to weakness of the temporal muscle, the shallow malar region to deficit of masseter function, and the small mandible to a diminished function of the mandible.

have become a common practice for the realignment of teeth and jaws during childhood.

Thorax and Lung

The growth of the ribs and thoracic cage is integral to the normal development of the lungs. The lungs develop as progressive arborizations from outbuddings of the foregut. The septation of the thoracic and abdominal cavities by the diaphragm allows the fetus to make respiratory movements. Adequate growth of the thoracic cage is important during the latter phases of lung development, when the lung progresses from a solid organ tissue to one with alveolar sacs capable of aeration. Restrictive crowding of the lungs during late fetal lung growth may result in the lung being incompletely developed by birth, causing respiratory insufficiency at birth. Deficient lung growth may be caused by several different causes, as summarized in Table 52.2. External constraint of an unusual degree, such as may occur within a bicornuate uterus, may cause thoracic restriction (Fig. 45.3). With oligohydramnios, the lack of fluid within the developing lung combined with early constraint to thoracic growth impairs normal lung development (Fig. 46.7).[58,59] Consequently, respiratory insufficiency is the predominant cause of death in newborn babies affected by the oligohydramnios deformation sequence. Crowding of the lung during growth may be intrinsic, as in diaphragmatic hernia, which allows variable amounts of the abdominal contents to gain access to the thoracic cavity, thereby limiting the capacity for normal lung growth. Hence, the newborn with a diaphragmatic hernia may die of respiratory insufficiency, even if diaphragmatic repair is performed promptly to displace the abdominal contents from the thoracic cage soon after birth. Because of this problem, fetal surgery for diaphragmatic hernia has helped to improve survival by allowing for more normal lung development. The thoracic cage is malleable and may show alterations of form in relation to constraint. If the fetus has its chin forced into the chest, for example, there may be both a small mandible and a mild "impression" on the chest wall.

Cardiovascular

The early heart tubes fuse to become one tube, which then undergoes further morphogenesis to become the four-chambered heart. The growth of specific ridges within the developing heart gives rise to the separations between the blood channels and the development of the valves. Thus the growth of the atrioventricular cushions assists in the separation of the atria and ventricles and the formation of the tricuspid and mitral valves. The growth of the conotruncal pads separates the single outlet truncus into the aorta and pulmonary arteries with the development of aortic and pulmonary valves. Throughout cardiac morphogenesis the direction and force of the streams of blood play a major role in the development of cardiac form. For example, the blood coming from the placenta through the ductus venosus flows across the right atrium and maintains the patency of the foramen ovale, directly shunting the blood into the left atrium. As soon as

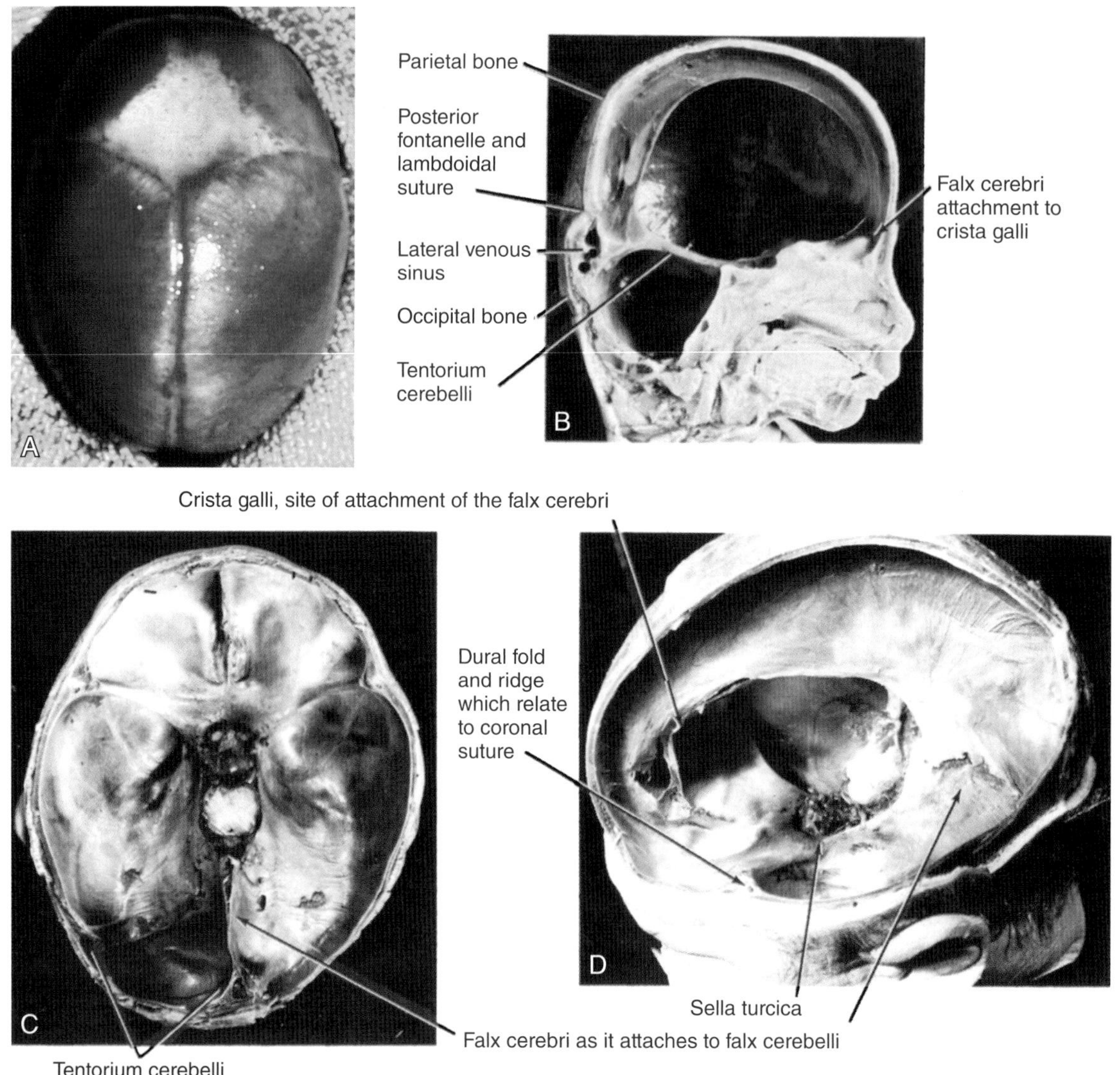

FIGURE 52.42 **A,** The calvarium in a 20-week fetus shows the anterior fontanelle and sutures. The dural reflections, which relate mechanically to the recesses in the developing brain, are shown in a 16-week fetus (**B**) and in a term baby (**C** and **D**). Note how the lines of growth stretch are evident in the alignment of collagen fibrils within the dura. (Courtesy Prof. Gian Töndury, University of Zürich, Zürich, Switzerland.)

placental blood flow ceases at birth, other changes occur, such as closure of the ductus arteriosus and the increase in blood flow to the pulmonary vascular bed. The direction and magnitude of blood flow changes result in the closure of the foramen ovale.

Any anatomic change in early heart development usually has a major effect on subsequent cardiac morphogenesis by changing the biomechanics within the developing heart. For example, a ventricular septal defect results in excessive shunting of blood into the right ventricle and the pulmonary system, thus causing enlargement of the right ventricle. The excessive pressure on the pulmonary circulation eventually causes increased vascular resistance, further increasing the load on the right ventricle, which may then begin to fail in its function. Early intervention, with

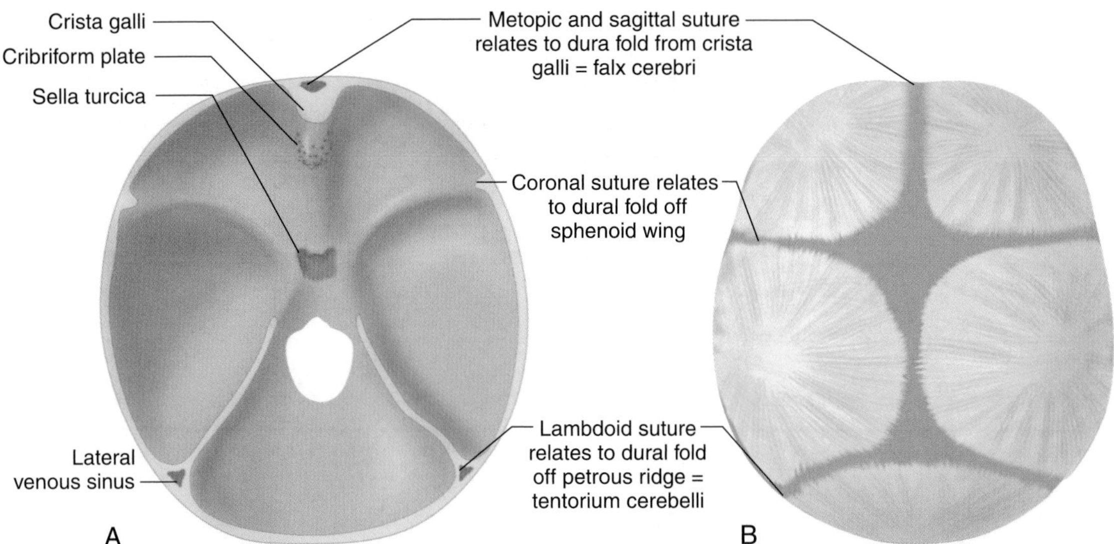

FIGURE 52.43 Conceptual drawing of a 17-week fetus, by which time the early calvarium is formed. **A,** The basilar view shows the sites of dural reflection from the crista galli, sphenoid wings, and petrous ridges. These dural reflections are the sites of passive sutural development, as shown on the right. **B,** The top view of the early calvarium shows how ossification begins in the central spots between the dural reflections and spreads centrifugally toward the sutures. (From Smith DW, Töndury G. Origins of the calvarium and its sutures. *Am J Dis Child.* 1978;132:662.)

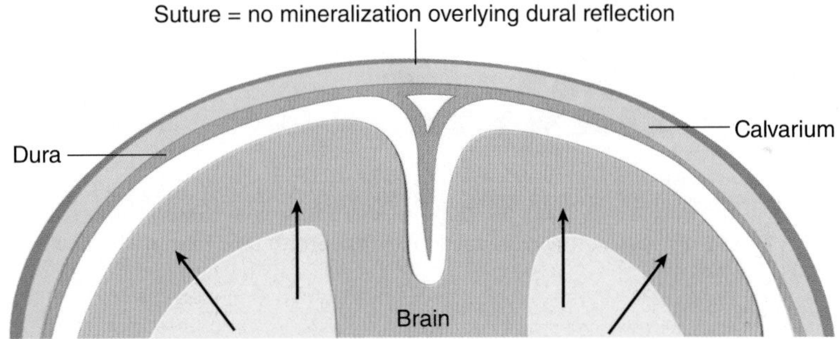

FIGURE 52.44 As long as there is continued growth stretch from the expanding brain, the sites over the dural reflections remain unossified, thereby forming the sutures.

closure of the ventricular septal defect, may prevent such biomechanical consequences, all of which may be interpreted as *deformations* in the cardiovascular system. Interference with the early flow patterns may be a primary cause for problems in cardiac morphogenesis. Lwigale et al. produced altered morphology and abolished contractions in chick embryos by placing them in a centrifuge for 18 hours during early cardiac morphogenesis.[60] These cardiac defects were presumed to be the consequence of alterations in cardiac flow patterns during this critical time in heart development. Similar alterations in chick heart morphogenesis have been induced by Clark, using mechanical alterations in early vascular flow patterns.[61,62] The peripheral blood vessels develop as a coalescence of multiple small lacunae into vessels. Initially there tends to be a general network of small vessels. The magnitude and direction of flow will result in enlargement of some of these minute vessels in a particular direction, whereas a diminished flow will result in regression of vessels. Hence the vascular patterns develop to a major extent in relation to the needs of a particular region and to its form. If there is

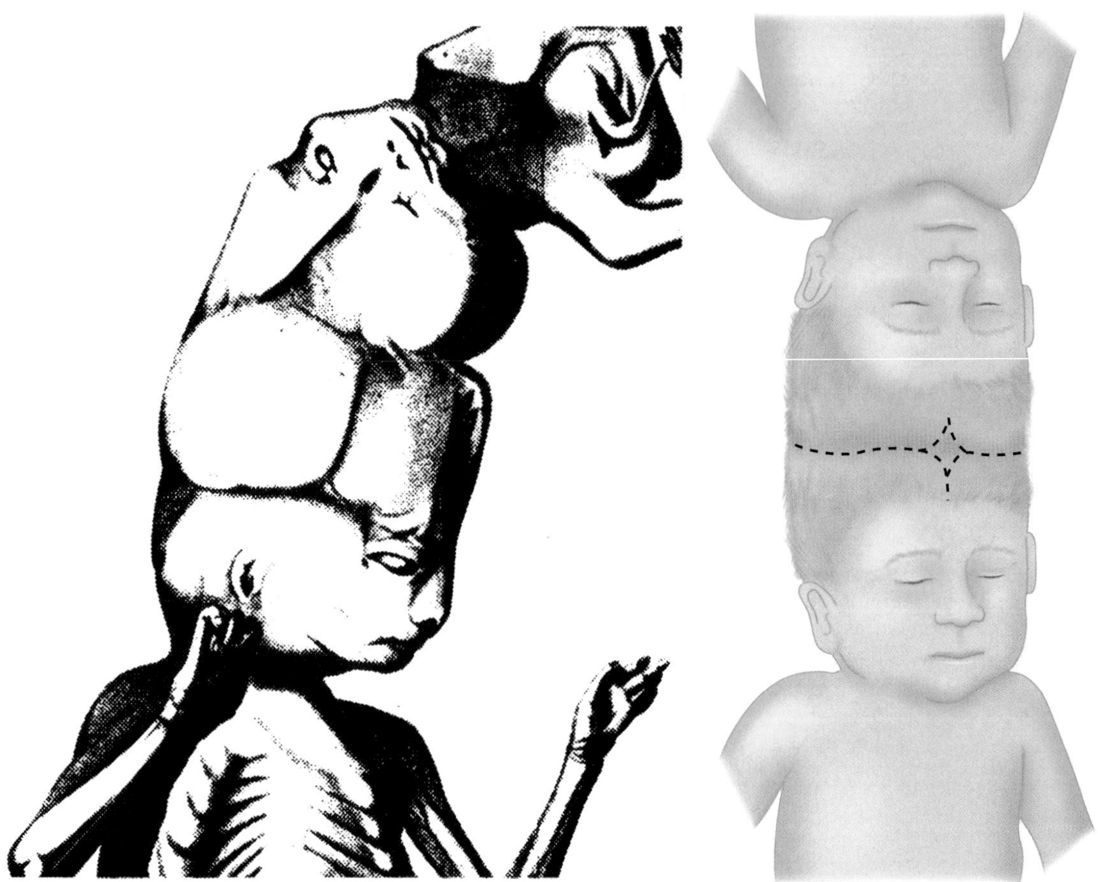

FIGURE 52.45 Conjoined twins provide an experiment of nature to demonstrate that the suture sites relate to the dural reflections. At the sites of juncture of the two brains, there are dural reflections, and at these locations sutures and fontanelles are observed in positions where they would not normally be present. (From Smith DW, Töndury G. Origins of the calvarium and its sutures. *Am J Dis Child*. 1978;132:662.)

hypoplasia of a region, the vascular channels in that region are generally smaller than usual.

Intestines

The endoderm outpouches in a forward direction as the foregut, and in a posterior direction as the hindgut. As the intestines enlarge, they extend beyond the abdominal wall into the allantoic sac and then later return to the abdominal cavity. This enlargement gives rise to multiple folding of the gut and to overall rotation of the midgut, such that the cecum ends up in the right lower quadrant. The capsule of the intestine, the peritoneum, follows this rotation and then becomes fixed to the inner abdominal wall at certain points. An incomplete rotation of the gut results in unusual mesenteric attachments and increases the liability toward volvulus of the midgut. Any obstruction of the intestine will alter mechanics within the gut, giving rise to distension of the proximal gut and changes in the bowel wall. The distal segment, being less distended, will be unusually small in caliber.

Urinary Tract and Kidneys

The early mesonephric ridges have a longitudinal series of nephron elements that drain into a common mesonephric duct. Toward the lower end of this duct an outpouching occurs, which is termed the *ureteral bud*. This induces the formation of glomeruli

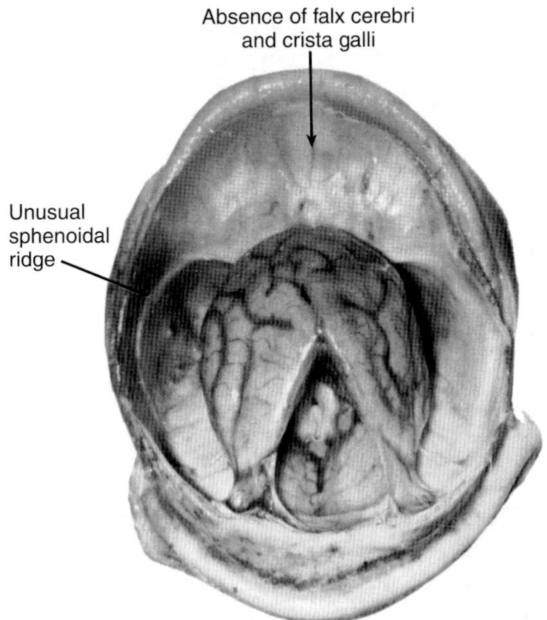

FIGURE 52.46 An instance of alobar holoprosencephaly. Because there was no interhemispheral fissure, there is no dural reflection at this site (falx cerebri), and as a consequence there is no metopic suture. There is also an aberrant alignment of the sphenoid wings relating to the altered brain impact in this location. This was associated with a comparable aberrant alignment of the coronal sutures. (From DeMeyer W, White PT. EEG in holoprosencephaly (arhinencephaly). *Arch Neurol.* 1964;11:507–520.)

and nephron elements in the adjacent metanephric blastema. The ureteral bud progressively arborizes, and each new bud induces a new group of glomeruli and nephrons that communicate with the ureteral buds. The ureteral bud becomes the ureter, and its multiple branches become the collecting ducts and distal tubules. The induced elements become the glomeruli and the proximal renal tubules. If there is any obstruction to the flow of urine, which usually begins by 8 to 9 weeks in the human fetus, the area proximal to the obstruction becomes dilated. If the flow from the whole kidney is obstructed, the pelvic drainage system of the kidney becomes dilated, which is termed *hydronephrosis*. If this occurs during early development, it may adversely affect renal morphogenesis, resulting in hypoplasia and the formation of cysts within the kidney. These are not true cysts but rather are dilations in the tubules that may appear as cysts on histologic sections of the kidney. Early obstruction to urine flow in the urethra results in the urethral obstruction malformation sequence, a series of consequences of the biomechanical effects of obstruction within the urinary tract.[26] Any renal system disorder that results in a lack of urine flow into the amniotic space will usually cause a deficit of amniotic fluid during late fetal life. It does not matter whether the lack of urine is caused by renal agenesis, hydronephrosis, or severe urethral obstruction; the consequences are the same and result in the oligohydramnios deformation sequence.

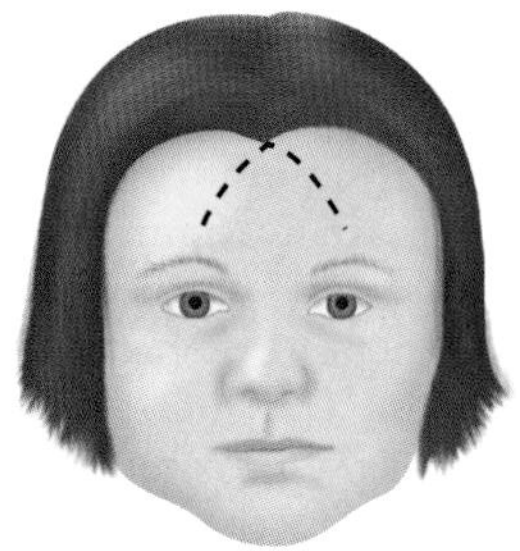

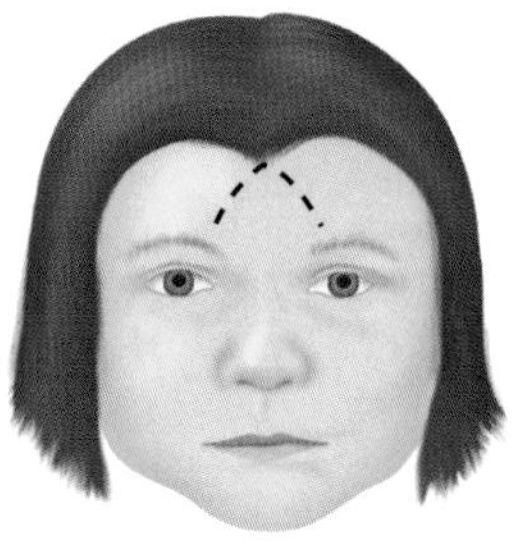

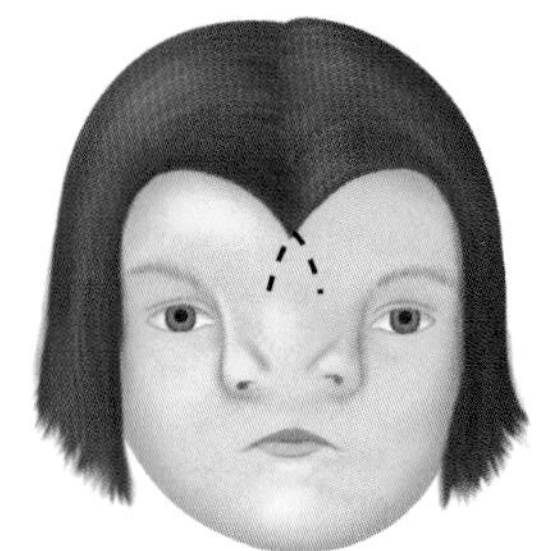

Periocular fields	Normal	Decreased	Normal
Interocular distance	Normal	Normal	Increased

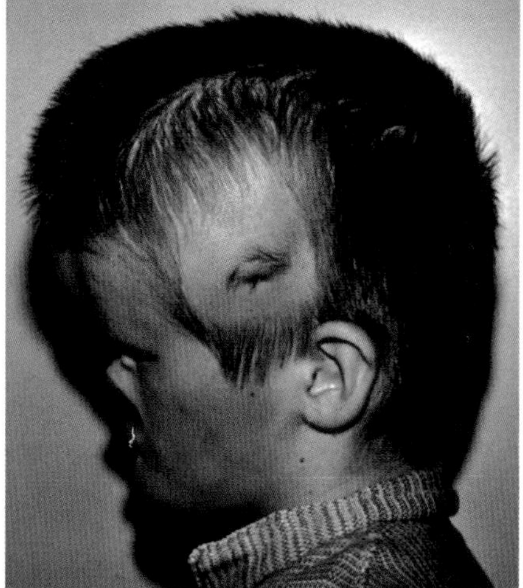

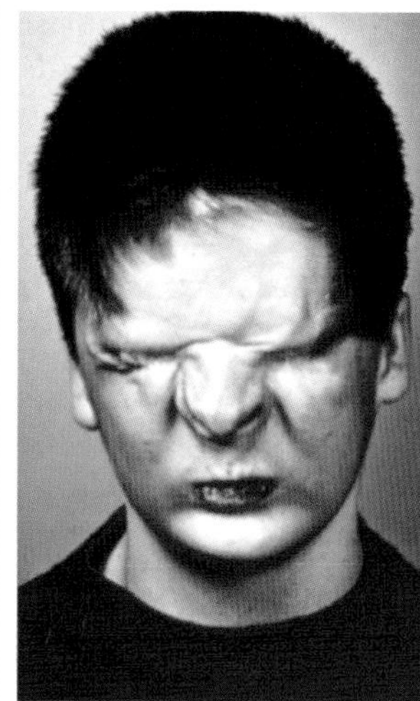

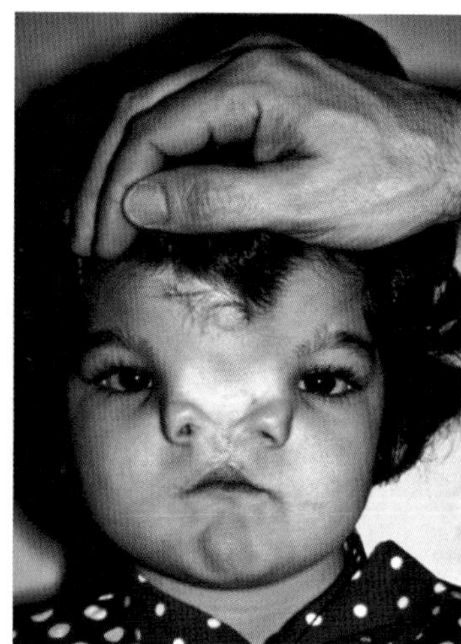

FIGURE 52.47 Zones of periocular hair growth suppression determine the frontal hair pattern, and with microphthalmia, hair extends onto the face, whereas ocular hypertelorism results in a widow's peak. A rudimentary eye projected to an unusual temporal location in the individual on the bottom left. At this site the early optic vesicle gave rise to the development of a small optic cup. Furthermore, there was the development of periocular muscles, lacrimal apparatus, and eyelids, plus the growth of hair at the eyebrow location and a zone of periocular hair growth suppression. (From Smith DW, Gong BT. Scalp-hair patterning: its origin and significance relative to early brain and upper facial development. *Teratology*. 1974;9:17.)

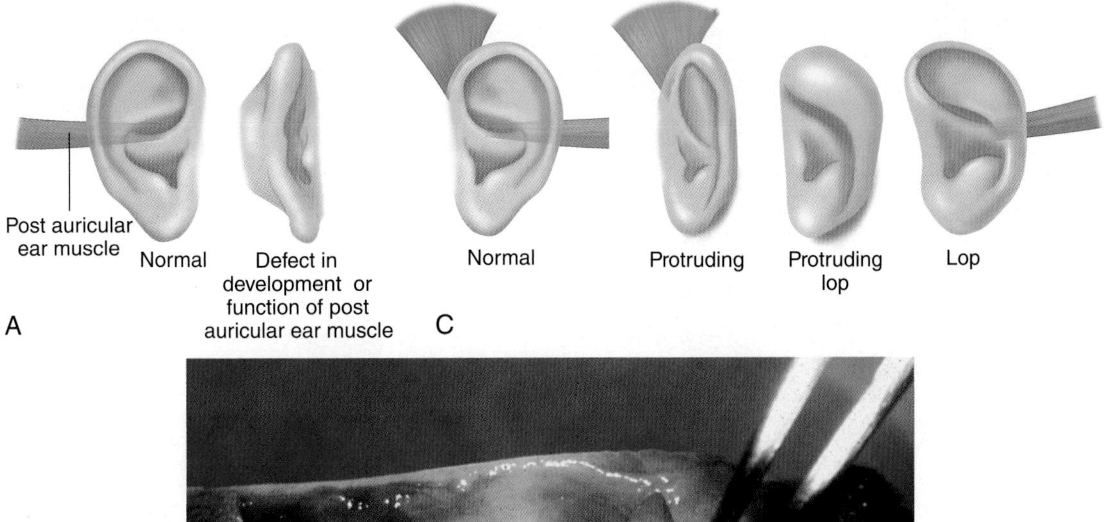

FIGURE 52.48 A, The posterior auricular muscle attaches from the concha of the ear to the mastoid region, thus holding the auricle toward the head. A protruding ear can result from absence or deficient function of the posterior auricular muscle. A lop ear is a secondary deformation caused by a defect in development of function of the superior auricular ear muscle, which attaches the superior auricle to the head. **B**, Photo from a 16-week fetus. **C**, Drawings summarize the relationship between the extrinsic ear muscles and ear form. (**B**, From Smith DW, Takashima H. Protruding auricle: a neuromuscular sign. *Lancet*. 1978;1:747. **C**, Courtesy Thomas Stebbins, University of Washington School of Medicine, Seattle, WA.)

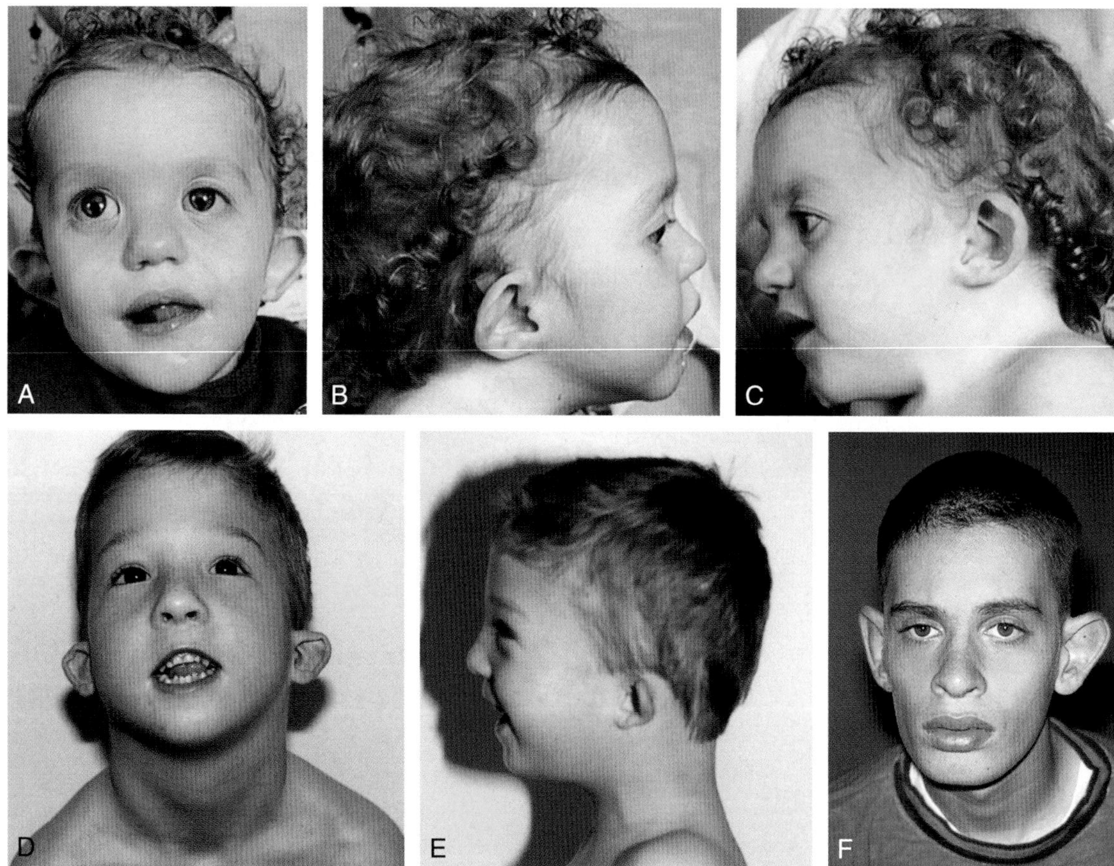

FIGURE 52.49 A–C, In CHARGE (coloboma, heart disease, atresia choanae, curtailed growth and development, genital hypoplasia, and ear anomalies and/or hearing loss) syndrome, asymmetric weakness of seventh nerve function leads to characteristic abnormal folding and prominence of the concha. **D** and **E**: In FG syndrome 1 (also called Opitz-Kaveggia syndrome), there is profound congenital hypotonia, which leads to small prominent cupped ears, whereas in fragile X syndrome (**F**), the ears tend to be large and prominent because of the combination of hypotonia and lax connective tissues.

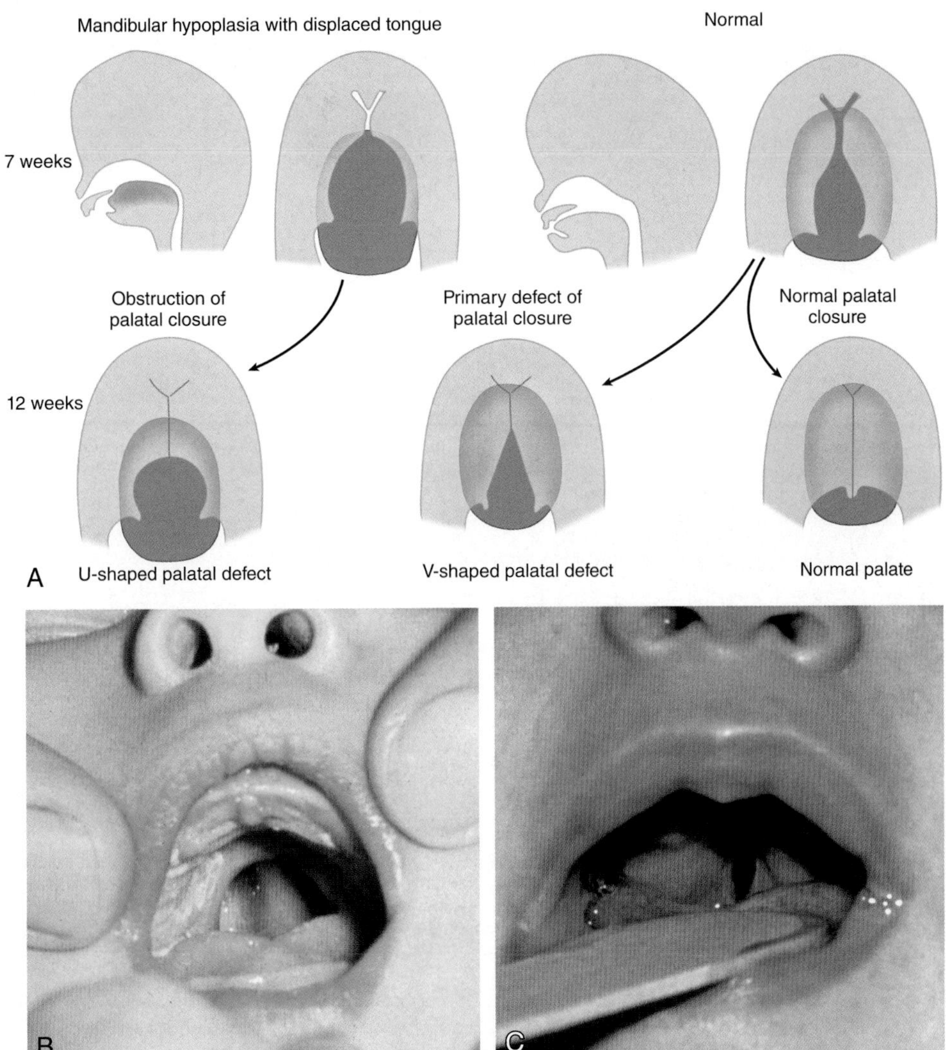

FIGURE 52.50 **A,** Pathways leading to defects of palatal closure as viewed in the lateral aspect and from above the palate. **B,** Lingual obstruction to closure of normal palatine shelves because of a small mandible with a retroplaced tongue, leading to a U-shaped palatal defect. Note that the retroplaced tongue has allowed the development of prominent rugous ridging in the anterior portion of the palate. **C,** Normal closure of the palatine shelves and the V-shaped palatine defect that results from a primary problem in their closure. (From Hanson JW, Smith DW. U-shaped palatal defect in the Robin anomalad: developmental and clinical relevance. *J Pediatr*. 1975;87:30.)

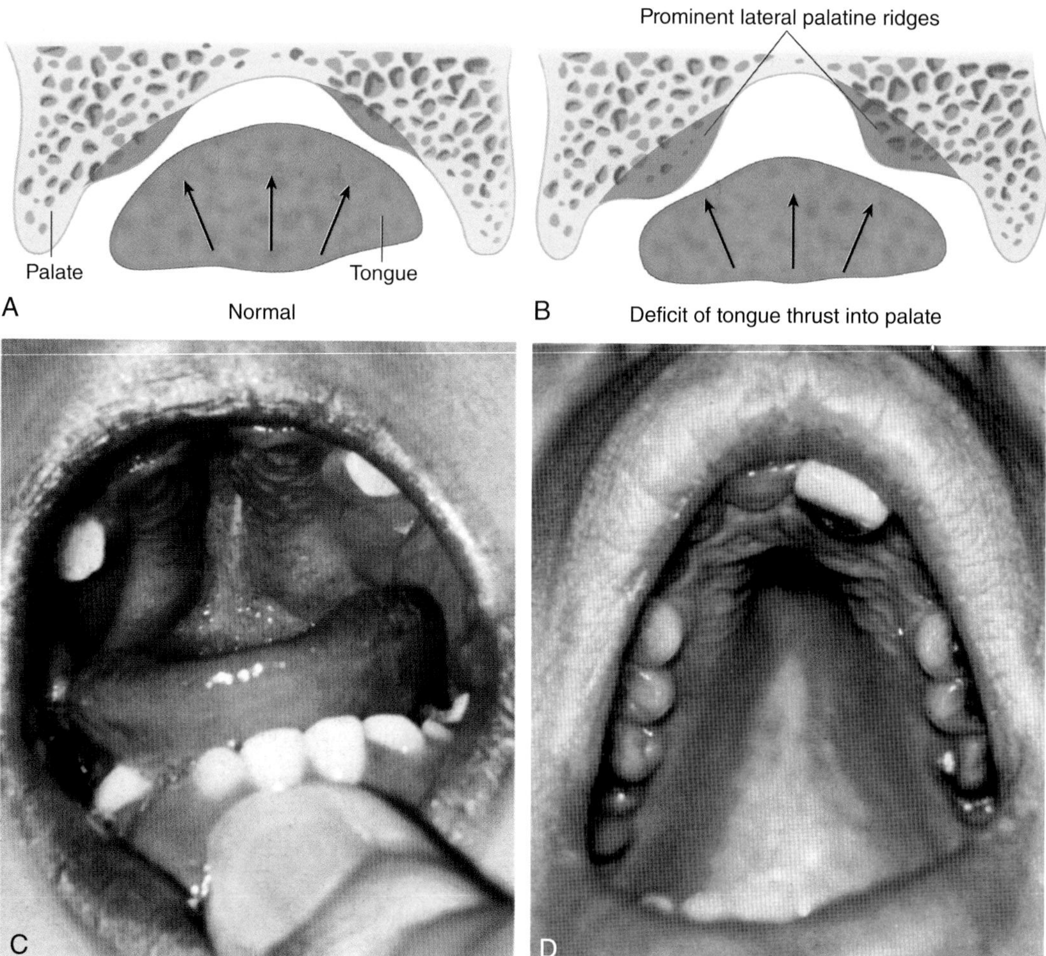

FIGURE 52.51 Cross-sectional depictions of palate and tongue in a normal infant (**A**) and in an infant with a deficit of tongue thrust into the hard palate (**B**), which allowed for the development of prominent lateral palatal ridges. **C,** Prominent lateral palatine shelves between the alveolar ridges and the center of the palate in this hypotonic infant indicated that the hypotonia was long-standing. **D,** Narrow palate in a intellectually disabled adult, the presumed consequences of the deficiency of normal forces relative to the growth and form of the maxilla. Such a narrow palate is unusual in intellectually disabled infants but is common in intellectually disabled older children.

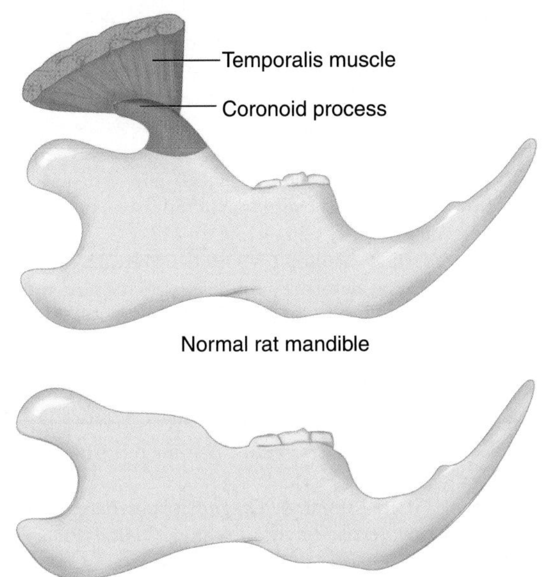

FIGURE 52.52 Early postnatal removal of the masseter muscle in the rat results in a lack of the coronoid process of the mandible, the bony protuberance that normally results from the tension of the masseter muscle at this site of attachment.

Table 52.2 CAUSES OF POOR FETAL LUNG GROWTH

General	Examples
Oligohydramnios	Renal agenesis
	Chronic amniotic leakage
External constraint	Small uterine cavity
	Bicornuate uterus
	Large uterine fibroids
Intrinsic constraint	Limited thoracic growth
	Thanatophoric dysplasia
	Thoracic mass
	Diaphragmatic hernia

References

1. Saldana L, Crespo L, Bensiamar F, et al. Mechanical forces regulate stem cell response to surface topography. *J Biomed Mater Res Part A*. 2013.
2. Thompson DAW. *On Growth and Form*. Cambridge, UK: Cambridge University Press; 2014.
3. Dingwall EJ. *Artificial Cranial Deformation*. London: J. Bale, sons & Danielsson, Ltd; 1931.
4. Graham JM Jr, Gomez M, Halberg A, et al. Management of deformational plagiocephaly: repositioning versus orthotic therapy. *J Pediatr*. 2005;146(2):258–262.
5. Graham JM Jr, Kreutzman J, Earl D, et al. Deformational brachycephaly in supine-sleeping infants. *J Pediatr*. 2005;146(2):253–257.
6. Watt A, Zammit D, Lee J, Gilardino M. Novel screening and monitoring techniques for deformational plagiocephaly: a systematic review. *Pediatrics*. 2022;149(2):e2021051736.
7. Gu Y, Li J, Li Z. Deformation of female foot binding in China. *J Clin Rheumatol*. 2013;19(7):418.
8. Cummings SR, Ling X, Stone K. Consequences of foot binding among older women in Beijing, China. *Am J Publ Hlth*. 1997;87(10):1677–1679.
9. Sanchez-Lara PA, Carmichael SL, Graham JM, et al. Fetal constraint as a potential risk factor for craniosynostosis. *Amer J Med Genet Part A*. 2010;152A(2):394–400.
10. Graham JM Jr, Kumar A. Diagnosis and management of extensive vertex birth molding. *Clin Pediatr (Phila)*. 2006;45(7):672–678.
11. Dunn PM. Congenital postural deformities. *Br Med Bull*. 1976;32(1):71–76.
12. Moh W, Graham JM Jr, Wadhawan I, et al. Extrinsic factors influencing fetal deformations and intrauterine growth restriction. *J Pregnancy*. 2012;750485
13. Hafez ESE. Reproductive failure in domestic mammals. In: Benirschke K, ed. *Comparative Aspects of Reproductive Failure*. New York: Springer-Verlag; 1967:44–95.
14. Yan S, Zhao Y, Zhang L, Yang L. Arch-related alteration in foot loading patterns affected by the increasing extent of body mass index in children: a follow-up study. *Gait Posture*. 2023;100:247–253.
15. Graham JM Jr, Smith DW. Parietal craniotabes in the neonate: its origin and relevance. *Journal of Pediatrics*. 1979;95:114–116.
16. Smith GE. The causation of the symmetrical thinning of the parietal bones in ancient Egyptians. *J Anat Physiol 41*. 1907(Pt 3):232–233.
17. Einspieler C, Prayer D, Marschik PB. Fetal movements: the origin of human behaviour. *Dev Med Child Neurol*. 2021;63(10):1142–1148.
18. Drachman DB, Coulombre AJ. Experimental clubfoot and arthrogryposis multiplex congenita. *Lancet*. 1962;2(7255):523–526.
19. Niles KM, Blaser S, Shannon P, Chitayat D. Fetal arthrogryposis multiplex congenita/fetal akinesia deformation sequence (FADS): aetiology, diagnosis, and management. *Prenat Diagn*. 2019;39(9):720–731.
20. Jago RH. Arthrogryposis following treatment of maternal tetanus with muscle relaxants. *Arch Dis Child*. 1970;45(240):277–279.
21. Moessinger AC. Fetal akinesia deformation sequence: an animal model. *Pediatrics*. 1983;72(6):857–863.
22. Hall JG. Oligohydramnios sequence revisited in relationship to arthrogryposis, with distinctive skin changes. *Am J Med Genet A*. 2014;164A(11):2775–2792.

23. Graham JM Jr, Stephens TD, Siebert JR, et al. Determinants in the morphogenesis of muscle tendon insertions. *J Pediatr*. 1982;101(5):825–831.
24. Smith DW. Commentary: redundant skin folds in the infant: their origin and relevance. *J Pediatr*. 1979;94(6):1021–1022.
25. Graham JM Jr, Smith DW. Dominantly inherited pterygium colli. *J Pediatr*. 1981;98(4):664–666.
26. Pagon RA, Smith DW, Shepard TH. Urethral obstruction malformation complex: a cause of abdominal muscle deficiency and the "prune belly. *J Pediatr*. 1979;94(6):900–906.
27. Stephan MJ, Smith DW, Ponzi JW, et al. Origin of scalp vertex aplasia cutis. *J Pediatr*. 1982;101(5):850–853.
28. Smith DW, Gong BT. Scalp hair patterning as a clue to early fetal brain development. *J Pediatr*. 1973;83(3): 374–380.
29. Furdon SA, Clark DA. Scalp hair characteristics in the newborn infant. *Adv Neonatal Care*. 2003;3(6):286–296.
30. Tirosh E, Jaffe M, Dar H. The clinical significance of multiple hair whorls and their association with unusual dermatoglyphics and dysmorphic features in mentally retarded Israeli children. *Eur J Pediatr*. 1987;146(6):568–570.
31. Mulvihill JJ, Smith DW. The genesis of dermatoglyphics. *J Pediatr*. 1969;75(4):579–589.
32. Popich GA, Smith DW. The genesis and significance of digital and palmar hand creases: preliminary report. *J Pediatr*. 1970;77(6):1017–1023.
33. Park JS, Shin DS, Jung W, et al. Improved analysis of palm creases. *Anat Cell Biol*. 2010;43(2):169–177.
34. Poush JR. Distal symphalangism: a report of two families. *J Hered*. 1991;82(3):233–238.
35. Demyer W, Zeman W, Palmer CG. The face predicts the brain: diagnostic significance of median facial anomalies for holoprosencephaly (arhinencephaly). *Pediatrics*. 1964;34:256–263.
36. Edison R, Muenke M. The interplay of genetic and environmental factors in craniofacial morphogenesis: holoprosencephaly and the role of cholesterol. *Congenit Anom (Kyoto)*. 2003;43(1):1–21.
37. Smith DW, Tondury G. Origin of the calvaria and its sutures. *Am J Dis Child*. 1978;132(7):662–666.
38. Raam MS, Solomon BD, Shalev SA, et al. Holoprosencephaly and craniosynostosis: a report of two siblings and review of the literature. *Am J Med Genet C Semin Med Genet*. 2010;154c(1):176–182.
39. Jones KL, Higginbottom MC, Smith DW. Determining role of the optic vesicle in orbital and periocular development and placement. *Pediatr Res*. 1980;14(5):703–708.
40. Gujar SK, Gandhi D. Congenital malformations of the orbit. *Neuroima Clin North Am*. 2011;21(3):585–602, viii.
41. Buchman SR, Bartlett SP, Wornom 3rd IL, et al. The role of pressure on regulation of craniofacial bone growth. *J Craniofac Surg*. 1994;5(1):2–10.
42. Sanchez-Lara PA, Graham JM Jr, Hing AV, et al. The morphogenesis of Wormian bones: a study of craniosynostosis and purposeful cranial deformation. *Am J Med Genet A*. 2007;143a(24):3243–3251.
43. Sanchez-Lara PA, Carmichael SL, Graham JM Jr, et al. the National Birth Defects Prevention Study. Fetal constraint as a potential risk factor for craniosynostosis. *Am J Med Genet Part A*. 2010;152A:394–400.
44. Ryoo HG, Kim SK, Cheon JE, et al. Slit ventricle syndrome and early-onset secondary craniosynostosis in an infant. *Am J Case Rept*. 2014;15:246–253.
45. Doorenbosch X, Molloy CJ, David DJ, et al. Management of cranial deformity following ventricular shunting. *Childs Nerv Syst*. 2009;25(7):871–874.
46. Kjaer I, Keeling JW, Fischer Hansen B, et al. Midline skeletodental morphology in holoprosencephaly. *Cleft Palate Craniofac J*. 2002;39(3):357–363.
47. Graham JM Jr, deSaxe M, Smith DW. Sagittal craniostenosis: fetal head constraint as one possible cause. *J Pediatr 95*. 1979(5 Pt 1):747–750.
48. Graham JM Jr, Kumar A. Diagnosis and management of extensive vertex birth molding. *Clinical Pediatrics*. 2006;45:672–678.
49. Coqueugniot H, Hublin JJ, Veillon F, et al. Early brain growth in *Homo erectus* and implications for cognitive ability. *Nature*. 2004;431(7006):299–302.
50. Aase JM. Structural defects as consequence of late intrauterine constraint: craniotabes, loose skin, and asymmetric ear size. *Semin Perinatol*. 1983;7(4):270–273.
51. Smith DW, Takashima H. Ear muscles and ear form. *Birth Defects Orig Article Ser*. 1980;16(4):299–302.
52. Hanson JW, Smith DW. U-shaped palatal defect in the Robin anomalad: developmental and clinical relevance. *J Pediatr*. 1975;87(1):30–33.
53. Evans KN, Sie KC, Hopper RA, et al. Robin sequence: from diagnosis to development of an effective management plan. *Pediatrics*. 2011;127(5):936–948.
54. Holder-Espinasse M, Abadie V, Cormier-Daire V, et al. Pierre Robin sequence: a series of 117 consecutive cases. *J Pediatr*. 2001;139(4):588–590.
55. Weaver KN, Sullivan BR, Balow SA, et al. Robin sequence without cleft palate: genetic diagnoses and management implications. *Am J Med Genet A*. 2022;188(1):160–177.
56. Varadarajan S, Balaji TM, Raj AT, et al. Genetic mutations associated with Pierre Robin syndrome/sequence: a systematic review. *Mol Syndromol*. 2021;12(2):69–86.
57. Hanson JW, Smith DW, Cohen JM Jr. Prominent lateral palatine ridges: developmental and clinical relevance. *J Pediatr*. 1976;89(1):54–58.
58. Thomas IT, Smith DW. Oligohydramnios, cause of the nonrenal features of Potter's syndrome, including pulmonary hypoplasia. *J Pediatr*. 1974;84(6):811–815.
59. ten Broek CM, Bots J, Varela-Lasheras I, et al. Amniotic fluid deficiency and congenital abnormalities both influence fluctuating asymmetry in developing limbs of human deceased fetuses. *Plos One*. 2013;8(11):e81824.
60. Lwigale PY, Thurmond JE, Norton WN, et al. Simulated microgravity and hypergravity attenuate heart tissue

development in explant culture. *Cells Tissues Organs.* 2000;167(2-3):171-183.

61. Sedmera D, Pexieder T, Rychterova V, et al. Remodeling of chick embryonic ventricular myoarchitecture under experimentally changed loading conditions. *Anatom Rec.* 1999;254(2):238-252.

62. Lindsey SE, Butcher JT, Yalcin HC. Mechanical regulation of cardiac development. *Front Physiol.* 2014;5:318.

Further Reading

Thompson D. *On Growth and Form. A New Edition,.* Cambridge, UK: Cambridge University Press; 1942.

INDEX

Page numbers followed by "*f*" indicate figures, "*t*" indicate tables, and "*b*" indicate boxes.

M